HCPCS Level II
Professional

2007

Acknowledgments

Brad Ericson, MPC, CPC, CPC-OS, *Product Manager*

Michael E. Desposito, *Director of Client Relations/Product Director*

Lynn Speirs, *Senior Director, Editorial/Desktop Publishing*

Karen Schmidt, BSN, *Technical Director*

Stacy Perry, *Manager, Desktop Publishing*

Lisa Singley, *Project Manager*

Wendy Gabbert, CPC, CPC-H, *Clinical/Technical Editor*

Regina Magnani, RHIT, *Clinical/Technical Editor*

Kerrie Hornsby, *Desktop Publishing Specialist*

Jean Parkinson, *Editor*

Technical Editors

Wendy Gabbert, CPC, CPC-H
Clinical/Technical Editor

Ms. Gabbert has more than 20 years of experience in the health care field. She has extensive background in CPT/HCPCS and ICD-9-CM coding. She served several years as a coding consultant. Her areas of expertise include physician and hospital CPT coding assessments, chargemaster reviews, and the Outpatient Prospective Payment System (OPPS). She is a member of the American Academy of Professional Coders (AAPC).

Regina Magnani, RHIT
Clinical/Technical Editor

Ms. Magnani has 25 years of experience in the health care industry in both health information management and patient financial services. Her areas of expertise include patient financial services, CPT/HCPCS and ICD-9-CM coding, the Outpatient Prospective Payment System (OPPS), and chargemaster development and maintenance. She is an active member of the Healthcare Financial Management Association (HFMA), the American Health Information Management Association (AHIMA), and the American Association of Heathcare Administrative Management (AAHAM).

Introduction

ORGANIZATION OF HCPCS

The Ingenix 2007 *HCPCS Level II* book contains mandated changes and new codes for use as of January 1, 2007. Deleted codes have also been indicated and cross-referenced to active codes when possible. New codes have been added to the appropriate sections, eliminating the time-consuming step of looking in two places for a code. However, keep in mind that the information in this book is a reproduction of the 2007 HCPCS; additional information on coverage issues may have been provided to Medicare contractors after publication. All contractors periodically update their systems and records throughout the year. If this book does not agree with your contractor, it is either because of a mid-year update or correction, or a specific local or regional coverage policy.

To make this year's HCPCS book even more useful, we have included codes noted in addendum B of the 2007 OPPS update as published in the *Federal Register* and from transmittals through 2006 that include codes not discussed in other CMS documents. The sources for these codes are often noted in blue beneath the description.

Index

Since HCPCS is organized by code number rather than by service or supply name, the index enables the coder to locate any code without looking through individual ranges of codes. Just look up the medical or surgical supply, service, orthotic, prosthetic, or generic or brand name drug in question to find the appropriate codes. This index also refers to many of the brand names by which these items are known.

Table of Drugs

The brand names listed are examples only and may not include all products available for that type of drug. Our table of drugs lists HCPCS codes from any available sections including A codes, C codes, J codes, S codes, and Q codes under brand and generic drug names with amount, route of administration, and code numbers. While we try to make the table comprehensive, it is not all-inclusive.

Color-coded Coverage Instructions

The Ingenix HCPCS Level II codebook provides colored symbols for each coverage and reimbursement instruction. A legend to these symbols is provided on the bottom of each two-page spread.

HOW TO USE INGENIX HCPCS LEVEL II BOOKS

> **Blue Color Bar—Special Coverage Instructions**
> A blue bar for "special coverage instructions" over a code means that special coverage instructions apply to that code. These special instructions are also typically given in the form of Medicare Pub.100 reference numbers. The appendixes provide the full text of the cited Medicare Pub.100 references.

A4211   Supplies for self-administered injections

> **Yellow Color Bar—Carrier Discretion**
> Issues that are left to "contractor discretion" are covered with a yellow bar. Contact the contractor for specific coverage information on those codes.

A4248   Chlorhexidine containing antiseptic, 1 ml

> **Red Color Bar—Not Covered by or Invalid for Medicare**
> Codes that are not covered by or are invalid for Medicare are covered by a red bar. The pertinent Medicare internet-only manuals (Pub. 100) reference numbers are also given explaining why a particular code is not covered. These numbers refer to the appendixes, where we have listed the Medicare references.

A4232   Syringe with needle for external insulin pump, sterile, 3cc

> The Ingenix HCPCS Level II codes follow the AMA CPT code book conventions to indicate new, revised, and deleted codes.
>
> - A black circle (●) precedes a new code.
> - A black triangle (▲) precedes a code with revised terminology or rules.
> - A circle (○) precedes a reissued code.
> - Codes deleted from the 2006 active codes appear with a strike-out.

●	A4461	Surgical dressing holder, non-reusable, each
▲	A4216	Sterile water, saline and/or dextrose, diluent/flush, 10 ml
○	J1740	Injection, ibandronate sodium, 1 mg
	~~A4359~~	~~Urinary suspensory without leg bag, each~~
		Use A5105

> **☑ Quantity Alert**
> Many codes in HCPCS report quantities that may not coincide with quantities available in the marketplace. For instance, a HCPCS code for an ostomy pouch with skin barrier reports each pouch, but the product is generally sold in a package of 10; "10" must be indicated in the quantity box on the CMS claim form to ensure proper reimbursement. This symbol indicates that care should be taken to verify quantities in this code.

☑   A4207   Syringe with needle, sterile 2 cc, each

♀ Female Only
This icon identifies procedures that should only be reported for female patients.

♂ Male Only
This icon identifies procedures that should only be reported for male patients.

Ⓐ Age Edit
This icon denotes codes intended for use with a specific age group, such as neonate, newborn, pediatric, and adult. Carefully review the code description to assure the code you report most appropriately reflects the patient's age.

Ⓜ Maternity
This icon identifies procedures that by definition should only be used for maternity patients generally between 12 and 55 years of age.

❶-❾ ASC Groupings
Codes designated as being paid by ASC groupings that were effective at the time of printing are denoted by the group number.

& DMEPOS
Use this icon to identify when to consult the CMS DMEPOS for payment of this durable medical item.

⊘ Skilled Nursing Facility (SNF)
Use this icon to identify certain items and services excluded from skilled nursing facility consolidated billing. These items may be billed directly to the Medicare contractor by the provider or supplier of the service or item.

Ingenix provides explanatory information in blue beneath many codes. These annotations help you better understand the code and its billing.

Drugs commonly reported with a code are listed underneath by brand or generic name.

"See" references help determine related or alternate codes for the supply or service.

CMS does not use consistent terminology when a code for a specific procedure is not listed. The code description may include any of the following terms: unlisted, not otherwise classified (NOC), unspecified, unclassified, other, and miscellaneous. If you are sure there is no code for the service or supply provided or used, be sure to provide adequate documentation to the payer. Check with the payer for more information.

A4280 — Adhesive skin support attachment for use with external breast prosthesis, each ♀

A4326 — Male external catheter specialty type with integral collection chamber, any type, each ♂

D8010 — Limited orthodontic treatment of the primary dentition Ⓐ

H1001 — Prenatal care, at-risk enhanced service; antepartum management Ⓜ

G0105 — Colorectal cancer screening; colonoscopy on individual at high risk ❷

A4600 — Sleeve for intermittent limb compression device, replacement only, each &

A4653 — Peritoneal dialysis catheter anchoring device, belt, each ⊘

J7191 — Factor VIII (anti-hemophilic factor (porcine), per IU
Use this code for Hyate:C. Medicare jurisdiction: local contractor.

J7193 — Factor IX (antihemophilic factor, purified, non-recombinant) per IU
Use this code for AlphaNine SD, Mononine.

S0147 — Injection, alglucosidase alfa, 20 mg
Use this code for Myozyme
See also code: C9234

A0999 — Unlisted ambulance service

OPPS Status Indicators

A-**Y** APC Status Indicators

Status indicators identify how individual HCPCS Level II codes are paid or not paid under the OPPS. The same status indicator is assigned to all the codes within an APC. Consult the payer or resource to learn which CPT codes fall within various APCs. Status indicators for HCPCS and their definitions are below:

A Indicates services that are paid under some other method such as the DMEPOS fee schedule or the physician fee schedule

B Indicates codes not allowed or paid under OPPS

C Indicates inpatient services that are not paid under the OPPS

E Indicates services for which payment is not allowed under the OPPS. In some instances, the service is not covered by Medicare. In other instances, Medicare does not use the code in question but does use another code to describe the service

F Indicates corneal tissue acquisition costs, certain CRNA services and hepatitis B vaccines that are paid at reasonable cost

G Indicates a current drug or biological for which payment is made under the transitional pass-through provisions

H Indicates either a device paid under pass-through provisions; or brachytherapy sources and radiopharmaceuticals that are paid at reasonable cost

K Indicates non-pass-through drugs and biologicals.

L Indicates influenza or pneumococcal pneumonia vaccine paid as of reasonable cost with no deductable or coinsurance

M Indicates that this code should not be reported by hospitals to their fiscal intermediary

N Indicates services that are incidental, with payment packaged into another service or APC group

P Indicates services paid only in partial hospitalization programs

S Indicates significant procedures for which payment is allowed under the hospital OPPS but to which the multiple procedure reduction does not apply

T Indicates surgical services for which payment is allowed under the hospital OPPS. Services with this payment indicator are the only ones to which the multiple procedure payment reduction applies.

V Indicates visits for which payment is allowed under the hospital OPPS

X Indicates ancillary services for which payment is allowed under the hospital OPPS

Y Indicates nonimplantable durable medical equipment (DME) that is billed by providers other than home health agencies to the DMERC

A	A4321	Therapeutic agent for urinary catheter irrigation
B	Q4005	Cast supplies, long arm cast, adult (11 years +), plaster
C	G0341	Percutaneous islet cell transplant, includes portal vein catheterization and infusion
E	A0021	Ambulance service, outside state per mile, transport (Medicaid only)
F	V2785	Processing, preserving and transporting corneal tissue
G	J0129	Injection, abatacept, 10 mg
H	A9505	Thallium Tl-201 thallous chloride, diagnostic, per millicurie
K	Q9954	Oral magnetic resonance contrast agent, per 100 ml
L	G0008	Administration of influenza virus vaccine when no physician fee schedule service on the same day
M	G0333	Dispense fee initial 30 day
N	A4220	Refill kit for implantable infusion pump
P	G0177	Training and educational services related to the care and treatment of patient's disabling mental health problems per session (45 minutes or more)
S	G0251	Linear accelerator based stereotactic radiosurgery, delivery including collimator changes and custom plugging, fractionated treatment, all lesions, per session, maximum five sessions per course of treatment
T	C9724	Endoscopic full-thickness plication in the gastric cardia using endoscopic plication system (EPS); includes endoscopy
V	G0101	Cervical or vaginal cancer screening; pelvic and clinical breast examination
X	Q0035	Cardiokymography
Y	A4222	Infusion supplies for external drug infusion pump, per cassette or bag (list drugs separately)

MED: This notation precedes an instruction pertaining to this code in the Centers for Medicare and Medicaid Services' (CMS) Publication 100 (Pub 100) electronic manual or in a National Coverage Determinatuion (NCD). These CMS sources, formerly called the Medicare Carriers Manual (MCM) and Coverage Issues Manual (CIM), present the rules for submitting these services to the federal government or its contractors and are included in the appendix of this book

A4300   Implantable access catheter, (e.g., venous, arterial, epidural subarachnoid, or peritoneal, etc.) external access

> **MED: 100-2, 15, 120**

AHA: American Hospital Association Coding Clinic for HCPCS citations help you find expanded information about specific codes and their usage.

A4290   Sacral nerve stimulation test lead, each

> **AHA: 1Q, '02, 9**

Current as of 11/22/2006

You may subscribe to an e-mail service to receive special reports when information in this book changes. Contact Customer Service at 1.800.INGENIX (464.3649), option 1.

ABOUT HCPCS CODES

Ingenix does not develop or maintain HCPCS Level II codes. The federal government does.

Any supplier or manufacturer can submit a request for coding modification to the HCPCS Level II national codes. A document explaining the HCPCS modification process, as well as a detailed format for submitting a recommendation for a modification to HCPCS Level II codes, is available on the HCPCS website at www.cms.hhs.gov/medhcpcsgeninfo/01_overview.asp. Besides the information requested in this format, a requestor should also submit any additional descriptive material, including the manufacturer's product literature and information that is believed would be helpful in furthering CMS's understanding of the medical features of the item for which a coding modification is being recommended. The HCPCS coding review process is an ongoing, continuous process.

Requests for coding modifications should be sent to the following address:

Alpha-Numeric HCPCS Coordinator
Center for Medicare Management
Centers for Medicare and Medicaid Services
C5-08-27
7500 Security Boulevard
Baltimore, MD 21244-1850

HOW TO USE HCPCS LEVEL II

Coders should keep in mind, however, that the insurance companies and government do not base payment solely on what was done for the patient. They need to know why the services were performed. In addition to using the HCPCS coding system for procedures and supplies, coders must also use the ICD-9-CM coding system to denote the diagnosis. This book will not discuss ICD-9-CM codes, which can be found in a current ICD-9-CM code book for diagnosis codes. To locate a HCPCS Level II code, follow these steps:

1. Identify the services or procedures the patient received.

    Example:

    Patient administered PSA exam.

2. Look up the appropriate term in the index.

    Example:

    Screening

    prostate

    Coding Tip: Coders who are unable to find the procedure or service in the index can look in the table of contents for the type of procedure or device to narrow the code choices. Also, coders should remember to check the unlisted procedure guidelines for additional choices.

3. Assign a tentative code.

    Example:

    Codes G0103

    Coding Tip: To the right of the terminology, there may be a single code or multiple codes, a cross-reference or an indication that the code has been deleted. Tentatively assign all codes listed.

4. Locate the code or codes in the appropriate section. When multiple codes are listed in the index, be sure to read the narrative of all codes listed to find the appropriate code based on the service performed.

    Example:

    G0103   Prostate cancer screening; prostate specific antigen test (PSA)

5. Check for color bars, symbols, notes, and references.

    Example:

    Ⓐ   G0103   Prostate cancer screening; prostate specific antigen test (PSA)   ♂

    MED: 100-3, 210.1; 100-4, 18, 50

6. Review the appendixes for the reference definitions and other guidelines for coverage issues that apply.

7. Determine whether any modifiers should be used.

8. Assign the code.

    Example:

    The code assigned is G0103.

CODING STANDARDS
Levels of Use

Coders may find that the same procedure is coded at two or even three levels. Which code is correct? There are certain rules to follow if this should occur.

When both a CPT and a HCPCS Level II code have virtually identical narratives for a procedure or service, the CPT code should be used. If, however, the narratives are not identical (for example, the CPT code narrative is generic, whereas the HCPCS Level II code is specific), the Level II code should be used.

Be sure to check for a national code when a CPT code description contains an instruction to include additional information, such as describing specific medication. For example, when billing Medicare or Medicaid for supplies, avoid using CPT code 99070, supplies and materials (except spectacles), provided by the physician over and above those usually included with the office visit or other services rendered (list drugs, trays, supplies, or materials provided). There are many HCPCS Level II codes that specify supplies in more detail.

Special Reports

Submit a special report with the claim when a new, unusual, or variable procedure is provided or a modifier is used. Include the following information:

*   A copy of the appropriate report (e.g., operative, x-ray), explaining the nature, extent, and need for the procedure

*   Documentation of the medical necessity of the procedure

*   Documentation of the time and effort necessary to perform the procedure

CMS Process to Request a Revision to the HCPCS Level II Codes

From the Centers for Medicare and Medicaid Website:

Anyone can submit a request for modifying the HCPCS level II national code set. A document explaining the HCPCS revision process, as well as a detailed format for submitting a request, is available on the HCPCS Website at http://www.cms.hhs.gov/medicare/hcpcs. Besides the information requested in this format, a requestor should also submit any additional descriptive material, including the manufacturer's product literature and information, that it thinks would be helpful in furthering our understanding of the medical features of the item for which a coding revision is being recommended. The HCPCS coding review process is an ongoing continuous process. Requests may be submitted at any time throughout the year. Requests that are received and complete by January 3 of the current year will be considered for inclusion in the next annual update (January 1st of the following year). Requests received on or after January 3, and requests received earlier that require additional evaluation, will be included in a later HCPCS update. There are three types of coding revisions to the HCPCS that can be requested:

1. That a permanent code be added

   When there is not a distinct code that describes a product, a code may be requested (1) if the FDA allows the product to be marketed in the United States and (2) if the product is not a drug, the product has been on the market for at least 3 months; if the product is a drug, there is no requirement to submit marketing data; and (3) the product represents 3 percent or more of the outpatient use for that type of product in the national market. If a request for a new code is approved, the addition of a new HCPCS codes does not mean that the item is necessarily covered by any insurer. Whether an item identified by a new code is covered is determined by the Medicare law, regulations, and medical review policies and not by the assignment of a code.

2. That the language used to describe an existing code be changed

   When there is an existing code, a recommendation to modify the code can be made when an interested party believes that the descriptor for the code needs to be modified to provide a better description of the category of products represented by the code.

3. That an existing code be deleted

   When an existing code becomes obsolete or is duplicative of another code, a request can be made to delete the code.

   When there is no currently existing code to describe a product, a miscellaneous code/not otherwise classified code may be appropriate. The use of a miscellaneous code permits a claims history to be established for an item that can be used to support the need for a national permanent code.

   Requests for coding revisions should be sent to the following:

   Alpha-Numeric HCPCS Coordinator
   Center for Medicare Management
   Centers for Medicare and Medicaid Services, C5-08-27
   7500 Security Boulevard
   Baltimore, MD 21244-1850.

CMS HCPCS WORKGROUP

The CMS HCPCS Workgroup is an internal workgroup comprised of representatives of the major components of CMS, the Medicaid State agencies, and the SADMERC. The SADMERC represents Medicare program operating needs with input from the four DMERCs which have responsibility for processing Durable Medical Equipment, Prosthetics, Orthotics and Supplies (DMEPOS) claims for the Medicare program. Coding decisions are coordinated with both public and private insurers. The CMS HCPCS workgroup considers each coding request, and beginning with the 2006 cycle,

will determine whether HCPCS coding requests warrant a change to the national permanent codes. Prior to the 2006 cycle, the National Panel was responsible for final decisions.

When a recommendation for a revision to the HCPCS is received, it is reviewed at a regularly scheduled meeting of the CMS HCPCS Workgroup. Ordinarily, the CMS HCPCS Workgroup meets monthly to discuss whether coding requests warrant a change to the national permanent codes.

Evaluating HCPCS Coding Requests

The CMS HCPCS workgroup applies the following criteria to determine whether there is a demonstrated need for a new or modified code or the need to remove a code:

1. When an existing code adequately describes the item in a coding request, then no new or modified code is established. An existing code adequately describes an item in a coding request when the existing code describes products with the following:

   - Functions similar to the item in the coding request.

   - No significant therapeutic distinctions from the item in the coding request.

2. When an existing code describes products that are almost the same in function with only minor distinctions from the item in the coding request, the item in the coding request may be grouped with that code and the code descriptor modified to reflect the distinctions.

3. A code is not established for an item that is used only in the inpatient setting or for an item that is not diagnostic or therapeutic in nature.

4. A new or modified code is not established for an item unless the FDA allows the item to be marketed. FDA approval documentation is required to be submitted with the coding request application for all non-drug items. For drugs, FDA approval documentation will be accepted up to March 31 following the application deadline as long as the application is otherwise complete and submitted by the deadline.

5. There must be sufficient claims activity or volume, as evidenced by 3 months of marketing activity for non-drug products, so that the adding of a new or modified code enhances the efficiency of the system and justifies the administrative burden of adding or modifying a code.

6. The determination to remove a code is based on the consideration of whether a code is obsolete (for example, products no longer are used, other more specific codes have been added) or duplicative and no longer useful (for example, new codes are established that better describe items identified by existing codes). In developing its decisions, the HCPCS Workgroup uses the criteria mentioned above. In deciding upon a recommendation, the workgroup does not include cost as a factor.

Opportunity for Public Input/Public Meeting Process for HCPCS

On December 21, 2000, the Congress passed the Medicare, Medicaid, and SCHIP Benefits Improvement and Protection Act of 2000 (BIPA), Pub. L. 106-554. Section 531(b) of BIPA mandated that we establish procedures that permit public consultation for coding and payment determinations for new DME under Medicare Part B of title XVIII of the Social Security Act (the Act). As part of HCPCS reform, CMS expanded the public meeting forum to include all public requests as of the 2005-2006 coding cycle. Accordingly, CMS hosts annual public meetings that provide a forum for interested parties to make oral presentations and/or to submit written comments in response to preliminary coding and pricing recommendations for new durable medical equipment that have been submitted using the Healthcare Common Procedure Coding System coding revision process. Agenda items for the meetings will be published in advance of the public meeting on the HCPCS Website at http://www.cms.hhs.gov/medicare/hcpcs . The agenda will include descriptions of the coding requests, the requestor, and the name of the product or service. This change will provide more opportunities for the public to become aware of coding changes under consideration, as well as opportunities for public input into decision-making.

The HCPCS coordinator schedules meetings with interested parties, at their request, as time permits, to discuss their recommendations regarding possible changes to the HCPCS level II codes. These meetings are held at the Central Office of CMS. In addition to representatives from the CMS HCPCS Workgroup, staff from Medicaid and Medicare coverage, payment and operations are invited to attend these meetings. These meetings are not related to the meetings mandated by section 531(b) of BIPA, they are also not decision making meetings or CMS HCPCS Workgroup meetings.

Final Decisions

The CMS HCPCS Workgroup is responsible for making the final decisions pertaining to additions, deletions, and revisions to the HCPCS codes. The CMS HCPCS Workgroup reviews all requests for coding changes and makes final decisions regarding the annual update to the national codes. The Workgroup sends letters to those who requested coding revisions to inform them of the Workgroup's decision regarding their coding requests. The decision letters include, but may not be limited to, the following types of responses:

1. A change to the national codes has been approved that reflects, completely or in part, your coding request.

2. Your request for a coding revision to this year's update has not been approved because the scope of your request necessitates that additional consideration be given to your request before the CMS HCPCS Workgroup reaches a final decision.

3. Your reported sales volume was insufficient to support your request for a revision to the national codes. To determine whether there is sufficient sales volume to warrant a permanent code, we ask requestors to submit 3 months of the most recent sales volume for non-drug items. There is not a requirement to submit marketing data for drugs.

4. Your request for a new national code has not been approved because there already is an existing permanent or temporary code that describes your product.

5. Your request for a code has not been approved because your product is not used by health care providers for diagnostic or therapeutic purposes.

6. Your request for a code has not been approved because the code you requested is for capital equipment.

7. Your request for a code has not been approved because your product is an integral part of another service and payment for that service includes payment for your product; therefore, your product may not be billed separately to Medicare.

8. Your request for a revision to the language that describes the current code has not been approved because it does not improve the code descriptor.

9. Your request for a new code has not been approved because your product is not primarily medical in nature (for example, generally not useful in the absence of an illness or injury).

10. Your request for a code has not been approved because your product is used exclusively in the inpatient hospital setting.

11. Your request for a code has not been approved because it is inappropriate for inclusion in the HCPCS Level II code set and request should be submitted independently to another coding authority (e.g. AMA for CPT coding, ADA for CDT coding, etc.)

Decision letters also inform the requestors that they may contact the entity in whose jurisdiction a claim is filed for assistance in answering any coding questions. For Medicare, contact the SADMERC. Under contract to CMS, the SADMERC is responsible for providing suppliers and manufacturers with assistance in determining which HCPCS code should be used to describe DMEPOS items for the purpose of billing Medicare. The SADMERC has a toll free help line for this purpose, (877) 735-1326, which is operational during the hours of 9 AM to 4 PM (EST) For Medicaid, contact the state Medicaid agency. For private insurance, contact the individual insurer. A requestor who is dissatisfied with the final decision may submit a new request asking the CMS HCPCS Workgroup to reconsider and re-evaluate the code request. At

that time, the requestor should include new information or additional explanations to support the request.

Reconsideration Process

CMS management is considering pilot-testing, a process by which denied applicants would be allowed an opportunity to have their application reconsidered during the same coding cycle. The basis for denial will be clearly delineated in a notice to the applicant and provided in a timely fashion. This pilot is expected to be introduced during the 2007 coding cycle.

HCPCS UPDATES

Permanent National Codes

The national codes are updated annually, according to the following schedule:

1. Coding requests have to be received by January 3 of the current year to be considered for the next January 1 update of the subsequent year. This means that completed requests must be received by no later than January 3 of the current year to be considered for inclusion in the January update of the following year unless January 3 falls on a weekend; then the due date is extended to the following Monday.

2. Computer tapes and instructions, that include an updated list of codes and identify which codes have been changed or deleted, are updated and sent to our contractors and Medicaid State agencies at least 60 days in advance of the January 1 implementation date for the annual update. In addition, the CMS HCPCS Workgroup's final decisions on all public requests for changes to the HCPCS coding system will be published on the official HCPCS web site at www.cms.hhs.gov/medicare/hcpcs in November of each year.

Temporary Codes

Temporary codes can be added, changed, or deleted on a quarterly basis. Once established, temporary codes are usually implemented within 90 days, the time needed to prepare and issue implementation instructions and to enter the new code into CMS's and the contractors' computer systems and initiate user education. This time is needed to allow for instructions such as bulletins and newsletters to be sent out to suppliers to provide them with information and assistance regarding the implementation of temporary CMS codes.

HCPCS/Medicare Website

CMS's Website, http://www.cms.hhs.gov/medicare/hcpcs lists all of the current HCPCS codes, an alphabetical index of HCPCS codes by type of service or product, and an alphabetical table of drugs for which there are level II codes. The Website also includes a list of applications submitted in the current coding cycle. Interested parties can submit comments regarding the agenda items to the CMS HCPCS Workgroup by sending an e-mail to CMS through this Website. These comments are included as part of the Workgroup's review as it considers the coding requests.

The newly established temporary codes and effective dates for their use are also posted on the HCPCS Website at http://www.cms.hhs.gov/medicare/hcpcs. This Website enables us to quickly disseminate information on coding requests and decisions.

Code Assignment Following Medicare National Coverage Determination

Pursuant to Sec. 1862 (l) (3) (C) (iv) of the Social Security Act (added by Section 731 (a) of the Medicare Modernization Act), the Centers for Medicare and Medicaid Services (CMS), has developed a process by which the CMS HCPCS Workgroup will identify an appropriate existing code category and/or establish a new code category to describe the item that is the subject of a National Coverage Determination (NCD). If the item is considered Durable Medical Equipment, Prosthetic, Orthotic or Supply (DMEPOS), the CMS will defer to the Statistical Analysis Durable Medical Equipment Regional Carrier (SADMERC) to determine the appropriate code category. Under contract to the CMS, the SADMERC assigns individual DMEPOS products to HCPCS code categories for the purpose of billing Medicare.

As a matter of meeting on-going Medicare program operating needs, processes have existed for some time by which items and services that are newly covered by Medicare are assigned to a new or existing code category. Effective July 1, 2004, the process outlined below has been used by CMS to comply with the requirements of Sec. 1862 (l).

1. Assignment of an Existing "Temporary" or "Permanent" Code: When the CMS determines that an item is already identified by an existing "temporary" or "permanent" (as described in A and B above) HCPCS code category, but was previously not covered, the CMS will assign the item to the existing code category, and ensure that the coverage indicator assigned to the code category accurately reflects Medicare policy regarding payment for the item. Sec. 731 of the MMA does not require that a new code category or a product specific code be created for an item simply because a new coverage determination was made, without regard to codes available in the existing code set.

2. Assignment of a New "Temporary" or "Permanent" Code: When the CMS determines that a new code category is appropriate, CMS will make every effort to establish, publish, and implement the new code at the time the final coverage determination is made.

3. Assignment of an Unclassified Code: Under certain circumstances, the assignment of an item to an unclassified code may be necessary. A number of unclassified codes already exist under various headings throughout the HCPCS Level II code set. When an item is newly covered, but usage is narrow and the item would be billed infrequently, it may be more of an administrative burden to revise the code set than to use an unclassified code along with other, existing processing methods. When a new "temporary" or "permanent" code is appropriate, but the change cannot be implemented and incorporated into billing and claims processing systems at the time the final NCD decision memorandum is released, an unclassified code may be assigned in the interim, until a new code can be implemented, in order to ensure that claims can be processed for the item. The timing of implementation of new "temporary" or "permanent" codes relative to the date of the coverage determination depends on a variety of factors, some of which are not within the direct control of the code set maintainers, for example:

- coding alternatives may require extensive research;

- the timing of the coverage determination may be such that the publication deadline for the next Quarterly Update is missed

- there is insufficient time between NCD and Quarterly Update to incorporate new codes into new policy and accompanying billing instructions, and into claims processing systems along with any edits needed to operationalize the new code.

CMS Revision November 30, 2005

Home health — *continued*
- infusion therapy, S9325-S9379, S9494-S9497, S9537-S9810
- insertion midline venous catheter, S5523
- nursing services, S9212-S9213
- postpartum hypertension, S9212
- services of
  - clinical social worker, G0155
  - occupational therapist, G0152
  - physical therapist, G0151
  - skilled nurse, G0154
  - speech/language pathologist, G0153
- transfusion, blood products, S9538
- wound care, S9097

Home uterine monitor, S9001

Hook
- electric, L7009
- mechanical, L6706-L6707

Hospice
- care, Q5001-Q5008, S9126, T2041-T2046
- evaluation and counseling services, G0337
- referral visit, S0255

Hospital
- call
  - dental, D9420
- observation
  - direct admit, G0379
  - per hour, G0378

Hot water bottle, E0220
Houdini security suit, E0700
House call, dental, D9410
Housing, supported, H0043-H0044
Hoyer patient lifts, E0621, E0625, E0630
H-Tron insulin pump, E0784
H-Tron Plus insulin pump, E0784
Hudson
- adult multi-vent venturi style mask, A4620
- nasal cannula, A4615
- oxygen supply tubing, A4616
- UC-BL type shoe insert, L3000

Humalog, J1815, J1817, S5550
Human insulin, J1815, J1817
Humidifer, E0550-E0560
- water chamber, A7046

Humira, J0135
Humulin insulin, J1815, J1817
H. Weniger finger orthosis
- cock-up splint
- combination Oppenheimer
  - with
    - knuckle bender no. 13, L3950
    - reverse knuckle no. 13B, L3952
- composite elastic no. 10, L3946
- dorsal wrist no. 8, L3938
  - with outrigger attachment no. 8A, L3940
- finger extension, with clock spring no. 5, L3928
- finger extension, with wrist support no.5A, L3930
- finger knuckle bender no. 11, L3948
- knuckle bender splint type no. 2, L3918
- knuckle bender, two segment no. 2B, L3922
- knuckle bender with outrigger no. 2, L3920
- Oppenheimer, L3924
- Palmer no. 7, L3936
- reverse knuckle bender no. 9, L3942
  - with outrigger no. 9A, L3944
- safety pin, modified no. 6A, L3934
- safety pin, spring wire no. 6, L3932
- spreading hand no. 14, L3954
- Thomas suspension no. 4, L3926

Hyaluronan or derivative, J7319
Hyaluronidase
- bovine, J3470
- ovine, up to 150 units, J3471

Hyaluronidase — *continued*
- ovine, up to 999 units, J3472
- recombinant, J3473

Hyate, J7191
Hybolin
- decanoate, J2321

Hycamtin, J9350
Hydralazine HCl, J0360
Hydrate, J1240
Hydration therapy, S9373-S9379
Hydraulic patient lift, E0630
Hydrocollator, E0225, E0239
Hydrocolloid dressing, A6234-A6241
Hydrocortisone
- acetate, J1700
- sodium phosphate, J1710
- sodium succinate, J1720

Hydrocortone
- acetate, J1700
- phosphate, J1710

Hydrogel dressing, A6242-A6248
Hydromorphone, J1170, S0092
Hydroxyurea, S0176
Hydroxyzine HCl, J3410
- pamoate, Q0177-Q0178

Hyoscyamine sulfate, J1980
Hyperbaric oxygen chamber, topical, A4575
Hyperstat IV, J1730
Hypertonic saline solution, J7130
Hypo-Let lancet device, A4258
Hypothermia
- intragastric, M0100

HypRho-D, J2790
Hyrexin-50, J1200
Hyzine-;50, J3410

I

I-125 sodium iothalamate, A9554
I-131
- sodium iodide, A9531
  - capsule, A9517, A9528
  - solution, A9529-A9530
- tositumomab, A9544-A9545

I&D
- Intraoral, D7511, D7521

Ibandronate sodium injection, J1740
Ibutilide fumarate, J1742
Ice cap or collar, E0230
Idamycin, J9211
Idarubicin HCl, J9211
Ifex, J9208
Ifosfamide, J9208
IL-2, J9015
Iletin insulin, J1815, J1817, S5552
Ilfeld, hip orthosis, L1650
Images, oral/facial, D0350
Imaging, C1770
- coil, MRI, C1770
- dynamic infrared blood perfusion (DIRI), C9723

Imatinib, S0088
Imiglucerase, J1785
Imitrex, J3030
Immune globulin
- IV preadministration-related services, G0332
- lyophilized IV, J1566
- nonlyophilized IV, J1567
- subcutaneous, J1562

Immunofluorescence
- direct, D0482
- indirect, D0483

Immunosuppressive drug, not otherwise classified, J7599
Impacted tooth, removal, D7220-D7241
Impaction
- tooth, treatment, D7283

Implant
- access system, A4301
- aqueous shunt, L8612
- auditory device
  - brainstem, S2235
  - middle ear, S2230
- breast, L8600

Implant — *continued*
- cochlear, L8614, L8619
- collagen, urinary tract, L8603
- contraceptive, J7306, S0180
- dental
  - chin, D7995
  - endodontic, D3460
  - endosteal/endosseous, D6010
  - eposteal/subperiosteal, D6040
  - facial, D7995
  - maintenance, D6080
  - other implant service, D6053-D6079
  - supported prosthetics, D6053-D6079
    - removal, D6100
    - repair, D6090, D6095
  - transosteal/tensosseous, D6050
- ganciclovir, J7310
- gastric electrical stimulation device, S2213
- gastric stimulation, S2213
- goserelin acetate, J9202
- hallux, L8642
- infusion pump, E0782, E0783
- injectable bulking agent, urinary tract, L8606
- interspinous process distraction device, C1821
- joint, L8630, L8641, L8658
- lacrimal duct, A4262, A4263
- levonorgestral, J7306
- maintenance procedures, D6080, D6100
- maxillofacial, D5913-D5937
- metacarpophalangeal joint, L8630
- metatarsal joint, L8641
- neurostimulator, pulse generator or receiver, E0755, L8685-L8688
- Norplant, J7306
- not otherwise specified, L8699
- ocular, L8610
- ossicular, L8613
- osteogenesis stimulator, E0749
- percutaneous access system, A4301
- removal, dental, D6100
- repair, dental, D6090
- vascular access portal, A4300
- vascular graft, L8670
- yttrium 90, S2095
- Zoladex, J9202

Implantation/reimplantation, tooth, D7270
- intentional reimplantation, D3470

Impregnated gauze dressing, A6222-A6230
Imuran, J7500, J7501
Inapsine, J1790
Incontinence
- appliances and supplies, A4310, A5051-A5093, A5102-A5114, A5120-A5200
- brief or diaper, T4521-T4524, T4543
- disposable/liner, T4535
- garment, A4520
- pediatric
  - brief or diaper, T4529-T4530
  - pull-on protection, T4531-T4532
- reusable
  - diaper or brief, T4539
  - pull-on protection, T4536
- treatment system, E0740
- underpad
  - disposable, T4541, T4542
  - reusable, T4537, T4540
- youth
  - brief or diaper, T4533
  - pull-on protection, T4534

Inderal, J1800
Indium 111
- capromab pendetide, A9507
- ibritumomab tiuxetan, A9542
- oxyquinoline, A9547
- pentetate, A9548
- satumomab pendetide, A4642

Infant safety, CPR, training, S9447

Infergen, J9212
Infliximab injection, J1745
Infusion
- catheter, C1752
- chemotherapy, OPPS
- IVIg service prior to administration, G0332
- IV, OPPS, C8957
- pump, C1772, C2626
  - ambulatory, with administrative equipment, E0781
  - epoprostenol, K0455
  - heparin, dialysis, E1520
  - implantable, E0782, E0783
  - implantable, refill kit, A4220
  - insulin, E0784
  - mechanical, reusable, E0779, E0780
  - nonprogrammable, C1891
  - supplies, A4221, A4222, A4230-A4232
  - Versa-Pole IV, E0776
- supplies, A4222, A4223
- therapy, home, S9347, S9497-S9504

Inhalation drugs
- acetylcysteine, J7608
- albuterol, J7609-J7611, J7613
- Alupent, J7668-J7669
- atropine, J7635-J7636
- Atrovent, J7644
- Azmacort, J7684
- aztreonam, S0143
- beclomethasone, J7622
- betamethasone, J7624
- bitolterol mesylate, J7628-J7629
- Brcanyl, J7680-J7681
- Brethine, J7680-J7681
- budesonide, J7626-J7627, J7633-J7634
- colistimethate sodium, S0142
- cromolyn sodium, J7631
- dexamethasone, J7637-J7638
- dornase alpha, J7639
- flunisolide, J7641
- formoterol, J7640
- Gastrocrom, J7631
- glycopyrolate, J7642-J7643
- iloprost, Q4080
- Intal, J7631
- ipratropium bromide, J7644-J7645
- isoetharine HCl, J7647-J7650
- isoproterenol HCl, J7657-J7660
- levalbuterol, J7607, J7612, J7614-J7615
- metaproterenol sulfate, J7667-J7670
- methacholine chloride, J7674
- Mucomyst, J7608
- Mucosil, J7608
- Nasalcrom, J7631
- NOC, J7699
- Pulmicort Respules, J7627
- terbutaline sulfate, J7680-J7681
- Tobi, J7682
- tobramycin, J7682, J7685
- Tornalate, J7628-J7629
- triamcinolone, J7683-J7684
- Xopenex, J7612, J7614

Initial
- ECG, Medicare, G0366-G0368
- physical exam, Medicare, G0344

Injectable bulking agent, urinary tract, L8606
Injection — *see also* Table of Drugs
- contrast material, during MRI, Q9952-Q9953
- dental service, D9610, D9630
- metatarsal neuroma, S2135
- supplies for self-administered, A4211

Injection adjustment, bariatric band, S2083
Inlay, dental
- fixed partial denture retainers
  - metallic, D6545-D6615
  - porcelain/ceramic, D6548-D6609
- metallic, D2510-D2530
- porcelain/ceramic, D2610-D2630

Wheelchair — *continued*
pediatric — *continued*
seat — *continued*
planar, E2292
power, accessories, E2300-E2399
gear box, E2369
motor, E2368
motor and gear box, E2370
reclining back, E1014
residual limb support, E1020
seat or back cushion, K0669
specially sized, E1220-E1230
support, E1020
tire, E2211, E2214, E2220-E2222, E2381-E2392
valve, E2393
transfer board or device, E0705
transport chair, E1037-E1038
van, nonemergency, A0130, S0209
wheel, E2394-E2395
WHFO, with inflatable air chamber, L3807
Whirlpool equipment, E1300-E1310
Wig, A9282
Win RhoSD, J2792
Wipes, A4245, A4247
Allkare protective barrier, A5120
Wire, guide, C1769
WIZZ-ard manual wheelchair, K0006
Wooden canes, E0100
Wound
cleanser, A6260
cover
alginate dressing, A6196-A6198

Wound — *continued*
cover — *continued*
collagen dressing, A6021-A6024
foam dressing, A6209-A6214
hydrocolloid dressing, A6234-A6239
hydrogel dressing, A6242-A6248
packing strips, A6407
specialty absorptive dressing, A6251-A6256
warming card, E0232
warming device, E0231
non-contact warming cover, A6000
dental, D7910-D7912
electrical stimulation, E0769
filler
alginate, A6199
foam, A6215
hydrocolloid, A6240-A6241
hydrogel, A6242-A6248
not elsewhere classified, A6261-A6262
healing
other growth factor preparation, S9055
Procuren, S9055
packing strips, A6407
pouch, A6154
warming device, E0231
cover, A6000
warming card, E0232

Wound — *continued*
therapy
negative pressure
supplies, A6550
Wrap
abdominal aneurysm, M0301
Wrist
brace, cock-up, L3908
disarticulation prosthesis, L6050, L6055
hand/finger orthosis (WHFO), E1805, E1825, L3800-L3954
Specialist Pre-Formed Ulnar Fracture Brace, L3982
Specialist Wrist/Hand Orthosis, L3999
Specialist Wrist-Hand-Thumb-orthosis, L3999
Splint, lace-up, L3800
Wrist-O-Prene Splint, L3800
Wrist-O-Prene Splint, L3800
Wycillin, J2510
Wydase, J3470

X

Xcaliber power wheelchair, K0014
Xenon Xe-133, A9558
Xolair, J2357
X-ray
dental, D0210-D0340
implant, D6190
equipment
portable, Q0092, R0070, R0075

Y

Y set tubing for peritoneal dialysis, A4719
Yttrium 90
ibritumomab tiuxeton, A9543
microsphere
brachytherapy, C2616
procedure, S2095

Z

Zalcitabine, S0141
Zanamivir, G9018, G9034
Zantac, J2780
Zenapax, J7513
Zetran, J3360
Zidovudine, J3485
ZIFT, S4014
Zinacef, J0697
Zinecard, J1190
Ziprasidone mesylate, J3486
Zithromax
I.V., J0456
oral, Q0144
Zofran, J2405
oral, S0181
Zoladex, J9202
Zoledronic acid, J3487
Zolicef, J0690
Zosyn, J2543
Zygomatic arch, fracture treatment, D7650, D7660, D7750, D7760
Zyprexa, S0166
Zyvok, J2020

TRANSPORTATION SERVICES INCLUDING AMBULANCE
A0000-A0999

This code range includes ground and air ambulance, nonemergency transportation (taxi, bus, automobile, wheelchair van), and ancillary transportation-related fees.

Ambulance Origin and Destination modifiers used with transportation service codes are single-digit modifiers used in combination in boxes 12 and 13 of CMS form 1491. The frst digit indicates the transport"s place of origin, and the destination is indicated by the second digit. The modifiers most commonly used are:

D	Diagnostic or therapeutic site other than "P" or "H"
E	Residential, domiciliary, custodial facility (nursing home, not skilled nursing facility)
G	Hospital-based dialysis facility (hospital or hospital-related)
H	Hospital
I	Site of transfer (for example, airport or helicopter pad) between types of ambulance
J	Non-hospital-based dialysis facility
N	Skilled nursing facility (SNF)
P	Physician"s offce (includes HMO non-hospital facility, clinic, etc.)
R	Residence
S	Scene of accident or acute event
X	Intermediate stop at physician"s offce enroute to the hospital (includes HMO non-hospital facility, clinic, etc.)

Note: Modifier X can only be used as a designation code in the second position of a modifier.

See Q3019, Q3020, and S0215. For Medicaid, see T codes and T modifiers.

Claims for transportation services fall under the jurisdiction of the local contractor.

E	A0021	Ambulance service, outside state per mile, transport (Medicaid only)
E	A0080	Nonemergency transportation, per mile — vehicle provided by volunteer (individual or organization), with no vested interest
E	A0090	Nonemergency transportation, per mile — vehicle provided by individual (family member, self, neighbor) with vested interest
E	A0100	Nonemergency transportation; taxi
E	A0110	Nonemergency transportation and bus, intra- or interstate carrier
E	A0120	Nonemergency transportation: mini-bus, mountain area transports, or other transportation systems
E	A0130	Nonemergency transportation: wheelchair van
E	A0140	Nonemergency transportation and air travel (private or commercial), intra- or interstate
E	A0160	Nonemergency transportation: per mile — caseworker or social worker
E	A0170	Transportation ancillary: parking fees, tolls, other
E	A0180	Nonemergency transportation: ancillary: lodging — recipient
E	A0190	Nonemergency transportation: ancillary: meals — recipient
E	A0200	Nonemergency transportation: ancillary: lodging — escort
E	A0210	Nonemergency transportation: ancillary: meals — escort

A	A0225	Ambulance service, neonatal transport, base rate, emergency transport, one way MED: 100-4,1,10.1.4.1
A	A0380	BLS mileage (per mile) See code(s): A0425 MED: 100-2,6,10; 100-4,1,10.1.4.1
A	A0382	BLS routine disposable supplies
A	A0384	BLS specialized service disposable supplies; defibrillation (used by ALS ambulances and BLS ambulances in jurisdictions where defibrillation is permitted in BLS ambulances)
A	A0390	ALS mileage (per mile) See code(s): A0425 MED: 100-4,1,10.1.4.1
A	A0392	ALS specialized service disposable supplies; defibrillation (to be used only in jurisdictions where defibrillation cannot be performed by BLS ambulances)
A	A0394	ALS specialized service disposable supplies; IV drug therapy
A	A0396	ALS specialized service disposable supplies; esophageal intubation
A	A0398	ALS routine disposable supplies

WAITING TIME TABLE

	Units		Time
1	1/2	to	1 hr.
2	1	to	11/2 hrs.
3	11/2	to	2 hrs.
4	2	to	21/2 hrs.
5	21/2	to	3 hrs.
6	3	to	31/2 hrs.
7	31/2	to	4 hrs.
8	4	to	41/2 hrs.
9	41/2	to	5 hrs.
10	5	to	51/2 hrs.

A	A0420	Ambulance waiting time (ALS or BLS), one-half (1/2) hour increments ⊘
A	A0422	Ambulance (ALS or BLS) oxygen and oxygen supplies, life sustaining situation ⊘
A	A0424	Extra ambulance attendant, ground (ALS or BLS) or air (fixed or rotary winged); (requires medical review) ⊘ Pertinent documentation to evaluate medical appropriateness should be included when this code is reported.
A	A0425	Ground mileage, per statute mile MED: 100-2,6,10; 100-4,1,10.1.4.1
A	A0426	Ambulance service, advanced life support, nonemergency transport, level 1 (ALS 1) MED: 100-2,6,10; 100-4,1,10.1.4.1
A	A0427	Ambulance service, advanced life support, emergency transport, level 1 (ALS 1 — emergency) MED: 100-2,6,10; 100-4,1,10.1.4.1
A	A0428	Ambulance service, basic life support, nonemergency transport (BLS) MED: 100-2,6,10; 100-4,1,10.1.4.1
A	A0429	Ambulance service, basic life support, emergency transport (BLS — emergency) MED: 100-2,6,10; 100-4,1,10.1.4.1

Special Coverage Instructions | Noncovered by Medicare | Carrier Discretion | ☑ Quality Alert | ● New Code | ○ Reinstated Code | ▲ Revised Code

Medical and Surgical Supplies

A0430 — A4248

[A]   A0430   Ambulance service, conventional air services, transport, one way (fixed wing)
MED: 100-2,6,10; 100-4,1,10.1.4.1

[A]   A0431   Ambulance service, conventional air services, transport, one way (rotary wing)
MED: 100-2,6,10; 100-4,1,10.1.4.1

[A]   A0432   Paramedic intercept (PI), rural area, transport furnished by a volunteer ambulance company which is prohibited by state law from billing third-party payers

[A]   A0433   Advanced life support, level 2 (ALS 2)

[A]   A0434   Specialty care transport (SCT)

[A]   A0435   Fixed wing air mileage, per statute mile

[A]   A0436   Rotary wing air mileage, per statute mile

~~A0800~~   ~~Ambulance transport provided between the hours of 7 p.m. and 7 a.m.~~

[E]   A0888   Noncovered ambulance mileage, per mile (e.g., for miles traveled beyond closest appropriate facility)
MED: 100-2,10,20

[E]   A0998   Ambulance response and treatment, no transport

[A]   A0999   Unlisted ambulance service   ⊘
Determine if an alternative HCPCS Level II or a CPT code better describes the service being reported. This code should be used only if a more specific code is unavailable.
MED: 100-2,10,10.1; 100-2,10,20; 100-4,1,10.1.4.1

MEDICAL AND SURGICAL SUPPLIES A4000-A8999

This section covers a wide variety of medical, surgical, and some durable medical equipment (DME) related supplies and accessories. DME-related supplies, accessories, maintenance, and repair required to ensure the proper functioning of this equipment is generally covered by Medicare under the prosthetic devices provision.

MISCELLANEOUS SUPPLIES

These codes are to be filed with the Medicare local contractor, unless otherwise noted (if incident to a physicians' services, not separately billable) unless they represent incidental services or supplies which are referred to the DME Medicare Administrative Contractor (DME MAC).

[E] ☑   A4206   Syringe with needle, sterile 1 cc, each
This code specifies a 1 cc syringe but is also used to report 3/10 cc or 1/2 cc syringes.

[E] ☑   A4207   Syringe with needle, sterile 2 cc, each

[E] ☑   A4208   Syringe with needle, sterile 3 cc, each

[E] ☑   A4209   Syringe with needle, sterile 5 cc or greater, each

[E]   A4210   Needle-free injection device, each
Sometimes covered by commercial payers with preauthorization and physician letter stating need (e.g., for insulin injection in young children).
MED: 100-3,280.1

[E]   A4211   Supplies for self-administered injections
When a drug that is usually injected by the patient (e.g., insulin or calcitonin) is injected by the physician, it is excluded from Medicare coverage unless administered in an emergency situation (e.g., diabetic coma).
MED: 100-2,15,50

[B]   A4212   Noncoring needle or stylet with or without catheter

[E]   A4213   Syringe, sterile, 20 cc or greater, each

[E]   A4215   Needle, sterile, any size, each

▲ [A] ☑   A4216   Sterile water, saline and/or dextrose, diluent/flush, 10 ml   ఉ
MED: 100-2,15,50

[A] ☑   A4217   Sterile water/saline, 500 ml   ఉ
MED: 100-2,15,50

[N]   A4218   Sterile saline or water, metered dose dispenser, 10 ml
MED: 100-4,4,230.1

[N]   A4220   Refill kit for implantable infusion pump
Implantable infusion pumps are covered by Medicare for 5-FUdR therapy for unresected liver or colorectal cancer and for opioid drug therapy for intractable pain. They are not covered by Medicare for heparin therapy for thromboembolic disease. Report drugs separately.
MED: 100-3,280.14

[Y]   A4221   Supplies for maintenance of drug infusion catheter, per week (list drug separately)   ఉ

[Y]   A4222   Infusion supplies for external drug infusion pump, per cassette or bag (list drugs separately)   ఉ

[E] ☑   A4223   Infusion supplies not used with external infusion pump, per cassette or bag (list drugs separately)

[Y] ☑   A4230   Infusion set for external insulin pump, nonneedle cannula type
Covered by some commercial payers as ongoing supply to preauthorized pump.
MED: 100-3,280.14

[Y] ☑   A4231   Infusion set for external insulin pump, needle type
Covered by some commercial payers as ongoing supply to preauthorized pump.
MED: 100-3,280.14

[E] ☑   A4232   Syringe with needle for external insulin pump, sterile, 3 cc
Covered by some commercial payers as ongoing supply to preauthorized pump.
MED: 100-3,280.14

[Y]   A4233   Replacement battery, alkaline (other than J cell), for use with medically necessary home blood glucose monitor owned by patient, each

[Y]   A4234   Replacement battery, alkaline, J cell, for use with medically necessary home blood glucose monitor owned by patient, each

[Y]   A4235   Replacement battery, lithium, for use with medically necessary home blood glucose monitor owned by patient, each

[Y]   A4236   Replacement battery, silver oxide, for use with medically necessary home blood glucose monitor owned by patient, each

[E] ☑   A4244   Alcohol or peroxide, per pint

[E] ☑   A4245   Alcohol wipes, per box

[E] ☑   A4246   Betadine or PhisoHex solution, per pint

[E] ☑   A4247   Betadine or iodine swabs/wipes, per box

[N] ☑   A4248   Chlorhexidine containing antiseptic, 1 ml

| Special Coverage Instructions | Noncovered by Medicare | Carrier Discretion | ☑ Quality Alert | ● New Code | ○ Reinstated Code | ▲ Revised Code |

2 — A Codes   [A] Age Edit   [M] Maternity Edit   ♀ Female Only   ♂ Male Only   [A] - [Y] APC Status Indicators   **2007 HCPCS**

Reference chart

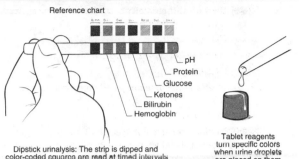

Dipstick urinalysis: The strip is dipped and color-coded squares are read at timed intervals (e.g., pH immediately; ketones at 15 sec., etc.). Results are compared against a reference chart

— pH
— Protein
— Glucose
— Ketones
— Bilirubin
— Hemoglobin

Tablet reagents turn specific colors when urine droplets are placed on them

E ☑ **A4250** Urine test or reagent strips or tablets (100 tablets or strips)
MED: 100-2,15,110

Y ☑ **A4253** Blood glucose test or reagent strips for home blood glucose monitor, per 50 strips   ら
Medicare covers glucose strips for diabetic patients using home glucose monitoring devices prescribed by their physicians.
MED: 100-3,40.2

Y ☑ **A4255** Platforms for home blood glucose monitor, 50 per box   ら
Some Medicare contractors cover monitor platforms for diabetic patients using home glucose monitoring devices prescribed by their physicians. Some commercial payers also provide this coverage to non-insulin dependent diabetics.
MED: 100-3,40.2

Y ☑ **A4256** Normal, low, and high calibrator solution/chips   ら
Some Medicare contractors cover calibration solutions or chips for diabetic patients using home glucose monitoring devices prescribed by their physicians. Some commercial payers also provide this coverage to non-insulin dependent diabetics.
MED: 100-3,40.2

Y ☑ **A4257** Replacement lens shield cartridge for use with laser skin piercing device, each   ら

Y ☑ **A4258** Spring-powered device for lancet, each   ら
Some Medicare contractors cover lancing devices for diabetic patients using home glucose monitoring devices prescribed by their physicians. Medicare jurisdiction: DME regional contractor. Some commercial payers also provide this coverage to non-insulin dependent diabetics.
MED: 100-3,40.2

Y ☑ **A4259** Lancets, per box of 100   ら
Medicare covers lancets for diabetic patients using home glucose monitoring devices prescribed by their physicians. Medicare jurisdiction: DME regional contractor. Some commercial payers also provide this coverage to non-insulin dependent diabetics.
MED: 100-3,40.2

E **A4261** Cervical cap for contraceptive use   ♀

N ☑ **A4262** Temporary, absorbable lacrimal duct implant, each
Always report concurrent to the implant procedure.

N ☑ **A4263** Permanent, long-term, nondissolvable lacrimal duct implant, each
Always report concurrent to the implant procedure.

Y ☑ **A4265** Paraffin, per lb.   ら
Medicare jurisdiction: DME regional contractor.
MED: 100-3,280.1

E **A4266** Diaphragm for contraceptive use   ♀

E ☑ **A4267** Contraceptive supply, condom, male, each
E ☑ **A4268** Contraceptive supply, condom, female, each   ♀
E ☑ **A4269** Contraceptive supply, spermicide (e.g., foam, gel), each   Ⓐ
N ☑ **A4270** Disposable endoscope sheath, each

Two part prosthesis

Adhesive skin support (A4280)

Any of several breast prostheses fits over skin support

Ⓐ **A4280** Adhesive skin support attachment for use with external breast prosthesis, each   Ⓐ♀ら

E **A4281** Tubing for breast pump, replacement   Ⓜ♀
E **A4282** Adapter for breast pump, replacement   Ⓜ♀
E **A4283** Cap for breast pump bottle, replacement   Ⓜ♀
E **A4284** Breast shield and splash protector for use with breast pump, replacement   Ⓜ♀
E **A4285** Polycarbonate bottle for use with breast pump, replacement   Ⓜ♀
E **A4286** Locking ring for breast pump, replacement   Ⓜ♀
B ☑ **A4290** Sacral nerve stimulation test lead, each
AHA: 1Q,'02,9

VASCULAR CATHETERS

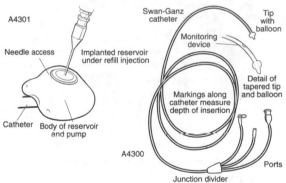

A4301

Needle access

Implanted reservoir under refill injection

Catheter   Body of reservoir and pump

Swan-Ganz catheter

Monitoring device

Tip with balloon

Detail of tapered tip and balloon

Markings along catheter measure depth of insertion

A4300

Junction divider

Ports

N **A4300** Implantable access catheter, (e.g., venous, arterial, epidural subarachnoid, or peritoneal, etc.) external access
MED: 100-2,15,120

N **A4301** Implantable access total catheter, port/reservoir (e.g., venous, arterial, epidural, subarachnoid, peritoneal, etc.)

N **A4305** Disposable drug delivery system, flow rate of 50 ml or greater per hour

▲ N **A4306** Disposable drug delivery system, flow rate of less than 50 ml per hour

Special Coverage Instructions   Noncovered by Medicare   Carrier Discretion   ☑ Quality Alert   ● New Code   ○ Reinstated Code   ▲ Revised Code

2007 HCPCS   **1**-**9** ASC Group   MED: Pub 100/NCD References   ら DMEPOS Paid   ⊘ SNF Excluded   **A Codes — 3**

Medical and Surgical Supplies

A4310 — A4355

INCONTINENCE APPLIANCES AND CARE SUPPLIES

Covered by Medicare when the medical record indicates incontinence is permanent, or of long and indefinite duration.

Medicare claims fall under the jurisdiction of the DME Medicare Administrative Contractor (DME MAC) for a permanent condition, and under the local contractor when provided in the physician's office for a temporary condition.

[A] **A4310** Insertion tray without drainage bag and without catheter (accessories only) ♻
MED: 100-2,15,120

[A] **A4311** Insertion tray without drainage bag with indwelling catheter, Foley type, two-way latex with coating (Teflon, silicone, silicone elastomer or hydrophilic, etc.) ♻
MED: 100-2,15,120

[A] **A4312** Insertion tray without drainage bag with indwelling catheter, Foley type, two-way, all silicone ♻
MED: 100-2,15,120

[A] **A4313** Insertion tray without drainage bag with indwelling catheter, Foley type, three-way, for continuous irrigation ♻
MED: 100-2,15,120

[A] **A4314** Insertion tray with drainage bag with indwelling catheter, Foley type, two-way latex with coating (Teflon, silicone, silicone elastomer or hydrophilic, etc.) ♻
MED: 100-2,15,120

[A] **A4315** Insertion tray with drainage bag with indwelling catheter, Foley type, two-way, all silicone ♻
MED: 100-2,15,120

[A] **A4316** Insertion tray with drainage bag with indwelling catheter, Foley type, three-way, for continuous irrigation ♻
MED: 100-2,15,120

[A] **A4320** Irrigation tray with bulb or piston syringe, any purpose ♻
MED: 100-2,15,120

[A] **A4321** Therapeutic agent for urinary catheter irrigation ♻
MED: 100-2,15,120

[A] ☑ **A4322** Irrigation syringe, bulb or piston, each ♻
MED: 100-2,15,120

▲ [A] ☑ **A4326** Male external catheter with integral collection chamber, any type, each ♂ ♻
MED: 100-2,15,120

[A] ☑ **A4327** Female external urinary collection device; metal cup, each ♀ ♻
MED: 100-2,15,120

[A] ☑ **A4328** Female external urinary collection device; pouch, each ♀ ♻
MED: 100-2,15,120

[A] ☑ **A4330** Perianal fecal collection pouch with adhesive, each ♻
MED: 100-2,15,120

[A] ☑ **A4331** Extension drainage tubing, any type, any length, with connector/adaptor, for use with urinary leg bag or urostomy pouch, each ♻
MED: 100-2,15,120

[A] ☑ **A4332** Lubricant, individual sterile packet, each ♻
MED: 100-2,15,120

[A] ☑ **A4333** Urinary catheter anchoring device, adhesive skin attachment, each ♻
MED: 100-2,15,120

[A] ☑ **A4334** Urinary catheter anchoring device, leg strap, each ♻
MED: 100-2,15,120

[A] **A4335** Incontinence supply; miscellaneous
MED: 100-2,15,120

[A] ☑ **A4338** Indwelling catheter; Foley type, two-way latex with coating (Teflon, silicone, silicone elastomer, or hydrophilic, etc.), each ♻
MED: 100-2,15,120

[A] ☑ **A4340** Indwelling catheter; specialty type, (e.g., Coude, mushroom, wing, etc.), each ♻
MED: 100-2,15,120

[A] ☑ **A4344** Indwelling catheter, Foley type, two-way, all silicone, each ♻
MED: 100-2,15,120

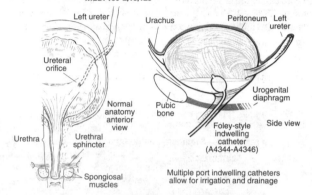

[A] ☑ **A4346** Indwelling catheter; Foley type, three-way for continuous irrigation, each ♻
MED: 100-2,15,120

~~**A4348** Male external catheter with integral collection compartment, extended wear, each (e.g., 2 per month)~~
See code(s) A4326

[A] ☑ **A4349** Male external catheter, with or without adhesive, disposable, each
MED: 100-2,15,120

[A] ☑ **A4351** Intermittent urinary catheter; straight tip, with or without coating (Teflon, silicone, silicone elastomer, or hydrophilic, etc.), each ♻
MED: 100-2,15,120

[A] ☑ **A4352** Intermittent urinary catheter; Coude (curved) tip, with or without coating (Teflon, silicone, silicone elastomeric, or hydrophilic, etc.), each ♻
MED: 100-2,15,120

[A] **A4353** Intermittent urinary catheter, with insertion supplies ♻
MED: 100-2,15,120

[A] **A4354** Insertion tray with drainage bag but without catheter ♻
MED: 100-2,15,120

[A] ☑ **A4355** Irrigation tubing set for continuous bladder irrigation through a three-way indwelling Foley catheter, each ♻
MED: 100-2,15,120

EXTERNAL URINARY SUPPLIES

Medicare claims fall under the jurisdiction of the DME Medicare Administrative Contractor (DME MAC) for a permanent condition, and under the local contractor when provided in the physician's office for a temporary condition.

| Special Coverage Instructions | Noncovered by Medicare | Carrier Discretion | ☑ Quality Alert | ● New Code | ○ Reinstated Code | ▲ Revised Code |

4 — A Codes   [A] Age Edit   [M] Maternity Edit   ♀ Female Only   ♂ Male Only   [A] - ☑ APC Status Indicators   *2007 HCPCS*

Ⓐ ☑ **A4356** External urethral clamp or compression device (not to be used for catheter clamp), each ♿
MED: 100-2,15,120

Ⓐ ☑ **A4357** Bedside drainage bag, day or night, with or without anti-reflux device, with or without tube, each ♿
MED: 100-2,15,120

Ⓐ ☑ **A4358** Urinary drainage bag, leg or abdomen, vinyl, with or without tube, with straps, each ♿
MED: 100-2,15,120

~~**A4359** Urinary suspensory without leg bag, each~~
Use A5105

OSTOMY SUPPLIES

Medicare claims fall under the jurisdiction of the DME Medicare Administrative Contractor (DME MAC) for a permanent condition, and under the local contractor when provided in the physician's office for a temporary condition.

Ⓐ ☑ **A4361** Ostomy faceplate, each ♿
MED: 100-2,15,120

Ⓐ ☑ **A4362** Skin barrier; solid, four by four or equivalent; each ♿
See code(s) A4461 or A4463

Ⓐ **A4363** Ostomy clamp, any type, replacement only, each ♿

Ⓐ ☑ **A4364** Adhesive, liquid, or equal, any type, per oz. ♿
MED: 100-2,15,120

Ⓐ ☑ **A4365** Adhesive remover wipes, any type, per 50 ♿
MED: 100-2,15,120

Ⓐ ☑ **A4366** Ostomy vent, any type, each ♿

Ⓐ ☑ **A4367** Ostomy belt, each ♿
MED: 100-2,15,120

Ⓐ ☑ **A4368** Ostomy filter, any type, each ♿

Ⓐ ☑ **A4369** Ostomy skin barrier, liquid (spray, brush, etc.), per oz. ♿
MED: 100-2,15,120

Ⓐ ☑ **A4371** Ostomy skin barrier, powder, per oz. ♿
MED: 100-2,15,120

Ⓐ ☑ **A4372** Ostomy skin barrier, solid 4x4 or equivalent, standard wear, with built-in convexity, each ♿
MED: 100-2,15,120

Barrier adheres to skin
Flange attaches to bag
Waste moves through hole in membrane
Faceplate flange and skin barrier combination (A4373)

Ⓐ ☑ **A4373** Ostomy skin barrier, with flange (solid, flexible or accordion), with built-in convexity, any size, each ♿
MED: 100-2,15,120

Ⓐ ☑ **A4375** Ostomy pouch, drainable, with faceplate attached, plastic, each ♿
MED: 100-2,15,120

Colostomy pouch with faceplate and drain (A4376)

Ⓐ ☑ **A4376** Ostomy pouch, drainable, with faceplate attached, rubber, each ♿
MED: 100-2,15,120

Ⓐ ☑ **A4377** Ostomy pouch, drainable, for use on faceplate, plastic, each ♿
MED: 100-2,15,120

Ⓐ ☑ **A4378** Ostomy pouch, drainable, for use on faceplate, rubber, each ♿
MED: 100-2,15,120

Ⓐ ☑ **A4379** Ostomy pouch, urinary, with faceplate attached, plastic, each ♿
MED: 100-2,15,120

Ⓐ ☑ **A4380** Ostomy pouch, urinary, with faceplate attached, rubber, each ♿
MED: 100-2,15,120

Ⓐ ☑ **A4381** Ostomy pouch, urinary, for use on faceplate, plastic, each ♿
MED: 100-2,15,120

Ⓐ ☑ **A4382** Ostomy pouch, urinary, for use on faceplate, heavy plastic, each ♿
MED: 100-2,15,120

Ⓐ ☑ **A4383** Ostomy pouch, urinary, for use on faceplate, rubber, each ♿
MED: 100-2,15,120

Ⓐ ☑ **A4384** Ostomy faceplate equivalent, silicone ring, each ♿
MED: 100-2,15,120

Ⓐ ☑ **A4385** Ostomy skin barrier, solid 4 x 4 or equivalent, extended wear, without built-in convexity, each ♿
MED: 100-2,15,120

Ⓐ ☑ **A4387** Ostomy pouch, closed, with barrier attached, with built-in convexity (one piece), each ♿
MED: 100-2,15,120

Ⓐ ☑ **A4388** Ostomy pouch, drainable, with extended wear barrier attached, (one piece), each ♿
MED: 100-2,15,120

Ⓐ ☑ **A4389** Ostomy pouch, drainable, with barrier attached, with built-in convexity (one piece), each ♿
MED: 100-2,15,120

Ⓐ ☑ **A4390** Ostomy pouch, drainable, with extended wear barrier attached, with built-in convexity (1 piece), each ♿
MED: 100-2,15,120

Ⓐ ☑ **A4391** Ostomy pouch, urinary, with extended wear barrier attached (1 piece), each ♿
MED: 100-2,15,120

Ⓐ ☑ **A4392** Ostomy pouch, urinary, with standard wear barrier attached, with built-in convexity (1 piece), each ♿
MED: 100-2,15,120

Ⓐ ☑ **A4393** Ostomy pouch, urinary, with extended wear barrier attached, with built-in convexity (1 piece), each ♿
MED: 100-2,15,120

Special Coverage Instructions | Noncovered by Medicare | Carrier Discretion | ☑ Quality Alert | ● New Code | ○ Reinstated Code | ▲ Revised Code

2007 HCPCS | 1-9 ASC Group | MED: Pub 100/NCD References | ♿ DMEPOS Paid | ○ SNF Excluded | A Codes — 5

Medical and Surgical Supplies

A4394 — A4455

▲ A ☑ **A4394** Ostomy deodorant, with or without lubricant, for use in ostomy pouch, per fluid ounce
MED: 100-2,15,120

A ☑ **A4395** Ostomy deodorant for use in ostomy pouch, solid, per tablet
MED: 100-2,15,120

A **A4396** Ostomy belt with peristomal hernia support
MED: 100-2,15,120

A ☑ **A4397** Irrigation supply; sleeve, each
MED: 100-2,15,120

A ☑ **A4398** Ostomy irrigation supply; bag, each
MED: 100-2,15,120

A **A4399** Ostomy irrigation supply; cone/catheter, including brush
MED: 100-2,15,120

A **A4400** Ostomy irrigation set
MED: 100-2,15,120

A ☑ **A4402** Lubricant, per oz.
MED: 100-2,15,120

A ☑ **A4404** Ostomy ring, each
MED: 100-2,15,120

A ☑ **A4405** Ostomy skin barrier, nonpectin-based, paste, per oz.
MED: 100-2,15,120

A ☑ **A4406** Ostomy skin barrier, pectin-based, paste, per oz.
MED: 100-2,15,120

A ☑ **A4407** Ostomy skin barrier, with flange (solid, flexible, or accordion), extended wear, with built-in convexity, 4 x 4 in. or smaller, each
MED: 100-2,15,120

A ☑ **A4408** Ostomy skin barrier, with flange (solid, flexible or accordion), extended wear, with built-in convexity, larger than 4 x 4 in., each
MED: 100-2,15,120

A ☑ **A4409** Ostomy skin barrier, with flange (solid, flexible or accordion), extended wear, without built-in convexity, 4 x 4 in. or smaller, each
MED: 100-2,15,120

A ☑ **A4410** Ostomy skin barrier, with flange (solid, flexible or accordion), extended wear, without built-in convexity, larger than 4 x 4 in., each
MED: 100-2,15,120

A **A4411** Ostomy skin barrier, solid 4x4 or equivalent, extended wear, with built-in convexity, each

A **A4412** Ostomy pouch, drainable, high output, for use on a barrier with flange (2 piece system), without filter, each

A ☑ **A4413** Ostomy pouch, drainable, high output, for use on a barrier with flange (two piece system), with filter, each
MED: 100-2,15,120

A ☑ **A4414** Ostomy skin barrier, with flange (solid, flexible or accordion), without built-in convexity, 4 x 4 in. or smaller, each
MED: 100-2,15,120

A ☑ **A4415** Ostomy skin barrier, with flange (solid, flexible or accordion), without built-in convexity, larger than 4 x 4 in., each
MED: 100-2,15,120

A ☑ **A4416** Ostomy pouch, closed, with barrier attached, with filter (one piece), each

A ☑ **A4417** Ostomy pouch, closed, with barrier attached, with built-in convexity, with filter (one piece), each

A ☑ **A4418** Ostomy pouch, closed; without barrier attached, with filter (one piece), each

A ☑ **A4419** Ostomy pouch, closed; for use on barrier with nonlocking flange, with filter (two piece), each

A ☑ **A4420** Ostomy pouch, closed; for use on barrier with locking flange (two piece), each

E **A4421** Ostomy supply; miscellaneous
Determine if an alternative HCPCS Level II or a CPT code better describes the service being reported. This code should be used only if a more specific code is unavailable.
MED: 100-2,15,120

A **A4422** Ostomy absorbent material (sheet/pad/crystal packet) for use in ostomy pouch to thicken liquid stomal output, each
MED: 100-2,15,120

A ☑ **A4423** Ostomy pouch, closed; for use on barrier with locking flange, with filter (two piece), each

A ☑ **A4424** Ostomy pouch, drainable, with barrier attached, with filter (one piece), each

A ☑ **A4425** Ostomy pouch, drainable; for use on barrier with nonlocking flange, with filter (two piece system), each

A ☑ **A4426** Ostomy pouch, drainable; for use on barrier with locking flange (two piece system), each

A ☑ **A4427** Ostomy pouch, drainable; for use on barrier with locking flange, with filter (two piece system), each

A ☑ **A4428** Ostomy pouch, urinary, with extended wear barrier attached, with faucet-type tap with valve (one piece), each

A ☑ **A4429** Ostomy pouch, urinary, with barrier attached, with built-in convexity, with faucet-type tap with valve (one piece), each

A ☑ **A4430** Ostomy pouch, urinary, with extended wear barrier attached, with built-in convexity, with faucet-type tap with valve (one piece), each

A ☑ **A4431** Ostomy pouch, urinary; with barrier attached, with faucet-type tap with valve (one piece), each

A ☑ **A4432** Ostomy pouch, urinary; for use on barrier with nonlocking flange, with faucet-type tap with valve (two piece), each

A ☑ **A4433** Ostomy pouch, urinary; for use on barrier with locking flange (two piece), each

A ☑ **A4434** Ostomy pouch, urinary; for use on barrier with locking flange, with faucet-type tap with valve (two piece), each

ADDITIONAL MISCELLANEOUS SUPPLIES

A ☑ **A4450** Tape, nonwaterproof, per 18 sq. in.
See also code A4452.
MED: 100-2,15,120

A ☑ **A4452** Tape, waterproof, per 18 sq. in.
See also code A4450.
MED: 100-2,15,120

A ☑ **A4455** Adhesive remover or solvent (for tape, cement or other adhesive), per oz.
MED: 100-2,15,120

Special Coverage Instructions　　　Noncovered by Medicare　　　Carrier Discretion　　　☑ Quality Alert　　● New Code　　○ Reinstated Code　▲ Revised Code

6 — A Codes　　　　　A Age Edit　　M Maternity Edit　♀ Female Only　　♂ Male Only　　A - ☑ APC Status Indicators　　　***2007 HCPCS***

E		A4458	Enema bag with tubing, reusable
●	A	A4461	Surgical dressing holder, nonreusable, each
		A4462	Abdominal dressing holder, each
●	A	A4463	Surgical dressing holder, reusable, each
	A	A4465	Nonelastic binder for extremity
	A	A4470	Gravlee jet washer

The Gravlee jet washer is a disposable device used to detect endometrial cancer. It is covered only in patients exhibiting clinical symptoms or signs suggestive of endometrial disease. Medicare jurisdiction: local contractor.

MED: 100-2,16,90; 100-3,230.5

A4480 VABRA aspirator ♀

The VABRA aspirator is a disposable device used to detect endometrial cancer. It is covered only in patients exhibiting clinical symptoms or signs suggestive of endometrial disease. Medicare jurisdiction: local contractor.

MED: 100-2,16,90; 100-3,230.6

A4481 ☑ Tracheostoma filter, any type, any size, each

MED: 100-2,15,120

A4483 Moisture exchanger, disposable, for use with invasive mechanical ventilation

MED: 100-2,15,120

A4490 ☑ Surgical stocking above knee length, each

MED: 100-2,15,100; 100-2,15,110; 100-3,280.1

A4495 ☑ Surgical stocking thigh length, each

MED: 100-2,15,100; 100-2,15,110; 100-3,280.1

A4500 ☑ Surgical stocking below knee length, each

MED: 100-2,15,100; 100-2,15,110; 100-3,280.1

A4510 ☑ Surgical stocking full-length, each

MED: 100-2,15,100; 100-2,15,110; 100-3,280.1

A4520 ☑ Incontinence garment, any type, (e.g., brief, diaper), each

MED: 100-3,280.1

A4550 Surgical trays

Medicare jurisdiction: local contractor.

A4554 ☑ Disposable underpads, all sizes (e.g., Chux's)

MED: 100-2,15,120; 100-3,280.1

A4556 ☑ Electrodes (e.g., apnea monitor), per pair

A4557 ☑ Lead wires (e.g., apnea monitor), per pair

▲ **A4558** Conductive gel or paste, for use with electrical device (e.g., TENS, NMES), per oz.

● **A4559** Coupling gel or paste, for use with ultrasound device, per ounce

A4561 Pessary, rubber, any type ♀

A4562 Pessary, nonrubber, any type ♀

Medicare jurisdiction: DME regional contractor.

A4565 Slings

Dressings applied by a physician are included as part of the professional service. Surgical dressings obtained by the patient to perform homecare as prescribed by the physician are covered.

A4570 Splint

Dressings applied by a physician are included as part of the professional service.

MED: 100-2,6,10; 100-2,15,100; 100-4,4,240

A4575 Topical hyperbaric oxygen chamber, disposable

MED: 100-3,20.29

A4580 Cast supplies (e.g., plaster)

See Q4001-Q4048.

MED: 100-2,6,10; 100-2,15,100; 100-4,4,240

A4590 Special casting material (e.g., fiberglass)

See Q4001-Q4048.

MED: 100-2,6,10; 100-2,15,100; 100-4,4,240

A4595 Electrical stimulator supplies, 2 lead, per month, (e.g. TENS, NMES)

MED: 100-3,160.13

● **A4600** Sleeve for intermittent limb compression device, replacement only, each

● **A4601** Lithium ion battery for nonprosthetic use, replacement

A4604 Tubing with integrated heating element for use with positive airway pressure device

A4605 ☑ Tracheal suction catheter, closed system, each

A4606 Oxygen probe for use with oximeter device, replacement

A4608 ☑ Transtracheal oxygen catheter, each

Medicare jurisdiction: DME regional contractor.

SUPPLIES FOR OXYGEN AND RELATED RESPIRATORY EQUIPMENT

A4611 Battery, heavy duty; replacement for patient-owned ventilator

Medicare jurisdiction: DME regional contractor.

A4612 Battery cables; replacement for patient-owned ventilator

Medicare jurisdiction: DME regional contractor.

A4613 Battery charger; replacement for patient-owned ventilator

Medicare jurisdiction: DME regional contractor.

A4614 Peak expiratory flow rate meter, hand held

A4615 Cannula, nasal

MED: 100-3,160.6; 100-4,20,100.2

A4616 ☑ Tubing (oxygen), per foot

MED: 100-3,160.6; 100-4,20,100.2

A4617 Mouthpiece

MED: 100-3,160.6; 100-4,20,100.2

A4618 Breathing circuits

MED: 100-3,160.6; 100-4,20,100.2

A4619 Face tent

MED: 100-3,160.6; 100-4,20,100.2

A4620 Variable concentration mask

MED: 100-3,160.6; 100-4,20,100.2

A4623 Tracheostomy, inner cannula

MED: 100-2,15,120; 100-3,20.9

A4624 ☑ Tracheal suction catheter, any type other than closed system, each

A4625 Tracheostomy care kit for new tracheostomy

MED: 100-2,15,120

A4626 ☑ Tracheostomy cleaning brush, each

MED: 100-2,15,120

A4627 Spacer, bag or reservoir, with or without mask, for use with metered dose inhaler

MED: 100-2,15,110

A4628 ☑ Oropharyngeal suction catheter, each

Special Coverage Instructions   Noncovered by Medicare   Carrier Discretion   ☑ Quality Alert   ● New Code   ○ Reinstated Code   ▲ Revised Code

2007 HCPCS   **1**-**9** ASC Group   **MED:** Pub 100/NCD References   ᕕ DMEPOS Paid   ⊘ SNF Excluded   **A Codes — 7**

Medical and Surgical Supplies

A4629 — A4724

Ⓐ   **A4629** Tracheostomy care kit for established tracheostomy   ♿
MED: 100-2,15,120

SUPPLIES FOR OTHER DURABLE MEDICAL EQUIPMENT

Ⓨ ☑   **A4630** Replacement batteries, medically necessary, transcutaneous electrical stimulator, owned by patient   ♿
MED: 100-3,160.7

~~**A4632** Replacement battery for external infusion pump, any type, each~~
See code(s) K0601-K0605

Ⓨ   **A4633** Replacement bulb/lamp for ultraviolet light therapy system, each   ♿

Ⓐ   **A4634** Replacement bulb for therapeutic light box, tabletop model

Ⓨ ☑   **A4635** Underarm pad, crutch, replacement, each   ♿
Medicare jurisdiction: DME regional contractor.
MED: 100-3,280.1

Ⓨ ☑   **A4636** Replacement, handgrip, cane, crutch, or walker, each   ♿
Medicare jurisdiction: DME regional contractor.
MED: 100-3,280.1

Ⓨ ☑   **A4637** Replacement, tip, cane, crutch, walker, each   ♿
Medicare jurisdiction: DME regional contractor.
MED: 100-3,280.1

Ⓨ ☑   **A4638** Replacement battery for patient-owned ear pulse generator, each   ♿

Ⓨ   **A4639** Replacement pad for infrared heating pad system, each   ♿

Ⓨ   **A4640** Replacement pad for use with medically necessary alternating pressure pad owned by patient   ♿
Medicare jurisdiction: DME regional contractor.
MED: 100-3,280.1; 100-8,5.1.1.2

SUPPLIES FOR RADIOLOGIC PROCEDURES

Ⓝ   **A4641** Radiopharmaceutical, diagnostic, not otherwise classified
Medicare jurisdiction: local contractor.
MED: 100-4,13,60.3; 100-4,13,60.3.1

Ⓗ ☑   **A4642** Indium In-111 satumomab pendetide, diagnostic, per study dose, up to 6 millicuries
Use this code for Oncoscint. Medicare jurisdiction: local contractor.
MED: 100-4,4,20.5; 100-4,4,230.1

Ⓐ   **A4649** Surgical supply; miscellaneous
Determine if an alternative HCPCS Level II or a CPT code better describes the service being reported. This code should be used only if a more specific code is unavailable. Medicare jurisdiction: local contractor.

Ⓐ ☑   **A4651** Calibrated microcapillary tube, each   ⊘
MED: 100-4,3,40.3

Ⓐ   **A4652** Microcapillary tube sealant   ⊘
MED: 100-4,3,40.3

Ⓐ ☑   **A4653** Peritoneal dialysis catheter anchoring device, belt, each   ⊘
MED: 100-4,3,40.3

Ⓐ ☑   **A4657** Syringe, with or without needle, each   ⊘
MED: 100-4,3,40.3

Ⓐ   **A4660** Sphygmomanometer/blood pressure apparatus with cuff and stethoscope   ⊘
MED: 100-4,3,40.3

Ⓐ   **A4663** Blood pressure cuff only   ⊘
MED: 100-4,3,40.3

Ⓔ   **A4670** Automatic blood pressure monitor   ⊘
MED: 100-3,20.19; 100-4,3,40.3

Ⓑ ☑   **A4671** Disposable cycler set used with cycler dialysis machine, each   ⊘
MED: 100-4,3,40.3

Ⓑ ☑   **A4672** Drainage extension line, sterile, for dialysis, each   ⊘
MED: 100-4,3,40.3

Ⓑ   **A4673** Extension line with easy lock connectors, used with dialysis   ⊘
MED: 100-4,3,40.3

Ⓑ ☑   **A4674** Chemicals/antiseptics solution used to clean/sterilize dialysis equipment, per 8 oz.   ⊘
MED: 100-4,3,40.3

Ⓐ ☑   **A4680** Activated carbon filter for hemodialysis, each   ⊘
MED: 100-3,230.7; 100-4,3,40.3

Ⓐ ☑   **A4690** Dialyzer (artificial kidneys), all types, all sizes, for hemodialysis, each   ⊘
MED: 100-4,3,40.3

Ⓐ ☑   **A4706** Bicarbonate concentrate, solution, for hemodialysis, per gallon   ⊘
MED: 100-4,3,40.3

Ⓐ ☑   **A4707** Bicarbonate concentrate, powder, for hemodialysis, per packet   ⊘
MED: 100-4,3,40.3

Ⓐ ☑   **A4708** Acetate concentrate solution, for hemodialysis, per gallon   ⊘
MED: 100-4,3,40.3

Ⓐ ☑   **A4709** Acid concentrate, solution, for hemodialysis, per gallon   ⊘
MED: 100-4,3,40.3

Ⓐ ☑   **A4714** Treated water (deionized, distilled, or reverse osmosis) for peritoneal dialysis, per gallon   ⊘
MED: 100-3,230.7; 100-4,3,40.3

Ⓐ   **A4719** Y set tubing for peritoneal dialysis   ⊘
MED: 100-4,3,40.3

Ⓐ ☑   **A4720** Dialysate solution, any concentration of dextrose, fluid volume greater than 249 cc, but less than or equal to 999 cc, for peritoneal dialysis   ⊘
MED: 100-4,3,40.3

Ⓐ ☑   **A4721** Dialysate solution, any concentration of dextrose, fluid volume greater than 999 cc, but less than or equal to 1999 cc, for peritoneal dialysis   ⊘
MED: 100-4,3,40.3

Ⓐ ☑   **A4722** Dialysate solution, any concentration of dextrose, fluid volume greater than 1999 cc, but less than or equal to 2999 cc, for peritoneal dialysis   ⊘
MED: 100-4,3,40.3

Ⓐ ☑   **A4723** Dialysate solution, any concentration of dextrose, fluid volume greater than 2999 cc, but less than or equal to 3999 cc, for peritoneal dialysis   ⊘
MED: 100-4,3,40.3

Ⓐ ☑   **A4724** Dialysate solution, any concentration of dextrose, fluid volume greater than 3999 cc, but less than or equal to 4999 cc, for peritoneal dialysis   ⊘
MED: 100-4,3,40.3

Special Coverage Instructions   Noncovered by Medicare   Carrier Discretion   ☑ Quality Alert   ● New Code   ○ Reinstated Code   ▲ Revised Code

A ☑ **A4725** Dialysate solution, any concentration of dextrose, fluid volume greater than 4999 cc, but less than or equal to 5999 cc, for peritoneal dialysis ⊘
MED: 100-4,3,40.3

A ☑ **A4726** Dialysate solution, any concentration of dextrose, fluid volume greater than 5999 cc ⊘
MED: 100-4,3,40.3

B ☑ **A4728** Dialysate solution, nondextrose containing, 500 ml ⊘
MED: 100-4,3,40.3

A ☑ **A4730** Fistula cannulation set for hemodialysis, each ⊘
MED: 100-4,3,40.3

A ☑ **A4736** Topical anesthetic, for dialysis, per gm ⊘
MED: 100-4,3,40.3

A ☑ **A4737** Injectable anesthetic, for dialysis, per 10 ml ⊘
MED: 100-4,3,40.3

A **A4740** Shunt accessory, for hemodialysis, any type, each ⊘
MED: 100-4,3,40.3

A ☑ **A4750** Blood tubing, arterial or venous, for hemodialysis, each ⊘
MED: 100-4,3,40.3

A **A4755** Blood tubing, arterial and venous combined, for hemodialysis, each ⊘
MED: 100-4,3,40.3

A ☑ **A4760** Dialysate solution test kit, for peritoneal dialysis, any type, each ⊘
MED: 100-4,3,40.3

A ☑ **A4765** Dialysate concentrate, powder, additive for peritoneal dialysis, per packet ⊘
MED: 100-4,3,40.3

A **A4766** Dialysate concentrate, solution, additive for peritoneal dialysis, per 10 ml ⊘
MED: 100-4,3,40.3

A **A4770** Blood collection tube, vacuum, for dialysis, per 50 ⊘
MED: 100-4,3,40.3

A ☑ **A4771** Serum clotting time tube, for dialysis, per 50 ⊘
MED: 100-4,3,40.3

A ☑ **A4772** Blood glucose test strips, for dialysis, per 50 ⊘
MED: 100-4,3,40.3

A ☑ **A4773** Occult blood test strips, for dialysis, per 50 ⊘
MED: 100-4,3,40.3

A ☑ **A4774** Ammonia test strips, for dialysis, per 50 ⊘
MED: 100-4,3,40.3

A ☑ **A4802** Protamine sulfate, for hemodialysis, per 50 mg ⊘
MED: 100-4,3,40.3

A ☑ **A4860** Disposable catheter tips for peritoneal dialysis, per 10 ⊘
MED: 100-4,3,40.3

A **A4870** Plumbing and/or electrical work for home hemodialysis equipment ⊘
MED: 100-4,3,40.3

A **A4890** Contracts, repair and maintenance, for hemodialysis equipment ⊘
MED: 100-2,15,110.2; 100-4,3,40.3

A ☑ **A4911** Drain bag/bottle, for dialysis, each ⊘

A **A4913** Miscellaneous dialysis supplies, not otherwise specified ⊘
Pertinent documentation to evaluate medical appropriateness should be included when this code is reported. Determine if an alternative HCPCS Level II or a CPT code better describes the service being reported. This code should be used only if a more specific code is unavailable.

A ☑ **A4918** Venous pressure clamp, for hemodialysis, each ⊘

A ☑ **A4927** Gloves, nonsterile, per 100 ⊘

A ☑ **A4928** Surgical mask, per 20 ⊘

A **A4929** Tourniquet for dialysis, each ⊘

A **A4930** Gloves, sterile, per pair ⊘

A **A4931** Oral thermometer, reusable, any type, each ⊘

E **A4932** Rectal thermometer, reusable, any type, each

ADDITIONAL OSTOMY SUPPLIES

Medicare claims fall under the jurisdiction of the DME Administrative Contractor (DME MAC), unless otherwise noted.

A ☑ **A5051** Ostomy pouch, closed; with barrier attached (one piece), each ⛭
MED: 100-2,15,120

A ☑ **A5052** Ostomy pouch, closed; without barrier attached (one piece), each ⛭
MED: 100-2,15,120

A ☑ **A5053** Ostomy pouch, closed; for use on faceplate, each ⛭
MED: 100-2,15,120

A ☑ **A5054** Ostomy pouch, closed; for use on barrier with flange (two piece), each ⛭
MED: 100-2,15,120

A **A5055** Stoma cap ⛭
MED: 100-2,15,120

A ☑ **A5061** Ostomy pouch, drainable; with barrier attached, (one piece), each ⛭
MED: 100-2,15,120

A ☑ **A5062** Ostomy pouch, drainable; without barrier attached (one piece), each ⛭
MED: 100-2,15,120

A ☑ **A5063** Ostomy pouch, drainable; for use on barrier with flange (two piece system), each ⛭
MED: 100-2,15,120

A ☑ **A5071** Ostomy pouch, urinary; with barrier attached (one piece), each ⛭
MED: 100-2,15,120

A ☑ **A5072** Ostomy pouch, urinary; without barrier attached (one piece), each ⛭
MED: 100-2,15,120

A ☑ **A5073** Ostomy pouch, urinary; for use on barrier with flange (two piece), each ⛭
MED: 100-2,15,120

A **A5081** Continent device; plug for continent stoma ⛭
MED: 100-2,15,120

A **A5082** Continent device; catheter for continent stoma ⛭
MED: 100-2,15,120

A **A5093** Ostomy accessory; convex insert ⛭
MED: 100-2,15,120

ADDITIONAL INCONTINENCE APPLIANCES/SUPPLIES

Medicare claims fall under the jurisdiction of the DME Administrative Contractor (DME MAC), unless otherwise noted.

Special Coverage Instructions | Noncovered by Medicare | Carrier Discretion | ☑ Quality Alert | ● New Code | ○ Reinstated Code | ▲ Revised Code

2007 HCPCS   **1**-**9** ASC Group   **MED:** Pub 100/NCD References   ⛭ DMEPOS Paid   ⊘ SNF Excluded   **A Codes — 9**

Medical and Surgical Supplies

A5102 — A6154

Ⓐ ☑ **A5102** Bedside drainage bottle, with or without tubing, rigid or expandable, each 🖐
MED: 100-2,15,120

▲ Ⓐ **A5105** Urinary suspensory; with or without leg bag, with or without tube, each 🖐
MED: 100-2,15,120

Ⓐ **A5112** Urinary leg bag; latex 🖐
MED: 100-2,15,120

Ⓐ ☑ **A5113** Leg strap; latex, replacement only, per set 🖐
MED: 100-2,15,120

Ⓐ ☑ **A5114** Leg strap; foam or fabric, replacement only, per set 🖐
MED: 100-2,15,120

SUPPLIES FOR EITHER INCONTINENCE OR OSTOMY APPLIANCES

For additional skin barrier codes see codes A4405-A4415.

Ⓐ **A5120** Skin barrier, wipes or swabs, each
MED: 100-2,15,120

Ⓐ ☑ **A5121** Skin barrier; solid, 6 x 6 or equivalent, each 🖐
MED: 100-2,15,120

Ⓐ ☑ **A5122** Skin barrier; solid, 8 x 8 or equivalent, each 🖐
MED: 100-2,15,120

Ⓐ **A5126** Adhesive or nonadhesive; disk or foam pad 🖐
MED: 100-2,15,120

Ⓐ ☑ **A5131** Appliance cleaner, incontinence and ostomy appliances, per 16 oz. 🖐
MED: 100-2,15,120

Ⓐ **A5200** Percutaneous catheter/tube anchoring device, adhesive skin attachment 🖐
MED: 100-2,15,120

DIABETIC SHOES, FITTING, AND MODIFICATIONS

According to Medicare, documentation from the prescribing physician must certify the diabetic patient has one of the following conditions: peripheral neuropathy with evidence of callus formation; history of preulcerative calluses; history of ulceration; foot deformity; previous amputation; or poor circulation. The footwear must be fitted and furnished by a podiatrist, pedorthist, orthotist, or prosthetist.

Ⓨ ☑ **A5500** For diabetics only, fitting (including follow-up) custom preparation and supply of off-the-shelf depth-inlay shoe manufactured to accommodate multi-density insert(s), per shoe
MED: 100-2,15,140

Ⓨ ☑ **A5501** For diabetics only, fitting (including follow-up) custom preparation and supply of shoe molded from cast(s) of patient's foot (custom molded shoe), per shoe
MED: 100-2,15,140

Ⓨ ☑ **A5503** For diabetics only, modification (including fitting) of off-the-shelf depth-inlay shoe or custom molded shoe with roller or rigid rocker bottom, per shoe
MED: 100-2,15,140

Ⓨ ☑ **A5504** For diabetics only, modification (including fitting) of off-the-shelf depth-inlay shoe or custom molded shoe with wedge(s), per shoe
MED: 100-2,15,140

Ⓨ ☑ **A5505** For diabetics only, modification (including fitting) of off-the-shelf depth-inlay shoe or custom molded shoe with metatarsal bar, per shoe
MED: 100-2,15,140

Ⓨ ☑ **A5506** For diabetics only, modification (including fitting) of off-the-shelf depth-inlay shoe or custom molded shoe with off-set heel(s), per shoe
MED: 100-2,15,140

Ⓨ ☑ **A5507** For diabetics only, not otherwise specified modification (including fitting) of off-the-shelf depth-inlay shoe or custom molded shoe, per shoe
MED: 100-2,15,140

Ⓨ ☑ **A5508** For diabetics only, deluxe feature of off-the-shelf depth-inlay shoe or custom-molded shoe, per shoe
MED: 100-2,15,140

Ⓔ **A5510** For diabetics only, direct formed, compression molded to patient's foot without external heat source, multiple-density insert(s) prefabricated, per shoe
MED: 100-2,15,140

Ⓨ **A5512** For diabetics only, multiple density insert, direct formed, molded to foot after external heat source of 230 degrees Fahrenheit or higher, total contact with patient's foot, including arch, base layer minimum of 1/4 inch material of shore a 35 durometer or 3/16 inch material of shore a 40 durometer (or higher), prefabricated, each 🖐

Ⓨ **A5513** For diabetics only, multiple density insert, custom molded from model of patient's foot, total contact with patient's foot, including arch, base layer minimum of 3/16 inch material of shore a 35 durometer or higher, includes arch filler and other shaping material, custom fabricated, each 🖐

DRESSINGS

Medicare claims for A6010-A6024 and A6154-A6404 fall under the jurisdiction of the local contractor if the supply or accessory is used for an implanted prosthetic device (e.g., pleural catheter) or implanted DME (e.g., infusion pump). Medicare claims for other uses of A6021-A6404 fall under the jurisdiction of the DME Medicare Administrative Contractor (DME MAC). The jurisdiction for Medicare claims containing all other codes falls to the DME MAC, unless otherwise noted.

Ⓔ **A6000** Noncontact wound-warming wound cover for use with the noncontact wound-warming device and warming card
MED: 100-2,16,20

Ⓐ ☑ **A6010** Collagen based wound filler, dry form, per gram of collagen 🖐
MED: 100-2,15,100

Ⓐ ☑ **A6011** Collagen based wound filler, gel/paste, per gram of collagen 🖐
MED: 100-2,15,100

Ⓐ ☑ **A6021** Collagen dressing, pad size 16 sq. in. or less, each 🖐
MED: 100-2,15,100; 100-4,4,240

Ⓐ ☑ **A6022** Collagen dressing, pad size more than 16 sq. in. but less than or equal to 48 sq. in., each 🖐
MED: 100-2,15,100; 100-4,4,240

Ⓐ ☑ **A6023** Collagen dressing, pad size more than 48 sq. in., each 🖐
MED: 100-2,15,100; 100-4,4,240

Ⓐ ☑ **A6024** Collagen dressing wound filler, per six in. 🖐
MED: 100-2,15,100; 100-4,4,240

Ⓔ ☑ **A6025** Gel sheet for dermal or epidermal application, (e.g., silicone, hydrogel, other), each

Ⓐ ☑ **A6154** Wound pouch, each 🖐
MED: 100-2,15,100

Special Coverage Instructions   Noncovered by Medicare   Carrier Discretion   ☑ Quality Alert   ● New Code   ○ Reinstated Code   ▲ Revised Code

10 — A Codes   Ⓐ Age Edit   Ⓜ Maternity Edit   ♀ Female Only   ♂ Male Only   Ⓐ - Ⓨ APC Status Indicators   *2007 HCPCS*

Ⓐ ☑ **A6196** Alginate or other fiber gelling dressing, wound cover, pad size 16 sq. in. or less, each dressing ㅗ
MED: 100-2,15,100; 100-4,4,240

Ⓐ ☑ **A6197** Alginate or other fiber gelling dressing, wound cover, pad size more than 16 sq. in. but less than or equal to 48 sq. in., each dressing ㅗ
MED: 100-2,15,100; 100-4,4,240

Ⓐ ☑ **A6198** Alginate or other fiber gelling dressing, wound cover, pad size more than 48 sq. in., each dressing ㅗ
MED: 100-2,15,100; 100-4,4,240

Ⓐ ☑ **A6199** Alginate or other fiber gelling dressing, wound filler, per 6 in. ㅗ
MED: 100-2,15,100; 100-4,4,240

Ⓐ ☑ **A6200** Composite dressing, pad size 16 sq. in. or less, without adhesive border, each dressing ㅗ
MED: 100-2,15,100; 100-4,4,240

Ⓐ ☑ **A6201** Composite dressing, pad size more than 16 sq. in. but less than or equal to 48 sq. in., without adhesive border, each dressing ㅗ
MED: 100-2,15,100; 100-4,4,240

Ⓐ ☑ **A6202** Composite dressing, pad size more than 48 sq. in., without adhesive border, each dressing ㅗ
MED: 100-2,15,100; 100-4,4,240

Ⓐ ☑ **A6203** Composite dressing, pad size 16 sq. in. or less, with any size adhesive border, each dressing ㅗ
MED: 100-2,15,100; 100-4,4,240

Ⓐ ☑ **A6204** Composite dressing, pad size more than 16 sq. in. but less than or equal to 48 sq. in., with any size adhesive border, each dressing ㅗ
MED: 100-2,15,100; 100-4,4,240

Ⓐ ☑ **A6205** Composite dressing, pad size more than 48 sq. in., with any size adhesive border, each dressing ㅗ
MED: 100-2,15,100; 100-4,4,240

Ⓐ ☑ **A6206** Contact layer, 16 sq. in. or less, each dressing
MED: 100-2,15,100; 100-4,4,240

Ⓐ ☑ **A6207** Contact layer, more than 16 sq. in. but less than or equal to 48 sq. in., each dressing ㅗ
MED: 100-2,15,100; 100-4,4,240

Ⓐ ☑ **A6208** Contact layer, more than 48 sq. in., each dressing
MED: 100-2,15,100; 100-4,4,240

Ⓐ ☑ **A6209** Foam dressing, wound cover, pad size 16 sq. in. or less, without adhesive border, each dressing ㅗ
MED: 100-2,15,100; 100-4,4,240

Ⓐ ☑ **A6210** Foam dressing, wound cover, pad size more than 16 sq. in. but less than or equal to 48 sq. in., without adhesive border, each dressing ㅗ
MED: 100-2,15,100; 100-4,4,240

Ⓐ ☑ **A6211** Foam dressing, wound cover, pad size more then 48 sq. in., without adhesive border, each dressing ㅗ
MED: 100-2,15,100; 100-4,4,240

Ⓐ ☑ **A6212** Foam dressing, wound cover, pad size 16 sq. in. or less, with any size adhesive border, each dressing ㅗ
MED: 100-2,15,100; 100-4,4,240

Ⓐ ☑ **A6213** Foam dressing, wound cover, pad size more than 16 sq. in. but less than or equal to 48 sq. in., with any size adhesive border, each dressing ㅗ
MED: 100-2,15,100; 100-4,4,240

Ⓐ ☑ **A6214** Foam dressing, wound cover, pad size more than 48 sq. in., with any size adhesive border, each dressing ㅗ
MED: 100-2,15,100; 100-4,4,240

Ⓐ ☑ **A6215** Foam dressing, wound filler, per gm
MED: 100-2,15,100; 100-4,4,240

Ⓐ ☑ **A6216** Gauze, nonimpregnated, nonsterile, pad size 16 sq. in. or less, without adhesive border, each dressing ㅗ
MED: 100-2,15,100; 100-4,4,240

Ⓐ ☑ **A6217** Gauze, nonimpregnated, nonsterile, pad size more than 16 sq. in. but less than or equal to 48 sq. in., without adhesive border, each dressing ㅗ
MED: 100-2,15,100; 100-4,4,240

Ⓐ ☑ **A6218** Gauze, nonimpregnated, nonsterile, pad size more than 48 sq. in., without adhesive border, each dressing
MED: 100-2,15,100; 100-4,4,240

Ⓐ ☑ **A6219** Gauze, nonimpregnated, pad size 16 sq. in. or less, with any size adhesive border, each dressing ㅗ
MED: 100-2,15,100; 100-4,4,240

Ⓐ ☑ **A6220** Gauze, nonimpregnated, pad size more than 16 sq. in. but less than or equal to 48 sq. in., with any size adhesive border, each dressing ㅗ
MED: 100-2,15,100; 100-4,4,240

Ⓐ ☑ **A6221** Gauze, nonimpregnated, pad size more than 48 sq. in., with any size adhesive border, each dressing
MED: 100-2,15,100; 100-4,4,240

Ⓐ ☑ **A6222** Gauze, impregnated with other than water, normal saline, or hydrogel, pad size 16 sq. in. or less, without adhesive border, each dressing ㅗ
MED: 100-2,15,100; 100-4,4,240

Ⓐ ☑ **A6223** Gauze, impregnated with other than water, normal saline, or hydrogel, pad size more than 16 sq. in. but less than or equal to 48 sq. in., without adhesive border, each dressing ㅗ
MED: 100-2,15,100; 100-4,4,240

Ⓐ ☑ **A6224** Gauze, impregnated with other than water, normal saline, or hydrogel, pad size more than 48 sq. in., without adhesive border, each dressing ㅗ
MED: 100-2,15,100; 100-4,4,240

Ⓐ ☑ **A6228** Gauze, impregnated, water or normal saline, pad size 16 sq. in. or less, without adhesive border, each dressing
MED: 100-2,15,100; 100-4,4,240

Ⓐ ☑ **A6229** Gauze, impregnated, water or normal saline, pad size more than 16 sq. in. but less than or equal to 48 sq. in., without adhesive border, each dressing ㅗ
MED: 100-2,15,100; 100-4,4,240

Ⓐ ☑ **A6230** Gauze, impregnated, water or normal saline, pad size more than 48 sq. in., without adhesive border, each dressing
MED: 100-2,15,100; 100-4,4,240

Ⓐ ☑ **A6231** Gauze, impregnated, hydrogel, for direct wound contact, pad size 16 sq. in. or less, each dressing ㅗ
MED: 100-2,15,100; 100-4,4,240

Ⓐ ☑ **A6232** Gauze, impregnated, hydrogel, for direct wound contact, pad size greater than 16 sq. in., but less than or equal to 48 sq. in., each dressing ㅗ
MED: 100-2,15,100; 100-4,4,240

Ⓐ ☑ **A6233** Gauze, impregnated, hydrogel for direct wound contact, pad size more than 48 sq. in., each dressing ㅗ
MED: 100-2,15,100; 100-4,4,240

Ⓐ ☑ **A6234** Hydrocolloid dressing, wound cover, pad size 16 sq. in. or less, without adhesive border, each dressing ㅗ
MED: 100-2,15,100; 100-4,4,240

Special Coverage Instructions   Noncovered by Medicare   Carrier Discretion   ☑ Quality Alert   ● New Code   ○ Reinstated Code   ▲ Revised Code

2007 HCPCS   ▊-▊ ASC Group   MED: Pub 100/NCD References   ㅗ DMEPOS Paid   ⊘ SNF Excluded   A Codes — 11

Medical and Surgical Supplies

A6235 — A6266

Ⓐ ☑ **A6235** Hydrocolloid dressing, wound cover, pad size more than 16 sq. in. but less than or equal to 48 sq. in., without adhesive border, each dressing 🔶
MED: 100-2,15,100; 100-4,4,240

Ⓐ ☑ **A6236** Hydrocolloid dressing, wound cover, pad size more than 48 sq. in., without adhesive border, each dressing 🔶
MED: 100-2,15,100; 100-4,4,240

Ⓐ ☑ **A6237** Hydrocolloid dressing, wound cover, pad size 16 sq. in. or less, with any size adhesive border, each dressing 🔶
MED: 100-2,15,100; 100-4,4,240

Ⓐ ☑ **A6238** Hydrocolloid dressing, wound cover, pad size more than 16 sq. in. but less than or equal to 48 sq. in., with any size adhesive border, each dressing 🔶
MED: 100-2,15,100; 100-4,4,240

Ⓐ ☑ **A6239** Hydrocolloid dressing, wound cover, pad size more than 48 sq. in., with any size adhesive border, each dressing 🔶
MED: 100-2,15,100; 100-4,4,240

Ⓐ ☑ **A6240** Hydrocolloid dressing, wound filler, paste, per fl. oz. 🔶
MED: 100-2,15,100; 100-4,4,240

Ⓐ ☑ **A6241** Hydrocolloid dressing, wound filler, dry form, per gm 🔶
MED: 100-2,15,100; 100-4,4,240

Ⓐ ☑ **A6242** Hydrogel dressing, wound cover, pad size 16 sq. in. or less, without adhesive border, each dressing 🔶
MED: 100-2,15,100; 100-4,4,240

Ⓐ ☑ **A6243** Hydrogel dressing, wound cover, pad size more than 16 sq. in. but less than or equal to 48 sq. in., without adhesive border, each dressing 🔶
MED: 100-2,15,100; 100-4,4,240

Ⓐ ☑ **A6244** Hydrogel dressing, wound cover, pad size more than 48 sq. in., without adhesive border, each dressing 🔶
MED: 100-2,15,100; 100-4,4,240

Ⓐ ☑ **A6245** Hydrogel dressing, wound cover, pad size 16 sq. in. or less, with any size adhesive border, each dressing 🔶
MED: 100-2,15,100; 100-4,4,240

Ⓐ ☑ **A6246** Hydrogel dressing, wound cover, pad size more than 16 sq. in. but less than or equal to 48 sq. in., with any size adhesive border, each dressing 🔶
MED: 100-2,15,100; 100-4,4,240

Ⓐ ☑ **A6247** Hydrogel dressing, wound cover, pad size more than 48 sq. in., with any size adhesive border, each dressing 🔶
MED: 100-2,15,100; 100-4,4,240

Ⓐ ☑ **A6248** Hydrogel dressing, wound filler, gel, per fl. oz. 🔶
MED: 100-2,15,100; 100-4,4,240

Ⓐ **A6250** Skin sealants, protectants, moisturizers, ointments, any type, any size
Surgical dressings applied by a physician are included as part of the professional service. Surgical dressings obtained by the patient to perform homecare as prescribed by the physician are covered.
MED: 100-2,15,100; 100-4,4,240

Ⓐ ☑ **A6251** Specialty absorptive dressing, wound cover, pad size 16 sq. in. or less, without adhesive border, each dressing 🔶
MED: 100-2,15,100; 100-4,4,240

Ⓐ ☑ **A6252** Specialty absorptive dressing, wound cover, pad size more than 16 sq. in. but less than or equal to 48 sq. in., without adhesive border, each dressing 🔶
MED: 100-2,15,100; 100-4,4,240

Ⓐ ☑ **A6253** Specialty absorptive dressing, wound cover, pad size more than 48 sq. in., without adhesive border, each dressing 🔶
MED: 100-2,15,100; 100-4,4,240

Ⓐ ☑ **A6254** Specialty absorptive dressing, wound cover, pad size 16 sq. in. or less, with any size adhesive border, each dressing 🔶
MED: 100-2,15,100; 100-4,4,240

Ⓐ ☑ **A6255** Specialty absorptive dressing, wound cover, pad size more than 16 sq. in. but less than or equal to 48 sq. in., with any size adhesive border, each dressing 🔶
MED: 100-2,15,100; 100-4,4,240

Ⓐ ☑ **A6256** Specialty absorptive dressing, wound cover, pad size more than 48 sq. in., with any size adhesive border, each dressing
MED: 100-2,15,100; 100-4,4,240

Ⓐ ☑ **A6257** Transparent film, 16 sq. in. or less, each dressing 🔶
Surgical dressings applied by a physician are included as part of the professional service. Surgical dressings obtained by the patient to perform homecare as prescribed by the physician are covered. Use this code for Polyskin, Tegaderm, and Tegaderm HP.
MED: 100-2,15,100; 100-4,4,240

Ⓐ ☑ **A6258** Transparent film, more than 16 sq. in. but less than or equal to 48 sq. in., each dressing 🔶
Surgical dressings applied by a physician are included as part of the professional service. Surgical dressings obtained by the patient to perform homecare as prescribed by the physician are covered.
MED: 100-2,15,100; 100-4,4,240

Ⓐ ☑ **A6259** Transparent film, more than 48 sq. in., each dressing 🔶
Surgical dressings applied by a physician are included as part of the professional service. Surgical dressings obtained by the patient to perform homecare as prescribed by the physician are covered.
MED: 100-2,15,100; 100-4,4,240

Ⓐ **A6260** Wound cleansers, any type, any size
Surgical dressings applied by a physician are included as part of the professional service. Surgical dressings obtained by the patient to perform homecare as prescribed by the physician are covered.
MED: 100-2,15,100; 100-4,4,240

Ⓐ ☑ **A6261** Wound filler, gel/paste, per fl. oz., not elsewhere classified
Surgical dressings applied by a physician are included as part of the professional service. Surgical dressings obtained by the patient to perform homecare as prescribed by the physician are covered.
MED: 100-2,15,100; 100-4,4,240

Ⓐ ☑ **A6262** Wound filler, dry form, per gm, not elsewhere classified
MED: 100-2,15,100; 100-4,4,240

Ⓐ ☑ **A6266** Gauze, impregnated, other than water, normal saline, or zinc paste, any width, per linear yd. 🔶
Surgical dressings applied by a physician are included as part of the professional service. Surgical dressings obtained by the patient to perform homecare as prescribed by the physician are covered.
MED: 100-2,15,100; 100-4,4,240

Special Coverage Instructions   Noncovered by Medicare   Carrier Discretion   ☑ Quality Alert   ● New Code   ○ Reinstated Code   ▲ Revised Code

Ⓐ ☑ A6402 Gauze, nonimpregnated, sterile, pad size 16 sq. in. or less, without adhesive border, each dressing ℔
Surgical dressings applied by a physician are included as part of the professional service. Surgical dressings obtained by the patient to perform homecare as prescribed by the physician are covered.
MED: 100-2,15,100; 100-4,4,240

Ⓐ ☑ A6403 Gauze, nonimpregnated, sterile, pad size more than 16 sq. in. but less than or equal to 48 sq. in., without adhesive border, each dressing ℔
Surgical dressings applied by a physician are included as part of the professional service. Surgical dressings obtained by the patient to perform homecare as prescribed by the physician are covered.
MED: 100-2,15,100; 100-4,4,240

Ⓐ ☑ A6404 Gauze, nonimpregnated, sterile, pad size more than 48 sq. in., without adhesive border, each dressing
MED: 100-2,15,100; 100-4,4,240

Ⓐ ☑ A6407 Packing strips, nonimpregnated, up to 2 in. in width, per linear yd. ℔

Ⓐ ☑ A6410 Eye pad, sterile, each ℔
MED: 100-2,15,100

Ⓐ ☑ A6411 Eye pad, nonsterile, each ℔
MED: 100-2,15,100

Ⓔ ☑ A6412 Eye patch, occlusive, each

Ⓐ ☑ A6441 Padding bandage, nonelastic, nonwoven/nonknitted, width greater than or equal to 3 in. and less than 5 in., per yd. ℔

Ⓐ ☑ A6442 Conforming bandage, nonelastic, knitted/woven, nonsterile, width less than 3 in., per yd. ℔

Ⓐ ☑ A6443 Conforming bandage, nonelastic, knitted/woven, nonsterile, width greater than or equal to 3 in. and less than 5 in., per yd. ℔

Ⓐ ☑ A6444 Conforming bandage, nonelastic, knitted/woven, nonsterile, width greater than or equal to 5 in., per yd. ℔

Ⓐ ☑ A6445 Conforming bandage, nonelastic, knitted/woven, sterile, width less than 3 in., per yd. ℔

Ⓐ ☑ A6446 Conforming bandage, nonelastic, knitted/woven, sterile, width greater than or equal to 3 in. and less than 5 in., per yd. ℔

Ⓐ ☑ A6447 Conforming bandage, nonelastic, knitted/woven, sterile, width greater than or equal to 5 in., per yd. ℔

Ⓐ ☑ A6448 Light compression bandage, elastic, knitted/woven, width less than 3 in., per yd. ℔

Ⓐ ☑ A6449 Light compression bandage, elastic, knitted/woven, width greater than or equal to three in. and less than five in., per yd. ℔

Ⓐ ☑ A6450 Light compression bandage, elastic, knitted/woven, width greater than or equal to five in., per yd. ℔

Ⓐ ☑ A6451 Moderate compression bandage, elastic, knitted/woven, load resistance of 1.25 to 1.34 foot pounds at 50% maximum stretch, width greater than or equal to three in. and less than five in., per yd ℔

Ⓐ ☑ A6452 High compression bandage, elastic, knitted/woven, load resistance greater than or equal to 1.35 foot pounds at 50% maximum stretch, width greater than or equal to three in. and less than five in., per yd. ℔

Ⓐ ☑ A6453 Self-adherent bandage, elastic, nonknitted/nonwoven, width less than three in., per yd. ℔

Ⓐ ☑ A6454 Self-adherent bandage, elastic, nonknitted/nonwoven, width greater than or equal to three in. and less than five in., per yd. ℔

Ⓐ ☑ A6455 Self-adherent bandage, elastic, nonknitted/nonwoven, width greater than or equal to 5 in., per yd. ℔

Ⓐ ☑ A6456 Zinc paste impregnated bandage, nonelastic, knitted/woven, width greater than or equal to 3 in. and less than 5 in., per yd. ℔

Ⓐ A6457 Tubular dressing with or without elastic, any width, per linear yard

Ⓐ A6501 Compression burn garment, bodysuit (head to foot), custom fabricated ℔
MED: 100-2,15,100

Ⓐ A6502 Compression burn garment, chin strap, custom fabricated ℔
MED: 100-2,15,100

Ⓐ A6503 Compression burn garment, facial hood, custom fabricated ℔
MED: 100-2,15,100

Ⓐ A6504 Compression burn garment, glove to wrist, custom fabricated ℔
MED: 100-2,15,100

Ⓐ A6505 Compression burn garment, glove to elbow, custom fabricated ℔
MED: 100-2,15,100

Ⓐ A6506 Compression burn garment, glove to axilla, custom fabricated ℔
MED: 100-2,15,100

Ⓐ A6507 Compression burn garment, foot to knee length, custom fabricated ℔
MED: 100-2,15,100

Ⓐ A6508 Compression burn garment, foot to thigh length, custom fabricated ℔
MED: 100-2,15,100

Ⓐ A6509 Compression burn garment, upper trunk to waist including arm openings (vest), custom fabricated ℔
MED: 100-2,15,100

Ⓐ A6510 Compression burn garment, trunk, including arms down to leg openings (leotard), custom fabricated ℔
MED: 100-2,15,100

Ⓐ A6511 Compression burn garment, lower trunk including leg openings (panty), custom fabricated ℔
MED: 100-2,15,100

Ⓐ A6512 Compression burn garment, not otherwise classified
MED: 100-2,15,100

Ⓑ A6513 Compression burn mask, face and/or neck, plastic or equal, custom fabricated

Ⓔ A6530 Gradient compression stocking, below knee, 18-30 mm Hg, each

Ⓐ A6531 Gradient compression stocking, below knee, 30-40 mm Hg, each
MED: 100-2,15,100

Ⓐ A6532 Gradient compression stocking, below knee, 40-50 mm Hg, each
MED: 100-2,15,100

Ⓔ A6533 Gradient compression stocking, thigh length, 18-30 mm Hg, each
MED: 100-2,15,130

Ⓔ A6534 Gradient compression stocking, thigh length, 30-40 mm Hg, each
MED: 100-2,15,130

Special Coverage Instructions   Noncovered by Medicare   Carrier Discretion   ☑ Quality Alert   ● New Code   ○ Reinstated Code   ▲ Revised Code

2007 HCPCS   ❶-❾ ASC Group   MED: Pub 100/NCD References   ℔ DMEPOS Paid   ⊘ SNF Excluded   A Codes — 13

E | A6535 | Gradient compression stocking, thigh length, 40-50 mm Hg, each
MED: 100-2,15,130

E | A6536 | Gradient compression stocking, full length/chap style, 18-30 mm Hg, each
MED: 100-2,15,130

E | A6537 | Gradient compression stocking, full length/chap style, 30-40 mm Hg, each
MED: 100-2,15,130

E | A6538 | Gradient compression stocking, full length/chap style, 40-50 mm Hg, each
MED: 100-2,15,130

E | A6539 | Gradient compression stocking, waist length, 18-30 mm Hg, each
MED: 100-2,15,130

E | A6540 | Gradient compression stocking, waist length, 30-40 mm Hg, each
MED: 100-2,15,130

E | A6541 | Gradient compression stocking, waist length, 40-50 mm Hg, each
MED: 100-2,15,130

E | A6542 | Gradient compression stocking, custom made
MED: 100-2,15,130

E | A6543 | Gradient compression stocking, lymphedema
MED: 100-2,15,130

E | A6544 | Gradient compression stocking, garter belt
MED: 100-2,15,130

E | A6549 | Gradient compression stocking, not otherwise specified
MED: 100-2,15,130

Y ☑ | A6550 | Wound care set, for negative pressure wound therapy electrical pump, includes all supplies and accessories

MISCELLANEOUS SUPPLIES

Y ☑ | A7000 | Canister, disposable, used with suction pump, each

Y ☑ | A7001 | Canister, nondisposable, used with suction pump, each

Y | A7002 | Tubing, used with suction pump, each

Y | A7003 | Administration set, with small volume nonfiltered pneumatic nebulizer, disposable

Y | A7004 | Small volume nonfiltered pneumatic nebulizer, disposable

Y | A7005 | Administration set, with small volume nonfiltered pneumatic nebulizer, nondisposable

Y | A7006 | Administration set, with small volume filtered pneumatic nebulizer

Y | A7007 | Large volume nebulizer, disposable, unfilled, used with aerosol compressor

Y | A7008 | Large volume nebulizer, disposable, prefilled, used with aerosol compressor

Y | A7009 | Reservoir bottle, nondisposable, used with large volume ultrasonic nebulizer

Y ☑ | A7010 | Corrugated tubing, disposable, used with large volume nebulizer, 100 ft.

Y ☑ | A7011 | Corrugated tubing, nondisposable, used with large volume nebulizer, 10 ft.

Y | A7012 | Water collection device, used with large volume nebulizer

Y | A7013 | Filter, disposable, used with aerosol compressor

Y | A7014 | Filter, nondisposable, used with aerosol compressor or ultrasonic generator

Y | A7015 | Aerosol mask, used with DME nebulizer

Y | A7016 | Dome and mouthpiece, used with small volume ultrasonic nebulizer

Y | A7017 | Nebulizer, durable, glass or autoclavable plastic, bottle type, not used with oxygen
MED: 100-3,280.1

Y ☑ | A7018 | Water, distilled, used with large volume nebulizer, 1000 ml

Y ☑ | A7025 | High frequency chest wall oscillation system vest, replacement for use with patient owned equipment, each

Y ☑ | A7026 | High frequency chest wall oscillation system hose, replacement for use with patient owned equipment, each

Y ☑ | A7030 | Full face mask used with positive airway pressure device, each

Y ☑ | A7031 | Face mask interface, replacement for full face mask, each

Y ☑ | A7032 | Cushion for use on nasal mask interface, replacement only, each

Y | A7033 | Pillow for use on nasal cannula type interface, replacement only, pair

Y | A7034 | Nasal interface (mask or cannula type) used with positive airway pressure device, with or without head strap

Y | A7035 | Headgear used with positive airway pressure device

Y | A7036 | Chinstrap used with positive airway pressure device

Y | A7037 | Tubing used with positive airway pressure device

Y | A7038 | Filter, disposable, used with positive airway pressure device

Y | A7039 | Filter, nondisposable, used with positive airway pressure device

A | A7040 | One way chest drain valve

A | A7041 | Water seal drainage container and tubing for use with implanted chest tube

A | A7042 | Implanted pleural catheter, each

A | A7043 | Vacuum drainage bottle and tubing for use with implanted catheter

Y | A7044 | Oral interface used with positive airway pressure device, each

Y | A7045 | Exhalation port with or without swivel used with accessories for positive airway devices, replacement only
MED: 100-3,230.17

Y ☑ | A7046 | Water chamber for humidifier, used with positive airway pressure device, replacement, each
MED: 100-3,230.17

A ☑ | A7501 | Tracheostoma valve, including diaphragm, each
MED: 100-2,15,120

A ☑ | A7502 | Replacement diaphragm/faceplate for tracheostoma valve, each
MED: 100-2,15,120

Special Coverage Instructions   Noncovered by Medicare   Carrier Discretion   ☑ Quality Alert   ● New Code   ○ Reinstated Code   ▲ Revised Code

14 — A Codes   A Age Edit   M Maternity Edit   ♀ Female Only   ♂ Male Only   A - Y APC Status Indicators   2007 HCPCS

A ☑ **A7503** Filter holder or filter cap, reusable, for use in a tracheostoma heat and moisture exchange system, each   ᵴ
MED: 100-2,15,120

A ☑ **A7504** Filter for use in a tracheostoma heat and moisture exchange system, each   ᵴ
MED: 100-2,15,120

A ☑ **A7505** Housing, reusable without adhesive, for use in a heat and moisture exchange system and/or with a tracheostoma valve, each   ᵴ
MED: 100-2,15,120

A ☑ **A7506** Adhesive disc for use in a heat and moisture exchange system and/or with tracheostoma valve, any type each   ᵴ
MED: 100-2,15,120

A ☑ **A7507** Filter holder and integrated filter without adhesive, for use in a tracheostoma heat and moisture exchange system, each   ᵴ
MED: 100-2,15,120

A ☑ **A7508** Housing and integrated adhesive, for use in a tracheostoma heat and moisture exchange system and/or with a tracheostoma valve, each   ᵴ
MED: 100-2,15,120

A ☑ **A7509** Filter holder and integrated filter housing, and adhesive, for use as a tracheostoma heat and moisture exchange system, each   ᵴ
MED: 100-2,15,120

A ☑ **A7520** Tracheostomy/laryngectomy tube, noncuffed, polyvinylchloride (PVC), silicone or equal, each   ᵴ
MED: 100-2,1,40

A ☑ **A7521** Tracheostomy/laryngectomy tube, cuffed, polyvinylchloride (PVC), silicone or equal, each   ᵴ
MED: 100-2,1,40

A ☑ **A7522** Tracheostomy/laryngectomy tube, stainless steel or equal (sterilizable and reusable), each   ᵴ
MED: 100-2,1,40

A ☑ **A7523** Tracheostomy shower protector, each

A ☑ **A7524** Tracheostoma stent/stud/button, each   ᵴ

A ☑ **A7525** Tracheostomy mask, each   ᵴ

A ☑ **A7526** Tracheostomy tube collar/holder, each   ᵴ

A ☑ **A7527** Tracheostomy/laryngectomy tube plug/stop, each

● Y **A8000** Helmet, protective, soft, prefabricated, includes all components and accessories   ᵴ

● Y **A8001** Helmet, protective, hard, prefabricated, includes all components and accessories   ᵴ

● Y **A8002** Helmet, protective, soft, custom fabricated, includes all components and accessories   ᵴ

● Y **A8003** Helmet, protective, hard, custom fabricated, includes all components and accessories   ᵴ

● Y **A8004** Soft interface for helmet, replacement only   ᵴ

ADMINISTRATIVE, MISCELLANEOUS & INVESTIGATIONAL A9000-A9999

This section of codes reports items such as nonprescription drugs, noncovered items/services, exercise equipment and, most notably, radiopharmaceutical diagnostic imaging agents.

B **A9150** Nonprescription drug
MED: 100-2,15,50

E ☑ **A9152** Single vitamin/mineral/trace element, oral, per dose, not otherwise specified

E ☑ **A9153** Multiple vitamins, with or without minerals and trace elements, oral, per dose, not otherwise specified

E **A9180** Pediculosis (lice infestation) treatment, topical, for administration by patient/caretaker

E **A9270** Noncovered item or service
Medicare jurisdiction: local or DME regional contractor.
MED: 100-2,16,20

E **A9275** Home glucose disposable monitor, includes test strips

● E **A9279** Monitoring feature/device, stand-alone or integrated, any type, includes all accessories, components and electronics, not otherwise classified

E **A9280** Alert or alarm device, not otherwise classified

E **A9281** Reaching/grabbing device, any type, any length, each

E **A9282** Wig, any type, each

E **A9300** Exercise equipment
MED: 100-2,15,110.1; 100-3,280.1

H ☑ **A9500** Technetium Tc-99m sestamibi, diagnostic, per study dose, up to 40 millicuries
Use this code for Cardiolite.
MED: 100-4,4,20.5; 100-4,4,230.1; 100-4,12,70; 100-4,13,20; 100-4,13,90

H ☑ **A9502** Technetium Tc-99m tetrofosmin, diagnostic, per study dose, up to 40 millicuries
Use this code for Myoview.
MED: 100-4,4,230.1; 100-4,12,70; 100-4,13,20; 100-4,13,90

N ☑ **A9503** Technetium Tc-99m medronate, diagnostic, per study dose, up to 30 millicuries
MED: 100-4,4,230.1; 100-4,12,70; 100-4,13,20; 100-4,13,90
AHA: 2Q,'02,9

N **A9504** Technetium Tc-99m apcitide, diagnostic, per study dose, up to 20 millicuries
Use this code for Acutect.
MED: 100-4,4,230.1; 100-4,12,70; 100-4,13,20; 100-4,13,90
AHA: 2Q,'02,9; 4Q,'01,5

H ☑ **A9505** Thallium Tl-201 thallous chloride, diagnostic, per millicurie
Use this code for Thallous Chloride USP.
MED: 100-4,4,230.1; 100-4,12,70; 100-4,13,20; 100-4,13,90
AHA: 2Q,'02,9

H ☑ **A9507** Indium In-111 capromab pendetide, diagnostic, per study dose, up to 10 millicuries
Use this code for Prostascint.
MED: 100-4,4,230.1; 100-4,12,70; 100-4,13,20; 100-4,13,90

H ☑ **A9508** Iodine I-131 iobenguane sulfate, diagnostic, per 0.5 millicurie
Use this code for MIBG.
MED: 100-4,4,230.1
AHA: 2Q,'02,9

N ☑ **A9510** Technetium Tc-99m disofenin, diagnostic, per study dose, up to 15 millicuries
MED: 100-4,4,230.1

N ☑ **A9512** Technetium Tc-99m pertechnetate, diagnostic, per millicurie
Use this code for TechneScan.
MED: 100-4,4,230.1

H ☑ **A9516** Iodine I-123 sodium iodide capsule(s), diagnostic, per 100 microcuries
MED: 100-4,4,230.1

H ☑ **A9517** Iodine I-131 sodium iodide capsule(s), therapeutic, per millicurie
MED: 100-4,4,230.1

Special Coverage Instructions   **Noncovered by Medicare**   **Carrier Discretion**   ☑ Quality Alert   ● New Code   ○ Reinstated Code   ▲ Revised Code

2007 HCPCS   1-9 ASC Group   **MED:** Pub 100/NCD References   ᵴ DMEPOS Paid   Ⓢ SNF Excluded   **A Codes — 15**

Administrative, Miscellaneous & Investigational

A9521 — A9566

H ☑ **A9521** Technetium Tc-99m exametazime, diagnostic, per study dose, up to 25 millicuries
Use this code for Ceretec.
MED: 100-4,4,230.1

H ☑ **A9524** Iodine I-131 iodinated serum albumin, diagnostic, per 5 microcuries
MED: 100-4,4,230.1; 100-4,12,70; 100-4,13,20; 100-4,13,90

H ☑ **A9526** Nitrogen N-13 ammonia, diagnostic, per study dose, up to 40 millicuries
MED: 100-3,220.6; 100-4,4,230.1; 100-4,13,60.3; 100-4,13,60.3.1; 100-4,13,60.3.2

● K **A9527** Iodine I-125, sodium iodide solution, therapeutic, per millicurie

H ☑ **A9528** Iodine I-131 sodium iodide capsule(s), diagnostic, per millicurie
MED: 100-4,4,230.1

N ☑ **A9529** Iodine I-131 sodium iodide solution, diagnostic, per millicurie
MED: 100-4,4,230.1

H ☑ **A9530** Iodine I-131 sodium iodide solution, therapeutic, per millicurie ⊘
MED: 100-4,4,230.1

N ☑ **A9531** Iodine I-131 sodium iodide, diagnostic, per microcurie (up to 100 microcuries)
MED: 100-4,4,230.1

N ☑ **A9532** Iodine I-125 serum albumin, diagnostic, per 5 microcuries
MED: 100-4,4,230.1

N **A9535** Injection, methylene blue, 1 ml

H **A9536** Technetium Tc-99m depreotide, diagnostic, per study dose, up to 35 millicuries
MED: 100-4,4,230.1

N **A9537** Technetium Tc-99m mebrofenin, diagnostic, per study dose, up to 15 millicuries
MED: 100-4,4,230.1

N **A9538** Technetium Tc-99m pyrophosphate, diagnostic, per study dose, up to 25 millicuries
MED: 100-4,4,230.1

H **A9539** Technetium Tc-99m pentetate, diagnostic, per study dose, up to 25 millicuries
MED: 100-4,4,230.1

N **A9540** Technetium Tc-99m macroaggregated albumin, diagnostic, per study dose, up to 10 millicuries
MED: 100-4,4,230.1

N **A9541** Technetium Tc-99m sulfur colloid, diagnostic, per study dose, up to 20 millicuries
MED: 100-4,4,230.1

H **A9542** Indium In-111 ibritumomab tiuxetan, diagnostic, per study dose, up to 5 millicuries ⊘
MED: 100-4,4,230.1

H **A9543** Yttrium Y-90 ibritumomab tiuxetan, therapeutic, per treatment dose, up to 40 millicuries ⊘
MED: 100-4,4,230.1

H **A9544** Iodine I-131 tositumomab, diagnostic, per study dose ⊘

H **A9545** Iodine I-131 tositumomab, therapeutic, per treatment dose ⊘

H **A9546** Cobalt Co-57/58, cyanocobalamin, diagnostic, per study dose, up to 1 microcurie

H **A9547** Indium In-111 oxyquinoline, diagnostic, per 0.5 millicurie
MED: 100-4,4,230.1

H **A9548** Indium In-111 pentetate, diagnostic, per 0.5 millicurie
MED: 100-4,4,230.1

~~A9549~~ ~~Technetium Tc-99m arcitumomab, diagnostic, per study dose, up to 25 millicuries~~
See code(s) A9568

H **A9550** Technetium Tc-99m sodium gluceptate, diagnostic, per study dose, up to 25 millicurie
MED: 100-4,4,230.1

H **A9551** Technetium Tc-99m succimer, diagnostic, per study dose, up to 10 millicuries
MED: 100-4,4,230.1

H **A9552** Fluorodeoxyglucose F-18 FDG, diagnostic, per study dose, up to 45 millicuries
MED: 100-4,4,230.1

H **A9553** Chromium Cr-51 sodium chromate, diagnostic, per study dose, up to 250 microcuries
MED: 100-4,4,230.1

N **A9554** Iodine I-125 sodium iothalamate, diagnostic, per study dose, up to 10 microcuries
MED: 100-4,4,230.1

H **A9555** Rubidium Rb-82, diagnostic, per study dose, up to 60 millicuries
Use this code for Cardiogen 82.
MED: 100-4,4,230.1

H **A9556** Gallium Ga-67 citrate, diagnostic, per millicurie
MED: 100-4,4,230.1

H **A9557** Technetium Tc-99m bicisate, diagnostic, per study dose, up to 25 millicuries
Use this code for Neurolite.
MED: 100-4,4,230.1

N **A9558** Xenon Xe-133 gas, diagnostic, per 10 millicuries
MED: 100-4,4,230.1

H **A9559** Cobalt Co-57 cyanocobalamin, oral, diagnostic, per study dose, up to 1 microcurie
Use this code for Cobatope 57, Rubratope 57.
MED: 100-4,4,230.1

H **A9560** Technetium Tc-99m labeled red blood cells, diagnostic, per study dose, up to 30 millicuries
MED: 100-4,4,230.1

N **A9561** Technetium Tc-99m oxidronate, diagnostic, per study dose, up to 30 millicuries
MED: 100-4,4,230.1

H **A9562** Technetium Tc-99m mertiatide, diagnostic, per study dose, up to 15 millicuries
Use this code for MAG-3.
MED: 100-4,4,230.1

H **A9563** Sodium phosphate P-32, therapeutic, per millicurie
MED: 100-4,4,230.1

H **A9564** Chromic phosphate P-32 suspension, therapeutic, per millicurie
Use this code for Phosphocol (P32).
MED: 100-4,4,230.1

H **A9565** Indium In-111 pentetreotide, diagnostic, per millicurie
Use this code for Octreoscan.
MED: 100-4,4,230.1

H **A9566** Technetium Tc-99m fanolesomab, diagnostic, per study dose, up to 25 millicuries
MED: 100-4,4,230.1

Special Coverage Instructions   Noncovered by Medicare   Carrier Discretion   ☑ Quality Alert   ● New Code   ○ Reinstated Code   ▲ Revised Code

Ⓗ   A9567   Technetium Tc-99m pentetate, diagnostic, aerosol, per study dose, up to 75 millicuries

● Ⓗ   A9568   Technetium Tc-99m arcitumomab, diagnostic, per study dose, up to 45 millicuries

Ⓗ ☑   A9600   Strontium Sr-89 chloride, therapeutic, per millicurie

       Medicare jurisdiction: local contractor.

       MED: 100-4,4,230.1

       AHA: 2Q,'02,9

Ⓗ ☑   A9605   Samarium Sm-153 lexidronamm, therapeutic, per 50 millicuries
       Use this code for Quadramet. Medicare jurisdiction: DME regional contractor.

       MED: 100-4,4,20.5; 100-4,4,230.1

       AHA: 2Q,'02,9

Ⓝ   A9698   Nonradioactive contrast imaging material, not otherwise classified, per study

       MED: 100-4,12,70; 100-4,13,20; 100-4,13,90

Ⓝ   A9699   Radiopharmaceutical, therapeutic, not otherwise classified

Ⓑ   A9700   Supply of injectable contrast material for use in echocardiography, per study

       MED: 100-4,12,30.4

       AHA: 4Q,'01,5

Ⓨ   A9900   Miscellaneous DME supply, accessory, and/or service component of another HCPCS code   ໕
       Medicare jurisdiction: local contractor if implanted DME; if other, regional contractor.

Ⓐ   A9901   DME delivery, set up, and/or dispensing service component of another HCPCS code
       Medicare jurisdiction: local contractor if implanted DME; if other, DME MAC.

Ⓨ   A9999   Miscellaneous DME supply or accessory, not otherwise specified

Special Coverage Instructions   Noncovered by Medicare   Carrier Discretion   ☑ Quality Alert   ● New Code   ○ Reinstated Code   ▲ Revised Code

2007 HCPCS   ❶-❾ ASC Group   MED: Pub 100/NCD References   ໕ DMEPOS Paid   ⊘ SNF Excluded   **A Codes — 17**

ENTERAL AND PARENTERAL THERAPY B4000-B9999

This section includes codes for supplies, formulae, nutritional solutions, and infusion pumps.

ENTERAL FORMULAE AND ENTERAL MEDICAL SUPPLIES

Certification of medical necessity is required for coverage. Submit a revision to the certification of medical necessity if the patient's daily volume changes by more than one liter; if there is a change in infusion method; or if there is a change from premix to home mix or parenteral to enteral therapy.

Y   **B4034** Enteral feeding supply kit; syringe, per day
MED: 100-2,15,120; 100-3,180.2; 100-4,20,100.2.2; 100-4,20,160.1

Y   **B4035** Enteral feeding supply kit; pump fed, per day
MED: 100-2,15,120; 100-3,180.2; 100-4,20,100.2.2; 100-4,20,160.1

Y   **B4036** Enteral feeding supply kit; gravity fed, per day
MED: 100-2,15,120; 100-3,180.2; 100-4,20,100.2.2; 100-4,20,160.1

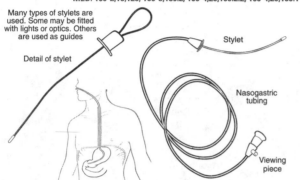

Many types of stylets are used. Some may be fitted with lights or optics. Others are used as guides

Detail of stylet

Stylet

Nasogastric tubing

Viewing piece

Y   **B4081** Nasogastric tubing with stylet
MED: 100-2,15,120; 100-3,180.2; 100-4,20,100.2.2; 100-4,20,160.1

Y   **B4082** Nasogastric tubing without stylet
MED: 100-2,15,120; 100-3,180.2; 100-4,20,100.2.2; 100-4,20,160.1

Y   **B4083** Stomach tube — Levine type
MED: 100-2,15,120; 100-3,180.2; 100-4,20,100.2.2

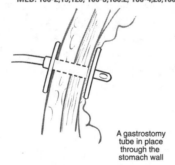

A gastrostomy tube in place through the stomach wall

Y   **B4086** Gastrostomy/jejunostomy tube, any material, any type, (standard or low profile), each

E   **B4100** Food thickener, administered orally, per oz.

Y ☑ **B4102** Enteral formula, for adults, used to replace fluids and electrolytes (e.g., clear liquids), 500 ml = 1 unit
MED: 100-3,180.2; 100-4,20,160.1

Y ☑ **B4103** Enteral formula, for pediatrics, used to replace fluids and electrolytes (e.g., clear liquids), 500 ml = 1 unit
MED: 100-3,180.2; 100-4,20,160.1

E ☑ **B4104** Additive for enteral formula (e.g., fiber)
MED: 100-3,180.2; 100-4,20,160.1

Y ☑ **B4149** Enteral formula, manufactured blenderized natural foods with intact nutrients, includes proteins, fats, carbohydrates, vitamins and minerals, may include fiber, administered through an enteral feeding tube, 100 calories = 1 unit
MED: 100-2,15,120; 100-3,180.2; 100-4,20,100.2.2; 100-4,20,160.1

Y   **B4150** Enteral formula, nutritionally complete with intact nutrients, includes proteins, fats, carbohydrates, vitamins and minerals, may include fiber, administered through an enteral feeding tube, 100 calories = 1 unit
Use this code for Enrich, Ensure, Ensure HN, Ensure Powder, Isocal, Lonalac Powder, Meritene, Meritene Powder, Osmolite, Osmolite HN, Portagen Powder, Sustacal, Renu, Sustagen Powder, Travasorb.
MED: 100-2,15,120; 100-3,180.2; 100-4,20,100.2.2; 100-4,20,160.1

Y   **B4152** Enteral formula, nutritionally complete, calorically dense (equal to or greater than 1.5 kcal/ml) with intact nutrients, includes proteins, fats, carbohydrates, vitamins and minerals, may include fiber, administered through an enteral feeding tube, 100 calories = 1 unit
Use this code for Magnacal, Isocal HCN, Sustacal HC, Ensure Plus, Ensure Plus HN.
MED: 100-2,15,120; 100-3,180.2; 100-4,20,100.2.2; 100-4,20,160.1

Y   **B4153** Enteral formula, nutritionally complete, hydrolyzed proteins (amino acids and peptide chain), includes fats, carbohydrates, vitamins and minerals, may include fiber, administered through an enteral feeding tube, 100 calories = 1 unit
Use this code for Criticare HN, Vivonex t.e.n. (Total Enteral Nutrition), Vivonex HN, Vital (Vital HN), Travasorb HN, Isotein HN, Precision HN, Precision Isotonic.
MED: 100-2,15,120; 100-3,180.2; 100-4,20,100.2.2; 100-4,20,160.1

Y   **B4154** Enteral formula, nutritionally complete, for special metabolic needs, excludes inherited disease of metabolism, includes altered composition of proteins, fats, carbohydrates, vitamins and/or minerals, may include fiber, administered through an enteral feeding tube, 100 calories = 1 unit
Use this code for Hepatic-aid, Travasorb Hepatic, Travasorb MCT, Travasorb Renal, Traum-aid, Tramacal, Aminaid.
MED: 100-2,15,120; 100-3,180.2; 100-4,20,100.2.2; 100-4,20,160.1

Y   **B4155** Enteral formula, nutritionally incomplete/modular nutrients, includes specific nutrients, carbohydrates (e.g., glucose polymers), proteins/amino acids (e.g., glutamine, arginine), fat (e.g., medium chain triglycerides) or combination, administered through an enteral feeding tube, 100 calories = 1 unit
Use this code for Propac, Gerval Protein, Promix, Casec, Moducal, Controlyte, Polycose Liquid or Powder, Sumacal, Microlipids, MCT Oil, Nutri-source.
MED: 100-2,15,120; 100-3,180.2; 100-4,20,100.2.2; 100-4,20,160.1

Y ☑ **B4157** Enteral formula, nutritionally complete, for special metabolic needs for inherited disease of metabolism, includes proteins, fats, carbohydrates, vitamins and minerals, may include fiber, administered through an enteral feeding tube, 100 calories = 1 unit
MED: 100-3,180.2; 100-4,20,160.1

Y ☑ **B4158** Enteral formula, for pediatrics, nutritionally complete with intact nutrients, includes proteins, fats, carbohydrates, vitamins and minerals, may include fiber and/or iron, administered through an enteral feeding tube, 100 calories = 1 unit
MED: 100-3,180.2; 100-4,20,160.1

Special Coverage Instructions   Noncovered by Medicare   Carrier Discretion   ☑ Quality Alert   ● New Code   ○ Reinstated Code   ▲ Revised Code

18 — B Codes   🅰 Age Edit   🅼 Maternity Edit   ♀ Female Only   ♂ Male Only   🅰 - ☑ APC Status Indicators   *2007 HCPCS*

☑ ☑ **B4159** Enteral formula, for pediatrics, nutritionally complete soy based with intact nutrients, includes proteins, fats, carbohydrates, vitamins and minerals, may include fiber and/or iron, administered through an enteral feeding tube, 100 calories = 1 unit   ᵬ
MED: 100-3,180.2; 100-4,20,160.1

☑ ☑ **B4160** Enteral formula, for pediatrics, nutritionally complete calorically dense (equal to or greater than 0.7 kcal/ml) with intact nutrients, includes proteins, fats, carbohydrates, vitamins and minerals, may include fiber, administered through an enteral feeding tube, 100 calories = 1 unit   ᵬ
MED: 100-3,180.2; 100-4,20,160.1

☑ ☑ **B4161** Enteral formula, for pediatrics, hydrolyzed/amino acids and peptide chain proteins, includes fats, carbohydrates, vitamins and minerals, may include fiber, administered through an enteral feeding tube, 100 calories = 1 unit   ᵬ
MED: 100-3,180.2; 100-4,20,160.1

☑ ☑ **B4162** Enteral formula, for pediatrics, special metabolic needs for inherited disease of metabolism, includes proteins, fats, carbohydrates, vitamins and minerals, may include fiber, administered through an enteral feeding tube, 100 calories = 1 unit   ᵬ
MED: 100-3,180.2; 100-4,20,160.1

PARENTERAL NUTRITION SOLUTIONS AND SUPPLIES

☑ **B4164** Parenteral nutrition solution; carbohydrates (dextrose), 50% or less (500 ml = 1 unit) — home mix   ᵬ
MED: 100-2,15,120; 100-3,180.2; 100-4,3,10.4; 100-4,20,100.2.2

☑ **B4168** Parenteral nutrition solution; amino acid, 3.5%, (500 ml = 1 unit) — home mix   ᵬ
MED: 100-2,15,120; 100-3,180.2; 100-4,3,10.4; 100-4,20,100.2.2

☑ **B4172** Parenteral nutrition solution; amino acid, 5.5% through 7%, (500 ml = 1 unit) — home mix   ᵬ
MED: 100-2,15,120; 100-3,180.2; 100-4,3,10.4; 100-4,20,100.2.2

☑ **B4176** Parenteral nutrition solution; amino acid, 7% through 8.5%, (500 ml = 1 unit) — home mix   ᵬ
MED: 100-2,15,120; 100-3,180.2; 100-4,3,10.4; 100-4,20,100.2.2

☑ **B4178** Parenteral nutrition solution; amino acid, greater than 8.5% (500 ml = 1 unit) — home mix   ᵬ
MED: 100-2,15,120; 100-3,180.2; 100-4,3,10.4; 100-4,20,100.2.2

☑ **B4180** Parenteral nutrition solution; carbohydrates (dextrose), greater than 50% (500 ml = 1 unit) — home mix   ᵬ
MED: 100-2,15,120; 100-3,180.2; 100-4,3,10.4; 100-4,20,100.2.2

☑ **B4185** Parenteral nutrition solution, per 10 grams lipids

☑ ☑ **B4189** Parenteral nutrition solution; compounded amino acid and carbohydrates with electrolytes, trace elements, and vitamins, including preparation, any strength, 10 to 51 grams of protein — premix   ᵬ
MED: 100-2,15,120; 100-3,180.2; 100-4,3,10.4; 100-4,20,100.2.2

☑ ☑ **B4193** Parenteral nutrition solution; compounded amino acid and carbohydrates with electrolytes, trace elements, and vitamins, including preparation, any strength, 52 to 73 grams of protein — premix   ᵬ
MED: 100-2,15,120; 100-3,180.2; 100-4,3,10.4; 100-4,20,100.2.2

☑ ☑ **B4197** Parenteral nutrition solution; compounded amino acid and carbohydrates with electrolytes, trace elements and vitamins, including preparation, any strength, 74 to 100 grams of protein — premix   ᵬ
MED: 100-2,15,120; 100-3,180.2; 100-4,3,10.4; 100-4,20,100.2.2

☑ ☑ **B4199** Parenteral nutrition solution; compounded amino acid and carbohydrates with electrolytes, trace elements and vitamins, including preparation, any strength, over 100 grams of protein — premix   ᵬ
MED: 100-2,15,120; 100-3,180.2; 100-4,3,10.4; 100-4,20,100.2.2

☑ **B4216** Parenteral nutrition; additives (vitamins, trace elements, heparin, electrolytes) — home mix, per day   ᵬ
MED: 100-2,15,120; 100-3,180.2; 100-4,3,10.4; 100-4,20,100.2.2

☑ **B4220** Parenteral nutrition supply kit; premix, per day   ᵬ
MED: 100-2,15,120; 100-3,180.2; 100-4,3,10.4; 100-4,20,100.2.2

☑ **B4222** Parenteral nutrition supply kit; home mix, per day   ᵬ
MED: 100-2,15,120; 100-3,180.2; 100-4,3,10.4; 100-4,20,100.2.2

☑ **B4224** Parenteral nutrition administration kit, per day   ᵬ
MED: 100-2,15,120; 100-3,180.2; 100-4,3,10.4; 100-4,20,100.2.2

☑ **B5000** Parenteral nutrition solution; compounded amino acid and carbohydrates with electrolytes, trace elements, and vitamins, including preparation, any strength, renal — Amirosyn RF, NephrAmine, RenAmine — premix   ᵬ
Use this code for Amirosyn-RF, NephrAmine, RenAmin.
MED: 100-2,15,120; 100-3,180.2; 100-4,3,10.4; 100-4,20,100.2.2

☑ **B5100** Parenteral nutrition solution; compounded amino acid and carbohydrates with electrolytes, trace elements, and vitamins, including preparation, any strength, hepatic — FreAmine HBC, HepatAmine — premix   ᵬ
Use this code for FreAmine HBC, HepatAmine.
MED: 100-2,15,120; 100-3,180.2; 100-4,3,10.4; 100-4,20,100.2.2

☑ **B5200** Parenteral nutrition solution; compounded amino acid and carbohydrates with electrolytes, trace elements, and vitamins, including preparation, any strength, stress — branch chain amino acids — premix   ᵬ
MED: 100-2,15,120; 100-3,180.2; 100-4,3,10.4; 100-4,20,100.2.2

ENTERAL AND PARENTERAL PUMPS

Submit documentation of the need for the infusion pump. Medicare will reimburse for the simplest model that meets the patient's needs.

☑ **B9000** Enteral nutrition infusion pump — without alarm   ᵬ
MED: 100-2,15,120; 100-3,180.2; 100-4,20,100.2.2

☑ **B9002** Enteral nutrition infusion pump — with alarm   ᵬ
MED: 100-2,15,120; 100-3,180.2; 100-4,20,100.2.2

☑ **B9004** Parenteral nutrition infusion pump, portable   ᵬ
MED: 100-2,15,120; 100-3,180.2; 100-4,3,10.4; 100-4,20,100.2.2

☑ **B9006** Parenteral nutrition infusion pump, stationary   ᵬ
MED: 100-2,15,120; 100-3,180.2; 100-4,3,10.4; 100-4,20,100.2.2

☑ **B9998** NOC for enteral supplies   ᵬ
MED: 100-2,15,120; 100-3,180.2; 100-4,3,10.4; 100-4,20,100.2.2

☑ **B9999** NOC for parenteral supplies   ᵬ
Determine if an alternative HCPCS Level II or a CPT code better describes the service being reported. This code should be used only if a more specific code is unavailable.
MED: 100-2,15,120; 100-3,180.2; 100-4,3,10.4; 100-4,20,100.2.2

Special Coverage Instructions   Noncovered by Medicare   Carrier Discretion   ☑ Quality Alert   ● New Code   ○ Reinstated Code   ▲ Revised Code

OUTPATIENT PPS C1000-C9999

This section reports drugs, biologicals, and devices codes that must be used by OPPS hospitals. Non-OPPS hospitals, Critical Access Hospitals (CAHs), Indian Health Service Hospitals (HIS), hospitals located in American Samoa, Guam, Saipan, or the Virgin Islands, and Maryland waiver hospitals may report these codes at their discretion. The codes can only be reported for facility (technical) services.

The C series of HCPCS may include device categories, new technology procedures, and drugs, biologicals and radiopharmaceuticals that do not have other HCPCS codes assigned. Some of these items and services are eligible for transitional pass-through payments for OPPS hospitals, have separate APC payments, or are items that are packaged. Hospitals are encouraged to report all appropriate C codes regardless of payment status.

~~C1178 Injection, busulfan, per 6 mg~~
See code(s) J0594

S C1300 **Hyperbaric oxygen under pressure, full body chamber, per 30 minute interval**
MED: 100-4,32,30.1

N C1713 **Anchor/screw for opposing bone-to-bone or soft tissue-to-bone (implantable)**
MED: 100-4,4,61.1
AHA: 3Q,'02,5; 1Q,'01,5

N C1714 **Catheter, transluminal atherectomy, directional**
MED: 100-4,4,61.1; 100-4,4,61.2
AHA: 4Q,'03,8; 3Q,'02,5; 1Q,'01,5

N C1715 **Brachytherapy needle** ⊘
MED: 100-4,4,61.1
AHA: 3Q,'02,5; 1Q,'01,5

K C1716 **Brachytherapy source, gold 198, per source** ⊘
MED: 100-4,4,61.1
AHA: 3Q,'02,5; 1Q,'01,5

K C1717 **Brachytherapy source, high dose rate iridium 192, per source** ⊘
MED: 100-4,4,61.1
AHA: 3Q,'02,5; 1Q,'01,5

K C1718 **Brachytherapy source, iodine 125, per source** ⊘
MED: 100-4,4,61.1
AHA: 1Q,'04,2; 3Q,'02,5; 1Q,'01,5

K C1719 **Brachytherapy source, nonhigh dose rate iridium 192, per source** ⊘
MED: 100-4,4,61.1
AHA: 3Q,'02,5; 1Q,'01,5

K C1720 **Brachytherapy source, palladium 103, per source** ⊘
MED: 100-4,4,61.1
AHA: 1Q,'04,2; 3Q,'02,5; 1Q,'01,5

N C1721 **Cardioverter-defibrillator, dual chamber (implantable)**
MED: 100-4,4,61.1; 100-4,4,61.2
AHA: 3Q,'02,5; 1Q,'01,5

N C1722 **Cardioverter-defibrillator, single chamber (implantable)**
MED: 100-4,4,61.1; 100-4,4,61.2
AHA: 3Q,'02,5; 1Q,'01,5

N C1724 **Catheter, transluminal atherectomy, rotational**
MED: 100-4,4,61.1; 100-4,4,61.2
AHA: 4Q,'03,8; 3Q,'02,5; 1Q,'01,5

N C1725 **Catheter, transluminal angioplasty, nonlaser (may include guidance, infusion/perfusion capability)**
MED: 100-4,4,61.1; 100-4,4,61.2
AHA: 4Q,'03,8; 3Q,'02,5; 1Q,'01,5

N C1726 **Catheter, balloon dilatation, nonvascular**
MED: 100-4,4,61.1
AHA: 3Q,'02,5; 1Q,'01,5

N C1727 **Catheter, balloon tissue dissector, nonvascular (insertable)**
MED: 100-4,4,61.1
AHA: 3Q,'02,5; 1Q,'01,5

○ N C1728 **Catheter, brachytherapy seed administration** ⊘
MED: 100-4,4,61.1
AHA: 3Q,'02,5; 1Q,'01,5

N C1729 **Catheter, drainage**
MED: 100-4,4,61.1
AHA: 3Q,'02,5; 1Q,'01,5

N C1730 **Catheter, electrophysiology, diagnostic, other than 3D mapping (19 or fewer electrodes)**
MED: 100-4,4,61.1; 100-4,4,61.2
AHA: 3Q,'02,5; 1Q,'01,5

N C1731 **Catheter, electrophysiology, diagnostic, other than 3D mapping (20 or more electrodes)**
MED: 100-4,4,61.1; 100-4,4,61.2
AHA: 3Q,'02,5; 1Q,'01,5

N C1732 **Catheter, electrophysiology, diagnostic/ablation, 3D or vector mapping**
MED: 100-4,4,61.1; 100-4,4,61.2
AHA: 1Q,'01,5

N C1733 **Catheter, electrophysiology, diagnostic/ablation, other than 3D or vector mapping, other than cool-tip**
MED: 100-4,4,61.1; 100-4,4,61.2
AHA: 3Q,'02,5; 1Q,'01,5

N C1750 **Catheter, hemodialysis/peritoneal, long-term**
MED: 100-4,4,61.1
AHA: 4Q,'03,8; 3Q,'02,5; 1Q,'01,5

N C1751 **Catheter, infusion, inserted peripherally, centrally or midline (other than hemodialysis)**
MED: 100-4,4,61.1; 100-4,4,61.2
AHA: 4Q,'03,8; 3Q,'02,5; 3Q,'01,5

N C1752 **Catheter, hemodialysis/peritoneal, short-term**
MED: 100-4,4,61.1
AHA: 4Q,'03,8; 3Q,'02,5; 1Q,'01,5

N C1753 **Catheter, intravascular ultrasound**
MED: 100-4,4,61.1
AHA: 4Q,'03,8; 3Q,'02,5; 1Q,'01,5

N C1754 **Catheter, intradiscal**
MED: 100-4,4,61.1
AHA: 4Q,'03,8; 3Q,'02,5; 1Q,'01,5

N C1755 **Catheter, intraspinal**
MED: 100-4,4,61.1
AHA: 4Q,'03,8; 3Q,'02,5; 1Q,'01,5

N C1756 **Catheter, pacing, transesophageal**
MED: 100-4,4,61.1
AHA: 4Q,'03,8; 3Q,'02,5; 1Q,'01,5

N C1757 **Catheter, thrombectomy/embolectomy**
MED: 100-4,4,61.1; 100-4,4,61.2
AHA: 4Q,'03,8; 3Q,'02,5; 1Q,'01,5

N C1758 **Catheter, ureteral**
MED: 100-4,4,61.1
AHA: 4Q,'03,8; 3Q,'02,5; 1Q,'01,6

N C1759 **Catheter, intracardiac echocardiography**
MED: 100-4,4,61.1
AHA: 4Q,'03,8; 3Q,'02,5; 1Q,'01,5; 3Q,'01,4

N C1760 **Closure device, vascular (implantable/insertable)**
MED: 100-4,4,61.1
AHA: 4Q,'03,8; 3Q,'02,5; 1Q,'01,6

N C1762 **Connective tissue, human (includes fascia lata)**
MED: 100-4,4,61.1
AHA: 3Q,'03,12; 4Q,'03,8; 3Q,'02,5; 1Q,'01,6

Special Coverage Instructions   Noncovered by Medicare   Carrier Discretion   ☑ Quality Alert   ● New Code   ○ Reinstated Code   ▲ Revised Code

N **C1763** Connective tissue, nonhuman (includes synthetic)
MED: 100-4,4,61.1
AHA: 3Q,'03,12; 4Q,'03,8; 3Q,'02,5; 1Q,'01,6

N **C1764** Event recorder, cardiac (implantable)
MED: 100-4,4,61.1
AHA: 4Q,'03,8; 3Q,'02,5; 1Q,'01,6

N **C1765** Adhesion barrier
MED: 100-4,4,61.1

N **C1766** Introducer/sheath, guiding, intracardiac electrophysiological, steerable, other than peel-away
MED: 100-4,4,61.1; 100-4,4,61.2
AHA: 3Q,'02,5; 3Q,'01,5

N **C1767** Generator, neurostimulator (implantable), nonrechargeable
MED: 100-4,4,61.1; 100-4,4,61.2
AHA: 4Q,'03,8; 1Q,'02,9; 3Q,'02,5

N **C1768** Graft, vascular
MED: 100-4,4,61.1
AHA: 4Q,'03,8; 3Q,'02,5; 1Q,'01,6

N **C1769** Guide wire
MED: 100-4,4,61.1
AHA: 4Q,'03,8; 3Q,'02,5; 1Q,'01,6; 3Q,'01,4

N **C1770** Imaging coil, magnetic resonance (insertable)
MED: 100-4,4,61.1
AHA: 4Q,'03,8; 3Q,'02,5; 1Q,'01,6

N **C1771** Repair device, urinary, incontinence, with sling graft
MED: 100-4,4,61.1
AHA: 4Q,'03,8; 3Q,'02,5; 1Q,'01,6

N **C1772** Infusion pump, programmable (implantable)
MED: 100-4,4,61.1; 100-4,4,61.2
AHA: 3Q,'02,5; 1Q,'01,6

N **C1773** Retrieval device, insertable (used to retrieve fractured medical devices)
MED: 100-4,4,61.1
AHA: 4Q,'03,8; 3Q,'02,5; 1Q,'01,6

N **C1776** Joint device (implantable)
MED: 100-4,4,61.1; 100-4,4,61.2
AHA: 3Q,'02,5; 1Q,'01,6; 3Q,'01,5

N **C1777** Lead, cardioverter-defibrillator, endocardial single coil (implantable)
MED: 100-4,4,61.1; 100-4,4,61.2
AHA: 3Q,'02,5; 1Q,'01,6

N **C1778** Lead, neurostimulator (implantable)
MED: 100-4,4,61.1
AHA: 3Q,'02,5; 1Q,'02,9

N **C1779** Lead, pacemaker, transvenous VDD single pass
MED: 100-4,4,61.1; 100-4,4,61.2
AHA: 3Q,'02,5; 1Q,'01,6

N **C1780** Lens, intraocular (new technology)
MED: 100-4,4,61.1
AHA: 3Q,'02,5; 1Q,'01,6

N **C1781** Mesh (implantable)
MED: 100-4,4,61.1
AHA: 3Q,'02,5; 1Q,'01,6

N **C1782** Morcellator
MED: 100-4,4,61.1
AHA: 3Q,'02,5; 1Q,'01,6

N **C1783** Ocular implant, aqueous drainage assist device
MED: 100-4,4,61.1

N **C1784** Ocular device, intraoperative, detached retina
MED: 100-4,4,61.1
AHA: 3Q,'02,5; 1Q,'01,6

N **C1785** Pacemaker, dual chamber, rate-responsive (implantable)
MED: 100-4,3,10.4; 100-4,4,61.1
AHA: 4Q,'03,8; 3Q,'02,5; 1Q,'01,6

N **C1786** Pacemaker, single chamber, rate-responsive (implantable)
MED: 100-2,1,40; 100-4,4,61.1; 100-4,4,61.2
AHA: 4Q,'03,8; 3Q,'02,5; 1Q,'01,6

N **C1787** Patient programmer, neurostimulator
MED: 100-4,4,61.1
AHA: 4Q,'03,8; 3Q,'02,5; 1Q,'01,6

N **C1788** Port, indwelling (implantable)
MED: 100-4,4,61.1; 100-4,4,61.2
AHA: 4Q,'03,8; 3Q,'02,5; 1Q,'01,6; 3Q,'01,4

N **C1789** Prosthesis, breast (implantable)
MED: 100-4,4,61.1
AHA: 4Q,'03,8; 3Q,'02,5; 1Q,'01,6

N **C1813** Prosthesis, penile, inflatable
MED: 100-4,4,61.1
AHA: 4Q,'03,8; 3Q,'02,5; 1Q,'01,6

N **C1814** Retinal tamponade device, silicone oil
MED: 100-4,4,61.1

N **C1815** Prosthesis, urinary sphincter (implantable)
MED: 100-4,4,61.1
AHA: 4Q,'03,8; 3Q,'02,5; 1Q,'01,6

N **C1816** Receiver and/or transmitter, neurostimulator (implantable)
MED: 100-4,4,61.1
AHA: 4Q,'03,8; 3Q,'02,5; 1Q,'01,6

N **C1817** Septal defect implant system, intracardiac
MED: 100-4,4,61.1
AHA: 4Q,'03,8; 3Q,'02,5; 1Q,'01,6

N **C1818** Integrated keratoprosthesis
MED: 100-4,4,61.1
AHA: 4Q,'03,4

N **C1819** Surgical tissue localization and excision device (implantable)
This code has been added, effective January 1, 2004.
MED: 100-4,4,61.1

H **C1820** Generator, neurostimulator (implantable), with rechargeable battery and charging system
MED: 100-4,4,10.12

● H **C1821** Interspinous process distraction device (implantable)

N **C1874** Stent, coated/covered, with delivery system
MED: 100-4,4,61.1; 100-4,4,61.2
AHA: 4Q,'03,8; 1Q,'01,6

N **C1875** Stent, coated/covered, without delivery system
MED: 100-4,4,61.1; 100-4,4,61.2
AHA: 4Q,'03,8; 1Q,'01,6

N **C1876** Stent, noncoated/noncovered, with delivery system
MED: 100-4,4,61.1; 100-4,4,61.2
AHA: 4Q,'03,8; 3Q,'02,5; 1Q,'01,6; 3Q,'01,4

N **C1877** Stent, noncoated/noncovered, without delivery system
MED: 100-4,4,61.1; 100-4,4,61.2
AHA: 4Q,'03,8; 3Q,'02,5; 1Q,'01,6; 3Q,'01,4

N **C1878** Material for vocal cord medialization, synthetic (implantable)
MED: 100-4,4,61.1
AHA: 3Q,'02,5; 1Q,'01,6

N **C1879** Tissue marker (implantable)
MED: 100-4,4,61.1
AHA: 4Q,'03,8; 3Q,'02,5; 1Q,'01,6

Special Coverage Instructions   Noncovered by Medicare   Carrier Discretion   ☑ Quality Alert   ● New Code   ○ Reinstated Code   ▲ Revised Code

N	**C1880**	Vena cava filter

MED: 100-4,4,61.1
AHA: 4Q,'03,8; 3Q,'02,5; 1Q,'01,6

N **C1881** Dialysis access system (implantable)
MED: 100-4,4,61.1
AHA: 4Q,'03,8; 3Q,'02,5; 1Q,'01,6

N **C1882** Cardioverter-defibrillator, other than single or dual chamber (implantable)
MED: 100-4,4,61.1; 100-4,4,61.2
AHA: 3Q,'02,5; 1Q,'01,5

N **C1883** Adaptor/extension, pacing lead or neurostimulator lead (implantable)
MED: 100-4,4,61.1
AHA: 1Q,'02,9; 3Q,'02,5; 1Q,'01,5

N **C1884** Embolization protective system
MED: 100-4,4,61.1

N **C1885** Catheter, transluminal angioplasty, laser
MED: 100-4,4,61.1; 100-4,4,61.2
AHA: 4Q,'03,8; 3Q,'02,5; 1Q,'01,5

N **C1887** Catheter, guiding (may include infusion/perfusion capability)
MED: 100-4,4,61.1; 100-4,4,61.2
AHA: 3Q,'02,5; 1Q,'01,5

N **C1888** Catheter, ablation, noncardiac, endovascular (implantable)
MED: 100-4,4,61.1

N **C1891** Infusion pump, nonprogrammable, permanent (implantable)
MED: 100-4,4,61.1; 100-4,4,61.2
AHA: 4Q,'03,8; 3Q,'02,5; 1Q,'01,6

N **C1892** Introducer/sheath, guiding, intracardiac electrophysiological, fixed-curve, peel-away
MED: 100-4,4,61.1; 100-4,4,61.2
AHA: 3Q,'02,5; 1Q,'01,6

N **C1893** Introducer/sheath, guiding, intracardiac electrophysiological, fixed-curve, other than peel-away
MED: 100-4,4,61.1; 100-4,4,61.2
AHA: 3Q,'02,5; 1Q,'01,6; 3Q,'01,4

N **C1894** Introducer/sheath, other than guiding, other than intracardiac electrophysiological, nonlaser
MED: 100-4,4,61.1; 100-4,4,61.2
AHA: 3Q,'02,5

N **C1895** Lead, cardioverter-defibrillator, endocardial dual coil (implantable)
MED: 100-4,4,61.1; 100-4,4,61.2
AHA: 3Q,'02,5; 1Q,'01,6

N **C1896** Lead, cardioverter-defibrillator, other than endocardial single or dual coil (implantable)
MED: 100-4,4,61.1; 100-4,4,61.2
AHA: 3Q,'02,5; 1Q,'01,6

N **C1897** Lead, neurostimulator test kit (implantable)
MED: 100-4,4,61.1
AHA: 1Q,'02,9; 3Q,'02,5; 1Q,'01,6

N **C1898** Lead, pacemaker, other than transvenous VDD single pass
MED: 100-4,4,61.1
AHA: 1Q,'01,6; 3Q,'01,4

N **C1899** Lead, pacemaker/cardioverter-defibrillator combination (implantable)
MED: 100-4,4,61.1; 100-4,4,61.2
AHA: 3Q,'02,5; 1Q,'01,6

N **C1900** Lead, left ventricular coronary venous system
MED: 100-4,4,61.1; 100-4,4,61.2

N **C2614** Probe, percutaneous lumbar discectomy
MED: 100-4,4,61.1

N **C2615** Sealant, pulmonary, liquid
MED: 100-4,4,61.1
AHA: 3Q,'02,5; 1Q,'01,6

K **C2616** Brachytherapy source, yttrium 90, per source ⊘
MED: 100-4,4,61.1
AHA: 3Q,'03,11; 3Q,'02,5

N **C2617** Stent, noncoronary, temporary, without delivery system
MED: 100-4,4,61.1; 100-4,4,61.2
AHA: 4Q,'03,8; 3Q,'02,5; 1Q,'01,6

N **C2618** Probe, cryoablation
MED: 100-4,4,61.1; 100-4,4,61.2
AHA: 4Q,'03,8; 3Q,'02,5; 1Q,'01,6

N **C2619** Pacemaker, dual chamber, nonrate-responsive (implantable)
MED: 100-4,4,61.1
AHA: 3Q,'02,5; 1Q,'01,6; 3Q,'01,4

N **C2620** Pacemaker, single chamber, non rate-responsive (implantable)
MED: 100-4,3,10.4; 100-4,4,61.1; 100-4,4,61.2
AHA: 4Q,'03,8; 3Q,'02,5; 1Q,'01,6

N **C2621** Pacemaker, other than single or dual chamber (implantable)
MED: 100-4,3,10.4; 100-4,4,61.1
AHA: 4Q,'03,8; 1Q,'01,6

N **C2622** Prosthesis, penile, non-inflatable
MED: 100-4,4,61.1
AHA: 4Q,'03,8; 3Q,'02,5; 1Q,'01,6

N **C2625** Stent, noncoronary, temporary, with delivery system
MED: 100-4,4,61.1; 100-4,4,61.2
AHA: 4Q,'03,8; 3Q,'02,5; 1Q,'01,6

N **C2626** Infusion pump, nonprogrammable, temporary (implantable)
MED: 100-4,4,61.1; 100-4,4,61.2
AHA: 3Q,'02,5; 1Q,'01,6

N **C2627** Catheter, suprapubic/cystoscopic
MED: 100-4,4,61.1
AHA: 4Q,'03,8; 3Q,'02,5; 1Q,'01,5

N **C2628** Catheter, occlusion
MED: 100-4,4,61.1; 100-4,4,61.2
AHA: 4Q,'03,8; 3Q,'02,6; 1Q,'01,5

N **C2629** Introducer/sheath, other than guiding, intracardiac electrophysiological, laser
MED: 100-4,4,61.1
AHA: 3Q,'02,5; 1Q,'01,6

N **C2630** Catheter, electrophysiology, diagnostic/ablation, other than 3D or vector mapping, cool-tip
MED: 100-4,4,61.1
AHA: 3Q,'02,5; 1Q,'01,5

N **C2631** Repair device, urinary, incontinence, without sling graft
MED: 100-4,4,61.1
AHA: 4Q,'03,8; 3Q,'02,5; 1Q,'01,6

C2632 Brachytherapy solution, Iodine-125, per mCi
See code(s) A9527

K **C2633** Brachytherapy source, cesium-131, per source ⊘
MED: 100-4,4,61.1

K **C2634** Brachytherapy source, high-activity, Iodine-125, greater than 1.01 mCi (NIST), per source ⊘
MED: 100-4,4,61.1
AHA: 2Q,'05,8

Outpatient PPS C1880 — C2634

Special Coverage Instructions | Noncovered by Medicare | Carrier Discretion | ☑ Quality Alert | ● New Code | ○ Reinstated Code | ▲ Revised Code

2007 HCPCS ❶-❾ ASC Group **MED:** Pub 100/NCD References ℶ DMEPOS Paid ⊘ SNF Excluded **C Codes — 23**

Outpatient PPS

C2635 — C9235

K　**C2635** Brachytherapy source, high-activity, Paladium-103, greater than 2.2 mCi (NIST), per source ⊘
MED: 100-4,4,61.1
AHA: 2Q,'05,8

K　**C2636** Brachytherapy linear source, paladium 103, per 1 mm ⊘
MED: 100-4,4,61.1

B　**C2637** Brachytherapy source, ytterbium-169, per source ⊘
AHA: 3Q,'05,7

S　**C8900** Magnetic resonance angiography with contrast, abdomen ⊘
MED: 100-4,13,40.1.2

S　**C8901** Magnetic resonance angiography without contrast, abdomen ⊘
MED: 100-4,13,40.1.2

S　**C8902** Magnetic resonance angiography without contrast followed by with contrast, abdomen ⊘
MED: 100-4,13,40.1.2

S　**C8903** Magnetic resonance imaging with contrast, breast; unilateral ⊘

S　**C8904** Magnetic resonance imaging without contrast, breast; unilateral ⊘

S　**C8905** Magnetic resonance imaging without contrast followed by with contrast, breast; unilateral ⊘

S　**C8906** Magnetic resonance imaging with contrast, breast; bilateral ⊘

S　**C8907** Magnetic resonance imaging without contrast, breast; bilateral ⊘

S　**C8908** Magnetic resonance imaging without contrast followed by with contrast, breast; bilateral ⊘

S　**C8909** Magnetic resonance angiography with contrast, chest (excluding myocardium) ⊘
MED: 100-4,13,40.1.2

S　**C8910** Magnetic resonance angiography without contrast, chest (excluding myocardium) ⊘
MED: 100-4,13,40.1.2

S　**C8911** Magnetic resonance angiography without contrast followed by with contrast, chest (excluding myocardium) ⊘
MED: 100-4,13,40.1.2

S　**C8912** Magnetic resonance angiography with contrast, lower extremity ⊘
MED: 100-4,13,40.1.2

S　**C8913** Magnetic resonance angiography without contrast, lower extremity ⊘
MED: 100-4,13,40.1.2

S　**C8914** Magnetic resonance angiography without contrast followed by with contrast, lower extremity ⊘
MED: 100-4,13,40.1.2

S　**C8918** Magnetic resonance angiography with contrast, pelvis ⊘
MED: 100-4,13,40.1.2
AHA: 4Q,'03,4

S　**C8919** Magnetic resonance angiography without contrast, pelvis ⊘
MED: 100-4,13,40.1.2
AHA: 4Q,'03,4

S　**C8920** Magnetic resonance angiography without contrast followed by with contrast, pelvis ⊘
MED: 100-4,13,40.1.2
AHA: 4Q,'03,4

C8950 Intravenous infusion for therapy/diagnosis; up to 1 hour
See CPT code(s) 90765-90768

C8951 Intravenous infusion for therapy/diagnosis; each additional hour (List separately in addition to C8950)
See CPT code(s) 90765-90768.

C8952 Therapeutic, prophylactic or diagnostic injection; intravenous push of each new substance/drug
See CPT code(s) 90774, 90775

C8953 Chemotherapy administration, intravenous; push technique
See CPT code(s) 96409-96411

C8954 Chemotherapy administration, intravenous; infusion technique, up to one hour
See CPT code(s) 96413-96417

C8955 Chemotherapy administration, intravenous; infusion technique, each additional hour (List separately in addition to C8954)
See CPT code(s) 96413-96417

S　**C8957** Prolonged IV infusion, requiring pump
MED: 100-4,4,230.2.1; 100-4,4,230.2.3

K　**C9003** Palivizumab-RSV-IgM, per 50 mg
Use this code for Palivizumab, Synagis.

N　**C9113** Injection, pantoprazole sodium, per vial
Use this code for Protonix.

K　**C9121** Injection, argatroban, per 5 mg
Use this code for Acova.

C9220 Sodium hyaluronate per 30 mg dose, for intra-articular injection
See code(s) J7319

C9221 Acellular dermal tissue matrix, per 16 sq. cm.
See code(s) J7344

C9222 Decellularized soft tissue scaffold, per 1 cc
See code(s) J7346

C9224 Injection, galsulfase, per 5 mg
See code(s) J1458

C9225 Injection, fluocinolone acetonide intravitreal implant, per 0.59 mg
See code(s) J7311

C9227 Injection, micafungin sodium, per 1 mg
See code(s) J2248

C9228 Injection, tigecycline, per 1 mg
See code(s) J3243

C9229 Injection, ibandronate sodium, per 1 mg
See code(s) J1740

C9230 Injection, abatacept, per 10 mg
See code(s) J0129

C9231 Injection, decitabine, per 1 mg

●　G　**C9232** Injection, idursulfase, 1 mg
Use this code for Elaprase.

●　G　**C9233** Injection, ranibizumab, 0.5 mg
Use this code for Lucentis.

●　K　**C9234** Injection, alglucosidase alfa, 10 mg
Use this code for Myozyme.
See also code: S0147.

●　K　**C9235** Injection, panitumumab, 10 mg
Use this code for Vectibix.

Special Coverage Instructions　　Noncovered by Medicare　　Carrier Discretion　　☑ Quality Alert　　● New Code　　○ Reinstated Code　　▲ Revised Code

24 — C Codes　　A Age Edit　　M Maternity Edit　　♀ Female Only　　♂ Male Only　　A - Y APC Status Indicators　　*2007 HCPCS*

● ⃣G C9350 Microporous collagen tube of nonhuman origin, per centimeter length

● ⃣G C9351 Acellular dermal tissue matrix of nonhuman origin, per square centimeter (Do not report C9351 in conjunction with J7345)

  ⃣A C9399 Unclassified drugs or biologicals

  ⃣T C9716 Creations of thermal anal lesions by radiofrequency energy

  ⃣S C9723 Dynamic infrared blood perfusion imaging (DIRI)

  ⃣T C9724 Endoscopic full-thickness plication in the gastric cardia using endoscopic plication system (EPS); includes endoscopy

  ⃣S C9725 Placement of endorectal intracavitary applicator for high intensity brachytherapy   ⊘
        AHA: 3Q,'05,7

  ⃣S C9726 Placement and removal (if performed) of applicator into breast for radiation therapy

● ⃣S C9727 Insertion of implants into the soft palate; minimum of three implants

---

Special Coverage Instructions   Noncovered by Medicare   Carrier Discretion   ☑ Quality Alert   ● New Code   ○ Reinstated Code ▲ Revised Code

2007 HCPCS   ⃣1-⃣9 ASC Group   **MED:** Pub 100/NCD References   ᵴ. DMEPOS Paid   ⊘ SNF Excluded   **C Codes — 25**

DENTAL PROCEDURES D0000-D9999

The D, or dental, codes are a separate category of national codes. The Current Dental Terminology (CDT-2007/2008) code set is copyrighted by the American Dental Association (ADA). CDT-2007/2008 is included in HCPCS Level II. Decisions regarding the modification, deletion, or addition of CDT-2007/2008 codes are made by the ADA and not the national panel responsible for the administration of HCPCS.

The Department of Health and Human Services has an agreement with the AMA pertaining to the use of the CPT codes for physician services; it also has an agreement with the ADA to include CDT-2007/2008 as a set of HCPCS Level II codes for use in billing for dental services.

DIAGNOSTIC D0100-D0999

CLINICAL ORAL EVALUATION

All dental codes fall under the jurisdiction of the Medicare local contractor.

▲ E **D0120** Periodic oral evaluation, established patient
This procedure is covered if its purpose is to identify a patient's existing infections prior to kidney transplantation.

E **D0140** Limited oral evaluation — problem focused

● **D0145** Oral evaluation for a patient under three years of age and counseling with primary caregiver

S **D0150** Comprehensive oral evaluation — new or established patient ⊘
This procedure is covered if its purpose is to identify a patient's existing infections prior to kidney transplantation.
MED: 100-2,15,150; 100-2,16,140; 100-3,260.6; 100-4,4,20.5

E **D0160** Detailed and extensive oral evaluation — problem focused, by report
Pertinent documentation to evaluate medical appropriateness should be included when this code is reported.

E **D0170** Re-evaluation — limited, problem focused (established patient; not postoperative visit)

E **D0180** Comprehensive periodontal evaluation — new or established patient
See also equivalent CPT E&M codes.

RADIOGRAPHS

E **D0210** Intraoral — complete series (including bitewings)
See code(s): 70320

E ☑ **D0220** Intraoral — periapical, first film
See code(s): 70300

E ☑ **D0230** Intraoral — periapical, each additional film
See code(s): 70310

S **D0240** Intraoral — occlusal film ⊘
MED: 100-2,15,150; 100-2,16,140; 100-4,4,20.5

S ☑ **D0250** Extraoral — first film ⊘
MED: 100-2,15,150; 100-2,16,140; 100-4,4,20.5

S ☑ **D0260** Extraoral — each additional film ⊘
MED: 100-2,15,150; 100-2,16,140; 100-4,4,20.5

S ☑ **D0270** Bitewing — single film ⊘
MED: 100-2,15,150; 100-2,16,140; 100-4,4,20.5

S ☑ **D0272** Bitewings — two films ⊘
MED: 100-2,15,150; 100-2,16,140; 100-4,4,20.5

● **D0273** Bitewings, three films

S ☑ **D0274** Bitewings — four films ⊘
MED: 100-2,15,150; 100-2,16,140; 100-4,4,20.5

S ☑ **D0277** Vertical bitewings — 7 to 8 films
MED: 100-2,15,150; 100-2,16,140; 100-4,4,20.5

E **D0290** Posterior-anterior or lateral skull and facial bone survey film
See code(s): 70150

E **D0310** Sialography
See code(s): 70390

E **D0320** Temporomandibular joint arthrogram, including injection
See code(s): 70332

E **D0321** Other temporomandibular joint films, by report
See code(s): 76499

E **D0322** Tomographic survey
MED: 100-3,260.6

E **D0330** Panoramic film
See code(s): 70320

E **D0340** Cephalometric film
See code(s): 70350

E **D0350** Oral/facial photographic images
This code excludes conventional radiographs.

● **D0360** Cone beam CT, craniofacial data capture

● **D0362** Cone beam, two-dimensional image reconstruction using existing data, includes multiple images

● **D0363** Cone beam, three-dimensional image reconstruction using existing data, includes multiple images

TEST AND LABORATORY EXAMINATIONS

E **D0415** Collection of microorganisms for culture and sensitivity
This procedure is covered if its purpose is to identify a patient's existing infections prior to kidney transplantation.
See code(s): D0410

B **D0416** Viral culture

B **D0421** Genetic test for susceptibility to oral diseases

E **D0425** Caries susceptibility tests
This procedure is covered by Medicare if its purpose is to identify a patient's existing infections prior to kidney transplantation.
See code(s): D0420

B **D0431** Adjunctive pre-diagnostic test that aids In detection of mucosal abnormalities including premalignant and malignant lesions, not to include cytology or biopsy procedures

S **D0460** Pulp vitality tests ⊘
This procedure is covered by Medicare if its purpose is to identify a patient's existing infections prior to kidney transplantation.
MED: 100-2,15,150; 100-2,16,140; 100-3,260.6; 100-4,4,20.5

E **D0470** Diagnostic casts

B **D0472** Accession of tissue, gross examination, preparation, and transmission of written report
MED: 100-2,15,150; 100-2,16,140; 100-3,260.6; 100-4,4,20.5

B **D0473** Accession of tissue, gross and microscopic examination, preparation and transmission of written report
MED: 100-2,15,150; 100-2,16,140; 100-3,260.6; 100-4,4,20.5

Special Coverage Instructions   Noncovered by Medicare   Carrier Discretion   ☑ Quality Alert   ● New Code   ○ Reinstated Code   ▲ Revised Code

2007 HCPCS   1-9 ASC Group   MED: Pub 100/NCD References   ℞ DMEPOS Paid   ⊘ SNF Excluded   D Codes — 27

D0120 — D0473

Dental Procedures

D0474 — D2544

B   **D0474** Accession of tissue, gross and microscopic examination, including assessment of surgical margins for presence of disease, preparation and transmission of written report

MED: 100-2,15,150; 100-2,16,140; 100-3,260.6; 100-4,4,20.5

B   **D0475** Decalcification procedure

MED: 100-4,4,20.5

B   **D0476** Special stains for microorganisms

MED: 100-4,4,20.5

B   **D0477** Special stains, not for microorganisms

MED: 100-4,4,20.5

B   **D0478** Immunohistochemical stains

MED: 100-4,4,20.5

B   **D0479** Tissue in-situ hybridization, including interpretation

MED: 100-4,4,20.5

▲ B   **D0480** Accession of exfoliative cytologic smears, microscopic examination, preparation and transmission of written report

MED: 100-2,15,150; 100-2,16,140; 100-3,260.6; 100-4,4,20.5

B   **D0481** Electron microscopy — diagnostic

MED: 100-4,4,20.5

B   **D0482** Direct immunofluorescence

MED: 100-4,4,20.5

B   **D0483** Indirect immunofluorescence

MED: 100-4,4,20.5

B   **D0484** Consultation on slides prepared elsewhere

MED: 100-4,4,20.5

B   **D0485** Consultation, including preparation of slides from biopsy material supplied by referring source

MED: 100-4,4,20.5

●   **D0486** Accession of brush biopsy sample, microscopic examination, preparation and transmission of written report

B   **D0502** Other oral pathology procedures, by report   ⊘

Pertinent documentation to evaluate medical appropriateness should be included when this code is reported. This procedure is covered by Medicare if its purpose is to identify a patient's existing infections prior to kidney transplantation.

MED: 100-2,15,150; 100-2,16,140; 100-3,260.6; 100-4,4,20.5

B   **D0999** Unspecified diagnostic procedure, by report   ⊘

Determine if an alternative HCPCS Level II or a CPT code better describes the service being reported. This code should be used only if a more specific code is unavailable.

MED: 100-2,15,150; 100-2,16,140; 100-3,260.6; 100-4,4,20.5

PREVENTIVE D1000-D1999

DENTAL PROPHYLAXIS

E   **D1110** Prophylaxis — adult   A

E   **D1120** Prophylaxis — child   A

TOPICAL FLUORIDE TREATMENT (OFFICE PROCEDURE)

~~**D1201** Topical application of fluoride (including prophylaxis) — child~~

E   **D1203** Topical application of fluoride (prophylaxis not included) — child   A

E   **D1204** Topical application of fluoride (prophylaxis not included) — adult   A

~~**D1205** Topical application of fluoride (including prophylaxis) — adult~~

●   **D1206** Topical fluoride varnish; therapeutic application for moderate to high caries risk patients

OTHER PREVENTIVE SERVICES

E   **D1310** Nutritional counseling for control of dental disease

MED: 100-2,16,10

E   **D1320** Tobacco counseling for the control and prevention of oral disease

MED: 100-2,16,10

E   **D1330** Oral hygiene instructions

MED: 100-2,16,10

E ☑   **D1351** Sealant — per tooth

SPACE MAINTENANCE (PASSIVE APPLIANCES)

S   **D1510** Space maintainer — fixed-unilateral   ⊘

MED: 100-2,16,140; 100-4,4,20.5

S   **D1515** Space maintainer — fixed-bilateral   ⊘

MED: 100-2,15,150; 100-2,16,140; 100-4,4,20.5

S   **D1520** Space maintainer — removable-unilateral   ⊘

MED: 100-2,15,150; 100-2,16,140; 100-4,4,20.5

S   **D1525** Space maintainer — removable-bilateral   ⊘

MED: 100-2,15,150; 100-2,16,140; 100-4,4,20.5

S   **D1550** Recementation of space maintainer   ⊘

MED: 100-2,15,150; 100-2,16,140; 100-4,4,20.5

●   **D1555** Removal of fixed space maintainer

E ☑   **D2140** Amalgam—one surface, primary or permanent

E ☑   **D2150** Amalgam—two surfaces, primary or permanent

E ☑   **D2160** Amalgam—three surfaces, primary or permanent

E ☑   **D2161** Amalgam—four or more surfaces, primary or permanent

RESIN RESTORATIONS

E ☑   **D2330** Resin-based composite — one surface, anterior

E ☑   **D2331** Resin-based composite — two surfaces, anterior

E ☑   **D2332** Resin-based composite — three surfaces, anterior

E ☑   **D2335** Resin-based composite — four or more surfaces or involving incisal angle (anterior)

E   **D2390** Resin-based composite crown, anterior

E   **D2391** Resin-based composite — one surface, posterior

E   **D2392** Resin-based composite — two surfaces, posterior

E   **D2393** Resin-based composite — three surfaces, posterior

E   **D2394** Resin-based composite — four or more surfaces, posterior

GOLD FOIL RESTORATIONS

E ☑   **D2410** Gold foil — one surface

E ☑   **D2420** Gold foil — two surfaces

E ☑   **D2430** Gold foil — three surfaces

INLAY/ONLAY RESTORATIONS

E ☑   **D2510** Inlay — metallic — one surface

E ☑   **D2520** Inlay — metallic — two surfaces

E ☑   **D2530** Inlay — metallic — three or more surfaces

E ☑   **D2542** Onlay — metallic — two surfaces

E ☑   **D2543** Onlay — metallic — three surfaces

E ☑   **D2544** Onlay — metallic — four or more surfaces

Special Coverage Instructions   Noncovered by Medicare   Carrier Discretion   ☑ Quality Alert   ● New Code   ○ Reinstated Code   ▲ Revised Code

28 — D Codes   A Age Edit   M Maternity Edit   ♀ Female Only   ♂ Male Only   A - ☑ APC Status Indicators   *2007 HCPCS*

E ☑ D2610 Inlay — porcelain/ceramic — one surface

E ☑ D2620 Inlay — porcelain/ceramic — two surfaces

E ☑ D2630 Inlay — porcelain/ceramic — three or more surfaces

E ☑ D2642 Onlay — porcelain/ceramic — two surfaces

E ☑ D2643 Onlay — porcelain/ceramic — three surfaces

E ☑ D2644 Onlay — porcelain/ceramic — four or more surfaces

E ☑ D2650 Inlay — resin-based composite composite/resin — one surface

E ☑ D2651 Inlay — resin-based composite composite/resin — two surfaces

E ☑ D2652 Inlay — resin-based composite composite/resin — three or more surfaces

E ☑ D2662 Onlay — resin-based composite composite/resin — two surfaces

E ☑ D2663 Onlay — resin-based composite composite/resin — three surfaces

E ☑ D2664 Onlay — resin-based composite composite/resin — four or more surfaces

CROWNS - SINGLE RESTORATION ONLY

E D2710 Crown — resin-based composite (indirect)

E D2712 Crown — 3/4 resin-based composite (indirect)

E D2720 Crown — resin with high noble metal

E D2721 Crown — resin with predominantly base metal

E D2722 Crown — resin with noble metal

E D2740 Crown — porcelain/ceramic substrate

E D2750 Crown — porcelain fused to high noble metal

E D2751 Crown — porcelain fused to predominantly base metal

E D2752 Crown — porcelain fused to noble metal

E D2780 Crown — 3/4 cast high noble metal

E D2781 Crown — 3/4 cast predominately base metal

E D2782 Crown — 3/4 cast noble metal

E D2783 Crown — 3/4 porcelain/ceramic

E D2790 Crown — full cast high noble metal

E D2791 Crown — full cast predominantly base metal

E D2792 Crown — full cast noble metal

E D2794 Crown — titanium

E D2799 Provisional crown
Do not use this code to report a temporary crown for routine prosthetic restoration.

OTHER RESTORATIVE SERVICES

E D2910 Recement inlay, onlay or partial coverage restoration

E D2915 Recement cast or prefabricated post and core

E D2920 Recement crown

E D2930 Prefabricated stainless steel crown — primary tooth

E D2931 Prefabricated stainless steel crown — permanent tooth

E D2932 Prefabricated resin crown

E D2933 Prefabricated stainless steel crown with resin window

E D2934 Prefabricated esthetic coated stainless steel crown — primary tooth

E D2940 Sedative filling

E D2950 Core buildup, including any pins

E D2951 Pin retention — per tooth, in addition to restoration

▲ E D2952 Post and core in addition to crown, indirectly fabricated

▲ E D2953 Each additional indirectly fabricated post, same tooth
Report in addition to code D2952.

E D2954 Prefabricated post and core in addition to crown

E D2955 Post removal (not in conjunction with endodontic therapy)

E D2957 Each additional prefabricated post — same tooth
Report in addition to code D2954.

E D2960 Labial veneer (resin laminate) — chairside

E D2961 Labial veneer (resin laminate) — laboratory

E D2962 Labial veneer (porcelain laminate) — laboratory

E D2971 Additional procedures to construct new crown under existing partial denture framework

E D2975 Coping

E D2980 Crown repair, by report
Pertinent documentation to evaluate medical appropriateness should be included when this code is reported.

S D2999 Unspecified restorative procedure, by report ⊘
Determine if an alternative HCPCS Level II or a CPT code better describes the service being reported. This code should be used only if a more specific code is unavailable.

MED: 100-2,15,150; 100-2,16,140; 100-4,4,20.5

ENDODONTICS D3000-D3999

PULP CAPPING

E D3110 Pulp cap — direct (excluding final restoration)

E D3120 Pulp cap — indirect (excluding final restoration)

PULPOTOMY

E D3220 Therapeutic pulpotomy (excluding final restoration) — removal of pulp coronal to the dentinocemental junction and application of medicament
Do not use this code to report the first stage of root canal therapy.

E D3221 Pulpal debridement, primary and permanent teeth

PULPAL THERAPY ON PRIMARY TEETH (INCLUDES PRIMARY TEETH WITH SUCCEDANEOUS TEETH AND PLACEMENT OF RESORBABLE FILLING)

E D3230 Pulpal therapy (resorbable filling) — anterior, primary tooth (excluding final restoration)

E D3240 Pulpal therapy (resorbable filling) — posterior, primary tooth (excluding final restoration)

ROOT CANAL THERAPY (INCLUDING TREATMENT PLAN, CLINICAL PROCEDURES, AND FOLLOW-UP CARE, INCLUDES PRIMARY TEETH WITHOUT SUCCEDANEOUS TEETH AND PERMANENT TEETH)

E D3310 Anterior (excluding final restoration)

E D3320 Bicuspid (excluding final restoration)

E D3330 Molar (excluding final restoration)

E D3331 Treatment of root canal obstruction; nonsurgical access

Special Coverage Instructions   Noncovered by Medicare   Carrier Discretion   ☑ Quality Alert   ● New Code   ○ Reinstated Code   ▲ Revised Code

2007 HCPCS   **1**-**9** ASC Group   **MED:** Pub 100/NCD References   ᕃ DMEPOS Paid   ⊘ SNF Excluded   **D Codes — 29**

D2610 — D3331

Dental Procedures

D3332 — D4342

E **D3332** Incomplete endodontic therapy; inoperable, unrestorable or fractured tooth

E **D3333** Internal root repair of perforation defects

E **D3346** Retreatment of previous root canal therapy — anterior

E **D3347** Retreatment of previous root canal therapy — bicuspid

E **D3348** Retreatment of previous root canal therapy — molar

E **D3351** Apexification/recalcification — initial visit (apical closure/calcific repair of perforations, root resorption, etc.)

E **D3352** Apexification/recalcification — interim medication replacement (apical closure/calcific repair of perforations, root resorption, etc.)

E **D3353** Apexification/recalcification — final visit (includes completed root canal therapy — apical closure/calcific repair of perforations, root resorption, etc.)

APICOECTOMY/PERIRADICULAR SERVICES

E **D3410** Apicoectomy/periradicular surgery — anterior

E **D3421** Apicoectomy/periradicular surgery — bicuspid (first root)

E **D3425** Apicoectomy/periradicular surgery — molar (first root)

E ☑ **D3426** Apicoectomy/periradicular surgery (each additional root)

E ☑ **D3430** Retrograde filling — per root

E ☑ **D3450** Root amputation — per root

S **D3460** Endodontic endosseous implant   ⊘
   MED: 100-2,15,150; 100-2,16,140; 100-4,4,20.5

E **D3470** Intentional reimplantation (including necessary splinting)

OTHER ENDODONTIC PROCEDURES

E **D3910** Surgical procedure for isolation of tooth with rubber dam

E **D3920** Hemisection (including any root removal), not including root canal therapy

E **D3950** Canal preparation and fitting of preformed dowel or post

S **D3999** Unspecified endodontic procedure, by report   ⊘
   Determine if an alternative HCPCS Level II or a CPT code better describes the service being reported. This code should be used only if a more specific code is unavailable.
   MED: 100-2,15,150; 100-2,16,140; 100-4,4,20.5

PERIODONTICS D4000-D4999

SURGICAL SERVICES (INCLUDING USUAL POSTOPERATIVE SERVICES)

E ☑ **D4210** Gingivectomy or gingivoplasty — four or more contiguous teeth or bounded teeth spaces per quadrant
   See code(s): 41820

E ☑ **D4211** Gingivectomy or gingivoplasty — one to three contiguous teeth or bounded teeth spaces per quadrant
   See also CPT code (64400-64530).

● **D4230** Anatomical crown exposure, four or more contiguous teeth per quadrant

● **D4231** Anatomical crown exposure, one to three teeth per quadrant

E ☑ **D4240** Gingival flap procedure, including root planing — four or more contiguous teeth or bounded teeth spaces per quadrant

E **D4241** Gingival flap procedure, including root planing — one to three contiguous teeth or bounded teeth spaces per quadrant
   See also D4240.

E **D4245** Apically positioned flap

E **D4249** Clinical crown lengthening — hard tissue

S ☑ **D4260** Osseous surgery (including flap entry and closure) — four or more contiguous teeth or bounded teeth spaces per quadrant   ⊘
   MED: 100-2,15,150; 100-2,16,140; 100-4,4,20.5

E **D4261** Osseous surgery (including flap entry and closure) — one to three contiguous teeth or bounded teeth spaces per quadrant
   See CPT code 41823.

S ☑ **D4263** Bone replacement graft — first site in quadrant   ⊘
   MED: 100-2,15,150; 100-2,16,140; 100-3,260.6; 100-4,4,20.5

S ☑ **D4264** Bone replacement graft — each additional site in quadrant (use if performed on same date of service as D4263)   ⊘
   MED: 100-2,15,150; 100-2,16,140; 100-3,260.6; 100-4,4,20.5

E ☑ **D4265** Biologic materials to aid in soft and osseous tissue regeneration

E ☑ **D4266** Guided tissue regeneration — resorbable barrier, per site

E ☑ **D4267** Guided tissue regeneration — nonresorbable barrier, per site (includes membrane removal)

S ☑ **D4268** Surgical revision procedure, per tooth
   MED: 100-2,15,150; 100-2,16,140

S **D4270** Pedicle soft tissue graft procedure   ⊘
   MED: 100-2,15,150; 100-2,16,140; 100-4,4,20.5

S **D4271** Free soft tissue graft procedure (including donor site surgery)   ⊘
   MED: 100-2,15,150; 100-2,16,140; 100-4,4,20.5

S **D4273** Subepithelial connective tissue graft procedures, per tooth   ⊘
   For tissue grafts, see CPT 15000 and related codes.
   MED: 100-2,15,150; 100-2,16,140; 100-3,260.6; 100-4,4,20.5

E **D4274** Distal or proximal wedge procedure (when not performed in conjunction with surgical procedures in the same anatomical area)

E **D4275** Soft tissue allograft
   For tissue grafts, see CPT 15000 and related codes.

E **D4276** Combined connective tissue and double pedicle graft, per tooth
   For tissue/pedicle grafts see CPT 15000 and related codes.

ADJUNCTIVE PERIODONTAL SERVICES

E **D4320** Provisional splinting — intracoronal

E **D4321** Provisional splinting — extracoronal

E ☑ **D4341** Periodontal scaling and root planing — four or more teeth per quadrant

E **D4342** Periodontal scaling and root planing — one to three teeth, per quadrant

Special Coverage Instructions   Noncovered by Medicare   Carrier Discretion   ☑ Quality Alert   ● New Code   ○ Reinstated Code   ▲ Revised Code

30 — D Codes   A Age Edit   M Maternity Edit   ♀ Female Only   ♂ Male Only   Ⓐ - ☑ APC Status Indicators   *2007 HCPCS*

S	D4355	Full mouth debridement to enable comprehensive evaluation and diagnosis ⊘

This procedure is covered by Medicare if its purpose is to identify a patient's existing infections prior to kidney transplantation. For debridement see CPT 11000 and related codes.

MED: 100-2,15,150; 100-2,16,140; 100-3,260.6; 100-4,4,20.5

S	D4381	Localized delivery of antimicrobial agents via a controlled release vehicle into diseased crevicular tissue, per tooth, by report ⊘

Pertinent documentation to evaluate medical appropriateness should be included when this code is reported.

MED: 100-2,15,150; 100-2,16,140; 100-3,260.6; 100-4,4,20.5

OTHER PERIODONTAL SERVICES

E	D4910	Periodontal maintenance
E	D4920	Unscheduled dressing change (by someone other than treating dentist)
E	D4999	Unspecified periodontal procedure, by report

Determine if an alternative HCPCS Level II or a CPT code better describes the service being reported. This code should be used only if a more specific code is unavailable.

PROSTHODONTICS (REMOVABLE) D5000-D5899

COMPLETE DENTURES (INCLUDING ROUTINE POST DELIVERY CARE)

E	D5110	Complete denture — maxillary
E	D5120	Complete denture — mandibular
E	D5130	Immediate denture — maxillary
E	D5140	Immediate denture — mandibular

PARTIAL DENTURES (INCLUDING ROUTINE POST DELIVERY CARE)

E	D5211	Maxillary partial denture — resin base (including any conventional clasps, rests and teeth)
E	D5212	Mandibular partial denture — resin base (including any conventional clasps, rests and teeth)
E	D5213	Maxillary partial denture — cast metal framework with resin denture bases (including any conventional clasps, rests and teeth)
E	D5214	Mandibular partial denture — cast metal framework with resin denture bases (including any conventional clasps, rests and teeth)
E	D5225	Maxillary partial denture — flexible base (including any clasps, rests and teeth)
E	D5226	Mandibular partial denture — flexible base (including any clasps, rests and teeth)
E	D5281	Removable unilateral partial denture — one piece cast metal (including clasps and teeth)

ADJUSTMENTS TO REMOVABLE PROSTHESES

E	D5410	Adjust complete denture — maxillary
E	D5411	Adjust complete denture — mandibular
E	D5421	Adjust partial denture — maxillary
E	D5422	Adjust partial denture — mandibular

REPAIRS TO COMPLETE DENTURES

E	D5510	Repair broken complete denture base
E	D5520	Replace missing or broken teeth — complete denture (each tooth)

REPAIRS TO PARTIAL DENTURES

E	D5610	Repair resin denture base
E	D5620	Repair cast framework
E	D5630	Repair or replace broken clasp
E ☑	D5640	Replace broken teeth — per tooth
E	D5650	Add tooth to existing partial denture
E	D5660	Add clasp to existing partial denture
E	D5670	Replace all teeth and acrylic on cast metal framework (maxillary)
E	D5671	Replace all teeth and acrylic on cast metal framework (mandibular)

DENTURE REBASE PROCEDURES

E	D5710	Rebase complete maxillary denture
E	D5711	Rebase complete mandibular denture
E	D5720	Rebase maxillary partial denture
E	D5721	Rebase mandibular partial denture

DENTURE RELINE PROCEDURES

E	D5730	Reline complete maxillary denture (chairside)
E	D5731	Reline complete mandibular denture (chairside)
E	D5740	Reline maxillary partial denture (chairside)
E	D5741	Reline mandibular partial denture (chairside)
E	D5750	Reline complete maxillary denture (laboratory)
E	D5751	Reline complete mandibular denture (laboratory)
E	D5760	Reline maxillary partial denture (laboratory)
E	D5761	Reline mandibular partial denture (laboratory)

OTHER REMOVABLE PROSTHETIC SERVICES

E	D5810	Interim complete denture (maxillary)
E	D5811	Interim complete denture (mandibular)
E	D5820	Interim partial denture (maxillary)
E	D5821	Interim partial denture (mandibular)
E	D5850	Tissue conditioning, maxillary
E	D5851	Tissue conditioning, mandibular
E	D5860	Overdenture — complete, by report

Pertinent documentation to evaluate medical appropriateness should be included when this code is reported.

E	D5861	Overdenture — partial, by report

Pertinent documentation to evaluate medical appropriateness should be included when this code is reported.

E	D5862	Precision attachment, by report

Pertinent documentation to evaluate medical appropriateness should be included when this code is reported.

E	D5867	Replacement of replaceable part of semi-precision or precision attachment (male or female component)
E	D5875	Modification of removable prosthesis following implant surgery
E	D5899	Unspecified removable prosthodontic procedure, by report

Determine if an alternative HCPCS Level II or a CPT code better describes the service being reported. This code should be used only if a more specific code is unavailable.

Special Coverage Instructions   Noncovered by Medicare   Carrier Discretion   ☑ Quality Alert   ● New Code   ○ Reinstated Code   ▲ Revised Code

2007 HCPCS   1-9 ASC Group   MED: Pub 100/NCD References   ᵇ DMEPOS Paid   ⊘ SNF Excluded   D Codes — 31

D4355 — D5899

Dental Procedures

D5911 — D6058

MAXILLOFACIAL PROSTHETICS D5900-D5999

[S] **D5911** Facial moulage (sectional)   ⊘
  MED: 100-2,15,120; 100-2,15,150; 100-4,4,20.5

[S] **D5912** Facial moulage (complete)   ⊘
  MED: 100-2,15,120; 100-4,4,20.5

[E] **D5913** Nasal prosthesis
  See code(s): 21087

[E] **D5914** Auricular prosthesis
  See code(s): 21086

[E] **D5915** Orbital prosthesis
  See code(s): L8611

[E] **D5916** Ocular prosthesis
  See also CPT code (21077, 65770, 66982-66985, 92330-92335, 92358, 92393).
  See code(s): V2623, V2629

[E] **D5919** Facial prosthesis
  See code(s): 21088

[E] **D5922** Nasal septal prosthesis
  See code(s): 30220

[E] **D5923** Ocular prosthesis, interim
  See code(s): 92330

[E] **D5924** Cranial prosthesis
  See code(s): 62143

[E] **D5925** Facial augmentation implant prosthesis
  See code(s): 21208

[E] **D5926** Nasal prosthesis, replacement
  See code(s): 21087

[E] **D5927** Auricular prosthesis, replacement
  See code(s): 21086

[E] **D5928** Orbital prosthesis, replacement
  See code(s): 67550

[E] **D5929** Facial prosthesis, replacement
  See code(s): 21088

[E] **D5931** Obturator prosthesis, surgical
  See code(s): 21079

[E] **D5932** Obturator prosthesis, definitive
  See code(s): 21080

[E] **D5933** Obturator prosthesis, modification
  See code(s): 21080

[E] **D5934** Mandibular resection prosthesis with guide flange
  See code(s): 21081

[E] **D5935** Mandibular resection prosthesis without guide flange
  See code(s): 21081

[E] **D5936** Obturator/prosthesis, interim
  See code(s): 21079

[E] **D5937** Trismus appliance (not for TMD treatment)
  MED: 100-2,15,120

[E] **D5951** Feeding aid   ⊘
  MED: 100-2,15,120; 100-2,16,140

[E] **D5952** Speech aid prosthesis, pediatric
  See code(s): 21084

[E] **D5953** Speech aid prosthesis, adult
  See code(s): 21084

[E] **D5954** Palatal augmentation prosthesis
  See code(s): 21082

[E] **D5955** Palatal lift prosthesis, definitive
  See code(s): 21083

[E] **D5958** Palatal lift prosthesis, interim
  See code(s): 21083

[E] **D5959** Palatal lift prosthesis, modification
  See code(s): 21083

[E] **D5960** Speech aid prosthesis, modification
  See code(s): 21084

[E] **D5982** Surgical stent
  For oral surgical stent see CPT code. Surgical stent. Periodontal stent, skin graft stent, columellar stent.
  See code(s): 21085

[S] **D5983** Radiation carrier   ⊘
  MED: 100-2,15,150; 100-2,16,140; 100-4,4,20.5

[S] **D5984** Radiation shield   ⊘
  MED: 100-2,15,150; 100-2,16,140; 100-4,4,20.5

[S] **D5985** Radiation cone locator   ⊘
  MED: 100-2,15,150; 100-2,16,140; 100-4,4,20.5

[E] **D5986** Fluoride gel carrier

[S] **D5987** Commissure splint   ⊘
  MED: 100-2,15,150; 100-2,16,140; 100-4,4,20.5; 100-4,4,240

[E] **D5988** Surgical splint. See also CPT.
  See also CPT code (21085)
  MED: 100-4,4,240

[E] **D5999** Unspecified maxillofacial prosthesis, by report
  Determine if an alternative HCPCS Level II or a CPT code better describes the service being reported. This code should be used only if a more specific code is unavailable.

IMPLANT SERVICES D6000-D6199

[E] **D6010** Surgical placement of implant body: endosteal implant
  See code(s): 21248

● **D6012** Surgical placement of interim implant body for transitional prosthesis: endosteal implant

[E] **D6040** Surgical placement: eposteal implant
  See code(s): 21245

[E] **D6050** Surgical placement: transosteal implant
  See code(s): 21244

[E] **D6053** Implant/abutment supported removable denture for completely edentulous arch
  MED: 100-2,15,150

[E] **D6054** Implant/abutment supported removable denture for partially edentulous arch
  MED: 100-2,15,150

[E] **D6055** Dental implant supported connecting bar
  MED: 100-2,15,150

[E] **D6056** Prefabricated abutment — includes placement
  MED: 100-2,15,150

[E] **D6057** Custom abutment — includes placement
  MED: 100-2,15,150

[E] **D6058** Abutment supported porcelain/ceramic crown
  MED: 100-2,15,150

Special Coverage Instructions   Noncovered by Medicare   Carrier Discretion   ☑ Quality Alert   ● New Code   ○ Reinstated Code   ▲ Revised Code

E D6059 Abutment supported porcelain fused to metal crown (high noble metal)
MED: 100-2,15,150

E D6060 Abutment supported porcelain fused to metal crown (predominantly base metal)
MED: 100-2,15,150

E D6061 Abutment supported porcelain fused to metal crown (noble metal)
MED: 100-2,15,150

E D6062 Abutment supported cast metal crown (high noble metal)
MED: 100-2,15,150

E D6063 Abutment supported cast metal crown (predominantly base metal)
MED: 100-2,15,150

E D6064 Abutment supported cast metal crown (noble metal)
MED: 100-2,15,150

E D6065 Implant supported porcelain/ceramic crown
MED: 100-2,15,150

E D6066 Implant supported porcelain fused to metal crown (titanium, titanium alloy, high noble metal)
MED: 100-2,15,150

E D6067 Implant supported metal crown (titanium, titanium alloy, high noble metal)
MED: 100-2,15,150

E D6068 Abutment supported retainer for porcelain/ceramic FPD
MED: 100-2,15,150

E D6069 Abutment supported retainer for porcelain fused to metal FPD (high noble metal)
MED: 100-2,15,150

E D6070 Abutment supported retainer for porcelain fused to metal FPD (predominately base metal)
MED: 100-2,15,150

E D6071 Abutment supported retainer for porcelain fused to metal FPD (noble metal)
MED: 100-2,15,150

E D6072 Abutment supported retainer for cast metal FPD (high noble metal)
MED: 100-2,15,150

E D6073 Abutment supported retainer for cast metal FPD (predominately base metal)
MED: 100-2,15,150

E D6074 Abutment supported retainer for cast metal FPD (noble metal)
MED: 100-2,15,150

E D6075 Implant supported retainer for ceramic FPD
MED: 100-2,15,150

E D6076 Implant supported retainer for porcelain fused to metal FPD (titanium, titanium alloy, or high noble metal)
MED: 100-2,15,150

E D6077 Implant supported retainer for cast metal FPD (titanium, titanium alloy, or high noble metal)
MED: 100-2,15,150

E D6078 Implant/abutment supported fixed denture for completely edentulous arch
MED: 100-2,15,150

E D6079 Implant/abutment supported fixed denture for partially edentulous arch
MED: 100-2,15,150

E D6080 Implant maintenance procedures, including removal of prosthesis, cleansing of prosthesis and abutments, reinsertion of prosthesis
MED: 100-2,15,150

E D6090 Repair implant supported prosthesis, by report
Pertinent documentation to evaluate medical appropriateness should be included when this code is reported.
See code(s): 21299

● D6091 Replacement of semi-precision or precision attachment (male or female component) of implant/abutment supported prosthesis, per attachment

● D6092 Recement implant/abutment supported crown

● D6093 Recement implant/abutment supported fixed partial denture

E D6094 Abutment supported crown (titanium)

E D6095 Repair implant abutment, by report
Pertinent documentation to evaluate medical appropriateness should be included when this code is reported.
See code(s): 21299

E D6100 Implant removal, by report
Pertinent documentation to evaluate medical appropriateness should be included when this code is reported.
See code(s): 21299

E D6190 Radiographic/surgical implant index, by report

E D6194 Abutment supported retainer crown for FPD (titanium)

E D6199 Unspecified implant procedure, by report
See code(s): 21299

E D6205 Pontic — indirect resin based composite

PROSTHODONTICS (FIXED) D6200-D6999

FIXED PARTIAL DENTURE PONTICS

E D6210 Pontic — cast high noble metal
Each abutment and each pontic constitute a unit in a prosthesis. An alloy of at least 60 percent gold (Au), palladium (Pd), or platinum (Pt) is considered a high noble metal.

E D6211 Pontic — cast predominantly base metal
Each abutment and each pontic constitute a unit in a prosthesis. An alloy of less than 25 percent gold (Au), palladium (Pd), or platinum (Pt) is considered a high noble metal.

E D6212 Pontic — cast noble metal
Each abutment and each pontic constitute a unit in a prosthesis. An alloy of at least 25 percent gold (Au), palladium (Pd), or platinum (Pt) is considered a high noble metal.

E D6214 Pontic — titanium

E D6240 Pontic — porcelain fused to high noble metal
Each abutment and each pontic constitute a unit in a prosthesis. An alloy of at least 60 percent gold (Au), palladium (Pd), or platinum (Pt) is considered a high noble metal.

Special Coverage Instructions   Noncovered by Medicare   Carrier Discretion   ☑ Quality Alert   ● New Code   ○ Reinstated Code   ▲ Revised Code

2007 HCPCS   ■-■ ASC Group   MED: Pub 100/NCD References   ᛒ DMEPOS Paid   Ⓢ SNF Excluded   **D Codes — 33**

Dental Procedures

D6241 — D6794

E **D6241** Pontic — porcelain fused to predominantly base metal
Each abutment and each pontic constitute a unit in a prosthesis. An alloy of less than 25 percent gold (Au), palladium (Pd), or platinum (Pt) is considered a high noble metal.

E **D6242** Pontic — porcelain fused to noble metal
Each abutment and each pontic constitute a unit in a prosthesis. An alloy of at least 60 percent gold (Au), palladium (Pd), or platinum (Pt) is considered a high noble metal.

E **D6245** Pontic — porcelain/ceramic
MED: 100-2,15,150

E **D6250** Pontic — resin with high noble metal
Each abutment and each pontic constitute a unit in a prosthesis. An alloy of at least 60 percent gold (Au), palladium (Pd), or platinum (Pt) is considered a high noble metal.

E **D6251** Pontic — resin with predominantly base metal
Each abutment and each pontic constitute a unit in a prosthesis. An alloy of less than 25 percent gold (Au), palladium (Pd), or platinum (Pt) is considered a high noble metal.

E **D6252** Pontic — resin with noble metal
Each abutment and each pontic constitute a unit in a prosthesis. An alloy of at least 25 percent gold (Au), palladium (Pd), or platinum (Pt) is considered a high noble metal.

E **D6253** Provisional pontic

E **D6545** Retainer — cast metal for resin bonded fixed prosthesis

E **D6548** Retainer — porcelain/ceramic for resin bonded fixed prosthesis
MED: 100-2,15,150

E **D6600** Inlay — porcelain/ceramic, two surfaces
MED: 100-2,15,150

E **D6601** Inlay — porcelain/ceramic, three or more surfaces
MED: 100-2,15,150

E **D6602** Inlay — cast high noble metal, two surfaces
MED: 100-2,15,150

E **D6603** Inlay — cast high noble metal, three or more surfaces
MED: 100-2,15,150

E **D6604** Inlay — cast predominantly base metal, two surfaces
MED: 100-2,15,150

E **D6605** Inlay — cast predominantly base metal, three or more surfaces
MED: 100-2,15,150

E **D6606** Inlay — cast noble metal, two surfaces
MED: 100-2,15,150

E **D6607** Inlay — cast noble metal, three or more surfaces
MED: 100-2,15,150

E **D6608** Onlay — porcelain/ceramic, two surfaces
MED: 100-2,15,150

E **D6609** Onlay — porcelain/ceramic, three or more surfaces
MED: 100-2,15,150

E **D6610** Onlay — cast high noble metal, two surfaces
MED: 100-2,15,150

E **D6611** Onlay — cast high noble metal, three or more surfaces
MED: 100-2,15,150

E **D6612** Onlay — cast predominantly base metal, two surfaces
MED: 100-2,15,150

E **D6613** Onlay — cast predominantly base metal, three or more surfaces
MED: 100-2,15,150

E **D6614** Onlay — cast noble metal, two surfaces
MED: 100-2,15,150

E **D6615** Onlay — cast noble metal, three or more surfaces
MED. 100-2,15,150

E **D6624** Inlay — titanium

E **D6634** Onlay — titanium

E **D6710** Crown — indirect resin based composite

FIXED PARTIAL DENTURE RETAINERS - CROWNS

E **D6720** Crown — resin with high noble metal
An alloy of at least 60 percent gold (Au), palladium (Pd), or platinum (Pt) is considered a high noble metal.

E **D6721** Crown — resin with predominantly base metal
An alloy of less than 25 percent gold (Au), palladium (Pd), or platinum (Pt) is considered a base metal.

E **D6722** Crown — resin with noble metal
An alloy of at least 25 percent gold (Au), palladium (Pd), or platinum (Pt) is considered a noble metal.

E **D6740** Crown — porcelain/ceramic
MED: 100-2,15,150

E **D6750** Crown — porcelain fused to high noble metal
An alloy of at least 60 percent gold (Au), palladium (Pd), or platinum (Pt) is considered a high noble metal.

E **D6751** Crown — porcelain fused to predominantly base metal
An alloy of less than 25 percent gold (Au), palladium (Pd), or platinum (Pt) is considered a base metal.

E **D6752** Crown — porcelain fused to noble metal
An alloy of at least 25 percent gold (Au), palladium (Pd), or platinum (Pt) is considered a noble metal.

E **D6780** Crown — 3/4 cast high noble metal
An alloy of at least 60 percent gold (Au), palladium (Pd), or platinum (Pt) is considered a high noble metal.

E **D6781** Crown — 3/4 cast predominately base metal
An alloy of less than 25 percent gold (Au), palladium (Pd), or platinum (Pt) is considered a base metal.
MED: 100-2,15,150

E **D6782** Crown — 3/4 cast noble metal
An alloy of at least 25 percent gold (Au), palladium (Pd), or platinum (Pt) is considered a noble metal.
MED: 100-2,15,150

E **D6783** Crown — 3/4 porcelain/ceramic
MED: 100-2,15,150

E **D6790** Crown — full cast high noble metal
An alloy of at least 60 percent gold (Au), palladium (Pd), or platinum (Pt) is considered a high noble metal.

E **D6791** Crown — full cast predominantly base metal
An alloy of less than 25 percent gold (Au), palladium (Pd), or platinum (Pt) is considered a base metal.

E **D6792** Crown — full cast noble metal
An alloy of at least 25 percent gold (Au), palladium (Pd), or platinum (Pt) is considered a noble metal.

E **D6793** Provisional retainer crown

E **D6794** Crown — titanium

Special Coverage Instructions   Noncovered by Medicare   Carrier Discretion   ☑ Quality Alert   ● New Code   ○ Reinstated Code ▲ Revised Code

34 — D Codes   A Age Edit   M Maternity Edit   ♀ Female Only   ♂ Male Only   A - Y APC Status Indicators   *2007 HCPCS*

OTHER FIXED PARTIAL DENTURE SERVICES

S **D6920** Connector bar ⊘
MED: 100-2,15,150; 100-2,16,140; 100-3,260.6; 100-4,4,20.5

E **D6930** Recement fixed partial denture

E **D6940** Stress breaker

E **D6950** Precision attachment

▲ E **D6970** Post and core in addition to fixed partial denture retainer, indirectly fabricated

~~D6971~~ ~~Cast post as part of fixed partial denture retainer~~

E **D6972** Prefabricated post and core in addition to fixed partial denture retainer

E **D6973** Core build up for retainer, including any pins

E **D6975** Coping — metal

▲ E **D6976** Each additional indirectly fabricated post, same tooth
Report this code in addition to codes D6970 or D6971.
MED: 100-2,15,150

E **D6977** Each additional prefabricated post — same tooth
Report this code in addition to code D6972.
MED: 100-2,15,150

E **D6980** Fixed partial denture repair, by report
Pertinent documentation to evaluate medical appropriateness should be included when this code is reported.

E **D6985** Pediatric partial denture, fixed Ⓐ

E **D6999** Unspecified, fixed prosthodontic procedure, by report
Determine if an alternative HCPCS Level II or a CPT code better describes the service being reported. This code should be used only if a more specific code is unavailable.

S **D7111** Extraction, coronal remnants — deciduous tooth
MED: 100-2,16,140; 100-4,4,20.5

S **D7140** Extraction, erupted tooth or exposed root (elevation and/or forceps removal)
MED: 100-2,16,140; 100-4,4,20.5

SURGICAL EXTRACTIONS (INCLUDES LOCAL ANESTHESIA AND ROUTINE POSTOPERATIVE CARE)

S **D7210** Surgical removal of erupted tooth requiring elevation of mucoperiosteal flap and removal of bone and/or section of tooth ⊘
MED: 100-2,15,150; 100-2,16,140; 100-4,4,20.5

S **D7220** Removal of impacted tooth — soft tissue ⊘
MED: 100-2,15,150; 100-2,16,140; 100-4,4,20.5

S **D7230** Removal of impacted tooth — partially bony ⊘
MED: 100-2,15,150; 100-2,16,140; 100-4,4,20.5

S **D7240** Removal of impacted tooth — completely bony ⊘
MED: 100-2,15,150; 100-2,16,140; 100-4,4,20.5

S **D7241** Removal of impacted tooth — completely bony, with unusual surgical complications ⊘
MED: 100-2,15,150; 100-2,16,140; 100-4,4,20.5

S **D7250** Surgical removal of residual tooth roots (cutting procedure) ⊘
MED: 100-2,15,150; 100-2,16,140; 100-4,4,20.5

OTHER SURGICAL PROCEDURES

S **D7260** Orolantral fistula closure ⊘
MED: 100-2,15,150; 100-2,16,140; 100-4,4,20.5

S **D7261** Primary closure of a sinus perforation
See equivalent CPT code for repair of mucous membranes.
MED: 100-2,16,140

E **D7270** Tooth reimplantation and/or stabilization of accidentally evulsed or displaced tooth

E **D7272** Tooth transplantation (includes reimplantation from one site to another and splinting and/or stabilization)

E **D7280** Surgical access of an unerupted tooth

E **D7282** Mobilization of erupted or malpositioned tooth to aid eruption

B **D7283** Placement of device to facilitate eruption of impacted tooth

E **D7285** Biopsy of oral tissue — hard (bone, tooth)
See code(s): 20220, 20225, 20240, 20245

E **D7286** Biopsy of oral tissue — soft
See code(s): 40808

E **D7287** Exfoliative cytological sample collection

B **D7288** Brush biopsy — transepithelial sample collection

E **D7290** Surgical repositioning of teeth

S **D7291** Transseptal fiberotomy/supra crestal fiberotomy, by report ⊘
Pertinent documentation to evaluate medical appropriateness should be included when this code is reported.
MED: 100-2,15,150; 100-2,16,140; 100-4,4,20.5

● **D7292** Surgical placement: temporary anchorage device (screw retained plate) requiring surgical flap

● **D7293** Surgical placement: temporary anchorage device requiring surgical flap

● **D7294** Surgical placement: temporary anchorage device without surgical flap

ALVEOLOPLASTY - SURGICAL PREPARATION OF RIDGE FOR DENTURES

▲ E ☑ **D7310** Alveoloplasty in conjunction with extractions—four or more teeth or tooth spaces, per quadrant
See code(s): 41874

E ☑ **D7311** Alveoloplasty in conjunction with extractions — one to three teeth or tooth spaces, per quadrant

E ☑ **D7320** Alveoloplasty not in conjunction with extractions—four or more teeth or tooth spaces, per quadrant
See code(s): 41870

B ☑ **D7321** Alveoloplasty not in conjunction with extractions — one to three teeth or tooth spaces, per quadrant

VESTIBULOPLASTY

E **D7340** Vestibuloplasty — ridge extension (second epithelialization)
See code(s): 40840, 40842, 40843, 40844

E **D7350** Vestibuloplasty — ridge extension (including soft tissue grafts, muscle reattachments, revision of soft tissue attachment and management of hypertrophied and hyperplastic tissue)
See code(s): 40845

SURGICAL EXCISION OF REACTIVE INFLAMMATORY LESIONS (SCAR TISSUE OR LOCALIZED CONGENITAL LESIONS)

E ☑ **D7410** Excision of benign lesion up to 1.25 cm

E **D7411** Excision of benign lesion greater than 1.25 cm
See CPT codes in the surgical section (11440&40520)

Dental Procedures

D6920 — D7411

Special Coverage Instructions   Noncovered by Medicare   Carrier Discretion   ☑ Quality Alert   ● New Code   ⊘ Reinstated Code   ▲ Revised Code

E D7412 Excision of benign lesion, complicated
See CPT code in the surgical section (10000&40000)

E D7413 Excision of malignant lesion up to 1.25 cm
See CPT code in the surgical section (11442)

E D7414 Excision of malignant lesion greater than 1.25 cm
See CPT codes in the surgical section (11442-11446)

E D7415 Excision of malignant lesion, complicated
See CPT codes in the surgical section (11440-11446 with modifier 22 for complicated)

E ☑ D7440 Excision of malignant tumor — lesion diameter up to 1.25 cm

E ☑ D7441 Excision of malignant tumor — lesion diameter greater than 1.25 cm

E ☑ D7450 Removal of benign odontogenic cyst or tumor — lesion diameter up to 1.25 cm

E ☑ D7451 Removal of benign odontogenic cyst or tumor — lesion diameter greater than 1.25 cm

E ☑ D7460 Removal of benign nonodontogenic cyst or tumor — lesion diameter up to 1.25 cm

E ☑ D7461 Removal of benign nonodontogenic cyst or tumor — lesion diameter greater than 1.25 cm

E D7465 Destruction of lesion(s) by physical or chemical method, by report
Pertinent documentation to evaluate medical appropriateness should be included when this code is reported.
See code(s): 41850

E ☑ D7471 Removal of lateral exostosis (maxilla or mandible)
See code(s): 21031, 21032

E D7472 Removal of torus palatinus
See CPT code in the surgical section (21029, 21030, 21031)

E D7473 Removal of torus mandibularis

E D7485 Surgical reduction of osseous tuberosity

E D7490 Radical resection of maxilla or mandible
See code(s): 21045

SURGICAL INCISION

E D7510 Incision and drainage of abscess — intraoral soft tissue
See code(s): 41800

B D7511 Incision and drainage of abscess — intraoral soft tissue — complicated (includes drainage of multiple fascial spaces)

E D7520 Incision and drainage of abscess — extraoral soft tissue
See code(s): 40800

B D7521 Incision and drainage of abscess — extraoral soft tissue — complicated (includes drainage of multiple fascial spaces)

E D7530 Removal of foreign body from mucosa, skin, or subcutaneous alveolar tissue
See code(s): 41805, 41828

E D7540 Removal of reaction-producing foreign bodies, musculoskeletal system
See code(s): 20520, 41800, 41806

E D7550 Partial ostectomy/sequestrectomy for removal of nonvital bone
See code(s): 20999

E D7560 Maxillary sinusotomy for removal of tooth fragment or foreign body
See code(s): 31020

TREATMENT OF FRACTURES - SIMPLE

E D7610 Maxilla — open reduction (teeth immobilized, if present)
See code(s): 21422

E D7620 Maxilla — closed reduction (teeth immobilized, if present)

E D7630 Mandible — open reduction (teeth immobilized, if present)

E D7640 Mandible — closed reduction (teeth immobilized, if present)

E D7650 Malar and/or zygomatic arch — open reduction

E D7660 Malar and/or zygomatic arch — closed reduction

E D7670 Alveolus — closed reduction, may include stabilization of teeth

E D7671 Alveolus — open reduction, may include stabilization of teeth

E D7680 Facial bones — complicated reduction with fixation and multiple surgical approaches

TREATMENT OF FRACTURES - COMPOUND

E D7710 Maxilla — open reduction
See code(s): 21346

E D7720 Maxilla — closed reduction
See code(s): 21345

E D7730 Mandible — open reduction
See code(s): 21461, 21462

E D7740 Mandible — closed reduction
See code(s): 21455

E D7750 Malar and/or zygomatic arch — open reduction
See code(s): 21360, 21365

E D7760 Malar and/or zygomatic arch — closed reduction
See code(s): 21355

E D7770 Alveolus — open reduction stabilization of teeth
See code(s): 21422

E D7771 Alveolus, closed reduction stabilization of teeth
See CPT code in the surgical section (21421)

E D7780 Facial bones — complicated reduction with fixation and multiple surgical approaches
See code(s): 21433, 21435

REDUCTION OF DISLOCATION AND MANAGEMENT OF OTHER TEMPOROMANDIBULAR JOINT DYSFUNCTIONS

Procedures which are an integral part of a primary procedure should not be reported separately.

E D7810 Open reduction of dislocation
See code(s): 21490

E D7820 Closed reduction of dislocation
See code(s): 21480

E D7830 Manipulation under anesthesia

E D7840 Condylectomy

E D7850 Surgical discectomy, with/without implant
See code(s): 21060

E D7852 Disc repair
See code(s): 21299

Special Coverage Instructions   Noncovered by Medicare   Carrier Discretion   ☑ Quality Alert   ● New Code   ○ Reinstated Code ▲ Revised Code

36 — D Codes   A Age Edit   M Maternity Edit   ♀ Female Only   ♂ Male Only   A - Y APC Status Indicators   *2007 HCPCS*

E	D7854	**Synovectomy**	
		See code(s): 21299	

E **D7856 Myotomy**
See code(s): 21299

E **D7858 Joint reconstruction**
See code(s): 21242, 21243

E **D7860 Arthrotomy**
MED: 100-2,15,150; 100-2,16,140

E **D7865 Arthroplasty**
See code(s): 21240

E **D7870 Arthrocentesis**
See code(s): 21060

E **D7871 Nonarthroscopic lysis and lavage**

E **D7872 Arthroscopy — diagnosis, with or without biopsy**
See code(s): 29800

E **D7873 Arthroscopy — surgical: lavage and lysis of adhesions**
See code(s): 29804

E **D7874 Arthroscopy — surgical: disc repositioning and stabilization**
See code(s): 29804

E **D7875 Arthroscopy — surgical: synovectomy**
See code(s): 29804

E **D7876 Arthroscopy — surgical: discectomy**
See code(s): 29804

E **D7877 Arthroscopy — surgical: debridement**
See code(s): 29804

E **D7880 Occlusal orthotic device, by report**
See code(s): 21499

E **D7899 Unspecified TMD therapy, by report**
Determine if an alternative HCPCS Level II or a CPT code better describes the service being reported. This code should be used only if a more specific code is unavailable.

See code(s): 21499

REPAIR OF TRAUMATIC WOUNDS

E ☑ **D7910 Suture of recent small wounds up to 5 cm**
See code(s): 12011, 12013

COMPLICATED SUTURING (RECONSTRUCTION REQUIRING DELICATE HANDLING OF TISSUES AND WIDE UNDERMINING FOR METICULOUS CLOSURE)

E **D7911 Complicated suture — up to 5 cm**
See code(s): 12051, 12052

E **D7912 Complicated suture — greater than 5 cm**
See code(s): 13132

OTHER REPAIR PROCEDURES

E **D7920 Skin graft (identify defect covered, location and type of graft)**

S **D7940 Osteoplasty — for orthognathic deformities** ⊘
MED: 100-2,15,150; 100-2,16,140; 100-4,4,20.5

E **D7941 Osteotomy — mandibular rami**
See code(s): 21193, 21195, 21196

E **D7943 Osteotomy — mandibular rami with bone graft; includes obtaining the graft**
See code(s): 21194

▲ E ☑ **D7944 Osteotomy—segmented or subapical**
See code(s): 21198, 21206

E **D7945 Osteotomy — body of mandible**
See code(s): 21193, 21194, 21195, 21196

E **D7946 LeFort I (maxilla — total)**
See code(s): 21147

E **D7947 LeFort I (maxilla — segmented)**
See code(s): 21145, 21146

E **D7948 LeFort II or LeFort III (osteoplasty of facial bones for midface hypoplasia or retrusion) — without bone graft**
See code(s): 21150

E **D7949 LeFort II or LeFort III — with bone graft**

▲ E **D7950 Osseous, osteoperiosteal, or cartilage graft of the mandible or maxilla—autogenous or nonautogenous, by report**
Pertinent documentation to evaluate medical appropriateness should be included when this code is reported.

See code(s): 21247

● **D7951 Sinus augmentation with bone or bone substitutes**

E ☑ **D7953 Bone replacement graft for ridge preservation — per site**

E **D7955 Repair of maxillofacial soft and/or hard tissue defect**
See code(s): 21299

E **D7960 Frenulectomy (frenectomy or frenotomy) — separate procedure**
See code(s): 40819, 41010, 41115

E **D7963 Frenuloplasty**

E ☑ **D7970 Excision of hyperplastic tissue — per arch**

E **D7971 Excision of pericoronal gingiva**
See code(s): 41821

E **D7972 Surgical reduction of fibrous tuberosity**

E **D7980 Sialolithotomy**
See code(s): 42330, 42335, 42340

E **D7981 Excision of salivary gland, by report**
Pertinent documentation to evaluate medical appropriateness should be included when this code is reported.

See code(s): 42408

E **D7982 Sialodochoplasty**
See code(s): 42500

E **D7983 Closure of salivary fistula**
See code(s): 42600

E **D7990 Emergency tracheotomy**
See code(s): 31605

E **D7991 Coronoidectomy**
See code(s): 21070

E **D7995 Synthetic graft — mandible or facial bones, by report**
Pertinent documentation to evaluate medical appropriateness should be included when this code is reported.

See code(s): 21299

Special Coverage Instructions	Noncovered by Medicare	Carrier Discretion	☑ Quality Alert	● New Code	○ Reinstated Code	▲ Revised Code

Dental Procedures

D7996 — D9612

[E] D7996 Implant — mandible for augmentation purposes (excluding alveolar ridge), by report
Pertinent documentation to evaluate medical appropriateness should be included when this code is reported.

See code(s): 21299

[E] D7997 Appliance removal (not by dentist who placed appliance), includes removal of archbar

● D7998 Intraoral placement of a fixation device not in conjunction with a fracture

[E] D7999 Unspecified oral surgery procedure, by report
Determine if an alternative HCPCS Level II or a CPT code better describes the service being reported. This code should be used only if a more specific code is unavailable.

See code(s): 21299

ORTHODONTICS D8000-D8999

[E] D8010 Limited orthodontic treatment of the primary dentition [A]

[E] D8020 Limited orthodontic treatment of the transitional dentition

[E] D8030 Limited orthodontic treatment of the adolescent dentition [A]

[E] D8040 Limited orthodontic treatment of the adult dentition [A]

[E] D8050 Interceptive orthodontic treatment of the primary dentition [A]

[E] D8060 Interceptive orthodontic treatment of the transitional dentition

[E] D8070 Comprehensive orthodontic treatment of the transitional dentition

[E] D8080 Comprehensive orthodontic treatment of the adolescent dentition [A]

[E] D8090 Comprehensive orthodontic treatment of the adult dentition [A]

MINOR TREATMENT TO CONTROL HARMFUL HABITS

[E] D8210 Removable appliance therapy

[E] D8220 Fixed appliance therapy

OTHER ORTHODONTIC SERVICES

[E] D8660 Preorthodontic treatment visit

[E] D8670 Periodic orthodontic treatment visit (as part of contract)

[E] D8680 Orthodontic retention (removal of appliances, construction and placement of retainer(s))

[E] D8690 Orthodontic treatment (alternative billing to a contract fee)

[E] D8691 Repair of orthodontic appliance

[E] D8692 Replacement of lost or broken retainer

● D8693 Rebonding or recementing; and/or repair, as required, of fixed retainers

[E] D8999 Unspecified orthodontic procedure, by report
Determine if an alternative HCPCS Level II or a CPT code better describes the service being reported. This code should be used only if a more specific code is unavailable.

ADJUNCTIVE GENERAL SERVICES D9110-D9999

UNCLASSIFIED TREATMENT

[N] D9110 Palliative (emergency) treatment of dental pain — minor procedure ⊘
MED: 100-2,15,150; 100-2,16,140

ANESTHESIA

[E] D9210 Local anesthesia not in conjunction with operative or surgical procedures
See code(s): 90784

[E] D9211 Regional block anesthesia

[E] D9212 Trigeminal division block anesthesia
See code(s): 64400

[E] D9215 Local anesthesia
See code(s): 90784

[E] ☑ D9220 Deep sedation/general anesthesia — first 30 minutes
See also CPT code 00172-00176.

[E] ☑ D9221 Deep sedation/general anesthesia — each additional 15 minutes
MED: 100-2,15,150; 100-2,16,140

[N] D9230 Analgesia, anxiolysis, inhalation of nitrous oxide ⊘
MED: 100-2,15,150; 100-2,16,140

[E] ☑ D9241 Intravenous conscious sedation/analgesia — first 30 minutes
See also CPT code 90784, 99141.

See code(s): 90784

[E] ☑ D9242 Intravenous conscious sedation/analgesia — each additional 15 minutes
See also CPT code 90784, 99141.

See code(s): 90784

[N] D9248 Nonintravenous conscious sedation

PROFESSIONAL CONSULTATION

▲ [E] D9310 Consultation—diagnostic service provided by dentist or physician other than requesting dentist or physician

PROFESSIONAL VISITS

[E] D9410 House/extended care facility call

[E] D9420 Hospital call
See also CPT E&M codes

[E] D9430 Office visit for observation (during regularly scheduled hours) — no other services performed
See also CPT E&M codes

[E] D9440 Office visit — after regularly scheduled hours
See code(s): 99050

[E] D9450 Case presentation, detailed and extensive treatment planning

DRUGS

▲ [E] D9610 Therapeutic parenteral drug, single administration
Pertinent documentation to evaluate medical appropriateness should be included when this code is reported.

See code(s): 90788, 90784

● D9612 Therapeutic parenteral drugs, two or more administrations, different medications

---

Special Coverage Instructions　　Noncovered by Medicare　　Carrier Discretion　　☑ Quality Alert　　● New Code　　○ Reinstated Code　▲ Revised Code

38 — D Codes　　　[A] Age Edit　　[M] Maternity Edit　♀ Female Only　♂ Male Only　[A] - [☑] APC Status Indicators　　*2007 HCPCS*

S   **D9630** Other drugs and/or medicaments, by report   ⊘
Determine if an alternative HCPCS Level II or a CPT code better describes the service being reported. This code should be used only if a more specific code is unavailable.
MED: 100-2,15,150; 100-2,16,140; 100-4,4,20.5

MISCELLANEOUS SERVICES

E   **D9910** Application of desensitizing medicament

E ☑ **D9911** Application of desensitizing resin for cervical and/or root surface, per tooth

E   **D9920** Behavior management, by report
Pertinent documentation to evaluate medical appropriateness should be included when this code is reported.

S   **D9930** Treatment of complications (postsurgical) — unusual circumstances, by report   ⊘
MED: 100-2,15,150; 100-2,16,140; 100-4,4,20.5

S   **D9940** Occlusal guard, by report   ⊘
Pertinent documentation to evaluate medical appropriateness should be included when this code is reported.
MED: 100-2,15,150; 100-2,16,140; 100-4,4,20.5

E   **D9941** Fabrication of athletic mouthguard
See code(s): 21089

E   **D9942** Repair and/or reline of occlusal guard

S   **D9950** Occlusion analysis — mounted case   ⊘
MED: 100-2,15,150; 100-2,16,140; 100-4,4,20.5

S   **D9951** Occlusal adjustment — limited   ⊘
MED: 100-2,15,150; 100-2,16,140; 100-4,4,20.5

S   **D9952** Occlusal adjustment — complete   ⊘
MED: 100-2,15,150; 100-2,16,140; 100-4,4,20.5

E   **D9970** Enamel microabrasion

E ☑ **D9971** Odontoplasty 1-2 teeth; includes removal of enamel projections

E ☑ **D9972** External bleaching — per arch

E ☑ **D9973** External bleaching — per tooth

E ☑ **D9974** Internal bleaching — per tooth

E   **D9999** Unspecified adjunctive procedure, by report
Determine if an alternative HCPCS Level II or a CPT code better describes the service being reported. This code should be used only if a more specific code is unavailable.
See code(s): 21499

Special Coverage Instructions   Noncovered by Medicare   Carrier Discretion   ☑ Quality Alert   ● New Code   ○ Reinstated Code   ▲ Revised Code

2007 HCPCS   **1**-**9** ASC Group   **MED:** Pub 100/NCD References   ᵬ DMEPOS Paid   ⊘ SNF Excluded   **D Codes — 39**

DURABLE MEDICAL EQUIPMENT E0100-E9999

E codes include durable medical equipment such as canes, crutches, walkers, commodes, decubitus care, bath and toilet aids, hospital beds, oxygen and related respiratory equipment, monitoring equipment, pacemakers, patient lifts, safety equipment, restraints, traction equipment, fracture frames, wheelchairs, and artificial kidney machines.

CANES

Ⓨ **E0100** Cane, includes canes of all materials, adjustable or fixed, with tip ♿
White canes for the blind are not covered under Medicare.
MED: 100-2,15,110.1; 100-3,280.1; 100-3,280.2

Ⓨ **E0105** Cane, quad or three-prong, includes canes of all materials, adjustable or fixed, with tips ♿
MED: 100-2,15,110.1; 100-3,280.1; 100-3,280.5

CRUTCHES

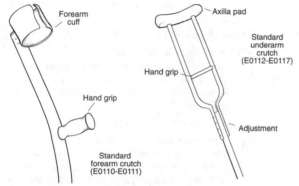

Forearm cuff
Axilla pad
Standard underarm crutch (E0112-E0117)
Hand grip
Hand grip
Standard forearm crutch (E0110-E0111)
Adjustment

Ⓨ ☑ **E0110** Crutches, forearm, includes crutches of various materials, adjustable or fixed, pair, complete with tips and handgrips ♿
MED: 100-2,15,110.1; 100-3,280.1

Ⓨ ☑ **E0111** Crutch, forearm, includes crutches of various materials, adjustable or fixed, each, with tip and handgrip ♿
MED: 100-2,15,110.1; 100-3,280.1

Ⓨ ☑ **E0112** Crutches, underarm, wood, adjustable or fixed, pair, with pads, tips and handgrips ♿
MED: 100-2,15,110.1; 100-3,280.1

Ⓨ ☑ **E0113** Crutch, underarm, wood, adjustable or fixed, each, with pad, tip and handgrip ♿
MED: 100-2,15,110.1; 100-3,280.1

Ⓨ **E0114** Crutches, underarm, other than wood, adjustable or fixed, pair, with pads, tips and handgrips ♿
MED: 100-2,15,110.1; 100-3,280.1

Ⓨ **E0116** Crutch, underarm, other than wood, adjustable or fixed, with PAD, tip, handgrip, with or without shock absorber, each ♿
MED: 100-2,15,110.1; 100-3,280.1

Ⓨ **E0117** Crutch, underarm, articulating, spring assisted, each ♿
MED: 100-2,15,110.1

Ⓔ ☑ **E0118** Crutch substitute, lower leg platform, with or without wheels, each
Medicare covers walkers if patient's ambulation is impaired.

Ⓨ **E0130** Walker, rigid (pickup), adjustable or fixed height
MED: 100-2,15,110.1; 100-3,280.1

Ⓨ **E0135** Walker, folding (pickup), adjustable or fixed height ♿
Medicare covers walkers if patient's ambulation is impaired.
MED: 100-2,15,110.1; 100-3,280.1

Ⓨ **E0140** Walker, with trunk support, adjustable or fixed height, any type ♿
MED: 100-2,15,110.1; 100-3,280.1

Ⓨ **E0141** Walker, rigid, wheeled, adjustable or fixed height ♿
Medicare covers walkers if patient's ambulation is impaired.
MED: 100-2,15,110.1; 100-3,280.1

Ⓨ **E0143** Walker, folding, wheeled, adjustable or fixed height ♿
Medicare covers walkers if patient's ambulation is impaired.
MED: 100-2,15,110.1; 100-3,280.1

Ⓨ **E0144** Walker, enclosed, four sided framed, rigid or folding, wheeled with posterior seat ♿
MED: 100-2,15,110.1; 100-3,280.1

Ⓨ **E0147** Walker, heavy duty, multiple braking system, variable wheel resistance ♿
Medicare covers safety roller walkers only in patients with severe neurological disorders or restricted use of one hand. In some cases, coverage will be extended to patients with a weight exceeding the limits of a standard wheeled walker.
MED: 100-2,15,110.1; 100-3,280.5

Ⓨ **E0148** Walker, heavy duty, without wheels, rigid or folding, any type, each ♿

Ⓨ **E0149** Walker, heavy duty, wheeled, rigid or folding, any type ♿

Ⓨ ☑ **E0153** Platform attachment, forearm crutch, each ♿

Ⓨ ☑ **E0154** Platform attachment, walker, each ♿

Ⓨ **E0155** Wheel attachment, rigid pick-up walker, per pair seat attachment, walker ♿

ATTACHMENTS

Ⓨ **E0156** Seat attachment, walker ♿

Ⓨ ☑ **E0157** Crutch attachment, walker, each ♿

Ⓨ ☑ **E0158** Leg extensions for walker, per set of four (4) ♿

Ⓨ ☑ **E0159** Brake attachment for wheeled walker, replacement, each ♿

COMMODES

Ⓨ **E0160** Sitz type bath or equipment, portable, used with or without commode ♿
Medicare covers sitz baths if medical record indicates that the patient has an infection or injury of the perineal area and the sitz bath is prescribed by the physician.
MED: 100-3,280.1

Ⓨ **E0161** Sitz type bath or equipment, portable, used with or without commode, with faucet attachment(s) ♿
Medicare covers sitz baths if medical record indicates that the patient has an infection or injury of the perineal area and the sitz bath is prescribed by the physician.
MED: 100-3,280.1

Ⓨ **E0162** Sitz bath chair ♿
Medicare covers sitz baths if medical record indicates that the patient has an infection or injury of the perineal area and the sitz bath is prescribed by the physician.
MED: 100-3,280.1

☐ Special Coverage Instructions ☐ Noncovered by Medicare ☐ Carrier Discretion ☑ Quality Alert ● New Code ○ Reinstated Code ▲ Revised Code

2007 HCPCS 1-9 ASC Group MED: Pub 100/NCD References ♿ DMEPOS Paid Ⓢ SNF Excluded **E Codes — 41**

Durable Medical Equipment

E0163 — E0198

▲ Ⓨ **E0163** **Commode chair, mobile or stationary, with fixed arms**   🦽
Medicare covers commodes for patients confined to their beds or rooms, for patients without indoor bathroom facilities, and to patients who cannot climb or descend the stairs necessary to reach the bathrooms in their homes.

MED: 100-2,15,110.1; 100-3,280.1

~~**E0164** **Commode chair, mobile, with fixed arms**~~
See code(s) E0163.

MED: 100-3,280.1

▲ Ⓨ **E0165** **Commode chair, mobile or stationary, with detachable arms**   🦽
Medicare covers commodes for patients confined to their beds or rooms, for patients without indoor bathroom facilities, and to patients who cannot climb or descend the stairs necessary to reach the bathrooms in their homes.

MED: 100-2,15,110.1; 100-3,280.1

~~**E0166** **Commode chair, mobile, with detachable arms**~~
See code(s) E0165.

MED: 100-3,280.1

▲ Ⓨ **E0167** **Pail or pan for use with commode chair, replacement only**   🦽
Medicare covers commodes for patients confined to their beds or rooms, for patients without indoor bathroom facilities, and to patients who cannot climb or descend the stairs necessary to reach the bathrooms in their homes.

MED: 100-3,280.1

Ⓨ **E0168** **Commode chair, extra wide and/or heavy duty, stationary or mobile, with or without arms, any type, each**   🦽

Ⓨ **E0170** **Commode chair with integrated seat lift mechanism, electric, any type**

Ⓨ **E0171** **Commode chair with integrated seat lift mechanism, non-electric, any type**

Ⓔ **E0172** **Seat lift mechanism placed over or on top of toilet, any type**

Ⓨ ☑ **E0175** **Foot rest, for use with commode chair, each**   🦽

DECUBITUS CARE EQUIPMENT

~~**E0180** **Pressure pad, alternating with pump**~~
See code(s) E0181, E0182.

MED: 100-3,280.1

▲ Ⓨ **E0181** **Powered pressure reducing mattress overlay/pad, alternating, with pump, includes heavy duty**   🦽
Medicare covers pads if physicians supervise their use in patients who have decubitus ulcers or susceptibility to them. Prior authorization is required by Medicare for this item.

MED: 100-3,280.1; 100-8,5,5.1.1.2

▲ Ⓨ **E0182** **Pump for alternating pressure pad, for replacement only**   🦽
Medicare covers pads if physicians supervise their use in patients who have decubitus ulcers or susceptibility to them. Prior authorization is required by Medicare for this item.

MED: 100-3,280.1; 100-8,5,5.1.1.2

Ⓨ **E0184** **Dry pressure mattress**   🦽
Medicare covers pads if physicians supervise their use in patients who have decubitus ulcers or susceptibility to them. Prior authorization is required by Medicare for this item.

MED: 100-3,280.1; 100-8,5,5.1.1.2

Ⓨ **E0185** **Gel or gel-like pressure pad for mattress, standard mattress length and width**   🦽
Medicare covers pads if physicians supervise their use in patients who have decubitus ulcers or susceptibility to them. Prior authorization is required by Medicare for this item.

MED: 100-3,280.1; 100-8,5,5.1.1.2

Ⓨ **E0186** **Air pressure mattress**   🦽
Medicare covers pads if physicians supervise their use in patients who have decubitus ulcers or susceptibility to them.

MED: 100-3,280.1

Ⓨ **E0187** **Water pressure mattress**   🦽
Medicare covers pads if physicians supervise their use in patients who have decubitus ulcers or susceptibility to them.

MED: 100-3,280.1

Ⓨ **E0188** **Synthetic sheepskin pad**   🦽
Medicare covers pads if physicians supervise their use in patients who have decubitus ulcers or susceptibility to them. Prior authorization is required by Medicare for this item.

MED: 100-3,280.1; 100-8,5,5.1.1.2

Ⓨ **E0189** **Lambswool sheepskin pad, any size**   🦽
Medicare covers pads if physicians supervise their use in patients who have decubitus ulcers or susceptibility to them. Prior authorization is required by Medicare for this item.

MED: 100-3,280.1; 100-8,5,5.1.1.2

▲ Ⓔ **E0190** **Positioning cushion/pillow/wedge, any shape or size, includes all components and accessories**

MED: 100-2,15,110.1

Ⓨ ☑ **E0191** **Heel or elbow protector, each**   🦽

Ⓨ **E0193** **Powered air flotation bed (low air loss therapy)**   🦽

Ⓨ **E0194** **Air fluidized bed**   🦽
An air fluidized bed is covered by Medicare if the patient has a stage 3 or stage 4 pressure sore and, without the bed, would require institutionalization. A physician's prescription is required.

MED: 100-3,280.8

Ⓨ **E0196** **Gel pressure mattress**   🦽
Medicare covers pads if physicians supervise their use in patients who have decubitus ulcers or susceptibility to them.

MED: 100-3,280.1

Ⓨ **E0197** **Air pressure pad for mattress, standard mattress length and width**   🦽
Medicare covers pads if physicians supervise their use in patients who have decubitus ulcers or susceptibility to them.

MED: 100-3,280.1

Ⓨ **E0198** **Water pressure pad for mattress, standard mattress length and width**   🦽
Medicare covers pads if physicians supervise their use in patients who have decubitus ulcers or susceptibility to them.

MED: 100-3,280.1

Special Coverage Instructions   Noncovered by Medicare   Carrier Discretion   ☑ Quality Alert   ● New Code   ○ Reinstated Code   ▲ Revised Code

42 — E Codes   Ⓐ Age Edit   Ⓜ Maternity Edit   ♀ Female Only   ♂ Male Only   Ⓐ - Ⓨ APC Status Indicators   *2007 HCPCS*

Y **E0199** Dry pressure pad for mattress, standard mattress length and width   ♻
Medicare covers pads if physicians supervise their use in patients who have decubitus ulcers or susceptibility to them.
MED: 100-3,280.1

HEAT/COLD APPLICATION

Y **E0200** Heat lamp, without stand (table model), includes bulb, or infrared element   ♻
MED: 100-2,15,110.1; 100-3,280.1

Y **E0202** Phototherapy (bilirubin) light with photometer   ♻

A **E0203** Therapeutic lightbox, minimum 10,000 lux, table top model

Y **E0205** Heat lamp, with stand, includes bulb, or infrared element   ♻
MED: 100-2,15,110.1; 100-3,280.1

Y **E0210** Electric heat pad, standard   ♻
MED: 100-3,280.1

Y **E0215** Electric heat pad, moist   ♻
MED: 100-3,280.1

Y **E0217** Water circulating heat pad with pump   ♻
MED: 100-3,280.1

Y **E0218** Water circulating cold pad with pump   ♻
MED: 100-3,280.1

Y **E0220** Hot water bottle   ♻

E **E0221** Infrared heating pad system   ♻
MED: 100-3,270.2

Y **E0225** Hydrocollator unit, includes pads   ♻
MED: 100-2,15,230; 100-3,280.1

Y **E0230** Ice cap or collar   ♻

E **E0231** Noncontact wound warming device (temperature control unit, AC adapter and power cord) for use with warming card and wound cover
MED: 100-2,16,20

E **E0232** Warming card for use with the noncontact wound warming device and noncontact wound warming wound cover
MED: 100-2,16,20

Y **E0235** Paraffin bath unit, portable (see medical supply code A4265 for paraffin)   ♻
MED: 100-2,15,230; 100-3,280.1

Y **E0236** Pump for water circulating pad   ♻
MED: 100-3,280.1

Y **E0238** Nonelectric heat pad, moist   ♻
MED: 100-3,280.1

Y **E0239** Hydrocollator unit, portable   ♻
MED: 100-2,15,230; 100-3,280.1

BATH AND TOILET AIDS

E **E0240** Bath/shower chair, with or without wheels, any size
MED: 100-3,280.1

E ☑ **E0241** Bathtub wall rail, each
MED: 100-2,15,110.1; 100-3,280.1

E **E0242** Bathtub rail, floor base
MED: 100-2,15,110.1; 100-3,280.1

E ☑ **E0243** Toilet rail, each
MED: 100-2,15,110.1; 100-3,280.1

E **E0244** Raised toilet seat
MED: 100-3,280.1

E **E0245** Tub stool or bench
MED: 100-3,280.1

E **E0246** Transfer tub rail attachment

E **E0247** Transfer bench for tub or toilet with or without commode opening
MED: 100-3,280.1

E **E0248** Transfer bench, heavy duty, for tub or toilet with or without commode opening
MED: 100-3,280.1

Y **E0249** Pad for water circulating heat unit   ♻
MED: 100-3,280.1

HOSPITAL BEDS AND ACCESSORIES

E **E0250** Hospital bed, fixed height, with any type side rails, with mattress   ♻
MED: 100-2,15,110.1; 100-3,280.7

E **E0251** Hospital bed, fixed height, with any type side rails, without mattress   ♻
MED: 100-2,15,110.1; 100-3,280.7

E **E0255** Hospital bed, variable height, hi-lo, with any type side rails, with mattress   ♻
MED: 100-2,15,110.1; 100-3,280.7

E **E0256** Hospital bed, variable height, hi-lo, with any type side rails, without mattress   ♻
MED: 100-2,15,110.1; 100-3,280.7

E **E0260** Hospital bed, semi-electric (head and foot adjustment), with any type side rails, with mattress   ♻
MED: 100-2,15,110.1; 100-3,280.7

E **E0261** Hospital bed, semi-electric (head and foot adjustment), with any type side rails, without mattress   ♻
MED: 100-2,15,110.1; 100-3,280.7

E **E0265** Hospital bed, total electric (head, foot, and height adjustments), with any type side rails, with mattress   ♻
MED: 100-2,15,110.1; 100-3,280.7

E **E0266** Hospital bed, total electric (head, foot, and height adjustments), with any type side rails, without mattress   ♻
MED: 100-2,15,110.1; 100-3,280.7

E **E0270** Hospital bed, institutional type includes: oscillating, circulating and stryker frame, with mattress
MED: 100-3,280.1

E **E0271** Mattress, inner spring   ♻
MED: 100-3,280.1; 100-3,280.7

E **E0272** Mattress, foam rubber   ♻
MED: 100-3,280.1; 100-3,280.7

E **E0273** Bed board
MED: 100-3,280.1

E **E0274** Over-bed table
MED: 100-3,280.1

Y **E0275** Bed pan, standard, metal or plastic   ♻
Reusable, autoclavable bedpans are covered by Medicare for bed-confined patients.
MED: 100-3,280.1

Y **E0276** Bed pan, fracture, metal or plastic   ♻
Reusable, autoclavable bedpans are covered by Medicare for bed-confined patients.
MED: 100-3,280.1

Special Coverage Instructions   Noncovered by Medicare   Carrier Discretion   ☑ Quality Alert   ● New Code   ○ Reinstated Code ▲ Revised Code

2007 HCPCS   **1**-**9** ASC Group   **MED:** Pub 100/NCD References   ♻ DMEPOS Paid   ⊘ SNF Excluded   **E Codes — 43**

Durable Medical Equipment

E0277 — E0441

Y **E0277** Powered pressure-reducing air mattress   🦽
     MED: 100-3,280.1

Y **E0280** Bed cradle, any type

E **E0290** Hospital bed, fixed height, without side rails, with mattress 🦽
     MED: 100-2,15,110.1; 100-3,280.7

Y **E0291** Hospital bed, fixed height, without side rails, without mattress 🦽
     MED: 100-2,15,110.1; 100-3,280.7

E **E0292** Hospital bed, variable height, hi-lo, without side rails, with mattress 🦽
     MED: 100-2,15,110.1; 100-3,280.7

Y **E0293** Hospital bed, variable height, hi-lo, without side rails, without mattress 🦽
     MED: 100-2,15,110.1; 100-3,280.7

E **E0294** Hospital bed, semi-electric (head and foot adjustment), without side rails, with mattress 🦽
     MED: 100-2,15,110.1; 100-3,280.7

Y **E0295** Hospital bed, semi-electric (head and foot adjustment), without side rails, without mattress 🦽
     MED: 100-2,15,110.1; 100-3,280.7

E **E0296** Hospital bed, total electric (head, foot, and height adjustments), without side rails, with mattress 🦽
     MED: 100-2,15,110.1; 100-3,280.7

Y **E0297** Hospital bed, total electric (head, foot, and height adjustments), without side rails, without mattress 🦽
     MED: 100-2,15,110.1; 100-3,280.7

Y **E0300** Pediatric crib, hospital grade, fully enclosed 🦽

Y **E0301** Hospital bed, heavy duty, extra wide, with weight capacity greater than 350 pounds, but less than or equal to 600 pounds, with any type side rails, without mattress 🦽
     MED: 100-3,280.7

Y **E0302** Hospital bed, extra heavy duty, extra wide, with weight capacity greater than 600 pounds, with any type side rails, without mattress 🦽
     MED: 100-3,280.7

E **E0303** Hospital bed, heavy duty, extra wide, with weight capacity greater than 350 pounds, but less than or equal to 600 pounds, with any type side rails, with mattress 🦽
     MED: 100-3,280.7

E **E0304** Hospital bed, extra heavy duty, extra wide, with weight capacity greater than 600 pounds, with any type side rails, with mattress 🦽
     MED: 100-3,280.7

    E0305 Bedside rails, half-length 🦽
     MED: 100-3,280.7

    E0310 Bedside rails, full-length 🦽
     MED: 100-3,280.7

E **E0315** Bed accessory: board, table, or support device, any type
     MED: 100-3,280.1

Y **E0316** Safety enclosure frame/canopy for use with hospital bed, any type 🦽

Y **E0325** Urinal; male, jug-type, any material ♂🦽
     MED: 100-3,280.1

Y **E0326** Urinal; female, jug-type, any material ♀🦽
     MED: 100-3,280.1

E **E0350** Control unit for electronic bowel irrigation/evacuation system

E **E0352** Disposable pack (water reservoir bag, speculum, valving mechanism and collection bag/box) for use with the electronic bowel irrigation/evacuation system

E **E0370** Air pressure elevator for heel

Y **E0371** Nonpowered advanced pressure reducing overlay for mattress, standard mattress length and width 🦽

Y **E0372** Powered air overlay for mattress, standard mattress length and width 🦽

Y **E0373** Nonpowered advanced pressure reducing mattress 🦽

OXYGEN AND RELATED RESPIRATORY EQUIPMENT

Y **E0424** Stationary compressed gaseous oxygen system, rental; includes container, contents, regulator, flowmeter, humidifier, nebulizer, cannula or mask, and tubing 🦽
For the first claim filed for home oxygen equipment or therapy, submit a certificate of medical necessity that includes the oxygen flow rate, anticipated frequency and duration of oxygen therapy, and physician signature. Medicare accepts oxygen therapy as medically necessary in cases documenting any of the following: erythocythemia with a hematocrit greater than 56 percent; a P pulmonale on EKG; or dependent edema consistent with congestive heart failure.
     MED: 100-3,240.2

E **E0425** Stationary compressed gas system, purchase; includes regulator, flowmeter, humidifier, nebulizer, cannula or mask, and tubing
     MED: 100-3,240.2

E **E0430** Portable gaseous oxygen system, purchase; includes regulator, flowmeter, humidifier, cannula or mask, and tubing
     MED: 100-3,240.2

Y **E0431** Portable gaseous oxygen system, rental; includes portable container, regulator, flowmeter, humidifier, cannula or mask, and tubing 🦽
     MED: 100-3,240.2

Y **E0434** Portable liquid oxygen system, rental; includes portable container, supply reservoir, humidifier, flowmeter, refill adaptor, contents gauge, cannula or mask, and tubing 🦽
     MED: 100-3,240.2

E **E0435** Portable liquid oxygen system, purchase; includes portable container, supply reservoir, flowmeter, humidifier, contents gauge, cannula or mask, tubing, and refill adapter
     MED: 100-3,240.2

Y **E0439** Stationary liquid oxygen system, rental; includes container, contents, regulator, flowmeter, humidifier, nebulizer, cannula or mask, and tubing 🦽
     MED: 100-3,240.2

E **E0440** Stationary liquid oxygen system, purchase; includes use of reservoir, contents indicator, regulator, flowmeter, humidifier, nebulizer, cannula or mask, and tubing
     MED: 100-3,240.2

Y ☑ **E0441** Oxygen contents, gaseous (for use with owned gaseous stationary systems or when both a stationary and portable gaseous system are owned), one month's supply = one unit 🦽
     MED: 100-3,240.2

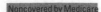 Special Coverage Instructions   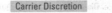 Noncovered by Medicare   Carrier Discretion   ☑ Quality Alert   ● New Code   ○ Reinstated Code   ▲ Revised Code

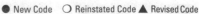

44 — E Codes   **A** Age Edit   **M** Maternity Edit   ♀ Female Only   ♂ Male Only   **A** - **Y** APC Status Indicators   *2007 HCPCS*

Y ☑ **E0442** Oxygen contents, liquid (for use with owned liquid stationary systems or when both a stationary and portable liquid system are owned), one month's supply = one unit   ♿
MED: 100-3,240.2

Y ☑ **E0443** Portable oxygen contents, gaseous (for use only with portable gaseous systems when no stationary gas or liquid system is used), one month's supply = one unit
MED: 100-3,240.2

Y ☑ **E0444** Portable oxygen contents, liquid (for use only with portable liquid systems when no stationary gas or liquid system is used), one month's supply = one unit   ♿
MED: 100-3,240.2

A **E0445** Oximeter device for measuring blood oxygen levels noninvasively

Y **E0450** Volume control ventilator, without pressure support mode, may include pressure control mode, used with invasive interface (e.g., tracheostomy tube)   ♿
MED: 100-3,280.1

Y **E0455** Oxygen tent, excluding croup or pediatric tents
MED: 100-3,240.2

Y **E0457** Chest shell (cuirass)   ♿

Y **E0459** Chest wrap   ♿

Y **E0460** Negative pressure ventilator; portable or stationary   ♿
MED: 100-3,280.1

Y **E0461** Volume control ventilator, without pressure support mode, may include pressure control mode, used with noninvasive interface (e.g., mask)   ♿
MED: 100-3,280.1

Y **E0462** Rocking bed, with or without side rails   ♿

Y **E0463** Pressure support ventilator with volume control mode, may include pressure control mode, used with invasive interface (e.g., tracheostomy tube)

Y **E0464** Pressure support ventilator with volume control mode, may include pressure control mode, used with noninvasive interface (e.g., mask)

Y **E0470** Respiratory assist device, bi-level pressure capability, without backup rate feature, used with noninvasive interface, e.g., nasal or facial mask (intermittent assist device with continuous positive airway pressure device)   ♿
MED: 100-3,280.1

Y **E0471** Respiratory assist device, bi-level pressure capability, with back-up rate feature, used with noninvasive interface, e.g., nasal or facial mask (intermittent assist device with continuous positive airway pressure device)   ♿
MED: 100-3,280.1

Y **E0472** Respiratory assist device, bi-level pressure capability, with backup rate feature, used with invasive interface, e.g., tracheostomy tube (intermittent assist device with continuous positive airway pressure device)   ♿
MED: 100-3,280.1

Y **E0480** Percussor, electric or pneumatic, home model   ♿
MED: 100-3,280.1

E **E0481** Intrapulmonary percussive ventilation system and related accessories
MED: 100-3,240.5

Y **E0482** Cough stimulating device, alternating positive and negative airway pressure   ♿

Y **E0483** High frequency chest wall oscillation air-pulse generator system, (includes hoses and vest), each   ♿

Y **E0484** Oscillatory positive expiratory pressure device, nonelectric, any type, each   ♿

Y **E0485** Oral device/appliance used to reduce upper airway collapsibility, adjustable or non-adjustable, prefabricated, includes fitting and adjustment

Y **E0486** Oral device/appliance used to reduce upper airway collapsibility, adjustable or non-adjustable, custom fabricated, includes fitting and adjustment

IPPB MACHINES

IPPB unit in use

Battery pack and controls

Nebulizer

Nebulizer reservoir

Oxygen supply tube

Intermittent Positive Pressure Breathing (IPPB) devices

Y **E0500** IPPB machine, all types, with built-in nebulization; manual or automatic valves; internal or external power source   ♿
MED: 100-3,280.1

HUMIDIFIERS/COMPRESSORS/NEBULIZERS FOR USE WITH OXYGEN IPPB EQUIPMENT

Y **E0550** Humidifier, durable for extensive supplemental humidification during ippb treatments or oxygen delivery   ♿
MED: 100-3,280.1

Y **E0555** Humidifier, durable, glass or autoclavable plastic bottle type, for use with regulator or flowmeter
MED: 100-3,280.1

Y **E0560** Humidifier, durable for supplemental humidification during IPPB treatment or oxygen delivery   ♿
MED: 100-3,280.1

Y **E0561** Humidifier, nonheated, used with positive airway pressure device   ♿

Y **E0562** Humidifier, heated, used with positive airway pressure device   ♿

Y **E0565** Compressor, air power source for equipment which is not self-contained or cylinder driven   ♿

Y **E0570** Nebulizer, with compressor   ♿
MED: 100-3,280.1

Y **E0571** Aerosol compressor, battery powered, for use with small volume nebulizer   ♿
MED: 100-3,280.1

Y **E0572** Aerosol compressor, adjustable pressure, light duty for intermittent use

Y **E0574** Ultrasonic/electronic aerosol generator with small volume nebulizer   ♿

Y **E0575** Nebulizer, ultrasonic, large volume   ♿
MED: 100-3,280.1

Y **E0580** Nebulizer, durable, glass or autoclavable plastic, bottle type, for use with regulator or flowmeter   ♿
MED: 100-3,280.1

Special Coverage Instructions   Noncovered by Medicare   Carrier Discretion   ☑ Quality Alert   ● New Code   ○ Reinstated Code   ▲ Revised Code

2007 HCPCS   1-9 ASC Group   **MED:** Pub 100/NCD References   ♿ DMEPOS Paid   ⊘ SNF Excluded   **E Codes — 45**

Durable Medical Equipment

E0585 — E0667

Y **E0585** Nebulizer, with compressor and heater   ♿
MED: 100-3,280.1

SUCTION PUMP/ROOM VAPORIZERS

Y **E0600** Respiratory suction pump, home model, portable or stationary, electric   ♿
MED: 100-3,280.1

Y **E0601** Continuous airway pressure (CPAP) device   ♿
MED: 100-3,240.4

Y **E0602** Breast pump, manual, any type   M ♀ ♿

A **E0603** Breast pump, electric (AC and/or DC), any type   M ♀

A **E0604** Breast pump, heavy duty, hospital grade, piston operated, pulsatile vacuum suction/release cycles, vacuum regulator, supplies, transformer, electric (AC and/or DC)   M ♀

Y **E0605** Vaporizer, room type   ♿
MED: 100-3,280.1

Y **E0606** Postural drainage board   ♿
MED: 100-3,280.1

MONITORING EQUIPMENT

Y **E0607** Home blood glucose monitor   ♿
Medicare covers home blood testing devices for diabetic patients when the devices are prescribed by the patients' physicians. Many commercial payers provide this coverage to non-insulin dependent diabetics as well.
MED: 100.3,230.16

PACEMAKER MONITOR

Y **E0610** Pacemaker monitor, self-contained, checks battery depletion, includes audible and visible check systems   ♿
MED: 100-3,20.8; 100-3,20.8.1; 100-3,20.8.2

Y **E0615** Pacemaker monitor, self-contained, checks battery depletion and other pacemaker components, includes digital/visible check systems   ♿
MED: 100-3,20.8; 100-3,20.8.1; 100-3,20.8.2

N **E0616** Implantable cardiac event recorder with memory, activator and programmer

Y **E0617** External defibrillator with integrated electrocardiogram analysis   ♿

A **E0618** Apnea monitor, without recording feature

A **E0619** Apnea monitor, with recording feature

Y **E0620** Skin piercing device for collection of capillary blood, laser, each   ♿

PATIENT LIFTS

Y **E0621** Sling or seat, patient lift, canvas or nylon   ♿
MED: 100-3,280.1

E **E0625** Patient lift, bathroom or toilet, not otherwise classified
MED: 100-3,280.1

Y **E0627** Seat lift mechanism incorporated into a combination lift-chair mechanism   ♿
See code(s): Q0080
MED: 100-3,280.4; 100-4,20,100; 100-4,20,130.2; 100-4,20,130.3; 100-4,20,130.4; 100-4,20,130.5

Y **E0628** Separate seat lift mechanism for use with patient owned furniture — electric   ♿
See code(s): Q0078
MED: 100-3,280.4; 100-4,20,100; 100-4,20,130.2; 100-4,20,130.3; 100-4,20,130.4; 100-4,20,130.5

Y **E0629** Separate seat lift mechanism for use with patient owned furniture — nonelectric   ♿
See code(s): Q0079
MED: 100-4,20,100; 100-4,20,130.2; 100-4,20,130.3; 100-4,20,130.4; 100-4,20,130.5

Y **E0630** Patient lift, hydraulic, with seat or sling   ♿
MED: 100-3,280.1

Y **E0635** Patient lift, electric, with seat or sling   ♿
MED: 100-3,280.1

Y **E0636** Multipositional patient support system, with integrated lift, patient accessible controls   ♿

E **E0637** Combination sit to stand system, any size including pediatric, with seatlift feature, with or without wheels   ♿
MED: 100-3,280.1

E **E0638** Standing frame system, one position (e.g., upright, supine or prone stander), any size including pediatric, with or without wheels   ♿
MED: 100-3,280.1

E **E0639** Patient lift, moveable from room to room with disassembly and reassembly, includes all components/accessories

E **E0640** Patient lift, fixed system, includes all components/accessories

E **E0641** Standing frame system, multi-position (e.g., three-way stander), any size including pediatric, with or without wheels

E **E0642** Standing frame system, mobile (dynamic stander), any size including pediatric

PNEUMATIC COMPRESSOR AND APPLIANCES

Y **E0650** Pneumatic compressor, nonsegmental home model   ♿
MED: 100-3,280.6

Y **E0651** Pneumatic compressor, segmental home model without calibrated gradient pressure   ♿
MED: 100-3,280.6

Y **E0652** Pneumatic compressor, segmental home model with calibrated gradient pressure   ♿
MED: 100-3,280.6

Y **E0655** Nonsegmental pneumatic appliance for use with pneumatic compressor, half arm   ♿
MED: 100-3,280.6

Y **E0660** Nonsegmental pneumatic appliance for use with pneumatic compressor, full leg   ♿
MED: 100-3,280.6

Y **E0665** Nonsegmental pneumatic appliance for use with pneumatic compressor, full arm   ♿
MED: 100-3,280.6

Y **E0666** Nonsegmental pneumatic appliance for use with pneumatic compressor, half leg   ♿
MED: 100-3,280.6

Y **E0667** Segmental pneumatic appliance for use with pneumatic compressor, full leg   ♿
MED: 100-3,280.6

Special Coverage Instructions   Noncovered by Medicare   Carrier Discretion   ☑ Quality Alert   ● New Code   ○ Reinstated Code   ▲ Revised Code

46 — E Codes   A Age Edit   M Maternity Edit   ♀ Female Only   ♂ Male Only   A - Y APC Status Indicators   2007 HCPCS

Y **E0668** Segmental pneumatic appliance for use with pneumatic compressor, full arm
MED: 100-3,280.6

Y **E0669** Segmental pneumatic appliance for use with pneumatic compressor, half leg
MED: 100-3,280.6

Y **E0671** Segmental gradient pressure pneumatic appliance, full leg
MED: 100-3,280.6

Y **E0672** Segmental gradient pressure pneumatic appliance, full arm
MED: 100-3,280.6

Y **E0673** Segmental gradient pressure pneumatic appliance, half leg
MED: 100-3,280.6

Y **E0675** Pneumatic compression device, high pressure, rapid inflation/deflation cycle, for arterial insufficiency (unilateral or bilateral system)

● Y **E0676** Intermittent limb compression device (includes all accessories), not otherwise specified

Y **E0691** Ultraviolet light therapy system panel, includes bulbs/lamps, timer and eye protection; treatment area two square feet or less

Y **E0692** Ultraviolet light therapy system panel, includes bulbs/lamps, timer and eye protection, four foot panel

Y **E0693** Ultraviolet light therapy system panel, includes bulbs/lamps, timer and eye protection, six foot panel

Y **E0694** Ultraviolet multidirectional light therapy system in six foot cabinet, includes bulbs/lamps, timer and eye protection

SAFETY EQUIPMENT

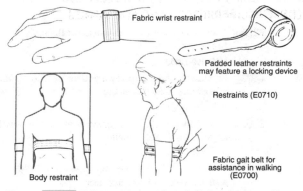

Fabric wrist restraint

Padded leather restraints may feature a locking device

Restraints (E0710)

Fabric gait belt for assistance in walking (E0700)

Body restraint

E **E0700** Safety equipment (e.g., belt, harness or vest)

~~E0701 Helmet with face guard and soft interface material, prefabricated~~
See code(s) A8000, A8001

B **E0705** Transfer board or device, any type, each

RESTRAINTS

E **E0710** Restraint, any type (body, chest, wrist or ankle)

TRANSCUTANEOUS AND/OR NEUROMUSCULAR ELECTRICAL NERVE STIMULATORS - TENS

▲ Y **E0720** Transcutaneous electrical nerve stimulation (TENS) device, two lead, localized stimulation
While TENS is covered when employed to control chronic pain, it is not covered for experimental treatment, as in motor function disorders like MS. Prior authorization is required by Medicare for this item.
MED: 100-3,40.5; 100-3,130.5; 100-3,130.6; 100-3,160.2; 100-3,160.7.1; 100-3,230.1; 100-8,5,5.1.1.2

▲ Y **E0730** Transcutaneous electrical nerve stimulation (TENS) device, four or more leads, for multiple nerve stimulation
While TENS is covered when employed to control chronic pain, it is not covered for experimental treatment, as in motor function disorders like MS. Prior authorization is required by Medicare for this item.
MED: 100-3,40.5; 100-3,130.5; 100-3,130.6; 100-3,160.2; 100-3,160.7.1; 100-3,230.1; 100-8,5,5.1.1.2

Y **E0731** Form-fitting conductive garment for delivery of TENS or NMES (with conductive fibers separated from the patient's skin by layers of fabric)
MED: 100-3,160.13

Y **E0740** Incontinence treatment system, pelvic floor stimulator, monitor, sensor and/or trainer
MED: 100-3,230.8

Y **E0744** Neuromuscular stimulator for scoliosis

Y **E0745** Neuromuscular stimulator, electronic shock unit
MED: 100-3,160.12

A **E0746** Electromyography (EMG), biofeedback device
Biofeedback therapy is covered by Medicare only for re-education of specific muscles or for treatment of incapacitating muscle spasm or weakness. Medicare jurisdiction: local contractor.
MED: 100-3,30.1; 100-3,30.1.1

Y **E0747** Osteogenesis stimulator, electrical, noninvasive, other than spinal applications
Medicare covers noninvasive osteogenic stimulation for nonunion of long bone fractures, failed fusion, or congenital pseudoarthroses.
MED: 100-3,150.2

Y **E0748** Osteogenesis stimulator, electrical, noninvasive, spinal applications
Medicare covers noninvasive osteogenic stimulation as an adjunct to spinal fusion surgery for patients at high risk of pseudoarthroses due to previously failed spinal fusion, or for those undergoing fusion of three or more vertebrae.
MED: 100-3,150.2

N **E0749** Osteogenesis stimulator, electrical, surgically implanted
Medicare covers invasive osteogenic stimulation for nonunion of long bone fractures or as an adjunct to spinal fusion surgery for patients at high risk of pseudoarthroses due to previously failed spinal fusion, or for those undergoing fusion of three or more vertebrae.
MED: 100-3,150.2; 100-4,4,20.5; 100-4,4,190

E **E0755** Electronic salivary reflex stimulator (intraoral/noninvasive)

Y **E0760** Osteogenesis stimulator, low intensity ultrasound, noninvasive
MED: 100-3,150.2

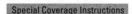

Special Coverage Instructions   Noncovered by Medicare   Carrier Discretion   ☑ Quality Alert   ● New Code   ○ Reinstated Code   ▲ Revised Code

2007 HCPCS   1-9 ASC Group   MED: Pub 100/NCD References   DMEPOS Paid   ⊘ SNF Excluded   **E Codes — 47**

Durable Medical Equipment

E0761 — E0945

Ⓔ   **E0761**   Nonthermal pulsed high frequency radiowaves, high peak power electromagnetic energy treatment device

Ⓑ   **E0762**   Transcutaneous electrical joint stimulation device system, includes all accessories

Ⓨ   **E0764**   Functional neuromuscular stimulator, transcutaneous stimulation of muscles of ambulation with computer control, used for walking by spinal cord injured, entire system, after completion of training program

Ⓨ   **E0765**   FDA approved nerve stimulator, with replaceable batteries, for treatment of nausea and vomiting   ♿

Ⓑ   **E0769**   Electrical stimulation or electromagnetic wound treatment device, not otherwise classified
       MED: 100-4,32,11.1

INFUSION SUPPLIES

Ⓨ   **E0776**   IV pole   ♿

Ⓨ   **E0779**   Ambulatory infusion pump, mechanical, reusable, for infusion 8 hours or greater   ♿

Ⓨ   **E0780**   Ambulatory infusion pump, mechanical, reusable, for infusion less than 8 hours   ♿

Ⓨ   **E0781**   Ambulatory infusion pump, single or multiple channels, electric or battery operated, with administrative equipment, worn by patient   ♿
       Medicare jurisdiction: DME local or regional contractor. Bill Medicare claims for regional contractor when the infusion is initiated in the physician's office but the patient does not return during the same day of business.
       MED: 100-3,280.14

Ⓝ   **E0782**   Infusion pump, implantable, nonprogrammable (includes all components, e.g., pump, catheter, connectors, etc.)   ♿
       Medicare jurisdiction: local contractor.
       MED: 100-3,280.14; 100-4,4,20.5; 100-4,4,190

Ⓝ   **E0783**   Infusion pump system, implantable, programmable (includes all components, e.g., pump, catheter, connectors, etc.)   ♿
       Medicare jurisdiction: local contractor.
       MED: 100-3,280.14; 100-4,4,20.5; 100-4,4,190

Ⓨ   **E0784**   External ambulatory infusion pump, insulin   ♿
       Covered by some commercial payers with preauthorization.
       MED: 100-3,280.14

Ⓝ   **E0785**   Implantable intraspinal (epidural/intrathecal) catheter used with implantable infusion pump, replacement   ♿
       Medicare jurisdiction: local contractor.
       MED: 100-3,280.14; 100-4,4,20.5; 100-4,4,190

Ⓝ   **E0786**   Implantable programmable infusion pump, replacement (excludes implantable intraspinal catheter)   ♿
       Medicare jurisdiction: local contractor.
       MED: 100-3,280.14

Ⓨ   **E0791**   Parenteral infusion pump, stationary, single or multichannel   ♿
       MED: 100-2,15,120; 100-3,180.2; 100-4,20,100.2.2

TRACTION - ALL TYPES

Ⓝ   **E0830**   Ambulatory traction device, all types, each
       MED: 100-3,280.1

TRACTION - CERVICAL

Ⓨ   **E0840**   Traction frame, attached to headboard, cervical traction   ♿
       MED: 100-3,280.1

Ⓨ   **E0849**   Traction equipment, cervical, free-standing stand/frame, pneumatic, applying traction force to other than mandible

Ⓨ   **E0850**   Traction stand, freestanding, cervical traction   ♿
       MED: 100-3,280.1

Ⓨ   **E0855**   Cervical traction equipment not requiring additional stand or frame   ♿

TRACTION - OVERDOOR

Ⓨ   **E0860**   Traction equipment, overdoor, cervical
       MED: 100-3,280.1

TRACTION - EXTREMITY

Ⓨ   **E0870**   Traction frame, attached to footboard, extremity traction (e.g., Buck's)   ♿
       MED: 100-3,280.1

Ⓨ   **E0880**   Traction stand, freestanding, extremity traction (e.g., Buck's)   ♿
       MED: 100-3,280.1

TRACTION - PELVIC

Ⓨ   **E0890**   Traction frame, attached to footboard, pelvic traction   ♿
       MED: 100-3,280.1

Ⓨ   **E0900**   Traction stand, freestanding, pelvic traction (e.g., Buck's)   ♿
       MED: 100-3,280.1

TRAPEZE EQUIPMENT, FRACTURE FRAME, AND OTHER ORTHOPEDIC DEVICES

Ⓨ   **E0910**   Trapeze bars, also known as Patient Helper, attached to bed, with grab bar   ♿
       MED: 100-3,280.1

Ⓨ   **E0911**   Trapeze bar, heavy duty, for patient weight capacity greater than 250 pounds, attached to bed, with grab bar

Ⓨ   **E0912**   Trapeze bar, heavy duty, for patient weight capacity greater than 250 pounds, free standing, complete with grab bar

Ⓨ   **E0920**   Fracture frame, attached to bed, includes weights   ♿
       MED: 100-3,280.1

Ⓨ   **E0930**   Fracture frame, freestanding, includes weights   ♿
       MED: 100-3,280.1

Ⓨ   **E0935**   Continuous passive motion exercise device for use on knee only   ♿
       MED: 100-3,280.1

● Ⓔ   **E0936**   Continuous passive motion exercise device for use other than knee

Ⓨ   **E0940**   Trapeze bar, freestanding, complete with grab bar   ♿
       MED: 100-3,280.1

Ⓨ   **E0941**   Gravity assisted traction device, any type   ♿
       MED: 100-3,280.1

Ⓨ   **E0942**   Cervical head harness/halter   ♿

Ⓨ   **E0944**   Pelvic belt/harness/boot   ♿

Ⓨ   **E0945**   Extremity belt/harness   ♿

Special Coverage Instructions   Noncovered by Medicare   Carrier Discretion   ☑ Quality Alert   ● New Code   ○ Reinstated Code   ▲ Revised Code

Ⓨ E0946 Fracture frame, dual with cross bars, attached to bed (e.g., Balken, Four Poster) ⧖
MED: 100-3,280.1

Ⓨ E0947 Fracture frame, attachments for complex pelvic traction ⧖
MED: 100-3,280.1

Ⓨ E0948 Fracture frame, attachments for complex cervical traction ⧖
MED: 100-3,280.1

Ⓐ E0950 Wheelchair accessory, tray, each ⧖
MED: 100-3,280.1

Ⓐ E0951 Heel loop/holder, any type, with or without ankle strap, each ⧖

Ⓐ E0952 Toe loop/holder, any type, each ⧖
MED: 100-3,280.1

Ⓨ ☑ E0955 Wheelchair accessory, headrest, cushioned, any type, including fixed mounting hardware, each ⧖

Ⓨ ☑ E0956 Wheelchair accessory, lateral trunk or hip support, any type, including fixed mounting hardware, each ⧖

Ⓨ ☑ E0957 Wheelchair accessory, medial thigh support, any type, including fixed mounting hardware, each ⧖

Ⓐ E0958 Manual wheelchair accessory, one-arm drive attachment, each ⧖
MED: 100-3,280.1

Ⓑ E0959 Manual wheelchair accessory, adapter for amputee, each ⧖
MED: 100-3,280.1

Ⓨ E0960 Wheelchair accessory, shoulder harness/straps or chest strap, including any type mounting hardware ⧖

Ⓑ E0961 Manual wheelchair accessory, wheel lock brake extension (handle), each ⧖
MED: 100-3,280.1

Ⓑ E0966 Manual wheelchair accessory, headrest extension, each ⧖
MED: 100-3,280.1

▲ Ⓨ ☑ E0967 Manual wheelchair accessory, hand rim with projections, any type, each ⧖
MED: 100-3,280.1

Ⓨ E0968 Commode seat, wheelchair ⧖
MED: 100-3,280.1

Ⓨ E0969 Narrowing device, wheelchair ⧖
MED: 100-3,280.1

Ⓑ E0970 No. 2 footplates, except for elevating legrest
See code(s): K0037, K0042
MED: 100-3,280.1

Ⓑ ☑ E0971 Manual wheelchair accessory, anti-tipping device, each
DME fee schedule reflects a base billing unit of each.
MED: 100-3,280.1

Ⓑ E0973 Wheelchair accessory, adjustable height, detachable armrest, complete assembly, each ⧖
MED: 100-3,280.1

Ⓑ E0974 Manual wheelchair accessory, anti-rollback device, each ⧖
MED: 100-3,280.1

E0977 Wedge cushion, wheelchair
See code(s): E2601, E2602.

Ⓑ E0978 Wheelchair accessory, positioning belt/safety belt/pelvic strap, each ⧖

Ⓨ E0980 Safety vest, wheelchair ⧖

Ⓨ ☑ E0981 Wheelchair accessory, seat upholstery, replacement only, each ⧖

Ⓨ ☑ E0982 Wheelchair accessory, back upholstery, replacement only, each ⧖

Ⓨ E0983 Manual wheelchair accessory, power add-on to convert manual wheelchair to motorized wheelchair, joystick control ⧖

Ⓨ E0984 Manual wheelchair accessory, power add-on to convert manual wheelchair to motorized wheelchair, tiller control ⧖

Ⓨ E0985 Wheelchair accessory, seat lift mechanism ⧖

Ⓨ ☑ E0986 Manual wheelchair accessory, push activated power assist, each ⧖

Ⓑ ☑ E0990 Wheelchair accessory, elevating leg rest, complete assembly, each ⧖
MED: 100-3,280.1

Ⓑ E0992 Manual wheelchair accessory, solid seat insert ⧖

Ⓨ ☑ E0994 Armrest, each ⧖
MED: 100-3,280.1

Ⓑ ☑ E0995 Wheelchair accessory, calf rest/pad, each ⧖
MED: 100-3,280.1

E0997 Caster with fork
See code(s) E2395, E2396
MED: 100-3,280.1

E0998 Caster without fork
See code(s) E2395
MED: 100-3,280.1

E0999 Pneumatic tire with wheel
See code(s) E2381-E2385
MED: 100-3,280.1

Ⓨ E1002 Wheelchair accessory, power seating system, tilt only ⧖

Ⓨ E1003 Wheelchair accessory, power seating system, recline only, without shear reduction ⧖

Ⓨ E1004 Wheelchair accessory, power seating system, recline only, with mechanical shear reduction ⧖

Ⓨ E1005 Wheelchair accessory, power seating system, recline only, with power shear reduction ⧖

Ⓨ E1006 Wheelchair accessory, power seating system, combination tilt and recline, without shear reduction ⧖

Ⓨ E1007 Wheelchair accessory, power seating system, combination tilt and recline, with mechanical shear reduction ⧖

Ⓨ E1008 Wheelchair accessory, power seating system, combination tilt and recline, with power shear reduction ⧖

Ⓨ ☑ E1009 Wheelchair accessory, addition to power seating system, mechanically linked leg elevation system, including pushrod and leg rest, each ⧖

Ⓨ ☑ E1010 Wheelchair accessory, addition to power seating system, power leg elevation system, including leg rest, pair ⧖

Ⓨ E1011 Modification to pediatric size wheelchair, width adjustment package (not to be dispensed with initial chair) ⧖
MED: 100-3,280.1

Ⓨ E1014 Reclining back, addition to pediatric size wheelchair ⧖
MED: 100-3,280.1

Special Coverage Instructions   Noncovered by Medicare   Carrier Discretion   ☑ Quality Alert   ● New Code   ○ Reinstated Code   ▲ Revised Code

2007 HCPCS   ❶-❾ ASC Group   MED: Pub 100/NCD References   ⧖ DMEPOS Paid   ⊘ SNF Excluded   E Codes — 49

Ⓨ	**E1015**	Shock absorber for manual wheelchair, each ♿
		MED: 100-3,280.1
Ⓨ	**E1016**	Shock absorber for power wheelchair, each ♿
		MED: 100-3,280.1
Ⓨ	**E1017**	Heavy duty shock absorber for heavy duty or extra heavy duty manual wheelchair, each ♿
		MED: 100-3,280.1
Ⓨ	**E1018**	Heavy duty shock absorber for heavy duty or extra heavy duty power wheelchair, each ♿
		MED: 100-3,280.1
Ⓨ	**E1020**	Residual limb support system for wheelchair ♿
		MED: 100-3,280.3
Ⓨ	**E1028**	Wheelchair accessory, manual swingaway, retractable or removable mounting hardware for joystick, other control interface or positioning accessory ♿
Ⓨ	**E1029**	Wheelchair accessory, ventilator tray, fixed ♿
Ⓨ	**E1030**	Wheelchair accessory, ventilator tray, gimbaled ♿

ROLLABOUT CHAIR

Ⓨ	**E1031**	Rollabout chair, any and all types with casters five inches or greater ♿
		MED: 100-3,280.1
Ⓨ	**E1035**	Multi-positional patient transfer system, with integrated seat, operated by care giver ♿
		MED: 100-2,15,110
Ⓨ	**E1037**	Transport chair, pediatric size ♿
		MED: 100-3,280.1
Ⓨ	**E1038**	Transport chair, adult size, patient weight capacity up to and including 300 pounds ♿
		MED: 100-3,280.1
Ⓨ	**E1039**	Transport chair, adult size, heavy duty, patient weight capacity greater than 300 pounds ♿

WHEELCHAIRS - FULLY RECLINING

Ⓐ	**E1050**	Fully reclining wheelchair; fixed full-length arms, swing-away, detachable, elevating legrests
		MED: 100-3,280.1
Ⓐ	**E1060**	Fully reclining wheelchair; detachable arms, desk or full-length, swing-away, detachable, elevating legrests
		MED: 100-3,280.1
Ⓐ	**E1070**	Fully reclining wheelchair; detachable arms, desk or full-length, swing-away, detachable footrests
		MED: 100-3,280.1
Ⓐ	**E1083**	Hemi-wheelchair; fixed full-length arms, swing-away, detachable, elevating legrests
		MED: 100-3,280.1
Ⓐ	**E1084**	Hemi-wheelchair; detachable arms, desk or full-length, swing-away, detachable, elevating legrests
		MED: 100-3,280.1
Ⓐ	**E1085**	Hemi-wheelchair; fixed full-length arms, swing-away, detachable footrests
		See code(s): K0002
		MED: 100-3,280.1
Ⓐ	**E1086**	Hemi-wheelchair; detachable arms, desk or full-length, swing-away, detachable footrests
		See code(s): K0002
		MED: 100-3,280.1
Ⓐ	**E1087**	High-strength lightweight wheelchair; fixed full-length arms, swing-away, detachable, elevating legrests
		MED: 100-3,280.1

Ⓐ	**E1088**	High-strength lightweight wheelchair; detachable arms, desk or full-length, swing-away, detachable, elevating legrests
		MED: 100-3,280.1
Ⓐ	**E1089**	High-strength lightweight wheelchair; fixed-length arms, swing-away, detachable footrests
		See code(s): K0004
		MED: 100-3,280.1
Ⓐ	**E1090**	High-strength lightweight wheelchair; detachable arms, desk or full-length, swing-away, detachable footrests
		See code(s): K0004
		MED: 100-3,280.1
Ⓐ	**E1092**	Wide, heavy-duty wheelchair; detachable arms, desk or full-length, swing-away, detachable, elevating legrests
		MED: 100-3,280.1
Ⓐ	**E1093**	Wide, heavy-duty wheelchair; detachable arms, desk or full-length arms, swing-away, detachable footrests
		MED: 100-3,280.1

WHEELCHAIR - SEMI-RECLINING

Ⓐ	**E1100**	Semi-reclining wheelchair; fixed full-length arms, swing-away, detachable, elevating legrests
		MED: 100-3,280.1
Ⓐ	**E1110**	Semi-reclining wheelchair; detachable arms, desk or full-length, elevating legrest
		MED: 100-3,280.1

WHEELCHAIR - STANDARD

Ⓐ	**E1130**	Standard wheelchair; fixed full-length arms, fixed or swing-away, detachable footrests
		See code(s): K0001
		MED: 100-3,280.1
Ⓐ	**E1140**	Wheelchair; detachable arms, desk or full-length, swing-away, detachable footrests
		See code(s): K0001
		MED: 100-3,280.1
Ⓨ	**E1150**	Wheelchair; detachable arms, desk or full-length, swing-away, detachable, elevating legrests ♿
		MED: 100-3,280.1
Ⓐ	**E1160**	Wheelchair; fixed full-length arms, swing-away, detachable, elevating legrests
		MED: 100-3,280.1
Ⓐ	**E1161**	Manual adult size wheelchair, includes tilt in space

WHEELCHAIR - AMPUTEE

Ⓐ	**E1170**	Amputee wheelchair; fixed full-length arms, swing-away, detachable, elevating legrests
		MED: 100-3,280.1
Ⓐ	**E1171**	Amputee wheelchair; fixed full-length arms, without footrests or legrests
		MED: 100-3,280.1
Ⓐ	**E1172**	Amputee wheelchair; detachable arms, desk or full-length, without footrests or legrests
		MED: 100-3,280.1
Ⓐ	**E1180**	Amputee wheelchair; detachable arms, desk or full-length, swing-away, detachable footrests
		MED: 100-3,280.1
Ⓐ	**E1190**	Amputee wheelchair; detachable arms, desk or full-length, swing-away, detachable, elevating legrests
		MED: 100-3,280.1

Special Coverage Instructions   Noncovered by Medicare   Carrier Discretion   ☑ Quality Alert   ● New Code   ○ Reinstated Code   ▲ Revised Code

Ⓐ **E1195** Heavy duty wheelchair; fixed full-length arms, swing-away, detachable, elevating legrests
MED: 100-3,280.1

Ⓐ **E1200** Amputee wheelchair; fixed full-length arms, swing-away, detachable footrests
MED: 100-3,280.1

WHEELCHAIR - SPECIAL SIZE

Ⓐ **E1220** Wheelchair; specially sized or constructed (indicate brand name, model number, if any, and justification)
MED: 100-3,280.3

Ⓐ **E1221** Wheelchair with fixed arm, footrests
MED: 100-3,280.3

Ⓐ **E1222** Wheelchair with fixed arm, elevating legrests
MED: 100-3,280.3

Ⓐ **E1223** Wheelchair with detachable arms, footrests
MED: 100-3,280.3

Ⓐ **E1224** Wheelchair with detachable arms, elevating legrests
MED: 100-3,280.3

Ⓨ **E1225** Wheelchair accessory, manual semi-reclining back, (recline greater than 15 degrees, but less than 80 degrees), each   ♿
MED: 100-3,280.3

Ⓑ **E1226** Wheelchair accessory, manual fully reclining back, (recline greater than 80 degrees), each   ♿
See also K0028
MED: 100-3,280.1

Ⓨ **E1227** Special height arms for wheelchair   ♿
MED: 100-3,280.3

Ⓨ **E1228** Special back height for wheelchair   ♿
MED: 100-3,280.3

Ⓨ **E1229** Wheelchair, pediatric size, not otherwise specified

Ⓨ **E1230** Power operated vehicle (three- or four-wheel nonhighway), specify brand name and model number   ♿
Prior authorization is required by Medicare for this item.
MED: 100-3,280.9; 100-8,5,5.1.1.2

Ⓨ **E1231** Wheelchair, pediatric size, tilt-in-space, rigid, adjustable, with seating system   ♿
MED: 100-3,280.1

Ⓨ **E1232** Wheelchair, pediatric size, tilt-in-space, folding, adjustable, with seating system   ♿
MED: 100-3,280.1

Ⓨ **E1233** Wheelchair, pediatric size, tilt-in-space, rigid, adjustable, without seating system   ♿
MED: 100-3,280.1

Ⓨ **E1234** Wheelchair, pediatric size, tilt-in-space, folding, adjustable, without seating system   ♿
MED: 100-3,280.1

Ⓨ **E1235** Wheelchair, pediatric size, rigid, adjustable, with seating system   ♿
MED: 100-3,280.1

Ⓨ **E1236** Wheelchair, pediatric size, folding, adjustable, with seating system   ♿
MED: 100-3,280.1

Ⓨ **E1237** Wheelchair, pediatric size, rigid, adjustable, without seating system   ♿
MED: 100-3,280.1

Ⓨ **E1238** Wheelchair, pediatric size, folding, adjustable, without seating system   ♿
MED: 100-3,280.1

Ⓨ **E1239** Power wheelchair, pediatric size, not otherwise specified

WHEELCHAIR - LIGHTWEIGHT

Ⓐ **E1240** Lightweight wheelchair; detachable arms, desk or full-length, swing-away, detachable, elevating legrest
MED: 100-3,280.1

Ⓐ **E1250** Lightweight wheelchair; fixed full-length arms, swing-away, detachable footrests
See code(s): K0003
MED: 100-3,280.1

Ⓐ **E1260** Lightweight wheelchair; detachable arms, desk or full-length, swing-away, detachable footrests
See code(s): K0003
MED: 100-3,280.1

Ⓐ **E1270** Lightweight wheelchair; fixed full-length arms, swing-away, detachable elevating legrests
MED: 100-3,280.1

WHEELCHAIR - HEAVY-DUTY

Ⓐ **E1280** Heavy-duty wheelchair; detachable arms, desk or full-length, elevating legrests
MED: 100-3,280.1

Ⓐ **E1285** Heavy-duty wheelchair; fixed full-length arms, swing-away, detachable footrests
See code(s): K0006
MED: 100-3,280.1

Ⓐ **E1290** Heavy-duty wheelchair; detachable arms, desk or full-length, swing-away, detachable footrests
See code(s): K0006
MED: 100-3,280.1

Ⓐ **E1295** Heavy-duty wheelchair; fixed full-length arms, elevating legrests
MED: 100-3,280.1

Ⓨ **E1296** Special wheelchair seat height from floor   ♿
MED: 100-3,280.3

Ⓨ **E1297** Special wheelchair seat depth, by upholstery   ♿
MED: 100-3,280.3

Ⓨ **E1298** Special wheelchair seat depth and/or width, by construction   ♿
MED: 100-3,280.3

WHIRLPOOL - EQUIPMENT

Ⓔ **E1300** Whirlpool, portable (overtub type)
MED: 100-3,280.1

Ⓨ **E1310** Whirlpool, nonportable (built-in type)   ♿
MED: 100-3,280.1

REPAIRS AND REPLACEMENT SUPPLIES

Ⓨ ☑ **E1340** Repair or nonroutine service for durable medical equipment requiring the skill of a technician, labor component, per 15 minutes
Medicare jurisdiction: local contractor if repair or implanted DME.
MED: 100-2,15,110.2

ADDITIONAL OXYGEN RELATED EQUIPMENT

Ⓨ **E1353** Regulator
MED: 100-3,240.2

Ⓨ **E1355** Stand/rack
MED: 100-3,240.2

Special Coverage Instructions   Noncovered by Medicare   Carrier Discretion   ☑ Quality Alert   ● New Code   ○ Reinstated Code   ▲ Revised Code

2007 HCPCS   **1-9** ASC Group   **MED:** Pub 100/NCD References   ♿ DMEPOS Paid   ⊘ SNF Excluded   **E Codes — 51**

Durable Medical Equipment

E1372 — E1840

Y **E1372** Immersion external heater for nebulizer &
MED: 100-3,240.2

Y **E1390** Oxygen concentrator, single delivery port, capable of delivering 85 percent or greater oxygen concentration at the prescribed flow rate &
MED: 100-3,240.2

Y ☑ **E1391** Oxygen concentrator, dual delivery port, capable of delivering 85 percent or greater oxygen concentration at the prescribed flow rate, each &
MED: 100-3,240.2

Y **E1392** Portable oxygen concentrator, rental &

Y **E1399** Durable medical equipment, miscellaneous &
Determine if an alternative HCPCS Level II or a CPT code better describes the service being reported. This code should be used only if a more specific code is unavailable. Medicare jurisdiction: local contractor if repair or implanted DME.

Y **E1405** Oxygen and water vapor enriching system with heated delivery &
MED: 100-3,240.2; 100-4,20,20; 100-4,20,20.4

Y **E1406** Oxygen and water vapor enriching system without heated delivery &
MED: 100-3,240.2; 100-4,20,20; 100-4,20,20.4

ARTIFICIAL KIDNEY MACHINES AND ACCESSORIES

For glucose monitors, see A4253-A4256. For supplies for ESRD, see procedure codes A4651-A4929.

A **E1500** Centrifuge, for dialysis ⊘

A **E1510** Kidney, dialysate delivery system kidney machine, pump recirculating, air removal system, flowrate meter, power off, heater and temp control with alarm, IV poles, pressure gauge, concentrate container ⊘

A **E1520** Heparin infusion pump for hemodialysis ⊘

A **E1530** Air bubble detector for hemodialysis, each, replacement ⊘

A **E1540** Pressure alarm for hemodialysis, each, replacement ⊘

A **E1550** Bath conductivity meter for hemodialysis, each ⊘

A **E1560** Blood leak detector for hemodialysis, each, replacement ⊘

A **E1570** Adjustable chair, for ESRD patients ⊘

A ☑ **E1575** Transducer protectors/fluid barriers, for hemodialysis, any size, per 10 ⊘

A **E1580** Unipuncture control system for hemodialysis ⊘

A **E1590** Hemodialysis machine ⊘

A **E1592** Automatic intermittent peritoneal dialysis system ⊘

A **E1594** Cycler dialysis machine for peritoneal dialysis ⊘

A **E1600** Delivery and/or installation charges for hemodialysis equipment ⊘

A **E1610** Reverse osmosis water purification system, for hemodialysis ⊘
MED: 100-3,230.7

A **E1615** Deionizer water purification system, for hemodialysis ⊘
MED: 100-3,230.7

A **E1620** Blood pump for hemodialysis, replacement ⊘

A **E1625** Water softening system, for hemodialysis ⊘
MED: 100-3,230.7

A **E1630** Reciprocating peritoneal dialysis system ⊘

A **E1632** Wearable artificial kidney, each ⊘

B ☑ **E1634** Peritoneal dialysis clamps, each ⊘

A **E1635** Compact (portable) travel hemodialyzer system ⊘

A ☑ **E1636** Sorbent cartridges, for hemodialysis, per 10 ⊘

A ☑ **E1637** Hemostats, each ⊘

A ☑ **E1639** Scale, each ⊘

A **E1699** Dialysis equipment, not otherwise specified
Determine if an alternative HCPCS Level II or a CPT code better describes the service being reported. This code should be used only if a more specific code is unavailable. Pertinent documentation to evaluate medical appropriateness should be included when this code is reported.

JAW MOTION REHABILITATION SYSTEM AND ACCESSORIES

Y **E1700** Jaw motion rehabilitation system &
Medicare jurisdiction: local contractor.

Y ☑ **E1701** Replacement cushions for jaw motion rehabilitation system, package of six &
Medicare jurisdiction: local contractor.

Y ☑ **E1702** Replacement measuring scales for jaw motion rehabilitation system, package of 200 &
Medicare jurisdiction: local contractor.

OTHER ORTHOPEDIC DEVICES

Y **E1800** Dynamic adjustable elbow extension/flexion device, includes soft interface material &

Y **E1801** Bi-directional static progressive stretch elbow device with range of motion adjustment, includes cuffs &

Y **E1802** Dynamic adjustable forearm pronation/supination device, includes soft interface material &

Y **E1805** Dynamic adjustable wrist extension/flexion device, includes soft interface material &

Y **E1806** Bi-directional static progressive stretch wrist device with range of motion adjustment, includes cuffs &

Y **E1810** Dynamic adjustable knee extension/flexion device, includes soft interface material &

Y **E1811** Bi-directional static progressive stretch knee device with range of motion adjustment, includes cuffs &

Y **E1812** Dynamic knee, extension/flexion device with active resistance control

Y **E1815** Dynamic adjustable ankle extension/flexion device, includes soft interface material &

Y **E1816** Bi-directional static progressive stretch ankle device with range of motion adjustment, includes cuffs &

Y **E1818** Bi-directional static progressive stretch forearm pronation/supination device with range of motion adjustment, includes cuffs &

Y **E1820** Replacement soft interface material, dynamic adjustable extension/flexion device &

Y **E1821** Replacement soft interface material/cuffs for bi-directional static progressive stretch device &

Y **E1825** Dynamic adjustable finger extension/flexion device, includes soft interface material &

Y **E1830** Dynamic adjustable toe extension/flexion device, includes soft interface material &

Y **E1840** Dynamic adjustable shoulder flexion/abduction/rotation device, includes soft interface material &

Special Coverage Instructions   Noncovered by Medicare   Carrier Discretion   ☑ Quality Alert   ● New Code   ○ Reinstated Code   ▲ Revised Code

52 — E Codes   Ⓐ Age Edit   Ⓜ Maternity Edit   ♀ Female Only   ♂ Male Only   Ⓐ - Ⓨ APC Status Indicators   *2007 HCPCS*

Ⓨ E1841 Multidirectional static progressive stretch shoulder device, with range of motion adjustability, includes cuffs

Ⓐ E1902 Communication board, nonelectronic augmentative or alternative communication device

Ⓨ E2000 Gastric suction pump, home model, portable or stationary, electric ⓑ

Ⓨ E2100 Blood glucose monitor with integrated voice synthesizer ⓑ
MED: 100.3,230.16

Ⓨ E2101 Blood glucose monitor with integrated lancing/blood sample ⓑ
MED: 100.3,230.16

Ⓨ E2120 Pulse generator system for tympanic treatment of inner ear endolymphatic fluid ⓑ

Ⓨ ☑ E2201 Manual wheelchair accessory, nonstandard seat frame, width greater than or equal to 20 inches and less than 24 inches ⓑ

Ⓨ ☑ E2202 Manual wheelchair accessory, nonstandard seat frame width, 24–27 in. ⓑ

Ⓨ ☑ E2203 Manual wheelchair accessory, nonstandard seat frame depth, 20 to less than 22 inches ⓑ

Ⓨ ☑ E2204 Manual wheelchair accessory, nonstandard seat frame depth, 22–25 in. ⓑ

Ⓨ E2205 Manual wheelchair accessory, handrim without projections, any type, replacement only, each

Ⓨ E2206 Manual wheelchair accessory, wheel Lock assembly, complete, each

Ⓨ E2207 Wheelchair accessory, crutch and cane holder, each

Ⓨ E2208 Wheelchair accessory, cylinder tank carrier, each

▲ Ⓨ E2209 Accessory, arm trough, with or without hand support, each

Ⓨ E2210 Wheelchair accessory, bearings, any type, replacement only, each

Ⓨ E2211 Manual wheelchair accessory, pneumatic propulsion tire, any size, each

Ⓨ E2212 Manual wheelchair accessory, tube for pneumatic propulsion tire, any size, each

Ⓨ E2213 Manual wheelchair accessory, insert for pneumatic propulsion tire (removable), any type, any size, each

Ⓨ E2214 Manual wheelchair accessory, pneumatic caster tire, any size, each

Ⓨ E2215 Manual wheelchair accessory, tube for pneumatic caster tire, any size, each

Ⓨ E2216 Manual wheelchair accessory, foam filled propulsion tire, any size, each

Ⓨ E2217 Manual wheelchair accessory, foam filled caster tire, any size, each

Ⓨ E2218 Manual wheelchair accessory, foam propulsion tire, any size, each

Ⓨ E2219 Manual wheelchair accessory, foam caster tire, any size, each

Ⓨ E2220 Manual wheelchair accessory, solid (rubber/plastic) propulsion tire, any size, each

Ⓨ E2221 Manual wheelchair accessory, solid (rubber/plastic) caster tire (removable), any size, each

Ⓨ E2222 Manual wheelchair accessory, solid (rubber/plastic) caster tire with integrated wheel, any size, each

Ⓨ E2223 Manual wheelchair accessory, valve, any type, replacement only, each

Ⓨ E2224 Manual wheelchair accessory, propulsion wheel excludes tire, any size, each

Ⓨ E2225 Manual wheelchair accessory, caster wheel excludes tire, any size, replacement only, each

Ⓨ E2226 Manual wheelchair accessory, caster fork, any size, replacement only, each

Ⓨ E2291 Back, planar, for pediatric size wheelchair including fixed attaching hardware

Ⓨ E2292 Seat, planar, for pediatric size wheelchair including fixed attaching hardware

Ⓨ E2293 Back, contoured, for pediatric size wheelchair including fixed attaching hardware

Ⓨ E2294 Seat, contoured, for pediatric size wheelchair including fixed attaching hardware

Ⓨ E2300 Power wheelchair accessory, power seat elevation system

Ⓨ E2301 Power wheelchair accessory, power standing system

Ⓨ E2310 Power wheelchair accessory, electronic connection between wheelchair controller and one power seating system motor, including all related electronics, indicator feature, mechanical function selection switch, and fixed mounting hardware ⓑ

Ⓨ E2311 Power wheelchair accessory, electronic connection between wheelchair controller and two or more power seating system motors, including all related electronics, indicator feature, mechanical function selection switch, and fixed mounting hardware ⓑ

~~E2320~~ ~~Power wheelchair accessory, hand or chin control interface, remote joystick or touchpad, proportional, including all related electronics, and fixed mounting hardware~~
See code(s) E2373, E2374

Ⓨ E2321 Power wheelchair accessory, hand control interface, remote joystick, nonproportional, including all related electronics, mechanical stop switch, and fixed mounting hardware ⓑ

Ⓨ E2322 Power wheelchair accessory, hand control interface, multiple mechanical switches, nonproportional, including all related electronics, mechanical stop switch, and fixed mounting hardware ⓑ

Ⓨ E2323 Power wheelchair accessory, specialty joystick handle for hand control interface, prefabricated ⓑ

Ⓨ E2324 Power wheelchair accessory, chin cup for chin control interface ⓑ

Ⓨ E2325 Power wheelchair accessory, sip and puff interface, nonproportional, including all related electronics, mechanical stop switch, and manual swingaway mounting hardware ⓑ

Ⓨ E2326 Power wheelchair accessory, breath tube kit for sip and puff interface ⓑ

Ⓨ E2327 Power wheelchair accessory, head control interface, mechanical, proportional, including all related electronics, mechanical direction change switch, and fixed mounting hardware ⓑ

Ⓨ E2328 Power wheelchair accessory, head control or extremity control interface, electronic, proportional, including all related electronics and fixed mounting hardware ⓑ

| Special Coverage Instructions | Noncovered by Medicare | Carrier Discretion | ☑ Quality Alert | ● New Code | ○ Reinstated Code | ▲ Revised Code |

2007 HCPCS   **❶-❾** ASC Group   **MED:** Pub 100/NCD References   ⓑ DMEPOS Paid   ⊘ SNF Excluded   **E Codes — 53**

Durable Medical Equipment

E2329 — E2504

Ⓨ **E2329** Power wheelchair accessory, head control interface, contact switch mechanism, nonproportional, including all related electronics, mechanical stop switch, mechanical direction change switch, head array, and fixed mounting hardware 🦽

Ⓨ **E2330** Power wheelchair accessory, head control interface, proximity switch mechanism, nonproportional, including all related electronics, mechanical stop switch, mechanical direction change switch, head array, and fixed mounting hardware 🦽

Ⓨ **E2331** Power wheelchair accessory, attendant control, proportional, including all related electronics and fixed mounting hardware

Ⓨ ☑ **E2340** Power wheelchair accessory, nonstandard seat frame width, 20–23 in. 🦽

Ⓨ ☑ **E2341** Power wheelchair accessory, nonstandard seat frame width, 24–27 in. 🦽

Ⓨ ☑ **E2342** Power wheelchair accessory, nonstandard seat frame depth, 20 or 21 in. 🦽

Ⓨ ☑ **E2343** Power wheelchair accessory, nonstandard seat frame depth, 22–25 in. 🦽

Ⓨ **E2351** Power wheelchair accessory, electronic interface to operate speech generating device using power wheelchair control interface 🦽

Ⓨ ☑ **E2360** Power wheelchair accessory, 22 NF nonsealed lead acid battery, each 🦽

Ⓨ **E2361** Power wheelchair accessory, 22 NF sealed lead acid battery, each, (e.g., gel cell, absorbed glassmat) 🦽

Ⓨ ☑ **E2362** Power wheelchair accessory, group 24 nonsealed lead acid battery, each 🦽

Ⓨ ☑ **E2363** Power wheelchair accessory, group 24 sealed lead acid battery, each (e.g., gel cell, absorbed glassmat) 🦽

Ⓨ ☑ **E2364** Power wheelchair accessory, U-1 nonsealed lead acid battery, each 🦽

Ⓨ ☑ **E2365** Power wheelchair accessory, U-1 sealed lead acid battery, each (e.g., gel cell, absorbed glassmat) 🦽

Ⓨ ☑ **E2366** Power wheelchair accessory, battery charger, single mode, for use with only one battery type, sealed or nonsealed, each 🦽

Ⓨ **E2367** Power wheelchair accessory, battery charger, dual mode, for use with either battery type, sealed or nonsealed, each

Ⓨ **E2368** Power wheelchair component, motor, replacement only

Ⓨ **E2369** Power wheelchair component, gear box, replacement only

Ⓨ **E2370** Power wheelchair component, motor and gear box combination, replacement only

Ⓨ **E2371** Power wheelchair accessory, group 27 sealed lead acid battery, (e.g., gel cell, absorbed glassmat), each

Ⓨ **E2372** Power wheelchair accessory, group 27 nonsealed lead acid battery, each

● Ⓨ **E2373** Power wheelchair accessory, hand or chin control interface, mini-proportional, compact, or short throw remote joystick or touchpad, proportional, including all related electronics and fixed mounting hardware 🦽

● Ⓨ **E2374** Power wheelchair accessory, hand or chin control interface, standard remote joystick (not including controller), proportional, including all related electronics and fixed mounting hardware, replacement only 🦽

● Ⓨ **E2375** Power wheelchair accessory, nonexpandable controller, including all related electronics and mounting hardware, replacement only 🦽

● Ⓨ **E2376** Power wheelchair accessory, expandable controller, including all related electronics and mounting hardware, replacement only 🦽

● Ⓨ **E2377** Power wheelchair accessory, expandable controller, including all related electronics and mounting hardware, upgrade provided at initial issue 🦽

● Ⓨ **E2381** Power wheelchair accessory, pneumatic drive wheel tire, any size, replacement only, each 🦽

● Ⓨ **E2382** Power wheelchair accessory, tube for pneumatic drive wheel tire, any size, replacement only, each 🦽

● Ⓨ **E2383** Power wheelchair accessory, insert for pneumatic drive wheel tire (removable), any type, any size, replacement only, each 🦽

● Ⓨ **E2384** Power wheelchair accessory, pneumatic caster tire, any size, replacement only, each 🦽

● Ⓨ **E2385** Power wheelchair accessory, tube for pneumatic caster tire, any size, replacement only, each 🦽

● Ⓨ **E2386** Power wheelchair accessory, foam filled drive wheel tire, any size, replacement only, each 🦽

● Ⓨ **E2387** Power wheelchair accessory, foam filled caster tire, any size, replacement only, each 🦽

● Ⓨ **E2388** Power wheelchair accessory, foam drive wheel tire, any size, replacement only, each 🦽

● Ⓨ **E2389** Power wheelchair accessory, foam caster tire, any size, replacement only, each 🦽

● Ⓨ **E2390** Power wheelchair accessory, solid (rubber/plastic) drive wheel tire, any size, replacement only, each 🦽

● Ⓨ **E2391** Power wheelchair accessory, solid (rubber/plastic) caster tire (removable), any size, replacement only, each 🦽

● Ⓨ **E2392** Power wheelchair accessory, solid (rubber/plastic) caster tire with integrated wheel, any size, replacement only, each 🦽

● Ⓨ **E2393** Power wheelchair accessory, valve for pneumatic tire tube, any type, replacement only, each 🦽

● Ⓨ **E2394** Power wheelchair accessory, drive wheel excludes tire, any size, replacement only, each 🦽

● Ⓨ **E2395** Power wheelchair accessory, caster wheel excludes tire, any size, replacement only, each 🦽

● Ⓨ **E2396** Power wheelchair accessory, caster fork, any size, replacement only, each 🦽

Ⓨ **E2399** Power wheelchair accessory, not otherwise classified interface, including all related electronics and any type mounting hardware 🦽

Ⓨ **E2402** Negative pressure wound therapy electrical pump, stationary or portable 🦽

Ⓨ ☑ **E2500** Speech generating device, digitized speech, using prerecorded messages, less than or equal to 8 minutes recording time 🦽
MED: 100-3,50.1

Ⓨ ☑ **E2502** Speech generating device, digitized speech, using prerecorded messages, greater than eight minutes but less than or equal to 20 minutes recording time 🦽
MED: 100-3,50.1

Ⓨ ☑ **E2504** Speech generating device, digitized speech, using prerecorded messages, greater than 20 minutes but less than or equal to 40 minutes recording time 🦽
MED: 100-3,50.1

Special Coverage Instructions   Noncovered by Medicare   Carrier Discretion   ☑ Quality Alert   ● New Code   ○ Reinstated Code   ▲ Revised Code

54 — E Codes   Ⓐ Age Edit   Ⓜ Maternity Edit   ♀ Female Only   ♂ Male Only   Ⓐ - Ⓨ APC Status Indicators   *2007 HCPCS*

Ⓨ ☑ **E2506** Speech generating device, digitized speech, using prerecorded messages, greater than 40 minutes recording time ⅃
MED: 100-3,50.1

Ⓨ **E2508** Speech generating device, synthesized speech, requiring message formulation by spelling and access by physical contact with the device ⅃
MED: 100-3,50.1

Ⓨ **E2510** Speech generating device, synthesized speech, permitting multiple methods of message formulation and multiple methods of device access ⅃
MED: 100-3,50.1

Ⓨ **E2511** Speech generating software program, for personal computer or personal digital assistant ⅃
MED: 100-3,50.1

Ⓨ **E2512** Accessory for speech generating device, mounting system ⅃
MED: 100-3,50.1

Ⓨ **E2599** Accessory for speech generating device, not otherwise classified
MED: 100-3,50.1

Ⓨ **E2601** General use wheelchair seat cushion, width less than 22 in., any depth

Ⓨ **E2602** General use wheelchair seat cushion, width 22 in. or greater, any depth

Ⓨ **E2603** Skin protection wheelchair seat cushion, width less than 22 in., any depth

Ⓨ **E2604** Skin protection wheelchair seat cushion, width 22 in. or greater, any depth

Ⓨ **E2605** Positioning wheelchair seat cushion, width less than 22 in., any depth

Ⓨ **E2606** Positioning wheelchair seat cushion, width 22 in. or greater, any depth

Ⓨ **E2607** Skin protection and positioning wheelchair seat cushion, width less than 22 in., any depth

Ⓨ **E2608** Skin protection and positioning wheelchair seat cushion, width 22 in. or greater, any depth

Ⓨ **E2609** Custom fabricated wheelchair seat cushion, any size

Ⓑ **E2610** Wheelchair seat cushion, powered

Ⓨ **E2611** General use wheelchair back cushion, width less than 22 in., any height, including any type mounting hardware

Ⓨ **E2612** General use wheelchair back cushion, width 22 in. or greater, any height, including any type mounting hardware

Ⓨ **E2613** Positioning wheelchair back cushion, posterior, width less than 22 in., any height, including any type mounting hardware

Ⓨ **E2614** Positioning wheelchair back cushion, posterior, width 22 in. or greater, any height, including any type mounting hardware

Ⓨ **E2615** Positioning wheelchair back cushion, posterior-lateral, width less than 22 in., any height, including any type mounting hardware

Ⓨ **E2616** Positioning wheelchair back cushion, posterior-lateral, width 22 in. or greater, any height, including any type mounting hardware

Ⓨ **E2617** Custom fabricated wheelchair back cushion, any size, including any type mounting hardware

Ⓨ **E2618** Wheelchair accessory, solid seat support base (replaces sling seat), for use with manual wheelchair or lightweight power wheelchair, includes any type mounting hardware

Ⓨ **E2619** Replacement cover for wheelchair seat cushion or back cushion, each

Ⓨ **E2620** Positioning wheelchair back cushion, planar back with lateral supports, width less than 22 in., any height, including any type mounting hardware

Ⓨ **E2621** Positioning wheelchair back cushion, planar back with lateral supports, width 22 in. or greater, any height, including any type mounting hardware

Ⓔ **E8000** Gait trainer, pediatric size, posterior support, includes all accessories and components

Ⓔ **E8001** Gait trainer, pediatric size, upright support, includes all accessories and components

Ⓔ **E8002** Gait trainer, pediatric size, anterior support, includes all accessories and components

Special Coverage Instructions   Noncovered by Medicare   Carrier Discretion   ☑ Quality Alert   ● New Code   ○ Reinstated Code   ▲ Revised Code

2007 HCPCS   Ⅰ-Ⅸ ASC Group   **MED:** Pub 100/NCD References   ⅃ DMEPOS Paid   ⊘ SNF Excluded   E Codes — 55

PROCEDURES/PROFESSIONAL SERVICES (TEMPORARY)
G0000-G9999

The G codes are used to identify professional health care procedures and services that would otherwise be coded in CPT but for which there are no CPT codes.

G codes fall under the jurisdiction of the local contractor.

[S] **G0008** Administration of influenza virus vaccine ⊘
MED: 100-2,6,10; 100-4,4,240

[S] **G0009** Administration of pneumococcal vaccine ⊘
MED: 100-2,6,10; 100-4,4,240

[B] **G0010** Administration of hepatitis B vaccine ⊘
MED: 100-2,6,10; 100-4,4,240

[A] **G0027** Semen analysis; presence and/or motility of sperm excluding huhner

[V] **G0101** Cervical or vaginal cancer screening; pelvic and clinical breast examination ♀⊘
G0101 can be reported with an E/M code when a separately identifiable E/M service was provided.
MED: 100-2,6,10; 100-4,4,240
AHA: 4Q,'02,8; 3Q,'01,6

[N] **G0102** Prostate cancer screening; digital rectal examination ♂⊘
MED: 100-2,6,10; 100-3,210.1; 100-4,4,240

▲ **[A]** **G0103** Prostate cancer screening; prostate specific antigen test (PSA) ♂⊘
MED: 100-2,6,10; 100-3,210.1; 100-4,4,240

[S] **G0104** Colorectal cancer screening; flexible sigmoidoscopy ⊘
Medicare covers colorectal screening for cancer via flexible sigmoidoscopy once every four years for patients 50 years or older.
MED: 100-2,6,10; 100-4,4,240; 100-4,18,60.1; 100-4,18,60.2; 100-4,18,60.2.1; 100-4,18,60.6

[T] **G0105** Colorectal cancer screening; colonoscopy on individual at high risk **2**⊘
An individual with ulcerative enteritis or a history of a malignant neoplasm of the lower gastrointestinal tract is considered at high-risk for colorectal cancer, as defined by CMS.
MED: 100-2,6,10; 100-4,4,240; 100-4,18,60.1; 100-4,18,60.2; 100-4,18,60.2.1; 100-4,18,60.6
AHA: 3Q,'01,6

[S] **G0106** Colorectal cancer screening; alternative to G0104, screening sigmoidoscopy, barium enema ⊘
MED: 100-2,6,10; 100-4,4,240; 100-4,18,60.1; 100-4,18,60.2; 100-4,18,60.2.1; 100-4,18,60.6

~~G0107~~ ~~Colorectal cancer screening; fecal-occult blood test, 1-3 simultaneous determinations~~
See CPT code(s) 82270

[A] **G0108** Diabetes outpatient self-management training services, individual, per 30 minutes ⊘
MED: 100-2,6,10; 100-4,4,240

[A] **G0109** Diabetes self-management training services, group session (2 or more), per 30 minutes ⊘
MED: 100-2,6,10; 100-4,4,240

[S] **G0117** Glaucoma screening for high risk patients furnished by an optometrist or ophthalmologist ⊘
MED: 100-2,15,280.1
AHA: 1Q,'02,4; 3Q,'01,12

[S] **G0118** Glaucoma screening for high risk patient furnished under the direct supervision of an optometrist or ophthalmologist ⊘
MED: 100-2,15,280.1
AHA: 1Q,'02,4; 3Q,'01,12

[S] **G0120** Colorectal cancer screening; alternative to G0105, screening colonoscopy, barium enema ⊘
MED: 100-2,6,10; 100-4,18,60.1; 100-4,18,60.2; 100-4,18,60.2.1; 100-4,18,60.6

[T] **G0121** Colorectal cancer screening; colonoscopy on individual not meeting criteria for high risk **4**⊘
MED: 100-2,6,10; 100-4,4,240; 100-4,18,60.1; 100-4,18,60.2; 100-4,18,60.2.1; 100-4,18,60.6
AHA: 1Q,'02,4; 3Q,'01,12

[E] **G0122** Colorectal cancer screening; barium enema
MED: 100-4,18,60.2; 100-4,18,60.2.1; 100-4,18,60.6

[A] **G0123** Screening cytopathology, cervical or vaginal (any reporting system), collected in preservative fluid, automated thin layer preparation, screening by cytotechnologist under physician supervision ♀⊘
See also P3000-P3001.
MED: 100-2,6,10; 100-3,190.2; 100-4,4,240

[B] **G0124** Screening cytopathology, cervical or vaginal (any reporting system), collected in preservative fluid, automated thin layer preparation, requiring interpretation by physician ♀⊘
See also P3000-P3001.
MED: 100-2,6,10; 100-3,190.2; 100-4,4,240

[T] **G0127** Trimming of dystrophic nails, any number ⊘
MED: 100-2,15,290

[B] **G0128** Direct (face-to-face with patient) skilled nursing services of a registered nurse provided in a comprehensive outpatient rehabilitation facility, each 10 minutes beyond the first 5 minutes ⊘

[P] **G0129** Occupational therapy requiring the skills of a qualified occupational therapist, furnished as a component of a partial hospitalization treatment program, per day

[X] **G0130** Single energy x-ray absorptiometry (SEXA) bone density study, one or more sites; appendicular skeleton (peripheral) (e.g., radius, wrist, heel)
MED: 100-2,6,10; 100-3,150.3; 100-4,4,240; 100-4,13,140

[B] **G0141** Screening cytopathology smears, cervical or vaginal, performed by automated system, with manual rescreening, requiring interpretation by physician ♀
MED: 100-2,6,10

[A] **G0143** Screening cytopathology, cervical or vaginal (any reporting system), collected in preservative fluid, automated thin layer preparation, with manual screening and rescreening by cytotechnologist under physician supervision ♀
MED: 100-2,6,10

[A] **G0144** Screening cytopathology, cervical or vaginal (any reporting system), collected in preservative fluid, automated thin layer preparation, with screening by automated system, under physician supervision ♀
MED: 100-2,6,10

[A] **G0145** Screening cytopathology, cervical or vaginal (any reporting system), collected in preservative fluid, automated thin layer preparation, with screening by automated system and manual rescreening under physician supervision ♀
MED: 100-2,6,10

Special Coverage Instructions   Noncovered by Medicare   Carrier Discretion   ☑ Quality Alert   ● New Code   ○ Reinstated Code   ▲ Revised Code

Procedures/Professional Services (Temporary)

G0147 — G0243

Ⓐ   G0147   Screening cytopathology smears, cervical or vaginal, performed by automated system under physician supervision   ♀ ⊘
     MED: 100-2,6,10

Ⓐ   G0148   Screening cytopathology smears, cervical or vaginal, performed by automated system with manual rescreening   ♀ ⊘
     MED: 100-2,6,10

Ⓑ ☑ G0151   Services of physical therapist in home health setting, each 15 minutes

Ⓑ ☑ G0152   Services of occupational therapist in home health setting, each 15 minutes

Ⓑ ☑ G0153   Services of speech and language pathologist in home health setting, each 15 minutes

Ⓑ ☑ G0154   Services of skilled nurse in home health setting, each 15 minutes

Ⓑ ☑ G0155   Services of clinical social worker in home health setting, each 15 minutes

Ⓑ ☑ G0156   Services of home health aide in home health setting, each 15 minutes

Ⓣ ☑ G0166   External counterpulsation, per treatment session   ⊘
     MED: 100-3,20.20; 100-4,4,20.5

Ⓑ   G0168   Wound closure utilizing tissue adhesive(s) only   ⊘
     AHA: 3Q,'01,13; 4Q,'01,12

Ⓢ   G0173   Linear accelerator based stereotactic radiosurgery, complete course of therapy In one session   ⊘
     MED: 100-4,4,220.3

Ⓥ   G0175   Scheduled interdisciplinary team conference (minimum of three exclusive of patient care nursing staff) with patient present
     MED: 100-4,4,160

Ⓟ   G0176   Activity therapy, such as music, dance, art or play therapies not for recreation, related to the care and treatment of patient's disabling mental health problems, per session (45 minutes or more)

Ⓟ   G0177   Training and educational services related to the care and treatment of patient's disabling mental health problems per session (45 minutes or more)

Ⓜ   G0179   Physician re-certification for Medicare-covered home health services under a home health plan of care (patient not present), including contacts with home health agency and review of reports of patient status required by physicians to affirm the initial implementation of the plan of care that meets patient's needs, per re-certification period   ⊘

Ⓜ   G0180   Physician certification for Medicare-covered home health services under a home health plan of care (patient not present), including contacts with home health agency and review of reports of patient status required by physicians to affirm the initial implementation of the plan of care that meets patient's needs, per certification period   ⊘

Ⓜ   G0181   Physician supervision of a patient receiving Medicare-covered services provided by a participating home health agency (patient not present) requiring complex and multidisciplinary care modalities involving regular physician development and/or revision of care plans, review of subsequent reports of patient status, review of laboratory and other studies, communication (including telephone calls) with other health care professionals involved in the patient's care, integration of new information into the medical treatment plan and/or adjustment of medical therapy, within a calendar month, 30 minutes or more   ⊘

Ⓜ   G0182   Physician supervision of a patient under a Medicare-approved hospice (patient not present) requiring complex and multidisciplinary care modalities involving regular physician development and/or revision of care plans, review of subsequent reports of patient status, review of laboratory and other studies, communication (including telephone calls) with other health care professionals involved in the patient's care, integration of new information into the medical treatment plan and/or adjustment of medical therapy, within a calendar month, 30 minutes or more   ⊘

Ⓣ   G0186   Destruction of localized lesion of choroid (for example, choroidal neovascularization); photocoagulation, feeder vessel technique (one or more sessions)   ⊘

Ⓐ   G0202   Screening mammography, producing direct digital image, bilateral, all views   ⊘
     MED: 100-2,6,10; 100-4,4,240
     AHA: 1Q,'02,3

Ⓐ   G0204   Diagnostic mammography, producing direct digital image, bilateral, all views
     AHA: 1Q,'03,7

Ⓐ   G0206   Diagnostic mammography, producing direct digital image, unilateral, all views
     AHA: 1Q,'03,7

Ⓔ   G0219   PET imaging whole body; melanoma for noncovered indications
     MED: 100-3,220.6
     AHA: 1Q,'02,10

Ⓔ   G0235   PET imaging, any site, not otherwise specified
     MED: 100-4,13,60.14

Ⓢ   G0237   Therapeutic procedures to increase strength or endurance of respiratory muscles, face-to-face, one-on-one, each 15 minutes (includes monitoring)

Ⓢ   G0238   Therapeutic procedures to improve respiratory function, other than described by G0237, one-on-one, face-to-face, per 15 minutes (includes monitoring)

Ⓢ   G0239   Therapeutic procedures to improve respiratory function or increase strength or endurance of respiratory muscles, two or more individuals (includes monitoring)

Stereotactic guidance

This procedure employs stereotactic guidance, image processing computers such as MRIs and SPECT, and a photon "knife" linear accelerator to address a brain lesion

G0243   ~~Multisource photon stereotactic radiosurgery, delivery including collimator changes and custom plugging, complete course of treatment, all lesions~~
     See CPT code(s) 77371

Special Coverage Instructions   Noncovered by Medicare   Carrier Discretion   ☑ Quality Alert   ● New Code   ○ Reinstated Code   ▲ Revised Code

58 — G Codes   Ⓐ Age Edit   Ⓜ Maternity Edit   ♀ Female Only   ♂ Male Only   Ⓐ - Ⓥ APC Status Indicators   *2007 HCPCS*

☑ **G0245** Initial physician evaluation and management of a diabetic patient with diabetic sensory neuropathy resulting in a loss of protective sensation (LOPS) which must include: (1) the diagnosis of LOPS, (2) a patient history, (3) a physical examination that consists of at least the following elements: (a) visual inspection of the forefoot, hindfoot, and toe web spaces, (b) evaluation of a protective sensation, (c) evaluation of foot structure and biomechanics, (d) evaluation of vascular status and skin integrity, and (e) evaluation and recommendation of footwear, and (4) patient education ⊘
MED: 100-3,70.2.1
AHA: 4Q,'02,9

☑ **G0246** Follow-up physician evaluation and management of a diabetic patient with diabetic sensory neuropathy resulting in a loss of protective sensation (LOPS) to include at least the following: (1) a patient history, (2) a physical examination that includes: (a) visual inspection of the forefoot, hindfoot, and toe web spaces, (b) evaluation of protective sensation, (c) evaluation of foot structure and biomechanics, (d) evaluation of vascular status and skin integrity, and (e) evaluation and recommendation of footwear, and (3) patient education ⊘
MED: 100-3,70.2.1
AHA: 4Q,'02,9

☑ **G0247** Routine foot care by a physician of a diabetic patient with diabetic sensory neuropathy resulting in a loss of protective sensation (LOPS) to include, the local care of superficial wounds (i.e., superficial to muscle and fascia) and at least the following if present: (1) local care of superficial wounds, (2) debridement of corns and calluses, and (3) trimming and debridement of nails ⊘
MED: 100-3,70.2.1
AHA: 4Q,'02,9

☒ **G0248** Demonstration, at initial use, of home INR monitoring for patient with mechanical heart valve(s) who meets Medicare coverage criteria, under the direction of a physician; includes: demonstrating use and care of the INR monitor, obtaining at least one blood sample, provision of instructions for reporting home INR test results, and documentation of patient ability to perform testing
MED: 100-3,210.1
AHA: 4Q,'02,9

☒ **G0249** Provision of test materials and equipment for home INR monitoring to patient with mechanical heart valve(s) who meets Medicare coverage criteria; includes provision of materials for use in the home and reporting of test results to physician; per four tests
MED: 100-3,210.1
AHA: 4Q,'02,9

Ⓜ **G0250** Physician review, interpretation and patient management of home INR testing for a patient with mechanical heart valve(s) who meets other coverage criteria; per four tests (does not require face-to-face service) ⊘
MED: 100-3,210.1
AHA: 4Q,'02,9

Ⓢ **G0251** Linear accelerator based stereotactic radiosurgery, delivery including collimator changes and custom plugging, fractionated treatment, all lesions, per session, maximum five sessions per course of treatment ⊘
MED: 100-4,4,220.3

Ⓔ **G0252** PET imaging, full and partial-ring PET scanners only, for initial diagnosis of breast cancer and/or surgical planning for breast cancer (e.g., initial staging of axillary lymph nodes)
MED: 100-3,220.6

Ⓔ **G0255** Current perception threshold/sensory nerve conduction test, (SNCT) per limb, any nerve
MED: 100-3,160.23
AHA: 4Q,'02,9

Ⓢ **G0257** Unscheduled or emergency dialysis treatment for an ESRD patient in a hospital outpatient department that is not certified as an ESRD facility
AHA: 1Q,'03,9; 4Q,'02,9

Ⓝ **G0259** Injection procedure for sacroiliac joint; arthrography
AHA: 4Q,'02,9

Ⓣ **G0260** Injection procedure for sacroiliac joint; provision of anesthetic, steroid and/or other therapeutic agent, with or without arthrography ❶
AHA: 4Q,'02,9

Ⓐ **G0265** Cryopreservation, freezing and storage of cells for therapeutic use, each cell line

Ⓐ **G0266** Thawing and expansion of frozen cells for therapeutic use, each aliquot

Ⓢ **G0267** Bone marrow or peripheral stem cell harvest, modification or treatment to eliminate cell type(s) (e.g., T-cells, metastatic carcinoma)

Ⓧ **G0268** Removal of impacted cerumen (one or both ears) by physician on same date of service as audiologic function testing ⊘
AHA: 1Q,'03,12

Ⓝ **G0269** Placement of occlusive device into either a venous or arterial access site, post surgical or interventional procedure (e.g., angioseal plug, vascular plug) ⊘

Ⓐ **G0270** Medical nutrition therapy; reassessment and subsequent intervention(s) following second referral in same year for change in diagnosis, medical condition or treatment regimen (including additional hours needed for renal disease), individual, face-to-face with the patient, each 15 minutes ⊘

Ⓐ **G0271** Medical nutrition therapy, reassessment and subsequent intervention(s) following second referral in same year for change in diagnosis, medical condition, or treatment regimen (including additional hours needed for renal disease), group (2 or more individuals), each 30 minutes ⊘

Ⓝ **G0275** Renal artery angiography (unilateral or bilateral) performed at the time of cardiac catheterization, includes catheter placement, injection of dye, flush aortogram and radiologic supervision and interpretation and production of images (list separately in addition to primary procedure) ⊘

Ⓝ **G0278** Iliac artery angiography performed at the same time of cardiac catheterization, includes catheter placement, injection of dye, radiologic supervision and interpretation and production of images (list separately in addition to primary procedure) ⊘

Ⓐ **G0281** Electrical stimulation, (unattended), to one or more areas, for chronic Stage III and Stage IV pressure ulcers, arterial ulcers, diabetic ulcers, and venous stasis ulcers not demonstrating measurable signs of healing after 30 days of conventional care, as part of a therapy plan of care
MED: 100-4,32,11.1
AHA: 1Q,'03,7; 2Q,'03,7

Special Coverage Instructions Noncovered by Medicare Carrier Discretion ☑ Quality Alert ● New Code ○ Reinstated Code ▲ Revised Code

2007 HCPCS ❶-❾ ASC Group **MED:** Pub 100/NCD References ⅃ DMEPOS Paid ⊘ SNF Excluded **G Codes — 59**

E G0282 Electrical stimulation, (unattended), to one or more areas, for wound care other than described in G0281 ⊘
MED: 100-3,270.1
AHA: 1Q,'03,7; 2Q,'03,7

A G0283 Electrical stimulation (unattended), to one or more areas for indication(s) other than wound care, as part of a therapy plan of care
AHA: 1Q,'03,7; 2Q,'03,7

S G0288 Reconstruction, computed tomographic angiography of aorta for surgical planning for vascular surgery

N G0289 Arthroscopy, knee, surgical, for removal of loose body, foreign body, debridement/shaving of articular cartilage (chondroplasty) at the time of other surgical knee arthroscopy in a different compartment of the same knee ⊘

T G0290 Transcatheter placement of a drug eluting intracoronary stent(s), percutaneous, with or without other therapeutic intervention, any method; single vessel
AHA: 3Q,'03,11; 4Q,'03,7; 4Q,'02,9

T G0291 Transcatheter placement of a drug eluting intracoronary stent(s), percutaneous, with or without other therapeutic intervention, any method; each additional vessel
AHA: 3Q,'03,11; 4Q,'03,7; 4Q,'02,9

X G0293 Noncovered surgical procedure(s) using conscious sedation, regional, general or spinal anesthesia in a medicare qualifying clinical trial, per day
AHA: 4Q,'02,9

X G0294 Noncovered procedure(s) using either no anesthesia or local anesthesia only, in a medicare qualifying clinical trial, per day
AHA: 4Q,'02,9

E G0295 Electromagnetic therapy, to one or more areas, for wound care other than described In G0329 or for other uses
MED: 100-3,270.1
AHA: 1Q,'03,7

T G0297 Insertion of single chamber pacing cardioverter defibrillator pulse generator
MED: 100-4,4,61.2

T G0298 Insertion of dual chamber pacing cardioverter defibrillator pulse generator
MED: 100-4,4,61.2

T G0299 Insertion or repositioning of electrode lead for single chamber pacing cardioverter defibrillator and insertion of pulse generator
MED: 100-4,4,61.2

T G0300 Insertion or repositioning of electrode lead(s) for dual chamber pacing cardioverter defibrillator and insertion of pulse generator
MED: 100-4,4,61.2

S ☑ G0302 Preoperative pulmonary surgery services for preparation for LVRS, complete course of services, to include a minimum of 16 days of services

S ☑ G0303 Preoperative pulmonary surgery services for preparation for LVRS, 10 to 15 days of services

S ☑ G0304 Preoperative pulmonary surgery services for preparation for LVRS, 1 to 9 days of services

S ☑ G0305 Postdischarge pulmonary surgery services after LVRS, minimum of 6 days of services

A G0306 Complete CBC, automated (HgB, HCT, RBC, WBC, without platelet count) and automated WBC differential count

A G0307 Complete CBC, automated (HgB, HCT, RBC, WBC; without platelet count)

A G0308 ESRD related services during the course of treatment, for patients under 2 years of age to include monitoring for the adequacy of nutrition, assessment of growth and development, and counseling of parents; with 4 or more face-to-face physician visits per month. A ⊘
MED: 100-2,11,130.1; 100-4,12,190

A G0309 ESRD related services during the course of treatment, for patients under 2 years of age to include monitoring for the adequacy of nutrition, assessment of growth and development, and counseling of parents; with 2 or 3 face-to-face physician visits per month. A ⊘
MED: 100-2,11,130.1; 100-4,12,190

A G0310 ESRD related services during the course of treatment, for patients under 2 years of age to include monitoring for the adequacy of nutrition, assessment of growth and development, and counseling of parents; with 1 face-to-face physician visit per month A ⊘
MED: 100-2,11,130.1

A G0311 ESRD related services during the course of treatment, for patients between 2 and 11 years of age to include monitoring for the adequacy of nutrition, assessment of growth and development, and counseling of parents; with 4 or more face-to-face physician visits per month A ⊘
MED: 100-2,11,130.1; 100-4,12,190

A G0312 ESRD related services during the course of treatment, for patients between 2 and 11 years of age to include monitoring for the adequacy of nutrition, assessment of growth and development, and counseling of parents; with 2 or 3 face-to-face physician visits per month A ⊘
MED: 100-2,11,130.1; 100-4,12,190

A G0313 ESRD related services during the course of treatment, for patients between 2 and 11 years of age to include monitoring for the adequacy of nutrition, assessment of growth and development, and counseling of parents; with 1 face-to-face physician visit per month A ⊘
MED: 100-2,11,130.1

A G0314 ESRD related services during the course of treatment, for patients between 12 and 19 years of age to include monitoring for the adequacy of nutrition, assessment of growth and development, and counseling of parents; with 4 or more face-to-face physician visits per month A ⊘
MED: 100-2,11,130.1; 100-4,12,190

A G0315 ESRD related services during the course of treatment, for patients between 12 and 19 years of age to include monitoring for the adequacy of nutrition, assessment of growth and development, and counseling of parents; with 2 or 3 face-to-face physician visits per month A ⊘
MED: 100-2,11,130.1; 100-4,12,190

A G0316 ESRD related services during the course of treatment, for patients between 12 and 19 years of age to include monitoring for the adequacy of nutrition, assessment of growth and development, and counseling of parents; with 1 face-to-face physician visit per month A ⊘
MED: 100-2,11,130.1

A G0317 ESRD related services during the course of treatment, for patients 20 years of age and over; with 4 or more face-to-face physician visits per month A ⊘
MED: 100-2,11,130.1; 100-4,12,190

Special Coverage Instructions   Noncovered by Medicare   Carrier Discretion   ☑ Quality Alert   ● New Code   ○ Reinstated Code   ▲ Revised Code

60 — G Codes   A Age Edit   M Maternity Edit   ♀ Female Only   ♂ Male Only   A - Y APC Status Indicators   *2007 HCPCS*

Ⓐ G0318 ESRD related services during the course of treatment, for patients 20 years of age and over; with 2 or 3 face-to-face physician visits per month Ⓐ⊘
MED: 100-2,11,130.1; 100-4,12,190

Ⓐ G0319 ESRD related services during the course of treatment, for patients 20 years of age and over; with 1 face-to-face physician visit per month Ⓐ⊘
MED: 100-2,11,130.1

Ⓐ G0320 ESRD related services for home dialysis patients per full month; for patients under 2 years of age to include monitoring for adequacy of nutrition, assessment of growth and development, and counseling of parents Ⓐ⊘
MED: 100-2,11,130.1

Ⓐ G0321 ESRD related services for home dialysis patients per full month; for patients 2 to 11 years of age to include monitoring for adequacy of nutrition, assessment of growth and development, and counseling of parents Ⓐ⊘
MED: 100-2,11,130.1

Ⓐ G0322 ESRD related services for home dialysis patients per full month; for patients 12 to 19 years of age to include monitoring for adequacy of nutrition, assessment of growth and development, and counseling of parents Ⓐ⊘
MED: 100-2,11,130.1

Ⓐ G0323 ESRD related services for home dialysis patients per full month; for patients 20 years of age and older Ⓐ⊘
MED: 100-2,11,130.1

Ⓐ G0324 End stage renal disease (ESRD) related services for home dialysis (less than full month), per day; for patients under two years of age Ⓐ⊘
MED: 100-2,11,130.1

Ⓐ G0325 End stage renal disease (ESRD) related services for home dialysis (less than full month), per day; for patients between two and 11 years of age Ⓐ⊘
MED: 100-2,11,130.1

Ⓐ G0326 End stage renal disease (ESRD) related services for home dialysis (less than full month), per day; for patients between 12 and 19 years of age Ⓐ⊘
MED: 100-2,11,130.1

Ⓐ G0327 End stage renal disease (ESRD) related services for home dialysis (less than full month), per day; for patients 20 years of age and over Ⓐ⊘
MED: 100-2,11,130.1

Ⓐ G0328 Colorectalcancer screening; fecal-occult blood test, immunoassay, 1–3 simultaneous determinations. ⊘
MED: 100-4,18,60.1; 100-4,18,60.2; 100-4,18,60.2.1; 100-4,18,60.6

Ⓐ G0329 Electromagnetic therapy, to one or more areas for chronic Stage III and Stage IV pressure ulcers, arterial ulcers, diabetic ulcers and venous stasis ulcers not demonstrating measurable signs of healing after 30 days of conventional care as part of a therapay plan of care ⊘
MED: 100-4,32,11.2

▲ Ⓢ G0332 Services for intravenous infusion of immunoglobulin prior to administration (this service is to be billed in conjunction with administration of immunoglobulin)

Ⓜ G0333 Pharmacy dispensing fee for inhalation drug(s); initial 30-day supply as a beneficiary

Ⓑ G0337 Hospice evaluation and counseling services, pre-election

Ⓢ G0339 Image guided robotic linear accelerator-based stereotactic radiosurgery, complete course of therapy in one session, or first session of fractionated treatment ⊘

Ⓢ G0340 Image guided robotic linear accelerator-based stereotactic radiosurgery, delivery including collimator changes and custom plugging, fractionated treatment, all lesions, per session, second through fifth sessions, maximum five sessions per course of treatment ⊘

Ⓒ G0341 Percutaneous islet cell transplant, includes portal vein catherization and infusion ⊘
MED: 100-3,260.3; 100-4,32,70

Ⓒ G0342 Laparoscopy for islet cell transplant, includes portal vein catherization and infusion ⊘
MED: 100-3,260.3; 100-4,32,70

Ⓒ G0343 Laparotomy for islet cell transplant, includes portal vein catherization and infusion ⊘
MED: 100-3,260.3; 100-4,32,70

Ⓥ G0344 Initial preventive physical examination; face-to-face visit, services limited to new beneficiary during the first six months of Medicare enrollment ⊘
MED: 100-4,12,30.6.1.1

Ⓣ G0364 Bone marrow aspiration performed with bone marrow biopsy through the same incision on the same date of service

Ⓢ G0365 Vessel mapping of vessels for hemodialysis access (services for preoperative vessel mapping prior to creation of hemodialysis access using an autogenous hemodialysis conduit, including arterial inflow and venous outflow)

Ⓑ G0366 Electrocardiogram, routine ECG with at least 12 leads; with interpretation and report, performed as a component of the initial preventive physical examination
MED: 100-4,12,30.6.1.1

Ⓢ G0367 Tracing only, without interpretation and report, performed as a component of the initial preventive examination ⊘
MED: 100-4,12,30.6.1.1

Ⓜ G0368 Interpretation and report only, performed as a component of the initial preventive examination ⊘
MED: 100-4,12,30.6.1.1

Ⓜ G0372 Physician service required to establish and document the need for a power mobility device ⊘

Ⓧ G0375 Smoking and tobacco use cessation counseling visit; intermediate, greater than 3 minutes up to 10 minutes ⊘
Medicare will cover G0375 and G0376 for a combined total of eight sessions per 12 month period.
MED: 100-4,32,12
AHA: 3Q,'05,9

Ⓧ G0376 Smoking and tobacco use cessation counseling visit; intensive, greater than 10 minutes ⊘
Medicare will cover G0375 and G0376 for a combined total of eight sessions per 12 month period.
MED: 100-4,32,12
AHA: 3Q,'05,9

Ⓠ G0378 Hospital observation service, per hour
MED: 100-2,6,20.5; 100-4,4,290.4.1

Ⓠ G0379 Direct admission of patient for hospital observation care
MED: 100-2,6,20.5; 100-4,4,290.4.1

Special Coverage Instructions   Noncovered by Medicare   Carrier Discretion   ☑ Quality Alert   ● New Code   ○ Reinstated Code   ▲ Revised Code

Procedures/Professional Services (Temporary)

G0380 — G8007

● ☑ **G0380** Level 1 hospital emergency visit provided in a type B department or facility of the hospital (the department or facility must meet at least one of the following requirements: (1) it is licensed by the state in which it is located under applicable state law as an emergency room or emergency department; (2) it is held out to the public (by name, posted signs, advertising, or other means) as a place that provides care for emergency medical conditions on an urgent basis without requiring a previously scheduled appointment; or (3) during the calendar year immediately preceding the calendar year in which a determination under this section is being made, based on a representative sample of patient visits that occurred during that calendar year, it provides at least one-third of all of its outpatient visits for the treatment of emergency medical conditions on an urgent basis without requiring a previously scheduled appointment)

● ☑ **G0381** Level 2 hospital emergency visit provided in a type B department or facility of the hospital (the department or facility must meet at least one of the following requirements: (1) it is licensed by the state in which it is located under applicable state law as an emergency room or emergency department; (2) it is held out to the public (by name, posted signs, advertising, or other means) as a place that provides care for emergency medical conditions on an urgent basis without requiring a previously scheduled appointment; or (3) during the calendar year immediately preceding the calendar year in which a determination under this section is being made, based on a representative sample of patient visits that occurred during that calendar year, it provides at least one-third of all of its outpatient visits for the treatment of emergency medical conditions on an urgent basis without requiring a previously scheduled appointment)

● ☑ **G0382** Level 3 hospital emergency visit provided in a type B department or facility of the hospital (the department or facility must meet at least one of the following requirements: (1) it is licensed by the state in which it is located under applicable state law as an emergency room or emergency department; (2) it is held out to the public (by name, posted signs, advertising, or other means) as a place that provides care for emergency medical conditions on an urgent basis without requiring a previously scheduled appointment; or (3) during the calendar year immediately preceding the calendar year in which a determination under this section is being made, based on a representative sample of patient visits that occurred during that calendar year, it provides at least one-third of all of its outpatient visits for the treatment of emergency medical conditions on an urgent basis without requiring a previously scheduled appointment)

● ☑ **G0383** Level 4 hospital emergency visit provided in a type B department or facility of the hospital (the department or facility must meet at least one of the following requirements: (1) it is licensed by the state in which it is located under applicable state law as an emergency room or emergency department; (2) it is held out to the public (by name, posted signs, advertising, or other means) as a place that provides care for emergency medical conditions on an urgent basis without requiring a previously scheduled appointment; or (3) during the calendar year immediately preceding the calendar year in which a determination under this section is being made, based on a representative sample of patient visits that occurred during that calendar year, it provides at least one-third of all of its outpatient visits for the treatment of emergency medical conditions on an urgent basis without requiring a previously scheduled appointment)

● ☑ **G0384** Level 5 hospital emergency visit provided in a type B department or facility of the hospital (the department or facility must meet at least one of the following requirements: (1) it is licensed by the state in which it is located under applicable state law as an emergency room or emergency department; (2) it is held out to the public (by name, posted signs, advertising, or other means) as a place that provides care for emergency medical conditions on an urgent basis without requiring a previously scheduled appointment; or (3) during the calendar year immediately preceding the calendar year in which a determination under this section is being made, based on a representative sample of patient visits that occurred during that calendar year, it provides at least one-third of all of its outpatient visits for the treatment of emergency medical conditions on an urgent basis without requiring a previously scheduled appointment)

● Ⓢ **G0389** Ultrasound B-scan and/or real time with image documentation; for abdominal aortic aneurysm (AAA) screening

● Ⓢ **G0390** Trauma response team associated with hospital critical care service

● Ⓣ **G0392** Transluminal balloon angioplasty, percutaneous; for maintenance of hemodialysis access, arteriovenous fistula or graft; arterial 🔟

● Ⓣ **G0393** Transluminal balloon angioplasty, percutaneous; for maintenance of hemodialysis access, arteriovenous fistula or graft; venous 🔟

● Ⓐ **G0394** Blood occult test (e.g., guaiac), feces, for single determination for colorectal neoplasm (e.g., patient was provided three cards or single triple card for consecutive collection)

Ⓢ ☑ **G3001** Administration and supply of tositumomab, 450 mg ⊘

PHYSICIAN'S VOLUNTARY REPORTING PROGRAM CODES

HCPCS codes G8006-G8186 are to be used for the physician's voluntary reporting program in which CMS seeks to analyze the quality of care provided to Medicare beneficiaries. Reporting of these codes is voluntary. Physicians should not charge for these codes. Unless otherwise indicated, report these codes in addition to office visit, home visit, nursing facility, and domiciliary evaluation and management codes. For additional information, please visit the following website: http://www.cms.hhs.gov/providers/p4p/

Ⓜ **G8006** Acute myocardial infarction: patient documented to have received aspirin at arrival

Ⓜ **G8007** Acute myocardial infarction: patient not documented to have received aspirin at arrival

Special Coverage Instructions　　　Noncovered by Medicare　　　Carrier Discretion　　　☑ Quality Alert　　　● New Code　　○ Reinstated Code　▲ Revised Code

62 — G Codes　　Ⓐ Age Edit　　Ⓜ Maternity Edit　　♀ Female Only　　♂ Male Only　　Ⓐ - ☑ APC Status Indicators　　***2007 HCPCS***

Ⓜ **G8008** Clinician documented that acute myocardial infarction patient was not an eligible candidate to receive aspirin at arrival measure

▲ Ⓜ **G8009** Acute myocardial infarction: patient documented to have received beta-blocker at arrival

Ⓜ **G8010** Acute myocardial infarction: patient not documented to have received beta-blocker at arrival

▲ Ⓜ **G8011** Clinician documented that acute myocardial infarction patient was not an eligible candidate for beta-blocker at arrival measure

Ⓜ **G8012** Pneumonia: patient documented to have received antibiotic within 4 hours of presentation

Ⓜ **G8013** Pneumonia: patient not documented to have received antibiotic within 4 hours of presentation

Ⓜ **G8014** Clinician documented that pneumonia patient was not an eligible candidate for antibiotic within 4 hours of presentation measure

▲ Ⓜ **G8015** Diabetic patient with most recent hemoglobin A1c level (within the last 6 months) documented as greater than 9%
Report this code in addition to office visit; office consult; home visit; nursing facility; or initial preventive physical exam evaluation and management codes.

▲ Ⓜ **G8016** Diabetic patient with most recent hemoglobin A1c level (within the last 6 months) documented as less than or equal to 9%
Report this code in addition to office visit; home visit; nursing facility; domiciliary; or initial preventive physical exam evaluation and management codes.

▲ Ⓜ **G8017** Clinician documented that diabetic patient was not eligible candidate for hemoglobin A1c measure
Report this code in addition to office visit; home visit; nursing facility; domiciliary; or initial preventive physical exam evaluation and management codes.

▲ Ⓜ **G8018** Clinician has not provided care for the diabetic patient for the required time for hemoglobin A1c measure (6 months)
Report this code in addition to office visit; home visit; nursing facility; domiciliary; or initial preventive physical exam evaluation and management codes.

Ⓜ **G8019** Diabetic patient with most recent low-density lipoprotein (within the last 12 months) documented as greater than or equal to 100 mg/dl

Ⓜ **G8020** Diabetic patient with most recent low-density lipoprotein (within the last 12 months) documented as less than 100 mg/dl

Ⓜ **G8021** Clinician documented that diabetic patient was not eligible candidate for low-density lipoprotein measure

Ⓜ **G8022** Clinician has not provided care for the diabetic patient for the required time for low-density lipoprotein measure (12 months)

▲ Ⓜ **G8023** Diabetic patient with most recent blood pressure (within the last 6 months) documented as equal to or greater than 140 systolic or equal to or greater than 80 mm Hg diastolic

▲ Ⓜ **G8024** Diabetic patient with most recent blood pressure (within the last 6 months) documented less than 140 systolic and less than 80 diastolic

▲ Ⓜ **G8025** Clinician documented that the diabetic patient was not eligible candidate for blood pressure measure

▲ Ⓜ **G8026** Clinician has not provided care for the diabetic patient for the required time for blood measure (within the last 6 months)

Ⓜ **G8027** Heart failure patient with left ventricular systolic dysfunction (LVSD) documented to be on either angiotensin-converting enzyme-inhibitor or angiotensin-receptor blocker (ACE-1 or ARB) therapy

Ⓜ **G8028** Heart failure patient with left ventricular systolic dysfunction (LVSD) not documented to be on either angiotensin-converting enzyme-inhibitor or angiotensin-receptor blocker (ACE-1 or ARB) therapy
Patients with LVEF <\ 40% or with moderately or severely depressed left ventricular systolic function.

Ⓜ **G8029** Clinician documented that heart failure patient was not an eligible candidate for either angiotensin-converting enzyme-inhibitor or angiotensin-receptor blocker (ACE-I or ARB) therapy measure
Patients with LVEF <\ 40% or with moderately or severely depressed left ventricular systolic function.

Ⓜ **G8030** Heart failure patient with left ventricular systolic dysfunction (LVSD) documented to be on beta-blocker therapy
Patients with LVEF <\ 40% or with moderately or severely depressed left ventricular systolic function.

Ⓜ **G8031** Heart failure patient with left ventricular systolic dysfunction (LVSD) not documented to be on beta-blocker therapy
Patients with LVEF <\ 40% or with moderately or severely depressed left ventricular systolic function.

Ⓜ **G8032** Clinician documented that heart failure patient was not eligible candidate for beta-blocker therapy measure
Patients with LVEF <\ 40% or with moderately or severely depressed left ventricular systolic function.

Ⓜ **G8033** Prior myocardial infarction—coronary artery disease patient documented to be on beta-blocker therapy

Ⓜ **G8034** Prior myocardial infarction—coronary artery disease patient not documented to be on beta-blocker therapy

▲ Ⓜ **G8035** Clinician documented that prior myocardial infarction—coronary artery disease patient was not eligible candidate for beta-blocker therapy measure or the patient had no prior myocardial infarction

Ⓜ **G8036** Coronary artery disease patient documented to be on antiplatelet therapy

Ⓜ **G8037** Coronary artery disease patient not documented to be on antiplatelet therapy

Ⓜ **G8038** Clinician documented that coronary artery disease patient was not eligible candidate for antiplatelet therapy measure

Ⓜ **G8039** Coronary artery disease—patient with low-density lipoprotein documented to be greater than 100 mg/dl

Ⓜ **G8040** Coronary artery disease—patient with low-density lipoprotein documented to be less than or equal to 100 mg/dl

Ⓜ **G8041** Clinician documented that coronary artery disease patient was not eligible candidate for low-density lipoprotein measure

Ⓜ **G8051** Patient (female) documented to have been assessed for osteoporosis
This code is for female patients age 75 years or older.

Ⓜ **G8052** Patient (female) not documented to have been assessed for osteoporosis
This code is for female patients age 75 years or older.

Special Coverage Instructions   Noncovered by Medicare   Carrier Discretion   ☑ Quality Alert   ● New Code   ○ Reinstated Code   ▲ Revised Code

Ⓜ **G8053** Clinician documented that (female) patient was not an eligible candidate for osteoporosis assessment measure

This code is for female patients age 75 years or older.

Ⓜ **G8054** Patient not documented for the assessment of falls within last 12 months
Report this code in addition to office visit; office consult; home visit; nursing facility; or initial preventive physical exam evaluation and management code. This code is for patients age 75 years or older.

Ⓜ **G8055** Patient documented for the assessment of falls within last 12 months
Report this code in addition to office visit; office consult; home visit; nursing facility; or initial preventive physical exam evaluation and management code. This code is for patients age 75 years or older.

Ⓜ **G8056** Clinician documented that patient was not an eligible candidate for the falls assessment measure within the last 12 months
Report this code in addition to office visit; office consult; home visit; nursing facility; or initial preventive physical exam evaluation and management code. This code is for patients age 75 years or older.

Ⓜ **G8057** Patient documented to have received hearing assessment
Report this code in addition to office visit; office consult; home visit; nursing facility; or initial preventive physical exam evaluation and management code. This code is for patients age 75 years or older.

Ⓜ **G8058** Patient not documented to have received hearing assessment
Report this code in addition to office visit; office consult; home visit; nursing facility; or initial preventive physical exam evaluation and management code. This code is for patients age 75 years or older.

Ⓜ **G8059** Clinician documented that patient was not an eligible candidate for hearing assessment measure
Report this code in addition to office visit; office consult; home visit; nursing facility; or initial preventive physical exam evaluation and management code. This code is for patients age 75 years or older.

Ⓜ **G8060** Patient documented for the assessment of urinary incontinence
Report this code in addition to office visit; office consult; home visit; nursing facility; or initial preventive physical exam evaluation and management code. This code is for patients age 75 years or older.

Ⓜ **G8061** Patient not documented for the assessment of urinary incontinence
Report this code in addition to office visit; office consult; home visit; nursing facility; or initial preventive physical exam evaluation and management code. This code is for patients age 75 years or older.

Ⓜ **G8062** Clinician documented that patient was not an eligible candidate for urinary incontinence assessment measure

Report this code in addition to office visit; office consult; home visit; nursing facility; or initial preventive physical exam evaluation and management code. This code is for patients age 75 years or older.

Ⓜ **G8075** End-stage renal disease patient with documented dialysis dose of URR greater than or equal to 65% (or Kt/V greater than or equal to 1.2)
Use with codes G0308-G0327, 90945, 90947.

Ⓜ **G8076** End-stage renal disease patient with documented dialysis dose of URR less than 65% (or Kt/V less than 1.2)
Use with codes G0308-G0327, 90945, 90947.

Ⓜ **G8077** Clinician documented that end-stage renal disease patient was not eligible candidate for URR or Kt/V measure
Use with codes G0308-G0327, 90945, 90947.

Ⓜ **G8078** End-stage renal disease patient with documented hematocrit greater than or equal to 33 (or hemoglobin greater than or equal to 11)
Use with codes G0308-G0327, 90945, 90947.

Ⓜ **G8079** End-stage renal disease patient with documented hematocrit less than 33 (or hemoglobin less than 11)
Use with codes G0308-G0327, 90945, 90947.

Ⓜ **G8080** Clinician documented that end-stage renal disease patient was not eligible candidate for hematocrit (hemoglobin) measure
Use with codes G0308-G0327, 90945, 90947.

Ⓜ **G8081** End-stage renal disease patient requiring hemodialysis vascular access documented to have received autogenous AV fistula
Use with codes G0308-G0327, 90945, 90947, 36818-36812, 36825.

Ⓜ **G8082** End-stage renal disease patient requiring hemodialysis documented to have received vascular access other than autogenous AV fistula
Use with codes G0308-G0327, 90945, 90947, 36818-36812, 36825.

Ⓜ **G8085** End-stage renal disease patient requiring hemodialysis vascular access was not an eligible candidate for autogenous AV fistula

Ⓜ **G8093** Newly diagnosed chronic obstructive pulmonary disease (COPD) patient documented to have received smoking cessation intervention, within 3 months of diagnosis

Report this code in addition to office visit; office consult; home visit; nursing facility; evaluation and management codes and smoking and tobacco use cessation counseling codes.

Ⓜ **G8094** Newly diagnosed chronic obstructive pulmonary disease (COPD) patient not documented to have received smoking cessation intervention, within 3 months of diagnosis
Report this code in addition to office visit; office consult; home visit; nursing facility; evaluation and management codes and smoking and toba

Ⓜ **G8099** Osteoporosis patient documented to have been prescribed calcium and vitamin D supplements

Ⓜ **G8100** Clinician documented that osteoporosis patient was not eligible candidate for calcium and vitamin D supplement measure

Ⓜ **G8103** Newly diagnosed osteoporosis patients documented to have been treated with antiresorptive therapy and/or PTH within three months of diagnosis

Ⓜ **G8104** Clinician documented that newly diagnosed osteoporosis patient was not an eligible candidate for antiresorptive therapy and/or PTH treatment measure within three months of diagnosis

Ⓜ **G8106** Within 6 months of suffering a nontraumatic fracture, female patient 65 years of age or older documented to have undergone bone mineral density testing or to have been prescribed a drug to treat or prevent osteoporosis

---

Special Coverage Instructions   Noncovered by Medicare   Carrier Discretion   ☑ Quality Alert   ● New Code   ○ Reinstated Code ▲ Revised Code

64 — G Codes   Ⓐ Age Edit   Ⓜ Maternity Edit   ♀ Female Only   ♂ Male Only   Ⓐ - Ⓨ APC Status Indicators   *2007 HCPCS*

Ⓜ   **G8107**   Clinician documented that female patient 65 years of age or older who suffered a nontraumatic fracture within the last 6 months was not an eligible candidate for measure to test bone mineral density or drug to treat or prevent osteoporosis

Ⓜ   **G8108**   Patient documented to have received influenza vaccination during influenza season
Use this code for patients age 50 years and older.

Ⓜ   **G8109**   Patient not documented to have received influenza vaccination during influenza season
Report this code in addition to office visit; office consult; nursing facility; domiciliary evaluation and management codes and influenza vaccine administration code. Use this code for patients age 50 years and older.

Ⓜ   **G8110**   Clinician documented that patient was not an eligible candidate for influenza vaccination measure
Report this code in addition to office visit; office consult; nursing facility; domiciliary evaluation and management codes and influenza vaccine administration code. Use this code for patients age 50 years and older.

Ⓜ   **G8111**   Patient (female) documented to have received a mammogram during the measurement year or prior year to the measurement year
Report this code in addition to office visit; office consult; home visit; nursing facility; domiciliary or initial preventive physical exam evaluation and management codes. Use this code for patients age 40 years and older.

Ⓜ   **G8112**   Patient (female) not documented to have received a mammogram during the measurement year or prior year to the measurement year
Report this code in addition to office visit; office consult; home visit; nursing facility; domiciliary or initial preventive physical exam evaluation and management codes. Use this code for patients age 40 years and older.

Ⓜ   **G8113**   Clinician documented that female patient was not an eligible candidate for mammography measure
Report this code in addition to office visit; office consult; home visit; nursing facility; domiciliary or initial preventive physical exam evaluation and management codes. Use this code for patients age 40 years and older.

Ⓜ   **G8114**   Clinician did not provide care to patient for the required time of mammography measure (i.e., measurement year or prior year)
Report this code in addition to office visit; office consult; home visit; nursing facility; domiciliary or initial preventive physical exam evaluation and management codes. Use this code for patients age 40 years and older.

Ⓜ   **G8115**   Patient documented to have received pneumococcal vaccination
Report this code in addition to office visit; office consult; home visit; nursing facility; domiciliary or initial preventive physical exam evaluation and management codes, and pneumococcal vaccination administration codes. Use this code for patients age 65 years and over.

Ⓜ   **G8116**   Patient not documented to have received pneumococcal vaccination
Report this code in addition to office visit; office consult; home visit; nursing facility; domiciliary or initial preventive physical exam evaluation and management codes, and pneumococcal vaccination administration codes. Use this code for patients age 65 years and over.

Ⓜ   **G8117**   Clinician documented that patient was not eligible candidate for pneumococcal vaccination measure
Report this code in addition to office visit; office consult; home visit; nursing facility; domiciliary or initial preventive physical exam evaluation and management codes, and pneumococcal vaccination administration codes. Use this code for patients age 65 years and over.

Ⓜ   **G8126**   Patient documented as being treated with antidepressant medication during the entire 12 week acute treatment phase
Report this code in addition to office visit and psychiatry evaluation and management codes. Use this code for patients age 18 and older.

Ⓜ   **G8127**   Patient not documented as being treated with antidepressant medication during the entire 12 week acute treatment phase
Report this code in addition to office visit and psychiatry evaluation and management codes. Use this code for patients age 18 and older.

▲ Ⓜ   **G8128**   Patient was not treated with antidepressant medication or was not an eligible candidate for completion of the entire 12 week acute treatment phase measure
Report this code in addition to office visit and psychiatry evaluation and management codes. Use this code for patients age 18 and older.

Ⓜ   **G8129**   Patient documented as being treated with antidepressant medication for at least 6 months continuous treatment phase
Report this code in addition to office visit and psychiatry evaluation and management codes. Use this code for patients age 18 and older.

Ⓜ   **G8130**   Patient not documented as being treated with antidepressant medication for at least 6 months continuous treatment phase
Report this code in addition to office visit and psychiatry evaluation and management codes. Use this code for patients age 18 and older.

Ⓜ   **G8131**   Clinician documented that patient was not an eligible candidate for antidepressant medication for continuous treatment phase
Report this code in addition to office visit and psychiatry evaluation and management codes. Use this code for patients age 18 and older.

▲ Ⓜ   **G8152**   Patient documented to have received antibiotic prophylaxis one hour prior to incision time (two hours for vancomycin)

▲ Ⓜ   **G8153**   Patient not documented to have received antibiotic prophylaxis one hour prior to incision time (two hours for vancomycin)

▲ Ⓜ   **G8154**   Clinician documented that patient was not an eligible candidate for antibiotic prophylaxis one hour prior to incision time (two hours for vancomycin) measure

Ⓜ   **G8155**   Patient with documented receipt of thromboembolism prophylaxis

Ⓜ   **G8156**   Patient without documented receipt of thromboembolism prophylaxis

Ⓜ   **G8157**   Clinician documented that patient was not an eligible candidate for thromboembolism prophylaxis measure

Ⓜ   **G8158**   Patient documented to have received coronary artery bypass graft with use of internal mammary artery
Report this code in addition to CPT codes 33533-33536.

Special Coverage Instructions   Noncovered by Medicare   Carrier Discretion   ☑ Quality Alert   ● New Code   ○ Reinstated Code   ▲ Revised Code

2007 HCPCS   🔟-🟨 ASC Group   MED: Pub 100/NCD References   ᕇ DMEPOS Paid   ⊘ SNF Excluded   G Codes — 65

Procedures/Professional Services (Temporary)

G8159 — G8208

Ⓜ **G8159** Patient documented to have received coronary artery bypass graft without use of internal mammary artery

Report this code in addition to CPT codes 33533-33536.

Ⓜ **G8160** Clinician documented that patient was not an eligible candidate for coronary artery bypass graft with use of internal mammary artery measure
Report this code in addition to CPT codes 33533-33536.

Ⓜ **G8161** Patient with isolated coronary artery bypass graft documented to have received pre-operative beta-blockade
Report this code in addition to CPT codes 33510-33514, 33516, and 33533-33536.

Ⓜ **G8162** Patient with isolated coronary artery bypass graft not documented to have received pre-operative beta-blockade
Report this code in addition to CPT codes 33510-33514, 33516, and 33533-33536.

Ⓜ **G8163** Clinician documented that patient with isolated coronary artery bypass graft was not an eligible candidate for pre-operative beta-blockade measure
Report this code in addition to CPT codes 33510-33514, 33516, and 33533-33536.

Ⓜ **G8164** Patient with isolated coronary artery bypass graft documented to have prolonged intubation
Report this code in addition to CPT codes 33510-33514, 33516, and 33533-33536.

Ⓜ **G8165** Patient with isolated coronary artery bypass graft not documented to have prolonged intubation
Report this code in addition to CPT codes 33510-33514, 33516, and 33533-33536.

Ⓜ **G8166** Patient with isolated coronary artery bypass graft documented to have required surgical re-exploration

Report this code in addition to CPT codes 33510-33514, 33516, and 33533-33536.

Ⓜ **G8167** Patient with isolated coronary artery bypass graft did not require surgical re-exploration
Report this code in addition to CPT codes 33510-33514, 33516, and 33533-33536.

Ⓜ **G8170** Patient with isolated coronary artery bypass graft documented to have been discharged on aspirin or clopidogrel

Ⓜ **G8171** Patient with isolated coronary artery bypass graft not documented to have been discharged on aspirin or clopidogrel

Ⓜ **G8172** Clinician documented that patient with isolated coronary artery bypass graft was not an eligible cadidate for antiplatelet therapy at discharge measure

Ⓜ **G8182** Clinician has not provided care for the cardiac patient for the required time for low-density lipoprotein measure (6 months)

Ⓜ **G8183** Patient with heart failure and atrial fibrillation documented to be on Warfarin therapy

Ⓜ **G8184** Clinician documented that patient with heart failure and atrial fibrillation was not an eligible candidate for Warfarin therapy measure

Ⓜ **G8185** Patient diagnosed with symptomatic osteoarthritis with documented annual assessment of function and pain

Ⓜ **G8186** Clinician documented that symptomatic osteoarthritis patient was not an eligible candidate for annual assessment of function and pain measure

LAST MINUTE CODE ADDITIONS

CMS released codes G8191-G8347 at the last minute. Some of the codes are duplicates and we have no other information about the codes or how they should be used. We will publish updated information on our Website when we receive it from CMS. Clients who have purchased updateable HCPCS books will receive new pages in the next update.

● **G8191** Clinician documented to have given order for prophylactic antibiotic to be given within one hour (if vancomycin, two hours) prior to surgical incision (or start of procedure when no incision is required)

● **G8192** Clinician documented to have given the prophylactic antibiotic within one hour (if vancomycin, two hours) prior to the surgical incision (or start of procedure when no incision is required)

● **G8193** Clinician did not document that an order for prophylactic antibiotic to be given within one hour (if vancomycin, two hours) prior to surgical incision (or start of procedure when no incision is required) was given

● **G8194** Clinician documented that Patient was not an eligible candidate for prophylactic antibiotic

● **G8195** Clinician documented to have given the prophylactic antibiotic within one hour (if vancomycin, two hours) prior to the surgical incision (or start of procedure when no incision is required)

● **G8196** Clinician did not document a prophylactic antibiotic was administered within one hour (if vancomycin, two hours) prior to surgical incision (or start of procedure when no incision is required)

● **G8197** Patient documented to have order for prophylactic antibiotic to be given within one hour (if vancomycin, two hours) prior to surgical incision (or start of procedure when no incision is required)

● **G8198** Patient documented to have order for cefazolin or cefuroxime for antimicrobial prophylaxis

● **G8199** Clinician documented to have given cefazolin or cefuroxime for antimicrobial prophylaxis

● **G8200** Order for cefazolin or cefuroxime for antimicrobial prophylaxis not documented

● **G8201** Patient was not an eligible candidate for cefazolin or cefuroxime for antimicrobial prophylaxis

● **G8202** Clinician documented an order was given to discontinue prophylactic antibiotics within 24 hours of surgical end time

● **G8203** Clinician documented that prophylactic antibiotics were discontinued within 24 hours of surgical end time

● **G8204** Clinician did not document an order was given to discontinue prophylactic antibiotics within 24 hours of surgical end time

● **G8205** Clinician documented that patient was not an eligible candidate for prophylactic antibiotic discontinuation within 24 hours of surgical end time

● **G8206** Clinician documented that prophylactic antibiotic was given

● **G8207** Clinician documented an order was given to discontinue prophylactic antibiotics within 48 hours of surgical end time

● **G8208** Clinician documented that prophylactic antibiotics were discontinued within 48 hours of surgical end time

---

Special Coverage Instructions | Noncovered by Medicare | Carrier Discretion | ☑ Quality Alert   ● New Code   ○ Reinstated Code   ▲ Revised Code

66 — G Codes   Ⓐ Age Edit   Ⓜ Maternity Edit   ♀ Female Only   ♂ Male Only   Ⓐ - Ⓨ APC Status Indicators   *2007 HCPCS*

- **G8209** Clinician did not document an order was given to discontinue prophylactic antibiotics within 48 hours of surgical end time

- **G8210** Clinician documented Patient was not an eligible candidate for discontinuation of prophylactic antibiotic discontinuation within 48 hours of surgical end time

- **G8211** Clinician documented that prophylactic antibiotic was given

- **G8212** Clinician documented an order was given for appropriate venous thromboembolism (VTE) prophylaxis to be given within 24 hrs prior to incision time or 24 hours after surgery end time

- **G8213** Clinician documented to have given VTE prophylaxis within 24 hrs prior to incision time or 24 hours after surgery end time

- **G8214** Clinician did not document an order was given for appropriate venous thromboembolism (VTE) prophylaxis to be given within 24 hrs prior to incision time or 24 hours after surgery end time

- **G8215** Clinician documented that Patient was not an eligible candidate for venous thromboembolism (VTE) prophylaxis to be given within 24 hours prior to incision time or 24 hours after surgery end time

- **G8216** Patient documented to have received DVT prophylaxis by end of hospital day two

- **G8217** Patient not documented to have received DVT prophylaxis by end of hospital day 2

- **G8218** Patient was not an eligible candidate for DVT prophylaxis by end of hospital day 2, including physician documentation that Patient is ambulatory

- **G8219** Patient documented to have received DVT prophylaxis by end of hospital day 2

- **G8220** Patient not documented to have received DVT prophylaxis by end of hospital day 2

- **G8221** Clinician documented that patient was not an eligible candidate for DVT prophylaxis by the end of hospital day 2, including physician documentation that patient is ambulatory

- **G8222** Patient documented to have been prescribed antiplatelet therapy at discharge

- **G8223** Patient not documented to have received prescription for antiplatelet therapy at discharge

- **G8224** Clinician documented that patient was not an eligible candidate for antiplatelet therapy at discharge, including identification from medical record that patient is on anticoagulation therapy

- **G8225** Patient documented to have been prescribed an anticoagulant at discharge

- **G8226** Patient not documented to have received prescription for anticoagulant therapy at discharge

- **G8227** Patient not documented to have permanent, persistent, or paroxysmal atrial fibrillation

- **G8228** Clinician documented that patient was not an eligible candidate for anticoagulant therapy at discharge

- **G8229** Patient documented to have been administered or considered for TPA

- **G8230** Patient not eligible for TPA administration, ischemic stroke symptom onset of more than 3 hours

- **G8231** Patient not documented to have received TPA or not documented to have been considered a candidate for TPA administration

- **G8232** Patient documented to have received dysphagia screening prior to taking any foods, fluids or medication by mouth

- **G8234** Patient not documented to have received dysphagia screening

- **G8235** Patient not receiving or ineligible to receive food, fluids or medication by mouth, or documentation of NPO (nothing by mouth) order

- **G8236** Clinician documented that patient was not an eligible candidate for dysphagia screening prior to taking any foods, fluids or medication by mouth

- **G8237** Patient documented to have received order for rehabilitation services or documentation of consideration for rehabilitation services

- **G8238** Patient not documented to have received order for or consideration for rehabilitation services

- **G8239** Internal carotid stenosis patient below 30%, reference to measurements of distal internal carotid diameter as the denominator for stenosis measurement not necessary

- **G8240** Internal carotid stenosis patient in the 30-99% range, and no documentation of reference to measurements of distal internal carotid diameter as the denominator for stenosis measurement

- **G8241** Clinician documented that patient whose final report of the carotid imaging study performed (neck MRA, neck CTA, neck duplex ultrasound, carotid angiogram), with characterization of an internal carotid stenosis in the 30-99% range, was not an eligible candidate for reference to measurements of distal internal carotid diameter as the denominator for stenosis measurement

- **G8242** Patient documented to have received CT or MRI with presence or absence of hemorrhage, mass lesion and acute infarction documented in the final report

- **G8243** Patient not documented to have received CT or MRI and the presence or absence of hemorrhage, mass lesion and acute infarction not documented in the final report

- **G8245** Clinician documented presence or absence alarm symptoms

- **G8246** Patient was not an eligible candidate for medical history review with assessment of new or changing moles

- **G8247** Patient with alarm symptom(s) documented to have had upper endoscopy performed or referral for upper endoscopy

- **G8248** Patient with at least one alarm symptom not documented to have had upper endoscopy or referral for upper endoscopy

- **G8249** Clinician documented that patient was not an eligible candidate for upper endoscopy

- **G8250** Patient with suspicion of Barrett's esophagus in endoscopy report and documented to have received an esophageal biopsy

- **G8251** Patient not documented to have received an esophageal biopsy when suspicion of Barrett's esophagus is indicated in the endoscopy report

- **G8252** Clinician documented that patient was not an eligible candidate for esophageal biopsy

- **G8253** Patient documented to have received an order for a barium swallow test

- **G8254** Patient with no documentation order for barium swallow test

---

Special Coverage Instructions   Noncovered by Medicare   Carrier Discretion   ☑ Quality Alert   ● New Code   ○ Reinstated Code   ▲ Revised Code

2007 HCPCS   ▮-▮ ASC Group   **MED:** Pub 100/NCD References   ᚑ DMEPOS Paid   ⊘ SNF Excluded   **G Codes — 67**

- G8255 Clinician documentation that patient was an eligible candidate for barium swallow test
- G8256 Clinician documented reconciliation of discharge medications with current medication list in medical record
- G8257 Clinician has not documented reconciliation of discharge medications with current medication list in medical record
- G8258 Patient was not an eligible candidate for discharge medications review
- G8259 Patient documented to have surrogate decision maker or advance care plan in medical record
- G8260 Patient not documented to have surrogate decision maker or advance care plan in medical record
- G8261 Clinician documented that patient was not an eligible candidate for surrogate decision maker or advance care plan
- G8262 Patient documented to have been assessed for presence or absence of urinary incontinence
- G8263 Patient not documented to have been assessed for presence or absence of urinary incontinence
- G8264 Clinician documented that patient was not an eligible candidate for an assessment of the presence or absence of urinary incontinence
- G8265 Patient documented to have received characterization of urinary incontinence
- G8266 Patient not documented to have received characterization of urinary incontinence
- G8267 Patient documented to have received a plan of care for urinary incontinence
- G8268 Patient not documented to have received plan of care for urinary incontinence
- G8269 Clinician has not provided care for the patient for the required time to develop plan of care for urinary incontinence
- G8270 Patient documented to have received screening for fall risk (2 or more falls in the past year or any fall with injury in the past year)
- G8271 Patient with no documentation of screening for fall risks (2 or more falls in the past year or any fall with injury in the past year)
- G8272 Clinician documentation that patient was not an eligible candidate for fall risk screening
- G8273 Clinician has not provided care for the patient for the required time to screen for fall risk
- G8274 Clinician has not documented presence or absence of alarm symptoms
- G8275 Patient documented to have medical history taken which included assessment of new or changing moles
- G8276 Patient not documented to have received medical history with assessment of new or changing moles
- G8277 Patient was not an eligible candidate for medical history review with assessment of new or changing moles
- G8278 Patient documented to have received complete physical skin exam
- G8279 Patient not documented to have received a complete physical skin exam
- G8280 Patient was not an eligible candidate for complete physical skin exam during the reporting year

- G8281 Patient documented to have received counseling to perform a self-examination
- G8282 Patient not documented to have received counseling to perform a self-examination
- G8283 Patient was not an eligible candidate for counseling to perform self-examination
- G8284 Patient documented to have received a prescription for pharmacologic therapy for osteoporosis
- G8285 Patient not documented to have received pharmacologic therapy
- G8286 Clinician documented that patient was not an eligible candidate for pharmacologic therapy
- G8287 Clinician has not provided care for the patient for the required time for the pharmacologic therapy measure
- G8288 Patient documented to have received calcium and vitamin D or counseling on both calcium and vitamin D use, and exercise
- G8289 Patient with no documentation of calcium and vitamin D use or counseling regarding both calcium and vitamin D use, or exercise
- G8290 Clinician documentation that patient was not an eligible candidate for calcium and vitamin D, and exercise during the reporting year
- G8291 Clinician has not provided care for the patient for the required time for the calcium, vitamin D, and exercise measure
- G8292 COPD patient with spirometry results documented
- G8293 COPD patient without spirometry results documented
- G8294 COPD patient was not eligible for spirometry results
- G8295 COPD patient documented to have received inhaled bronchodilator therapy
- G8296 COPD patient not documented to have inhaled bronchodilator therapy prescribed
- G8297 COPD patient was not eligible for inhaled bronchodilator therapy
- G8298 Patient documented to have received optic nerve head evaluation
- G8299 Patient not documented to have received optic nerve head evaluation
- G8300 Clinician documented that patient was not an eligible candidate for optic nerve head evaluation during the reporting year
- G8301 Clinician has not provided care for the primary open-angle glaucoma patient for the required time for optic nerve head evaluation measure
- G8302 Patient documented to have a specific target intraocular pressure range goal
- G8303 Patient not documented to have a specific target intraocular pressure range goal
- G8304 Clinician documented that patient was not an eligible candidate for a specific target intraocular pressure range goal
- G8305 Clinician has not provided care for the primary open-angle glaucoma patient for the required time for treatment range goal documentation measurement
- G8306 Primary open-angle glaucoma patient with intraocular pressure above the target range goal documented to have received plan of care

Special Coverage Instructions   Noncovered by Medicare   Carrier Discretion   ☑ Quality Alert   ● New Code   ○ Reinstated Code   ▲ Revised Code

68 — G Codes   Ⓐ Age Edit   Ⓜ Maternity Edit   ♀ Female Only   ♂ Male Only   Ⓐ - ☑ APC Status Indicators   *2007 HCPCS*

- G8307 Primary open-angle glaucoma patient with intraocular pressure at or below goal, no plan of care necessary

- G8308 Primary open-angle glaucoma patient with intraocular pressure above the target range goal, and not documented to have received plan of care during the reporting year

- G8309 Patient documented to have been prescribed/recommended antioxidant vitamin or mineral supplement

- G8310 Patient not documented to have been prescribed/recommended at least one antioxidant vitamin or mineral supplement during the reporting year

- G8311 Clinician documentation that patient was not an eligible candidate for antioxidant vitamin or mineral supplement during the reporting year

- G8312 Clinician has not provided care for the age-related macular degeneration patient for the required time for antioxidant supplement prescription/recommended measure

- G8313 Patient documented to have received macular exam, including documentation of the presence or absence of macular thickening or hemorrhage and the Level of macular degeneration severity

- G8314 Patient not documented to have received macular exam with documentation of presence or absence of macular thickening or hemorrhage and no documentation of Level of macular degeneration severity

- G8315 Clinician documentation that patient was not an eligible candidate for macular examination during the reporting year

- G8316 Clinician has not provided care for the age-related macular degeneration patient for the required time for macular examination measurement

- G8317 Patient documented to have visual functional status assessed

- G8318 Patient documented not to have visual functional status assessed

- G8319 Clinician documented that patient was not an eligible candidate for assessment of visual functional status

- G8320 Clinician has not provided care for the cataract patient for the required time for assessment of visual functional status measurement

- G8321 Patient documented to have had pre-surgical axial length, corneal power measurement and method of intraocular lens power calculation

- G8322 Patient not documented to have had pre-surgical axial length, corneal power measurement and method of intraocular lens power calculation

- G8323 Clinician documentation that patient was not an eligible candidate for pre-surgical axial length, corneal power measurement and method of intraocular lens power calculation

- G8324 Clinician has not provided care for the cataract patient for the required time for pre-surgical measurement and intraocular lens power calculation measure

- G8325 Patient documented to have received fundus evaluation within six months prior to cataract surgery

- G8326 Patient not documented to have received fundus evaluation within six months prior to cataract surgery

- G8327 Patient was not an eligible candidate for pre-surgical fundus evaluation

- G8328 Clinician has not provided care for the cataract patient for the required time for fundus evaluation measurement

- G8329 Patient documented to have received dilated macular or fundus exam with level of severity of retinopathy and the presence or absence of macular edema documented

- G8330 Patient not documented to have received dilated macular or fundus exam with level of severity of retinopathy and the presence or absence of macular edema not documented

- G8331 Clinician documentation that patient was not an eligible candidate for dilated macular or fundus exam during the reporting year

- G8332 Clinician has not provided care for the diabetic retinopathy patient for the required time for macular edema and retinopathy measurement

- G8333 Patient documented to have had findings of macular or fundus exam communicated to the physician managing the diabetes care

- G8334 Documentation of findings of macular or fundus exam not communicated to the physician managing the patient's ongoing diabetes care

- G8335 Clinician documentation that patient was not an eligible candidate for the findings of their macular or fundus exam being communicated to the physician managing their diabetes care during the reporting year

- G8336 Clinician has not provided care for the diabetic retinopathy patient for the required time for physician communication measurement

- G8337 Clinician documented that communication was sent to the physician managing ongoing care of patient that a fracture occurred and that the patient was or should be tested or treated for osteoporosis

- G8338 Clinician has not documented that communication was sent to the physician managing ongoing care of patient that a fracture occurred and that the patient was or should be tested or treated for osteoporosis

- G8339 Patient was not an eligible candidate for communication with the physician managing the patient's ongoing care that a fracture occurred and that the patient was or should be tested or treated for osteoporosis

- G8340 Patient documented to have had central DEXA performed and results documented or central DEXA ordered or pharmacologic therapy prescribed

- G8341 Patient not documented to have had central DEXA measurement or pharmacologic therapy

- G8342 Clinician documented that patient was not an eligible candidate for central DEXA measurement or prescribing pharmacologic

- G8343 Clinician has not provided care for the patient for the required time for central DEXA measurement or pharmacological therapy measure

- G8344 Patient documented to have had central DEXA ordered or performed and results documented or pharmacological therapy prescribed

- G8345 Patient not documented to have had central DEXA measurement ordered or performed or pharmacologic therapy

- G8346 Clinician documented that patient was not an eligible candidate for central DEXA measurement or pharmacologic therapy

Special Coverage Instructions   Noncovered by Medicare   Carrier Discretion   ☑ Quality Alert   ● New Code   ○ Reinstated Code   ▲ Revised Code

2007 HCPCS   ∎-❾ ASC Group   **MED:** Pub 100/NCD References   ᕃ DMEPOS Paid   ⊘ SNF Excluded   **G Codes — 69**

● G8347 Clinician has not provided care for the patient for the required time for central DEXA measurement or pharmacological therapy measure

B G9001 Coordinated care fee, initial rate ⊘

B G9002 Coordinated care fee, maintenance rate ⊘

B G9003 Coordinated care fee, risk adjusted high, initial ⊘

B G9004 Coordinated care fee, risk adjusted low, initial ⊘

B G9005 Coordinated care fee, risk adjusted maintenance ⊘

B G9006 Coordinated care fee, home monitoring ⊘

B G9007 Coordinated care fee, schedule team conference ⊘

B G9008 Coordinated care fee, physician coordinated care oversight services ⊘

B G9009 Coordinated care fee, risk adjusted maintenance, Level 3 ⊘

B G9010 Coordinated care fee, risk adjusted maintenance, Level 4 ⊘

B G9011 Coordinated care fee, risk adjusted maintenance, Level 5 ⊘

B G9012 Coordinated care fee, risk adjusted maintenance, other specified care management ⊘

E G9013 ESRD demo basic bundle Level I

E G9014 ESRD demo expanded bundle including venous access and related services

E G9016 Smoking cessation counseling, individual, in the absence of or in addition to any other evaluation and management service, per session (6–10 minutes) [demonstration project code only] ⊘

A G9017 Amantadine HCl, oral, generic name, 100 mg (for use in a Medicare-approved demonstration project)

A G9018 Zanamivir, inhalation powder, administered through inhaler, generic, 10 mg (for use in a Medicare-approved demonstration project)
This code was developed in anticipation of a generic drug.

A G9019 Oseltamivir phosphate, oral, generic, 75 mg (for use in a Medicare-approved demonstration project)
This code was developed in anticipation of a generic drug.

A G9020 Rimantadine HCl, oral, generic, 100 mg (for use in a Medicare-approved demonstration project)

A G9033 Amantadine HCl, oral, brand name, 100 mg (for use in a Medicare-approved demonstration project)

A G9034 Zanamivir, inhalation powder, administered through inhaler, brand name, 10 mg (for use in a Medicare-approved demonstration project)

A G9035 Oseltamivir phosphate, oral, brand name, 75 mg (for use in a Medicare-approved demonstration project)

A G9036 Rimantadine HCl, oral, brand name, 100 mg (for use in a Medicare-approved demonstration project)

▲ A G9041 Low vision rehabilitation services, qualified occupational therapist, direct face-to-face one-on one, each 15 minutes

▲ A G9042 Low vision rehabilitation services, certified orientation and mobility specialist, direct face-to-face one-on-one, each 15 minutes

▲ A G9043 Low vision rehabilitation services, certified low vision therapist, direct face-to-face one-on-one, each 15 minutes

▲ A G9044 Low vision rehabilitation services, qualified rehabilitation teacher, direct face-to-face one-on-one, each 15 minutes

M G9050 Oncology; primary focus of visit; work-up, evaluation, or staging at the time of cancer diagnosis or recurrence (for use in a Medicare-approved demonstration project

M G9051 Oncology; primary focus of visit; treatment decision-making after disease is staged or restaged, discussion of treatment options, supervsing/coordinating active cancer directed therapy or managing consequences of cancer directed therapy (for use in a Medicare-approved demonstration project)

M G9052 Oncology; primary focus of visit; surveillance for disease recurrence for patient who has completed definitive cancer-directed therapy and currently lacks evidence of recurrent disease; cancer directed therapy might be considered in the future (for use in a Medicare-approved demonstration project)

M G9053 Oncology; primary focus of visit; expectant management of patient with evidence of cancer for whom no cancer directed therapy is being administered or arranged at present; cancer directed therapy might be considered in the future (for use in a Medicare-approved demonstration project)

M G9054 Oncology; primary focus of visit; supervising, coordinating or managing care of patient with terminal cancer or for whom other medical illness prevents further cancer treatment; includes symptom management, end-of-life care planning, management of palliative therapies (for use in a Medicare-approved demonstration project)

M G9055 Oncology; primary focus of visit; other, unspecified service not otherwise listed (for use in a Medicare-approved demonstration project)

M G9056 Oncology; practice guidelines; management adheres to guidelines (for use in a Medicare-approved demonstration project)

M G9057 Oncolocy; practice guidelines; management differs from guidelines as a result of patient enrollment in an institutional review board approved clinical trial (for use in a Medicare-approved demonstration project)

M G9058 Oncology; practice guidelines; management differs from guidelines because the treating physician disagrees with guideline recommendations (for use in a Medicare-approved demonstration project)

M G9059 Oncology; practice guidelines; management differs from guidelines because the patient, after being offered treatment consistent with guidelines, has opted for alternative treatment or management, including no treatment (for use in a Medicare-approved demonstration project)

M G9060 Oncology; practice guidelines; management differs from guidelines for reason(s) associated with patient comorbid illness or performance status not factored into guidelines (for use in a Medicare-approved demonstration project)

M G9061 Oncology; practice guidelines; patient's condition not addressed by available guidelines (for use in a Medicare-approved demonstration project)

M G9062 Oncology; practice guidelines; management differs from guidelines for other reason(s) not listed (for use in a Medicare-approved demonstration project)

Special Coverage Instructions   Noncovered by Medicare   Carrier Discretion   ☑ Quality Alert   ● New Code   ○ Reinstated Code   ▲ Revised Code

70 — G Codes   A Age Edit   M Maternity Edit   ♀ Female Only   ♂ Male Only   A - ☑ APC Status Indicators   *2007 HCPCS*

Ⓜ G9063 Oncology; disease status; limited to nonsmall cell lung cancer; extent of disease initially established as stage I (prior to neoadjuvant therapy, if any) with no evidence of disease progression, recurrence, or metastases (for use in a Medicare-approved demonstration project)

Ⓜ G9064 Oncology; disease status; limited to nonsmall cell lung cancer; extent of disease initially establised as stage II (prior to neoadjuvant therapy, if any) with no evidence of disease progression, recurrence, or metastases (for use in a Medicare-approved demonstration project)

Ⓜ G9065 Oncology; disease status; limited to nonsmall cell lung cancer; extent of disease initially established as stage III A (prior to neoadjuvant therapy, if any) with no evidence of disease progression, recurrence, or metastases (for use in a Medicare-approved demonstration project)

Ⓜ G9066 Oncology; disease status; limited to nonsmall cell lung cancer; stage III B-IV at diagnosis, metastatic, locally recurrent, or progressive (for use in a Medicare approved demonstration project)

▲ Ⓜ G9067 Oncology; disease status; limited to non-small cell lung cancer; extent of disease unknown, staging in progress, or not listed (for use in a Medicare-approved demonstration project)

Ⓜ G9068 Oncology; disease status; limited to small cell and combined small cell/nonsmall cell; extent of disease initially established as limited with no evidence of disease progression, recurrence, or metastases (for use in a Medicare-approved demonstration project)

Ⓜ G9069 Oncology; disease status; small cell lung cancer, limited to small cell and combined small cell/nonsmall cell; extensive stage at diagnosis, metastatic, locally recurrent, or progressive (for use in a Medicare-approved demonstration project)

▲ Ⓜ G9070 Oncology; disease status; small cell lung cancer, limited to small cell and combined small cell/non-small; extent of Disease unknown, staging in progress, or not listed (for use in a Medicare-approved demonstration project)

Ⓜ G9071 Oncology; disease status; invasive female breast cancer (does not include ductal carcinoma in situ); adenocarcinoma as predominant cell type; stage I or stage IIA-IIB; or T3, N1, M0; and ER and/or PR positive; with no evidence of disease progression, recurrence, or metastases (for use in a Medicare-approved demonstration project)

Ⓜ G9072 Oncology; disease status; invasive female breast cancer (does not include ductal carcinoma in situ); adenocarcinoma as predominant cell type; stage I, or stage IIA-IIB; or T3, N1, M0; and ER and PR negative; with no evidence of disease progression, recurrence, or metstases (for use in a Medicare-approved demonstration project)

Ⓜ G9073 Oncology; disease status; invasive female breast cancer (does not include ductal carcinoma in situ); adenocarcinoma as predominant cell type; stage IIIA-IIIB; and not T3, N1, M0; and ER and/or PR positive; with no evidence of disease progression, recurrence, or metastases (for use in a Medicare-approved demonstration project)

Ⓜ G9074 Oncology; disease status; invasive female breast cancer (does not include ductal carcinoma in situ); adenocarcinoma as predominant cell type; stage IIIA-IIIB; and not T3, N1, M0; and ER and PR negative; with no evidence of disease progression, recurrence, or metastases (for use in a Medicare-approved demonstration project)

Ⓜ G9075 Oncology; disease status; invasive female breast cancer (does not include ductal carcinoma in situ); adenocarcinoma as predominant cell type; M1 at diagnosis, metstatic locally recurrent, or progressive (for use in a Medicare-approved demonstration project)

~~G9076~~ ~~Oncology; disease status; invasive female breast cancer (does not include ductal carcinoma insitu); adenocarcinoma as predominant cell type; extent of disease unknown, under evaluation, pre-surgical or not listed (for use in a Medicare-approved demonstration project)~~

Ⓜ G9077 Oncology; disease status; prostate cancer, limited to adenocarcinoma as predominant cell type; T1-T2C and Gleason 2-7 and PSA < or equal to 20 at diagnosis with no evidence of disease progression, recurrence, or metastases (for use in a Medicare-approved demonstration project)

Ⓜ G9078 Oncology; disease status; prostate cancer, cell type; T2 or T3a gleason 8-10 or PSA > 20 at diagnosis with no evidence of disease progression, recurrence, or metastases

Ⓜ G9079 Oncology; disease status; prostate cancer, limited to adencarcinoma as predominant cell type; T3B-T4, any N; any T, N1 at diagnosis with no evidence of disease progression, recurrence, or metastases (for use in a Medicare-approved demonstration project)

Ⓜ G9080 Oncology; disease status; prostate cancer, limited to adenocarcinoma; after initial treatment with rising PSA or failure of PSA decline (for use in a Medicare-approved demonstration project)

~~G9081~~ ~~Oncology; disease status; prostate cancer, limited to adenocarcinoma, non-castrate, incompletely castrate; clinical metastases or M1 at diagnosis (for use in a Medicare-approved demonstration project)~~

~~G9082~~ ~~Oncology; disease status; prostate cancer, limited to adenocarcinoma; castrate; clinical metastases or M1 at diagnosis (for use in a Medicare-approved demonstration project)~~

▲ Ⓜ G9083 Oncology; disease status; prostate cancer, limited to adenocarcinoma; extent of disease unknown, staging in progress, or not listed (for use in a Medicare-approved demonstration project)

Ⓜ G9084 Oncology; disease status; colon cancer, limited to invasive cancer, adenocarcinoma as predominant cell type; extent of disease initially established as T1-3, N0, M0 with no evidence of disease progression, recurrence or metastases (for use in a Medicare-approved demonstration project)

Ⓜ G9085 Oncology; disease status; colon cancer, limited to invasive cancer, adenocarcinoma as predominant cell type; extent of disease initially established as T4, N0, M0 with no evidence of disease progression, recurrence, or metastases (for use in a Medicare-approved demonstration project)

Special Coverage Instructions   Noncovered by Medicare   Carrier Discretion   ☑ Quality Alert   ● New Code   ○ Reinstated Code   ▲ Revised Code

2007 HCPCS   🔟-🔟 ASC Group   MED: Pub 100/NCD References   ⅙ DMEPOS Paid   ⊘ SNF Excluded   G Codes — 71

Ⓜ **G9086** Oncology; disease status; colon cancer, limited to invasive cancer, adenocarcinoma as predominant cell type; extent of disease initially established as T1-4, N1-2, M0 with no evidence of disease progression, recurrrence, or metastases (for use in a Medicare-approved demonstration project)

Ⓜ **G9087** Oncology; disease status; colon cancer, limited to invasive cancer, adenocarcinoma as predominant cell type; M1 at diagnosis, metastatic locally recurrent, or progressive with current clinical, radiologic, or biochemical evidence of disease (for use in a Medicare-approved demonstration project)

Ⓜ **G9088** Oncology; disease status; colon cancer, limited to invasive cancer, adenocarcinoma as predominant cell type; M1 at diagnosis, metastatic, locally recurrent, or progressive without current clincal, radiologic, or biochemical evidence of disease (for use in a Medicare-approved demonstration project)

▲ Ⓜ **G9089** Oncology; disease status; colon cancer, limited to invasive cancer; adenocarcinoma as predominant cell type; extent of disease unknown, staging in progress, or not listed (for use in a Medicare-approved demonstration project)

Ⓜ **G9090** Oncology; disease status; rectal cancer, limited to invasive cancer, adenocarcinoma as predominant cell type; extent of disease initially established as T1-2, N0, M0 (prior to neoadjuvant therapy, if any) with no evidence of disease progression, recurrence, or metastases (for use in a Medicare-approved demonstration project)

Ⓜ **G9091** Oncology; disease status; rectal cancer, limited to invasive cancer, adenocarcinoma as predominant cell type; extent of disease initially established as T3, N0, M0 (prior to neoadjuvant therapy, if any) with no evidence of disease progression, recurrence, or metastases (for use in a Medicare-approved demonstration project)

Ⓜ **G9092** Oncology; disease status; rectal cancer, limited to invasive cancer, adenocarcinoma as predominant cell type; extent of disease initially established as T1-3, N1-2, M0 (prior to neoadjuvant therapy, if any) with no evidence of disease progression, recurrence or metastases (for use in a Medicare-approved demonstration project)

Ⓜ **G9093** Oncology; disease status; rectal cancer, limited to invasive cancer, adenocarcinoma as predominant cell type; extent of disease initially established as T4, any N, M0 (prior to neoadjuvant therapy, if any) with no evidence of disease progression, recurrence, or metastases (for use in a Medicare-approved demonstration project)

Ⓜ **G9094** Oncology; disease status; rectal cancer, limited to invasive cancer, adenocarcinoma as predominant cell type; M1 at diagnosis, meetastatic, locally recurrent, or progressive (for use in a Mediare-approved demonstration project)

▲ Ⓜ **G9095** Oncology; disease status; rectal cancer, limited to invasive cancer; adenocarcinoma as predominant cell type; extent of disease unknown, staging in progress, or not listed (for use in a Medicare-approved demonstration project)

Ⓜ **G9096** Oncology; disease status; esophageal cancer, limited to adenocarcinoma or squamous cell carcinoma as predominant cell type; extent of disease initially established as T1-T3, N0-N1 or NX (prior to neoadjuvant therapy, if any) with no evidence of disease progression, recurrence, or metastases (for use in a Medicare-approved demonstration project)

Ⓜ **G9097** Oncology; disease status; esophageal cancer, limited to adenocarcinoma or squamous cell carcinoma as predominant cell type; extent of disease initially established as T4, any N, M0 (prior to neoadjuvant therapy, if any) with no evidence of disease progression, recurrence, or metastases (for use in a Medicare-approved demonstration project)

Ⓜ **G9098** Oncology; disease status; esophageal cancer, limited to adenocarcinoma or squamous cell carcinoma as predominant cell type; M1 at diagnosis, metastatic, locally recurrent, or progressive (for use in a Medicare-approved demonstration project)

▲ Ⓜ **G9099** Oncology; disease status; esophageal cancer, limited to adenocarcinoma or squamous cell carcinoma as predominant cell type; extent of disease unknown, staging in progress, or not listed (for use in a Medicare-approved demonstration project)

Ⓜ **G9100** Oncology; disease status; gastric cancer, limited to adenocarcinoma as predominant cell type; post R0 resection (with or without neoadjuvant therapy) with no evidence of disease recurrence, progression, or metastases (for use in a Medicare-approved demonstration project)

Ⓜ **G9101** Oncology; disease status; gastric cancer, limited to adenocarcinoma as predominant cell type; post R1 or R2 resection (with or without neoadjuvant therapy) with no evidence of disease progression, or metastases (for use in a Medicare-approved demonstration project)

Ⓜ **G9102** Oncology; disease status; gastric cancer, limited to adenocarcinoma as predominant cell type; clinical or pathologic M0, unresectable with no evidence of disease progression, or metastases (for use in a Medicare-approved demonstration project)

Ⓜ **G9103** Oncology; disease status; gastric cancer, limited to adenocarcinoma as predominant cell type; clinical or pathologic M1 at diagnosis, metastatic, locally recurrent, or progressive (for use in a Medicare-approved demonstration project)

▲ Ⓜ **G9104** Oncology; disease status; gastric cancer, limited to adenocarcinoma as predominant cell type; extent of disease unknown, staging in progress, or not listed (for use in a Medicare-approved demonstration project)

Ⓜ **G9105** Oncology; disease status; pancreatic cancer, limited to adenocarcinoma as predominant cell type; post R0 resection without evidence of disease progression, recurrence, or metastases (for use in a Medicare-approved demonstration project)

Ⓜ **G9106** Oncology; disease status; pancreatic cancer, limited to adenocarcinoma; post R1 or R2 resection with no evidence of disease progression, or metastases (for use in a Medicare-approved demonstration project)

Ⓜ **G9107** Oncology; disease status; pancreatic cancer, limited to adenocarcinoma; unresectable at diagnosis, M1 at diagnosis, metastatic, locally recurrent, or progressive (for use in a Medicare-approved demonstration project)

▲ Ⓜ **G9108** Oncology; disease status; pancreatic cancer, limited to adenocarcinoma; extent of disease unknown, staging in progress, or not listed (for use in a Medicare-approved demonstration project)

Special Coverage Instructions   Noncovered by Medicare   Carrier Discretion   ☑ Quality Alert   ● New Code   ○ Reinstated Code   ▲ Revised Code

72 — G Codes   Ⓐ Age Edit   Ⓜ Maternity Edit   ♀ Female Only   ♂ Male Only   Ⓐ - ☑ APC Status Indicators   *2007 HCPCS*

Ⓜ G9109 Oncology; disease status; head and neck cancer, limited to cancers of oral cavity, pharynx and larynx with squamous cell as predominant cell type; extent of disease initially established as T1-T2 and N0, M0 (prior to neoadjuvant therapy, if any) with no evidence of disease progression, recurrence, or metastases (for use in a Medicare-approved demonstration project)

Ⓜ G9110 Oncology; disease status; head and neck cancer, limited to cancers of oral cavity, pharynx and larynx with squamous cell as predominant cell type; extent of disease initially established as T3-4 and/or N1-3, M0 (prior to neoadjuvant therapy, if any) with no evidence of disease progression, recurrence, or metastatses (for use in a Medicare-approved demonstration project)

Ⓜ G9111 Oncology; disease status; head and neck cancer, limited to cancers of oral cavity, pharynx and larynx with squamous cell as predominant cell type; M1 at diagnosis, metastatic, locally recurrent, or progressive (for use in a Medicare-approved demonstration project)

▲ Ⓜ G9112 Oncology; disease status; head and neck cancer, limited to cancers of oral cavity, pharynx and larynx with squamous cell as predominant cell type; extent of disease unknown, staging in progress, or not listed (for use in a Medicare-approved demonstration project)

Ⓜ G9113 Oncology; disease status; ovarian cancer, limited to epithelial cancer; pathologic state 1A-B (Grade 1) without evidence of disease progression, recurrence, or metastases (for use in a Medicare-approved demonstration project)

Ⓜ G9114 Oncology; disease status; ovarian cancer, limited to epithelial cancer; pathologic stage IA-B (grade 2-3); or stage IC (all grades); or stage II; without evidence of disease progression, recurrence, or metastases (for use in a Medicare-approved demonstration project)

Ⓜ G9115 Oncology; disease status; ovarian cancer, limited to epithelial cancer; pathologic stage III-IV; without evidence of progression, recurrence, or metastases (for use in a Medicare-approved demonstration project)

Ⓜ G9116 Oncology; disease status; ovarian cancer, limited to epithelial cancer; evidence of disease progression, or recurrence, and/or platinum resistance (for use in a Medicare-approved demonstration project)

▲ Ⓜ G9117 Oncology; disease status; ovarian cancer, limited to epithelial cancer; extent of disease unknown, staging in progress, or not listed (for use in a Medicare-approved demonstration project)

G9118 ~~Oncology; disease status; non-Hodgkin's lymphoma, limited to follicular lymphoma, mantle cell lymphoma, diffuse large B-cell lymphoma, small lymphocytic lymphoma; stage I, II at diagnosis, not relapsed, not refractory (for use in a Medicare-approved demonstration project)~~

G9119 ~~Oncology; disease status; non-Hodgkin's lymphoma, limited to follicular lymphoma, mantle cell lymphoma, diffuse large B-cell lymphoma, small lymphocytic lymphoma; stage III, IV not relapsed, not refractory (for use in a Medicare-approved demonstration project)~~

G9120 ~~Oncology; disease status; non-Hodgkin's lymphoma, limited to follicular lymphoma, diffuse large B-cell lymphoma; histologically transformed from follicular lymphoma to diffuse large B-cell lymphoma (for use in a Medicare-approved demonstration project)~~

G9121 ~~Oncology; disease status; non-Hodgkin's lymphoma, limited to follicular lymphoma, mantle cell lymphoma, diffuse large B-cell lymphoma, small lymphocytic lymphoma; relapsed/refractory (for use in a Medicare-approved demonstration project)~~

G9122 ~~Oncology; disease status; non-Hodgkin's lymphoma, limited to follicular lymphoma, mantle cell lymphoma, diffuse large B-cell lymphoma, small lymphocytic lymphoma; diagnostic evaluation, stage not determined, evaluation of possible relapse or non-response to therapy, or not listed (for use in a Medicare-approved demonstration project)~~

Ⓜ G9123 Oncology; disease status; chronic myelogenous leukemia, limited to Philadelphia chromosome positive and/or BCR-ABL positive; chronic phase not in hematologic, cytogenetic, or molecular remission (for use in a Medicare-approved demonstration project)

Ⓜ G9124 Oncology; disease status; chronic myelogenous leukemia, limited to Philadelphia chromosome positive and /or BCR-ABL positive; accelerated phase not in hematologic cytogenetic, or molecular remission (for use in a Medicare-approved demonstration project)

Ⓜ G9125 Oncology; disease status; chronic myelogenous leukemia, limited to Philadelphia chromosome positive and /or BCR-ABL positive; blast phase not in hematologic, cytogenetic, or molecular remission (for use in a Medicare-approved demonstration project)

Ⓜ G9126 Oncology; disease status; chronic myelogenous leukemia, limited to Philadelphia chromosome positive and /or BCR-ABL positive; in hematologic, cytogenetic, or molecular remission (for use in a Medicare-approved demonstration project)

G9127 ~~Oncology; disease status; chronic myelogenous leukemia, limited to Philadelphia chromosome positive and /or BCR-ABL positive; extent of disease unknown, under evaluation, not listed (for use in a Medicare-approved demonstration project)~~

Ⓜ G9128 Oncology; disease status; limited to multiple myeloma, systemic disease; smoldering, stage I (for use in a Medicare-approved demonstration project)

Ⓜ G9129 Oncology; disease status; limited to multiple myeloma, systemic disease; stage II or higher (for use in a Medicare-approved demonstration project)

▲ Ⓜ G9130 Oncology; disease status; limited to multiple myeloma, systemic disease; extent of disease unknown, staging in progress, or not listed (for use in a medicare-approved demonstration project)

● G9131 Oncology; disease status; invasive female breast cancer (does not include ductal carcinoma in situ); adenocarcinoma as predominant cell type; extent of disease unknown, staging in progress, or not listed (for use in a Medicare-approved demonstration project)

● G9132 Oncology; disease status; prostate cancer, limited to adenocarcinoma; hormone-refractory/androgen-independent (e.g., rising PSA on anti-androgen therapy or post-orchiectomy); clinical metastases (for use in a Medicare-approved demonstration project)

● G9133 Oncology; disease status; prostate cancer, limited to adenocarcinoma; hormone-responsive; clinical metastases or m1 at diagnosis (for use in a Medicare-approved demonstration project)

Special Coverage Instructions   Noncovered by Medicare   Carrier Discretion   ☑ Quality Alert   ● New Code   ○ Reinstated Code   ▲ Revised Code

2007 HCPCS   ❶-❾ ASC Group   **MED:** Pub 100/NCD References   ⅊ DMEPOS Paid   ⊘ SNF Excluded   G Codes — 73

Procedures/Professional Services (Temporary)

G9134 — G9139

●   G9134   Oncology; disease status; non-hodgkin's lymphoma, any cellular classification; Stage I, II at diagnosis, not relapsed, not refractory (for use in a Medicare-approved demonstration project)

●   G9135   Oncology; disease status; non-hodgkin's lymphoma, any cellular classification; Stage III, IV, not relapsed, not refractory (for use in a Medicare-approved demonstration project)

●   G9136   Oncology; disease status; non-Hodgkin's lymphoma, transformed from original cellular diagnosis to a second cellular classification (for use in a Medicare-approved demonstration project)

●   G9137   Oncology; disease status; non-Hodgkin's lymphoma, any cellular classification; relapsed/refractory (for use in a Medicare-approved demonstration project)

●   G9138   Oncology; disease status; non-Hodgkin's lymphoma, any cellular classification; diagnostic evaluation, Stage not determined, evaluation of possible relapse or non-response to therapy, or not listed (for use in a Medicare-approved demonstration project)

●   G9139   Oncology; disease status; chronic myelogenous leukemia, limited to Philadelphia chromosome positive and/or bcr-abl positive; extent of disease unknown, staging in progress, not listed (for use in a Medicare-approved demonstration project)

Special Coverage Instructions   Noncovered by Medicare   Carrier Discretion   ☑ Quality Alert   ● New Code   ○ Reinstated Code ▲ Revised Code

74 — G Codes   A Age Edit   M Maternity Edit   ♀ Female Only   ♂ Male Only   A - Y APC Status Indicators   2007 HCPCS

ALCOHOL AND DRUG ABUSE TREATMENT SERVICES
H0001-H2037

The H codes are used by those state Medicaid agencies that are mandated by state law to establish separate codes for identifying mental health services that include alcohol and drug treatment services.

H0001 Alcohol and/or drug assessment

H0002 Behavioral health screening to determine eligibility for admission to treatment program

H0003 Alcohol and/or drug screening; laboratory analysis of specimens for presence of alcohol and/or drugs

H0004 Behavioral health counseling and therapy, per 15 minutes

H0005 Alcohol and/or drug services; group counseling by a clinician

H0006 Alcohol and/or drug services; case management

H0007 Alcohol and/or drug services; crisis intervention (outpatient)

H0008 Alcohol and/or drug services; subacute detoxification (hospital inpatient)

H0009 Alcohol and/or drug services; acute detoxification (hospital inpatient)

H0010 Alcohol and/or drug services; subacute detoxification (residential addiction program inpatient)

H0011 Alcohol and/or drug services; acute detoxification (residential addiction program inpatient)

H0012 Alcohol and/or drug services; subacute detoxification (residential addiction program outpatient)

H0013 Alcohol and/or drug services; acute detoxification (residential addiction program outpatient)

H0014 Alcohol and/or drug services; ambulatory detoxification

H0015 Alcohol and/or drug services; intensive outpatient (treatment program that operates at least 3 hours/day and at least 3 days/week and is based on an individualized treatment plan), including assessment, counseling; crisis intervention, and activity therapies or education

H0016 Alcohol and/or drug services; medical/somatic (medical intervention in ambulatory setting)

H0017 Behavioral health; residential (hospital residential treatment program), without room and board, per diem

H0018 Behavioral health; short-term residential (nonhospital residential treatment program), without room and board, per diem

H0019 Behavioral health; long-term residential (nonmedical, nonacute care in a residential treatment program where stay is typically longer than 30 days), without room and board, per diem

H0020 Alcohol and/or drug services; methadone administration and/or service (provision of the drug by a licensed program)

H0021 Alcohol and/or drug training service (for staff and personnel not employed by providers)

H0022 Alcohol and/or drug intervention service (planned facilitation)

H0023 Behavioral health outreach service (planned approach to reach a targeted population)

H0024 Behavioral health prevention information dissemination service (one-way direct or nondirect contact with service audiences to affect knowledge and attitude)

H0025 Behavioral health prevention education service (delivery of services with target population to affect knowledge, attitude and/or behavior)

H0026 Alcohol and/or drug prevention process service, community-based (delivery of services to develop skills of impactors)

H0027 Alcohol and/or drug prevention environmental service (broad range of external activities geared toward modifying systems in order to mainstream prevention through policy and law)

H0028 Alcohol and/or drug prevention problem identification and referral service (e.g., student assistance and employee assistance programs), does not include assessment

H0029 Alcohol and/or drug prevention alternatives service (services for populations that exclude alcohol and other drug use e.g., alcohol free social events)

H0030 Behavioral health hotline service

H0031 Mental health assessment, by nonphysician

H0032 Mental health service plan development by nonphysician

H0033 Oral medication administration, direct observation

H0034 Medication training and support, per 15 minutes

H0035 Mental health partial hospitalization, treatment, less than 24 hours

H0036 Community psychiatric supportive treatment, face-to-face, per 15 minutes

H0037 Community psychiatric supportive treatment program, per diem

H0038 Self-help/peer services, per 15 minutes

H0039 Assertive community treatment, face-to-face, per 15 minutes

H0040 Assertive community treatment program, per diem

H0041 Foster care, child, nontherapeutic, per diem   Ⓐ

H0042 Foster care, child, nontherapeutic, per month   Ⓐ

H0043 Supported housing, per diem

H0044 Supported housing, per month

H0045 Respite care services, not in the home, per diem

H0046 Mental health services, not otherwise specified

H0047 Alcohol and/or other drug abuse services, not otherwise specified

H0048 Alcohol and/or other drug testing: collection and handling only, specimens other than blood

● **H0049** Alcohol and/or drug screening

● **H0050** Alcohol and/or drug service, brief intervention, per 15 minutes

H1000 Prenatal care, at-risk assessment   Ⓜ ♀

H1001 Prenatal care, at-risk enhanced service; antepartum management   Ⓜ ♀

H1002 Prenatal care, at risk enhanced service; care coordination   Ⓜ ♀

H1003 Prenatal care, at-risk enhanced service; education   Ⓜ ♀

H1004 Prenatal care, at-risk enhanced service; follow-up home visit   Ⓜ ♀

Special Coverage Instructions   Noncovered by Medicare   Carrier Discretion   ☑ Quality Alert   ● New Code   ○ Reinstated Code   ▲ Revised Code

2007 HCPCS   **1**-**9** ASC Group   **MED:** Pub 100/NCD References   ⅃ DMEPOS Paid   ⦰ SNF Excluded   **H Codes — 75**

Alcohol and Drug Abuse Treatment Services

H1005 — H2037

H1005 Prenatal care, at-risk enhanced service package (includes H1001–H1004) 　M ♀

H1010 Nonmedical family planning education, per session

H1011 Family assessment by licensed behavioral health professional for state defined purposes

H2000 Comprehensive multidisciplinary evaluation

H2001 Rehabilitation program, per 1/2 day

H2010 Comprehensive medication services, per 15 minutes

H2011 Crisis intervention service, per 15 minutes

H2012 Behavioral health day treatment, per hour

H2013 Psychiatric health facility service, per diem

H2014 Skills training and development, per 15 minutes

H2015 Comprehensive community support services, per 15 minutes

H2016 Comprehensive community support services, per diem

H2017 Psychosocial rehabilitation services, per 15 minutes

H2018 Psychosocial rehabilitation services, per diem

H2019 Therapeutic behavioral services, per 15 minutes

H2020 Therapeutic behavioral services, per diem

H2021 Community-based wrap-around services, per 15 minutes

H2022 Community-based wrap-around services, per diem

H2023 Supported employment, per 15 minutes

H2024 Supported employment, per diem

H2025 Ongoing support to maintain employment, per 15 minutes

H2026 Ongoing support to maintain employment, per diem

H2027 Psychoeducational service, per 15 minutes

H2028 Sexual offender treatment service, per 15 minutes

H2029 Sexual offender treatment service, per diem

H2030 Mental health clubhouse services, per 15 minutes

H2031 Mental health clubhouse services, per diem

H2032 Activity therapy, per 15 minutes

H2033 Multisystemic therapy for juveniles, per 15 minutes

H2034 Alcohol and/or drug abuse halfway house services, per diem

H2035 Alcohol and/or other drug treatment program, per hour

H2036 Alcohol and/or other drug treatment program, per diem

H2037 Developmental delay prevention activities, dependent child of client, per 15 minutes 　A

Special Coverage Instructions　　Noncovered by Medicare　　Carrier Discretion　　☑ Quality Alert　　● New Code　　○ Reinstated Code　▲ Revised Code

76 — H Codes　　　　A Age Edit　　M Maternity Edit　♀ Female Only　♂ Male Only　　A - Y APC Status Indicators　　*2007 HCPCS*

DRUGS ADMINISTERED OTHER THAN ORAL METHOD
J0000-J9999

J codes include drugs that ordinarily cannot be self-administered, chemotherapy drugs, immunosuppressive drugs, inhalation solutions, and other miscellaneous drugs and solutions.

EXCEPTION: ORAL IMMUNOSUPPRESSIVE DRUGS

J codes fall under the jurisdiction of the DME Regional office for Medicare, unless incidental or otherwise noted.

N ☑ **J0120** Injection, tetracycline, up to 250 mg
MED: 100-2,15,50

K ☑ **J0128** Injection, abarelix, 10 mg
Use this code for Plenaxis.

● G ☑ **J0129** Injection, abatacept, 10 mg
Use this code for Orencia

K ☑ **J0130** Injection abciximab, 10 mg
Use this code for ReoPro.
MED: 100-2,15,50

K **J0132** Injection, acetylcysteine, 100 mg
Use this code for Acetadote.

N **J0133** Injection, acyclovir, 5 mg
Use this code for Zovirax.
MED: 100-4,4,230.1

K ☑ **J0135** Injection, adalimumab, 20 mg
Use this code for Humira.

K ☑ **J0150** Injection, adenosine for therapeutic use, 6 mg (not to be used to report any adenosine phosphate compounds, instead use A9270)
Use this code for Adenocard, Adenoscan.
MED: 100-2,15,50; 100-4,4,230.1
AHA: 2Q,'02,10

K ☑ **J0152** Injection, adenosine for diagnostic use, 30 mg (not to be used to report any adenosine phosphate compounds; instead use A9270)
MED: 100-4,4,230.1

N ☑ **J0170** Injection, adrenalin, epinephrine, up to 1 ml ampule
Use this code for Adrenalin Chloride, Epipen, Sus-Phrine.
MED: 100-2,15,50

K ☑ **J0180** Injection, agalsidase beta, 1 mg
Use this code for Fabrazyme.

K ☑ **J0190** Injection, biperiden lactate, per 5 mg
MED: 100-2,15,50

N **J0200** Injection, alatrofloxacin mesylate, 100 mg
MED: 100-2,15,50.5

K ☑ **J0205** Injection, alglucerase, per 10 units
Use this code for Ceredase.
MED: 100-2,15,50

K ☑ **J0207** Injection, amifostine, 500 mg
Use this code for Ethyol.
MED: 100-2,15,50

K ☑ **J0210** Injection, methyldopate HCl, up to 250 mg
Use this code for Aldomet.
MED: 100-2,15,50

K ☑ **J0215** Injection, alefacept, 0.5 mg
Use this for Amevive.
MED: 100-4,4,230.1

K ☑ **J0256** Injection, alpha 1-proteinase inhibitor — human, 10 mg
Use this code for Prolastin, Zemira.
MED: 100-2,15,50

B ☑ **J0270** Injection, alprostadil, 1.25 mcg (code may be used for Medicare when drug administered under direct supervision of a physician, not for use when drug is self-administered)
Use this code for Alprostadil, Caverject, Edex, Prostin VR Pediatric.
MED: 100-2,15,50

B **J0275** Alprostadil urethral suppository (code may be used for Medicare when drug administered under direct supervision of a physician, not for use when drug is self-administered)
Use this code for Muse.
MED: 100-2,15,50

N **J0278** Injection, amikacin sulfate, 100 mg
Use this code for Amikin.

N ☑ **J0280** Injection, aminophyllin, up to 250 mg
MED: 100-2,15,50

N ☑ **J0282** Injection, amiodarone HCl, 30 mg
Use this code for Cordarone IV.
MED: 100-2,15,50

N ☑ **J0285** Injection, amphotericin B, 50 mg
Use this for Abelcent, Amphocin, Fungizonef.
MED: 100-2,15,50

K **J0287** Injection, amphotericin B lipid complex, 10 mg
MED: 100-2,15,50

K **J0288** Injection, amphotericin B cholesteryl sulfate complex, 10 mg
Use this code for Amphotec.
MED: 100-2,15,50

K **J0289** Injection, amphotericin B liposome, 10 mg
Use this code for Ambisome.
MED: 100-2,15,50

N ☑ **J0290** Injection, ampicillin sodium, 500 mg
MED: 100-2,15,50

N ☑ **J0295** Injection, ampicillin sodium/sulbactam sodium, per 1.5 g
Use this code for Unasyn.
MED: 100-2,15,50

N ☑ **J0300** Injection, amobarbital, up to 125 mg
Use this code for Amytal.
MED: 100-2,15,50

N ☑ **J0330** Injection, succinylcholine chloride, up to 20 mg
Use this code for Anectine, Quelicin.
MED: 100-2,15,50

● G ☑ **J0348** Injection, anidulafungin, 1 mg
Use this code for Eraxis.

K ☑ **J0350** Injection, anistreplase, per 30 units
Use this code for Eminase.
MED: 100-2,15,50

N ☑ **J0360** Injection, hydralazine HCl, up to 20 mg
MED: 100-2,15,50

● K ☑ **J0364** Injection, apomorphine hydrochloride, 1 mg
Use this code for Apokyn.

K **J0365** Injection, aprotonin, 10,000 kiu
Use this code for Trasylol.
MED: 100-2,15,50; 100-4,4,230.1

Special Coverage Instructions | Noncovered by Medicare | Carrier Discretion | ☑ Quality Alert | ● New Code | ○ Reinstated Code | ▲ Revised Code

2007 HCPCS | 1-9 ASC Group | MED: Pub 100/NCD References | � DMEPOS Paid | ⊘ SNF Excluded | J Codes — 77

Drugs Administered Other Than Oral Method

J0380 — J0698

K ☑ **J0380** Injection, metaraminol bitartrate, per 10 mg
Use this code for Aramine.
MED: 100-2,15,50

N ☑ **J0390** Injection, chloroquine HCl, up to 250 mg
Use this code for Aralen.
MED: 100-2,15,50

K ☑ **J0395** Injection, arbutamine HCl, 1 mg
MED: 100-2,15,50

N ☑ **J0456** Injection, azithromycin, 500 mg
Use this code for Zithromax.
MED: 100-2,15,50.5

N ☑ **J0460** Injection, atropine sulfate, up to 0.3 mg
Use this code for Atropen.
MED: 100-2,15,50

N ☑ **J0470** Injection, dimercaprol, per 100 mg
Use this code for BAL in oil.
MED: 100-2,15,50

K ☑ **J0475** Injection, baclofen, 10 mg
Use this code for Lioresal.
MED: 100-2,15,50; 100-4,4,230.1

K ☑ **J0476** Injection, baclofen, 50 mcg for intrathecal trial
Use this code for Lioresal for intrathecal trial.
MED: 100-2,15,50; 100-4,4,230.1

K **J0480** Injection, basiliximab, 20 mg
Use this code for Simulect.
MED: 100-2,15,50; 100-4,4,230.1; 100-4,4,240

N ☑ **J0500** Injection, dicyclomine HCl, up to 20 mg
Use this code for Bentyl.
MED: 100-2,15,50

N ☑ **J0515** Injection, benztropine mesylate, per 1 mg
Use this code for Cogentin.
MED: 100-2,15,50

N ☑ **J0520** Injection, bethanechol chloride, Mytonachol or Urecholine, up to 5 mg
MED: 100-2,15,50

N ☑ **J0530** Injection, penicillin G benzathine and penicillin G procaine, up to 600,000 units
Use this code for Bicillin C-R.
MED: 100-2,15,50

N ☑ **J0540** Injection, penicillin G benzathine and penicillin G procaine, up to 1,200,000 units
Use this code for Bicillin C-R, Bicillin C-R 900/300.
MED: 100-2,15,50

N ☑ **J0550** Injection, penicillin G benzathine and penicillin G procaine, up to 2,400,000 units
Use this code for Bicillin C-R.
MED: 100-2,15,50

N ☑ **J0560** Injection, penicillin G benzathine, up to 600,000 units
Use this code for Bicillin L-A, Permapen.
MED: 100-2,15,50

N ☑ **J0570** Injection, penicillin G benzathine, up to 1,200,000 units
Use this code for Bicillin L-A, Permapen.
MED: 100-2,15,50

N ☑ **J0580** Injection, penicillin G benzathine, up to 2,400,000 units
Use this code for Bicillin L-A, Permapen.
MED: 100-2,15,50

K ☑ **J0583** Injection, bivalirudin, 1 mg
Use this code for Angiomax.

K ☑ **J0585** Botulinum toxin type A, per unit
Use this code for Botox.
MED: 100-2,15,50

K ☑ **J0587** Botulinum toxin type B, per 100 units
Use this code for Myobloc.
MED: 100-2,15,50
AHA: 2Q,'02,8

N **J0592** Injection, buprenorphine HCl, 0.1 mg
Use this code for Buprenex.
MED: 100-2,15,50

● K ☑ **J0594** Injection, busulfan, 1 mg
Use this code for Busulfex.

N ☑ **J0595** Injection, butorphanol tartrate, 1 mg
Use this code for Stadol.

K ☑ **J0600** Injection, edetate calcium disodium, up to 1000 mg
Use this code for Calcium Disodium Versenate, Calcium EDTA.
MED: 100-2,15,50

N ☑ **J0610** Injection, calcium gluconate, per 10 ml
MED: 100-2,15,50

N ☑ **J0620** Injection, calcium glycerophosphate and calcium lactate, per 10 ml
MED: 100-2,15,50

N ☑ **J0630** Injection, calcitonin-salmon, up to 400 units
Use this code for Calcimar, Miacalcin.
MED: 100-2,15,50

N **J0636** Injection, calcitriol, 0.1 mcg
Use this code for Calcijex.
MED: 100-2,15,50

K **J0637** Injection, caspofungin acetate, 5 mg
Use this code for Cancidas.

N ☑ **J0640** Injection, leucovorin calcium, per 50 mg
MED: 100-2,15,50

N ☑ **J0670** Injection, mepivacaine HCl, per 10 ml
Use this code for Carbocaine, Polocaine, Isocaine HCl.
MED: 100-2,15,50

N ☑ **J0690** Injection, cefazolin sodium, 500 mg
Use this code for Ancef, Kefzol.
MED: 100-2,15,50

N **J0692** Injection, cefepime HCl, 500 mg
Use this code for Maxipime.

N ☑ **J0694** Injection, cefoxitin sodium, 1 g
Use this code for Mefoxin.

See code(s): Q0090
MED: 100-2,15,50

N ☑ **J0696** Injection, ceftriaxone sodium, per 250 mg
Use this code for Rocephin.
MED: 100-2,15,50

N ☑ **J0697** Injection, sterile cefuroxime sodium, per 750 mg
MED: 100-2,15,50

N ☑ **J0698** Cefotaxime sodium, per g
Use this code for Claforan.
MED: 100-2,15,50

Special Coverage Instructions   Noncovered by Medicare   Carrier Discretion   ☑ Quality Alert   ● New Code   ○ Reinstated Code   ▲ Revised Code

78 — J Codes   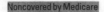 Ⓐ Age Edit   Ⓜ Maternity Edit   ♀ Female Only   ♂ Male Only   Ⓐ - ☑ APC Status Indicators   *2007 HCPCS*

N ☑ **J0702** Injection, betamethasone acetate and betamethasone sodium phosphate, per 3 mg
Use this code for Celestone Soluspan.
MED: 100-2,15,50

N ☑ **J0704** Injection, betamethasone sodium phosphate, per 4 mg
Use this code for Adbeon.
MED: 100-2,15,50

K **J0706** Injection, caffeine citrate, 5 mg
Use this code for Cafcit.
AHA: 2Q,'02,8

N ☑ **J0710** Injection, cephapirin sodium, up to 1 g
MED: 100-2,15,50

N ☑ **J0713** Injection, ceftazidime, per 500 mg
Use this code for Ceptaz, Fortaz, Tazicef.
MED: 100-2,15,50

N ☑ **J0715** Injection, ceftizoxime sodium, per 500 mg
Use this code for Cefizox.
MED: 100-2,15,50

N ☑ **J0720** Injection, chloramphenicol sodium succinate, up to 1 g
Use this code for Chloromycetin.
MED: 100-2,15,50

N ☑ **J0725** Injection, chorionic gonadotropin, per 1,000 USP units
Use this code for Corgonject-5, Novarel, Pregnyl.
MED: 100-2,15,50

K ☑ **J0735** Injection, clonidine HCl, 1 mg
Use this code for Catapres, Duraclon.
MED: 100-2,15,50

K ☑ **J0740** Injection, cidofovir, 375 mg
Use this code for Vistide.
MED: 100-2,15,50

N ☑ **J0743** Injection, cilastatin sodium imipenem, per 250 mg
Use this code for Primaxin I.M., Primaxin I.V.
MED: 100-2,15,50

N **J0744** Injection, ciprofloxacin for intravenous infusion, 200 mg
Use this code for Cipro.

N ☑ **J0745** Injection, codeine phosphate, per 30 mg
MED: 100-2,15,50

N ☑ **J0760** Injection, colchicine, per 1 mg
MED: 100-2,15,50

N ☑ **J0770** Injection, colistimethate sodium, up to 150 mg
Use this code for Coly-Mycin M.
MED: 100-2,15,50

N ☑ **J0780** Injection, prochlorperazine, up to 10 mg
Use this code for Compazine, Cotranzine, Compa-Z, Ultrazine-10.
MED: 100-2,15,50

K **J0795** Injection, corticorelin ovine triflutate, 1 mcg
MED: 100-2,15,50; 100-4,4,230.1

K ☑ **J0800** Injection, corticotropin, up to 40 units
Use this code for H.P. Acthar.
MED: 100-2,15,50

K ☑ **J0835** Injection, cosyntropin, per 0.25 mg
Use this code for Cortrosyn.
MED: 100-2,15,50

K ☑ **J0850** Injection, cytomegalovirus immune globulin intravenous (human), per vial
Use this code for Cytogam.
MED: 100-2,15,50; 100-4,4,240

K ☑ **J0878** Injection, daptomycin, 1 mg
Use this code for Cubicin.

K **J0881** Injection, darbepoetin alfa, 1 mcg (non-ESRD use)
Use this code for Aranesp.
MED: 100-2,6,10; 100-4,4,230.1; 100-4,4,240

A **J0882** Injection, darbepoetin alfa, 1 mcg (for ESRD on dialysis) ⊘
Use this code for Aranesp.
MED: 100-2,6,10; 100-4,4,240

K **J0885** Injection, epoetin alfa, (for non-ESRD use), 1000 units
Use this code for Epogen, Procrit.
MED: 100-2,6,10; 100-2,15,50; 100-4,4,230.1; 100-4,4,240

A **J0886** Injection, epoetin alfa, 1000 units (for ESRD on dialysis) ⊘
Use this code for Epogen, Procrit.
MED: 100-2,6,10; 100-4,4,240

● G ☑ **J0894** Injection, decitabine, 1 mg
Use this code for Dacogen.

K ☑ **J0895** Injection, deferoxamine mesylate, 500 mg
Use this code for Desferal.
See code(s): Q0087
MED: 100-2,15,50

N ☑ **J0900** Injection, testosterone enanthate and estradiol valerate, up to 1 cc
Use this code for Deladumone, Andrest 90-4, Andro-Estro 90-4, Androgyn L.A., Delatestadiol, Dua-Gen L.A., Duoval P.A., Estra-Testrin, TEEV, Testadiate, Testradiol 90/4, Valertest No. 1, Valertest No. 2, Deladumone OB, Ditate-DS.
MED: 100-2,15,50

N ☑ **J0945** Injection, brompheniramine maleate, per 10 mg
Use this code for Histaject, Cophene-B, Dehist, Nasahist B, ND Stat, Oraminic II, Sinusol-B.
MED: 100-2,15,50

N ☑ **J0970** Injection, estradiol valerate, up to 40 mg
Use this code for Clinagen LA, Delestrogen, Gynogen L.A. 10, Gynogen L.A. 20, Gynogen L.A. 40.
MED: 100-2,15,50

N ☑ **J1000** Injection, depo-estradiol cypionate, up to 5 mg
Use this code for Estradiol Cypionate, depGynogen, Depogen.
MED: 100-2,15,50

N ☑ **J1020** Injection, methylprednisolone acetate, 20 mg
Use this code for Depo-Medrol.
MED: 100-2,15,50; 100-4,4,240

N ☑ **J1030** Injection, methylprednisolone acetate, 40 mg
Use this code for Depo-Medrol, depMedalone 40, Sano-Drol.
MED: 100-2,15,50; 100-4,4,240

N ☑ **J1040** Injection, methylprednisolone acetate, 80 mg
Use this code for Cortimed, Depmedalone, Depo-Medrol, depMedalone 80, Duro Cort, Methylcotolone, Pri-Methylate, Sano-Drol.
MED: 100-2,15,50; 100-4,4,240

Special Coverage Instructions   Noncovered by Medicare   Carrier Discretion   ☑ Quality Alert   ● New Code   ○ Reinstated Code   ▲ Revised Code

2007 HCPCS   **1**-**9** ASC Group   MED: Pub 100/NCD References   ዄ DMEPOS Paid   ⊘ SNF Excluded   J Codes — 79

Drugs Administered Other Than Oral Method

J1051 — J1364

N J1051 Injection, medroxyprogesterone acetate, 50 mg
Use this code for Depo-Provera.
MED: 100-2,15,50

E ☑ J1055 Injection, medroxyprogesterone acetate for contraceptive use, 150 mg ♀
Use this code for Depo-Provera.

E J1056 Injection, medroxyprogesterone acetate/estradiol cypionate, 5 mg/25 mg ♀
Use this code for Lunelle monthly contraceptive.

N ☑ J1060 Injection, testosterone cypionate and estradiol cypionate, up to 1 ml
Use this code for Depo-Testadiol, Duo-Span, Duo-Span II.
MED: 100-2,15,50

N ☑ J1070 Injection, testosterone cypionate, up to 100 mg
Use this code for depAndro 100, Depo Testosterone Cypionate, Deptestrogen.
MED: 100-2,15,50

N ☑ J1080 Injection, testosterone cypionate, 1 cc, 200 mg
Use this code for Depandrante, Depo-Testosterone, Virilon.
MED: 100-2,15,50

N J1094 Injection, dexamethasone acetate, 1 mg
Use this code for Cortastat LA, Dalalone L.A., Decadron LA, Dexamethasone Acetate Anhydrous, Dexone LA.
MED: 100-2,15,50

N ☑ J1100 Injection, dexamethasone sodium phosphate, 1 mg
Use this code for Cortastat, Dalalone, Decadron Phosphate.
MED: 100-2,15,50

N ☑ J1110 Injection, dihydroergotamine mesylate, per 1 mg
Use this code for D.H.E. 45.
MED: 100-2,15,50

N ☑ J1120 Injection, acetazolamide sodium, up to 500 mg
Use this code for Diamox.
MED: 100-2,15,50

N ☑ J1160 Injection, digoxin, up to 0.5 mg
Use this code for Lanoxin.
MED: 100-2,15,50

K J1162 Injection, digoxin immune fab (ovine), per vial
Use this code for Digibind, Digifab.
MED: 100-2,15,50; 100-4,4,230.1

N ☑ J1165 Injection, phenytoin sodium, per 50 mg
Use this code for Dilantin.
MED: 100-2,15,50

N ☑ J1170 Injection, hydromorphone, up to 4 mg
Use this code for Dilaudid, Dilaudid-HP.
MED: 100-2,15,50

N ☑ J1180 Injection, dyphylline, up to 500 mg
Use this code for Lufyllin, Dilor.
MED: 100-2,15,50

K ☑ J1190 Injection, dexrazoxane HCl, per 250 mg
Use this code for Zinecard.
MED: 100-2,15,50; 100-4,4,230.1

N ☑ J1200 Injection, diphenhydramine HCl, up to 50 mg
Use this code for Benadryl, Benahist 10, Benahist 50, Benoject-10, Benoject-50, Bena-D 10, Bena-D 50, Nordryl, Dihydrex, Dimine, Diphenacen-50, Hyrexin-50, Truxadryl, Wehdryl.
MED: 100-2,15,50
AHA: 1Q,'02,2

K ☑ J1205 Injection, chlorothiazide sodium, per 500 mg
Use this code for Diuril Sodium.
MED: 100-2,15,50

N ☑ J1212 Injection, DMSO, dimethyl sulfoxide, 50%, 50 ml
Use this code for Rimso. DMSO is covered only as a treatment of interstitial cystitis.
MED: 100-2,15,50; 100-3,230.12

N ☑ J1230 Injection, methadone HCl, up to 10 mg
Use this code for Dolophine HCl.
MED: 100-2,15,50

N ☑ J1240 Injection, dimenhydrinate, up to 50 mg
Use this code for Dramamine, Dinate, Dommanate, Dramanate, Dramilin, Dramocen, Dramoject, Dymenate, Hydrate, Marmine, Wehamine.
MED: 100-2,15,50

N ☑ J1245 Injection, dipyridamole, per 10 mg
Use this code for Persantine IV.
MED: 100-2,15,50

N ☑ J1250 Injection, dobutamine HCl, per 250 mg
Use this code for Dobutrex.
MED: 100-2,15,50

K ☑ J1260 Injection, dolasetron mesylate, 10 mg
Use this code for Anzemet.
MED: 100-2,15,50

N J1265 Injection, dopamine HCl, 40 mg
Use this code for Intropin.
MED: 100-4,4,230.1

N J1270 Injection, doxercalciferol, 1 mcg
Use this code for Hectorol.

N ☑ J1320 Injection, amitriptyline HCl, up to 20 mg
Use this code for Elavil, Enovil, Tryptanol.
MED: 100-2,15,50

● K ☑ J1324 Injection, enfuvirtide, 1 mg
Use this code for Fuzeon.

N ☑ J1325 Injection, epoprostenol, 0.5 mg
Use this code for Flolan. See K0455 for infusion pump for epoprosterol.
MED: 100-2,15,50

K ☑ J1327 Injection, eptifibatide, 5 mg
Use this code for Integrilin.
MED: 100-2,15,50

K ☑ J1330 Injection, ergonovine maleate, up to 0.2 mg
Medicare jurisdiction: local contractor. Use this code for Ergotrate Maleate.
MED: 100-2,15,50

N ☑ J1335 Injection, ertapenem sodium, 500 mg
Use this code for Invanz.

N ☑ J1364 Injection, erythromycin lactobionate, per 500 mg
MED: 100-2,15,50

Special Coverage Instructions   Noncovered by Medicare   Carrier Discretion   ☑ Quality Alert   ● New Code   ○ Reinstated Code ▲ Revised Code

80 — J Codes   A Age Edit   M Maternity Edit   ♀ Female Only   ♂ Male Only   A - ☑ APC Status Indicators   *2007 HCPCS*

N ☑ **J1380** Injection, estradiol valerate, up to 10 mg
Use this code for Delestrogen, Dioval, Dioval XX, Dioval 40, Duragen-10, Duragen-20, Duragen-40, Estradiol L.A., Estradiol L.A. 20, Estradiol L.A. 40, Gynogen L.A. 10, Gynogen L.A. 20, Gynogen L.A. 40, Valergen 10, Valergen 20, Valergen 40, Estra-L 20, Estra-L 40, L.A.E. 20.
MED: 100-2,15,50

N ☑ **J1390** Injection, estradiol valerate, up to 20 mg
Use this code for Delestrogen, Dioval, Dioval XX, Dioval 40, Duragen-10, Duragen-20, Duragen-40, Estradiol L.A., Estradiol L.A. 20, Estradiol L.A. 40, Gynogen L.A. 10, Gynogen L.A. 20, Gynogen L.A. 40, Valergen 10, Valergen 20, Valergen 40, Estra-L 20, Estra-L 40, L.A.E. 20.
MED: 100-2,15,50

K ☑ **J1410** Injection, estrogen conjugated, per 25 mg
Use this code for Natural Estrogenic Substance, Premarin Intravenous, Primestrin Aqueous.
MED: 100-2,15,50

K **J1430** Injection, ethanolamine oleate, 100 mg
Use this code for Ethamiolin.
MED: 100-2,15,50; 100-4,4,230.1

N ☑ **J1435** Injection, estrone, per 1 mg
Use this code for Estone Aqueous, Estragyn, Estro-A, Estrone, Estronol, Theelin Aqueous, Estone 5, Kestrone 5.
MED: 100-2,15,50

K ☑ **J1436** Injection, etidronate disodium, per 300 mg
Use this code for Didronel.
MED: 100-2,15,50

K ☑ **J1438** Injection, etanercept, 25 mg (code may be used for Medicare when drug administered under the direct supervision of a physician, not for use when drug is self-administered)
Use this code for Enbrel.
MED: 100-2,15,50

K ☑ **J1440** Injection, filgrastim (G-CSF), 300 mcg
Use this code for Neupogen.
MED: 100-2,15,50

K ☑ **J1441** Injection, filgrastim (G-CSF), 480 mcg
Use this code for Neupogen.
MED: 100-2,15,50

N ☑ **J1450** Injection, fluconazole, 200 mg
Use this code for Diflucan.
MED: 100-2,15,50.5

K **J1451** Injection, fomepizole, 15 mg
Use this code for Antizol.
MED: 100-2,15,50; 100-4,4,230.1

K ☑ **J1452** Injection, fomivirsen sodium, intraocular, 1.65 mg
Use this code for Vitavene.
MED: 100-2,15,50.4; 100-2,15,50.4.2

K ☑ **J1455** Injection, foscarnet sodium, per 1,000 mg
Use this code for Foscavir.
MED: 100-2,15,50

N ☑ **J1457** Injection, gallium nitrate, 1 mg
Use this code for Ganite.

● K ☑ **J1458** Injection, galsulfase, 1 mg
Use this code for Naglazyme.

K ☑ **J1460** Injection, gamma globulin, intramuscular, 1 cc
Use this code for Baygam, Gammar, Gamastan, Flebogamma.
MED: 100-2,15,50

B ☑ **J1470** Injection, gamma globulin, intramuscular, 2 cc
Use this code for Gammar, Gamastan.
MED: 100-2,15,50

B ☑ **J1480** Injection, gamma globulin, intramuscular, 3 cc
Use this code for Gammar, Gamastan.
MED: 100-2,15,50

B ☑ **J1490** Injection, gamma globulin, intramuscular, 4 cc
Use this code for Gammar, Gamastan.
MED: 100-2,15,50

B ☑ **J1500** Injection, gamma globulin, intramuscular, 5 cc
Use this code for Gammar, Gamastan.
MED: 100-2,15,50

B ☑ **J1510** Injection, gamma globulin, intramuscular, 6 cc
Use this code for Gammar, Gamastan.
MED: 100-2,15,50

B ☑ **J1520** Injection, gamma globulin, intramuscular, 7 cc
Use this code for Gammar, Gamastan.
MED: 100-2,15,50

B ☑ **J1530** Injection, gamma globulin, intramuscular, 8 cc
Use this code for Gammar, Gamastan.
MED: 100-2,15,50

B ☑ **J1540** Injection, gamma globulin, intramuscular, 9 cc
Use this code for Gammar, Gamastan.
MED: 100-2,15,50

B ☑ **J1550** Injection, gamma globulin, intramuscular, 10 cc
Use this code for Gammar, Gamastan.
MED: 100-2,15,50

B ☑ **J1560** Injection, gamma globulin, intramuscular, over 10 cc
Use this code for Gammar, Gamastan.
MED: 100-2,15,50

● K **J1562** Injection, immune globulin, subcutaneous, 100 mg
Use this code for Vivaglobin.

K ☑ **J1565** Injection, respiratory syncytial virus immune globulin, intravenous, 50 mg
Use this code for Respigam.
MED: 100-2,15,50

K **J1566** Injection, immune globulin, intravenous, lyophilized (e.g., powder), 500 mg
MED: 100-2,15,50; 100-4,4,230.1

K **J1567** Injection, immune globulin, intravenous, non-lyophilized (e.g., liquid), 500 mg
MED: 100-2,15,50; 100-4,4,230.1

N ☑ **J1570** Injection, ganciclovir sodium, 500 mg
Use this code for Cytovene.
MED: 100-2,15,50

N ☑ **J1580** Injection, garamycin, gentamicin, up to 80 mg
Use this code for Gentamicin Sulfate, Jenamicin.
MED: 100-2,15,50

N ☑ **J1590** Injection, gatifloxacin, 10 mg
Use this code for Tequin.

N ☑ **J1595** Injection, glatiramer acetate, 20 mg
Use this code for Copaxone.
MED: 100-2,15,50

N ☑ **J1600** Injection, gold sodium thiomalate, up to 50 mg
Use this code for Myochrysine.
MED: 100-2,15,50

Special Coverage Instructions   Noncovered by Medicare   Carrier Discretion   ☑ Quality Alert   ● New Code   ○ Reinstated Code   ▲ Revised Code

Drugs Administered Other Than Oral Method

J1610 — J1890

K ☑ **J1610** Injection, glucagon HCl, per 1 mg
Use this code for Glucagen.
MED: 100-2,15,50

K ☑ **J1620** Injection, gonadorelin HCl, per 100 mcg
Use this code for Factrel, Lutrepulse.
MED: 100-2,15,50; 100-4,4,230.1

K ☑ **J1626** Injection, granisetron HCl, 100 mcg
Use this code for Kytril.
MED: 100-2,15,50

N ☑ **J1630** Injection, haloperidol, up to 5 mg
Use this code for Haldol.
MED: 100-2,15,50

N ☑ **J1631** Injection, haloperidol decanoate, per 50 mg
Use this code for Haldol Decanoate-50.
MED: 100-2,15,50

K **J1640** Injection, hemin, 1 mg
Use this code for Panhematin.
MED: 100-2,15,50; 100-4,4,230.1

N ☑ **J1642** Injection, heparin sodium, (heparin lock flush), per 10 units
Use this code for Hep-Lock, Hep-Lock U/P.
MED: 100-2,15,50

N ☑ **J1644** Injection, heparin sodium, per 1,000 units
Use this code for Heparin Sodium, Liquaemin Sodium.
MED: 100-2,15,50

N ☑ **J1645** Injection, dalteparin sodium, per 2500 IU
Use this code for Fragmin.
MED: 100-2,15,50

N ☑ **J1650** Injection, enoxaparin sodium, 10 mg
Use this code for Lovenox.

N **J1652** Injection, fondaparinux sodium, 0.5 mg
Use this code for Atrixtra.
MED: 100-2,15,50

K ☑ **J1655** Injection, tinzaparin sodium, 1000 IU
Use this code for Innohep.

K ☑ **J1670** Injection, tetanus immune globulin, human, up to 250 units
Use this code for Baytet.
MED: 100-2,15,50

B **J1675** Injection, histrelin acetate, 10 mcg
MED: 100-2,15,50

N ☑ **J1700** Injection, hydrocortisone acetate, up to 25 mg
Use this code for Hydrocortone Acetate.
MED: 100-2,15,50

N ☑ **J1710** Injection, hydrocortisone sodium phosphate, up to 50 mg
Use this code for Hydrocortone Phosphate.
MED: 100-2,15,50

N ☑ **J1720** Injection, hydrocortisone sodium succinate, up to 100 mg
Use this code for Solu-Cortef, A-Hydrocort.
MED: 100-2,15,50

K ☑ **J1730** Injection, diazoxide, up to 300 mg
Use this code for Hyperstat IV.
MED: 100-2,15,50

● G **J1740** Injection, ibandronate sodium, 1 mg
Use this code for Boniva.

K ☑ **J1742** Injection, ibutilide fumarate, 1 mg
Use this code for Corvert.
MED: 100-2,15,50

K ☑ **J1745** Injection, infliximab, 10 mg
Use this code for Remicade.
MED: 100-2,15,50

K **J1751** Injection, iron dextran 165, 50 mg
MED: 100-4,4,230.1

K **J1752** Injection, iron dextran 267, 50 mg
MED: 100-4,4,230.1

K **J1756** Injection, iron sucrose, 1 mg
Use this code for Venofer.

K ☑ **J1785** Injection, imiglucerase, per unit
Use this code for Cerezyme.
MED: 100-2,15,50

N ☑ **J1790** Injection, droperidol, up to 5 mg
Use this code for Inapsine.
MED: 100-2,15,50

N ☑ **J1800** Injection, propranolol HCl, up to 1 mg
Use this code for Inderal.
MED: 100-2,15,50

E ☑ **J1810** Injection, droperidol and fentanyl citrate, up to 2 ml ampule
Use this code for Innovar.
MED: 100-2,15,50
AHA: 2Q,'02,8

N **J1815** Injection, insulin, per 5 units
Use this code for Humalog, Humulin, Iletin, Insulin Lispo, Novo Nordisk, NPH, Pork insulin, Regular insulin, Ultralente, Velosulin, Humulin R, Iletin II Regular Port, Insulin Purified Pork, Relion, Lente Iletin I, Novolin R, Humulin R U-500.
MED: 100-2,15,50; 100-3,280.14

N **J1817** Insulin for administration through DME (i.e., insulin pump) per 50 units
Use this code for Humalog, Humulin, Vesolin BR, Iletin II NPH Pork, Lantus, Lispro-PFC, Novolin, Novolog, Novolog Flexpen, Novolog Mix, Relion Novolin.

E ☑ **J1825** Injection, interferon beta-1a, 33 mcg
Use this code for Avonex, Rebif.

K ☑ **J1830** Injection interferon beta-1b, 0.25 mg (code may be used for Medicare when drug administered under direct supervision of a physician, not for use when drug is self-administered)
Use this code for Actimmune and Betaseron.
MED: 100-2,15,50

K ☑ **J1835** Injection, itraconazole, 50 mg
Use this code for Sporonox IV.

N ☑ **J1840** Injection, kanamycin sulfate, up to 500 mg
Use this code for Kantrex, Klebcil.
MED: 100-2,15,50

N ☑ **J1850** Injection, kanamycin sulfate, up to 75 mg
Use this code for Kantrex, Klebcil.
MED: 100-2,15,50

N ☑ **J1885** Injection, ketorolac tromethamine, per 15 mg
Use this code for Toradol.
MED: 100-2,15,50

N ☑ **J1890** Injection, cephalothin sodium, up to 1 g
Use this code for Cephalothin Sodium, Keflin.
MED: 100-2,15,50

Special Coverage Instructions   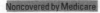Noncovered by Medicare   Carrier Discretion   ☑ Quality Alert   ● New Code   ○ Reinstated Code   ▲ Revised Code

K ☑ **J1931** Injection, laronidase, 0.1 mg
Use this code for Aldurazyme.

N ☑ **J1940** Injection, furosemide, up to 20 mg
Use this code for Lasix, Furomide M.D., Furocot.
MED: 100-2,15,50

K **J1945** Injection, lepirudin, 50 mg
Use this code for Refludan.
MED: 100-2,15,50; 100-4,4,230.1

K ☑ **J1950** Injection, leuprolide acetate (for depot suspension), per 3.75 mg
Use this code for Lupron Depot.
MED: 100-2,15,50

B ☑ **J1955** Injection, levocarnitine, per 1 g
Use this code for Carnitor, L-Carnitine.
MED: 100-2,15,50

N ☑ **J1956** Injection, levofloxacin, 250 mg
Use this code for Levaquin.
MED: 100-2,15,50

N ☑ **J1960** Injection, levorphanol tartrate, up to 2 mg
Use this code for Levo-Dromoran.
MED: 100-2,15,50

N **J1980** Injection, hyoscyamine sulfate, up to 0.25 mg
Use this code for Levsin.
MED: 100-2,15,50

N ☑ **J1990** Injection, chlordiazepoxide HCl, up to 100 mg
Use this code for Librium.
MED: 100-2,15,50

N ☑ **J2001** Injection, lidocaine HCl for intravenous infusion, 10 mg
Use this code for Xylocaine.
MED: 100-2,15,50

N ☑ **J2010** Injection, lincomycin HCl, up to 300 mg
Use this code for Lincocin, Bactramycin.
MED: 100-2,15,50

K ☑ **J2020** Injection, linezolid, 200 mg
Use this code for Zyvok.
AHA: 2Q,'02,8

N ☑ **J2060** Injection, lorazepam, 2 mg
Use this code for Ativan.
MED: 100-2,15,50

N ☑ **J2150** Injection, mannitol, 25% in 50 ml
Use this code for Osmitrol.
MED: 100-2,15,50

● K **J2170** Injection, mecasermin, 1 mg
Use this code for Iplex, Increlex.

N ☑ **J2175** Injection, meperidine HCl, per 100 mg
Use this code for Demerol.
MED: 100-2,15,50

N ☑ **J2180** Injection, meperidine and promethazine HCl, up to 50 mg
Use this code for Mepergan Injection.
MED: 100-2,15,50

K ☑ **J2185** Injection, meropenem, 100 mg

N ☑ **J2210** Injection, methylergonovine maleate, up to 0.2 mg
Use this code for Methergine.
MED: 100-2,15,50

● G ☑ **J2248** Injection, micafungin sodium, 1 mg
Use this code for Mycamine.

N ☑ **J2250** Injection, midazolam HCl, per 1 mg
Use this code for Versed.
MED: 100-2,15,50

N ☑ **J2260** Injection, milrinone lactate, 5 mg
Use this code for Primacor.
MED: 100-2,15,50

N ☑ **J2270** Injection, morphine sulfate, up to 10 mg
Use this code for Infumorph.
MED: 100-2,15,50

N ☑ **J2271** Injection, morphine sulfate, 100 mg
Use this code for Infumorph.
MED: 100-2,15,50; 100-3,280.14

N ☑ **J2275** Injection, morphine sulfate (preservative-free sterile solution), per 10 mg
Use this code for Astramorph PF, Duramorph, Infumorph.
MED: 100-2,15,50; 100-3,280.14

G **J2278** Injection, ziconotide, 1 mcg
MED: 100-4,4,230.1

N ☑ **J2280** Injection, moxifloxacin, 100 mg
Use this code for Avelox.

N ☑ **J2300** Injection, nalbuphine HCl, per 10 mg
Use this code for Nubain.
MED: 100-2,15,50

N ☑ **J2310** Injection, naloxone HCl, per 1 mg
Use this code for Narcan.
MED: 100-2,15,50

● K ☑ **J2315** Injection, naltrexone, depot form, 1 mg
Use this code for Vivitrol.

N ☑ **J2320** Injection, nandrolone decanoate, up to 50 mg
Use this code for Deca-Durabolin, Hybolin Decanoate, Decolone-50, Neo-Durabolic, Pri-Andriol LA.
MED: 100-2,15,50

N ☑ **J2321** Injection, nandrolone decanoate, up to 100 mg
Use this code for Deca-Durabolin, Hybolin Decanoate, Decolone-100, Neo-Durabolic, Anabolin LA 100, Androlone-D 100, Nandrobolic L.A.
MED: 100-2,15,50

N ☑ **J2322** Injection, nandrolone decanoate, up to 200 mg
Use this code for Deca-Durabolin, Neo-Durabolic.
MED: 100-2,15,50

K **J2325** Injection, nesiritide, 0.1 mg
Use this code for Natrecor.
MED: 100-2,15,50; 100-4,4,230.1

K ☑ **J2353** Injection, octreotide, depot form for intramuscular injection, 1 mg
Use this code for Sandostatin LAR.

N ☑ **J2354** Injection, octreotide, nondepot form for subcutaneous or intravenous injection, 25 mcg
Use this code for Sandostatin.

K ☑ **J2355** Injection, oprelvekin, 5 mg
Use this code for Neumega.
MED: 100-2,15,50

K ☑ **J2357** Injection, omalizumab, 5 mg
Use this code for Xolair.

N ☑ **J2360** Injection, orphenadrine citrate, up to 60 mg
Use this code for Antiflex, Mio Rel, Myophen, Norflex, Banflex, Flexoject, Flexon, K-Flex, Myolin, Neocyten, O-Flex, Orphenate.
MED: 100-2,15,50

Special Coverage Instructions   Noncovered by Medicare   Carrier Discretion   ☑ Quality Alert   ● New Code   ○ Reinstated Code   ▲ Revised Code

2007 HCPCS   1-9 ASC Group   MED: Pub 100/NCD References   ℔ DMEPOS Paid   ⊘ SNF Excluded   J Codes — 83

Drugs Administered Other Than Oral Method

J2370 — J2780

N ☑ **J2370** Injection, phenylephrine HCl, up to 1 ml
Use this code for Neo-Synephrine.
MED: 100-2,15,50

N ☑ **J2400** Injection, chloroprocaine HCl, per 30 ml
Use this code for Nesacaine, Nesacaine-MPF.
MED: 100-2,15,50

K ☑ **J2405** Injection, ondansetron HCl, per 1 mg
Use this code for Zofran.
MED: 100-2,15,50

N ☑ **J2410** Injection, oxymorphone HCl, up to 1 mg
Use this code for Numorphan, Numorphan H.P.,
Oxymorphone HCl.
MED: 100-2,15,50

K **J2425** Injection, palifermin, 50 mcg

K ☑ **J2430** Injection, pamidronate disodium, per 30 mg
Use this code for Aredia, Argatroban.
MED: 100-2,15,50; 100-4,4,230.1

N ☑ **J2440** Injection, papaverine HCl, up to 60 mg
MED: 100-2,15,50

N ☑ **J2460** Injection, oxytetracycline HCl, up to 50 mg
Use this code for Terramycin IM.
MED: 100-2,15,50

K ☑ **J2469** Injection, palonosetron HCl, 25 mcg
Use this code for Aloxi.

N **J2501** Injection, paricalcitol, 1 mcg
Use this code For Zemplar.
MED: 100-2,15,50

G **J2503** Injection, pegaptanib sodium, 0.3 mg
Use this code for Mucagen.
MED: 100-4,4,230.1

K **J2504** Injection, pegademase bovine, 25 IU
Use this code for Adagen.
MED: 100-2,15,50; 100-4,4,230.1

K ☑ **J2505** Injection, pegfilgrastim, 6 mg
Use this code for Neulasta.

N ☑ **J2510** Injection, penicillin G procaine, aqueous, up to 600,000
units
Use this code for Wycillin, Duracillin A.S., Pfizerpen A.S.,
Crysticillin 300 A.S., Crysticillin 600 A.S.
MED: 100-2,15,50

N **J2513** Injection, pentastarch, 10% solution, 100 ml
MED: 100-2,15,50; 100-4,4,230.1

N ☑ **J2515** Injection, pentobarbital sodium, per 50 mg
Use this code for Nembutal Sodium Solution.
MED: 100-2,15,50

N ☑ **J2540** Injection, penicillin G potassium, up to 600,000
units
Use this code for Pfizerpen.
MED: 100-2,15,50

N ☑ **J2543** Injection, piperacillin sodium/tazobactam sodium, 1
g/0.125 g (1.125 g)
Use this code for Zosyn.
MED: 100-2,15,50

B ☑ **J2545** Pentamidine isethionate, inhalation solution, per 300
mg, administered through a DME
Use this code for Nebupent, PentacaRinat, Pentam 300.
See code(s): Q0077
MED: 100-2,15,50

N ☑ **J2550** Injection, promethazine HCl, up to 50 mg
Use this code for Anergan 25, Anergan 50, Antinaus,
Phenazine 25, Phenazine 50, Phenergan, Prorex-25,
Prorex-50, Prothazine, V-Gan 25, V-Gan 50.
MED: 100-2,15,50

N ☑ **J2560** Injection, phenobarbital sodium, up to 120 mg
Use this code for Luminal Sodium, Nembutal Sodium.
MED: 100-2,15,50

N ☑ **J2590** Injection, oxytocin, up to 10 units
Use this code for Pitocin, Syntocinon.
MED: 100-2,15,50

N ☑ **J2597** Injection, desmopressin acetate, per 1 mcg
Use this code for DDAVP.
MED: 100-2,15,50

N ☑ **J2650** Injection, prednisolone acetate, up to 1 ml
Use this code for Colotone, Key-Pred 25, Key-Pred 50,
Predacort, Predcor-25, Predcor-50, Predoject-50,
Predalone-50, Predicort-50.
MED: 100-2,15,50; 100-4,4,240

N ☑ **J2670** Injection, tolazoline HCl, up to 25 mg
Use this code for Priscoline HCl.
MED: 100-2,15,50

N **J2675** Injection, progesterone, per 50 mg
Use this code for Gesterone, Gestrin.
MED: 100-2,15,50

N ☑ **J2680** Injection, fluphenazine decanoate, up to 25 mg
Use this code for Prolixin Decanoate.
MED: 100-2,15,50

N ☑ **J2690** Injection, procainamide HCl, up to 1 g
Use this code for Pronestyl.
MED: 100-2,15,50

N ☑ **J2700** Injection, oxacillin sodium, up to 250 mg
Use this code for Bactocill, Prostaphlin.
MED: 100-2,15,50

N ☑ **J2710** Injection, neostigmine methylsulfate, up to 0.5 mg
Use this code for Prostigmin.
MED: 100-2,15,50

N ☑ **J2720** Injection, protamine sulfate, per 10 mg
MED: 100-2,15,50

N ☑ **J2725** Injection, protirelin, per 250 mcg
Use this code for Relefact TRH, Thypinone, Thyrel TRH.
MED: 100-2,15,50

N ☑ **J2730** Injection, pralidoxime chloride, up to 1 g
Use this code for Protopam Chloride.
MED: 100-2,15,50

N ☑ **J2760** Injection, phentolamine mesylate, up to 5 mg
Use this code for Regitine.
MED: 100-2,15,50

N ☑ **J2765** Injection, metoclopramide HCl, up to 10 mg
Use this code for Ocatmide PFS, Reglan.
MED: 100-2,15,50

K ☑ **J2770** Injection, quinupristin/dalfopristin, 500 mg
(150/350)
Use this code for Synercid.
MED: 100-2,15,50

N ☑ **J2780** Injection, ranitidine HCl, 25 mg
Use this code for Zantac.
MED: 100-2,15,50

Special Coverage Instructions   Noncovered by Medicare   Carrier Discretion   ☑ Quality Alert   ● New Code   ○ Reinstated Code ▲ Revised Code

84 — J Codes    A Age Edit   M Maternity Edit ♀ Female Only ♂ Male Only A - ☑ APC Status Indicators   2007 HCPCS

K ☑ **J2783** Injection, rasburicase, 0.5 mg
Use this code for Elitek.

K **J2788** Injection, Rho D immune globulin, human, minidose, 50 mcg
Use this code for RhoGam, BAYRho-D, HYPRho-D, MICRhoGAM Ultra-Filtered.
MED: 100-2,15,50

K ☑ **J2790** Injection, Rho D immune globulin, human, full dose, 300 mcg
Use this code for Gamulin RH, HypRho-D, BayRho-D, RhoGam, Rhophylac.
MED: 100-2,15,50

K ☑ **J2792** Injection, Rho D immune globulin, intravenous, human, solvent detergent, 100 IU
Use this code for BAYRho-D, Rhophylac, WINRho SDF.
MED: 100-2,15,50

K ☑ **J2794** Injection, risperidone, long acting, 0.5 mg
Use this code for Risperidal Costa Long Acting.

N ☑ **J2795** Injection, ropivacaine HCl, 1 mg
Use this code for Naropin.

N ☑ **J2800** Injection, methocarbamol, up to 10 ml
Use this code for Robaxin, Carbacot, Methocarbamol, Relaxin.
MED: 100-2,15,50

N **J2805** Injection, sincalide, 5 mcg

N ☑ **J2810** Injection, theophylline, per 40 mg
MED: 100-2,15,50

K ☑ **J2820** Injection, sargramostim (GM-CSF), 50 mcg
Use this code for Leukine, Prokine.
MED: 100-2,15,50

K **J2850** Injection, secretin, synthetic, human, 1 mcg
MED: 100-2,15,50

N ☑ **J2910** Injection, aurothioglucose, up to 50 mg
Use this code for Solganal.
MED: 100-2,15,50

~~**J2912** Injection, sodium chloride, 0.9%, per 2 ml~~

N **J2916** Injection, sodium ferric gluconate complex in sucrose injection, 12.5 mg
Use this code for Ferrlecit, Sodium Ferric Gluconate Complex.
MED: 100-2,15,50.2

N ☑ **J2920** Injection, methylprednisolone sodium succinate, up to 40 mg
Use this code for Solu-Medrol, A-methaPred.
MED: 100-2,15,50; 100-4,4,240

N ☑ **J2930** Injection, methylprednisolone sodium succinate, up to 125 mg
Use this code for Solu-Medrol, A-methaPred.
MED: 100-2,15,50; 100-4,4,240

K ☑ **J2940** Injection, somatrem, 1 mg
Use this code for Protropin.
MED: 100-2,15,50
AHA: 2Q,'02,8

K ☑ **J2941** Injection, somatropin, 1 mg
Use this code for Humatrope, Genotropin Nutropin, Biotropin, Genotropin, Genotropin Miniquick, Norditropin, Nutropin, Nutropin AQ, Saizen, Saizen Somatropin RDNA Origin, Serostim, Serostim RDNA Origin, Zorbtive.
MED: 100-2,15,50
AHA: 2Q,'02,8

N ☑ **J2950** Injection, promazine HCl, up to 25 mg
Use this code for Sparine, Prozine-50.
MED: 100-2,15,50

K ☑ **J2993** Injection, reteplase, 18.1 mg
Use this code for Retavase
MED: 100-2,15,50

K ☑ **J2995** Injection, streptokinase, per 250,000 IU
Use this code for Kabikinase, Streptase.
MED: 100-2,15,50

K ☑ **J2997** Injection, alteplase recombinant, 1 mg
Use this code for Activase, Cathflo.
MED: 100-2,15,50

N ☑ **J3000** Injection, streptomycin, up to 1 g
Use this code for Streptomycin Sulfate.
MED: 100-2,15,50

N ☑ **J3010** Injection, fentanyl citrate, 0.1 mg
Use this code for Sublimaze.
MED: 100-2,15,50

K ☑ **J3030** Injection, sumatriptan succinate, 6 mg (code may be used for Medicare when drug administered under the direct supervision of a physician, not for use when drug is self-administered)
Use this code for Imitrex.
MED: 100-2,15,50

N ☑ **J3070** Injection, pentazocine, 30 mg
Use this code for Talwin.
MED: 100-2,15,50

K ☑ **J3100** Injection, tenecteplase, 50 mg
Use this code for TNKase.
AHA: 2Q,'02,8

N ☑ **J3105** Injection, terbutaline sulfate, up to 1 mg
Use this code for Brethine, Bricanyl Subcutaneous. For terbutaline in inhalation solution, see K0525 and K0526.
MED: 100-2,15,50

B ☑ **J3110** Injection, teriparatide, 10 mcg
Use this code for Forteo.

N ☑ **J3120** Injection, testosterone enanthate, up to 100 mg
Use this code for Everone, Delatest, Delatestryl, Andropository 100, Testone LA 100.
MED: 100-2,15,50

N ☑ **J3130** Injection, testosterone enanthate, up to 200 mg
Use this code for Everone, Delatestryl, Andro L.A. 200, Andryl 200, Durathate-200, Testone LA 200, Testrin PA.
MED: 100-2,15,50

N ☑ **J3140** Injection, testosterone suspension, up to 50 mg
Use this code for Andronaq 50, Testosterone Aqueous, Testaqua, Testoject-50, Histerone 50, Histerone 100.
MED: 100-2,15,50

N ☑ **J3150** Injection, testosterone propionate, up to 100 mg
Use this code for Testex.
MED: 100-2,15,50

N ☑ **J3230** Injection, chlorpromazine HCl, up to 50 mg
Use this code for Thorazine.
MED: 100-2,15,50

K ☑ **J3240** Injection, thyrotropin alpha, 0.9 mg, provided in 1.1 mg vial
Use this code for Thyrogen, Thytropar.
MED: 100-2,15,50

● G ☑ **J3243** Injection, tigecycline, 1 mg
Use this code for Tygacil.

Special Coverage Instructions | Noncovered by Medicare | Carrier Discretion | ☑ Quality Alert | ● New Code | ○ Reinstated Code | ▲ Revised Code

2007 HCPCS | **1**-**9** ASC Group | MED: Pub 100/NCD References | ℞ DMEPOS Paid | ⊘ SNF Excluded | J Codes — 85

Drugs Administered Other Than Oral Method

J3246 — J3535

K ☑ **J3246** Injection, tirofiban HCl, 0.25mg
Use this code for Aggrastat.

N ☑ **J3250** Injection, trimethobenzamide HCl, up to 200 mg
Use this code for Tigan, Ticon, Tiject-20, Arrestin.
MED: 100-2,15,50

N ☑ **J3260** Injection, tobramycin sulfate, up to 80 mg
Use this code for Nebcin.
MED: 100-2,15,50

N ☑ **J3265** Injection, torsemide, 10 mg/ml
Use this code for Demadex, Torsemide.
MED: 100-2,15,50

N ☑ **J3280** Injection, thiethylperazine maleate, up to 10 mg
Use this code for Norzine, Torecan.
MED: 100-2,15,50

K **J3285** Injection, treprostinil, 1 mg
Use this code for Remodulin.
MED: 100-4,4,230.1

N ☑ **J3301** Injection, triamcinolone acetonide, per 10 mg
Use this code for Kenalog-10, Kenalog-40, Tri-Kort, Kenaject-40, Cenacort A-40, Triam-A, Trilog. For triamcinolone in inhalation solution, see K0527 and K0528.
MED: 100-2,15,50

N ☑ **J3302** Injection, triamcinolone diacetate, per 5 mg
Use this code for Aristocort, Aristocort Intralesional, Aristocort Forte, Amcort, Trilone, Cenacort Forte.
MED: 100-2,15,50

N ☑ **J3303** Injection, triamcinolone hexacetonide, per 5 mg
Use this code for Aristospan Intralesional, Aristospan Intra-articular.
MED: 100-2,15,50

K ☑ **J3305** Injection, trimetrexate glucoronate, per 25 mg
Use this code for Neutrexin.
MED: 100-2,15,50

N ☑ **J3310** Injection, perphenazine, up to 5 mg
Use this code for Trilafon.
MED: 100-2,15,50

K **J3315** Injection, triptorelin pamoate, 3.75 mg
Use this code for Trelstar Depot, Trelstar Depot Plus Debioclip Kit, Trelstar LA.
MED: 100-2,15,50

K ☑ **J3320** Injection, spectinomycin dihydrochloride, up to 2 g
Use this code for Trobicin.
MED: 100-2,15,50

K ☑ **J3350** Injection, urea, up to 40 g
Use this code for Ureaphil.
MED: 100-2,15,50

K **J3355** Injection, urofollitropin, 75 IU
Use this code for Metrodin, Bravelle.
MED: 100-2,15,50; 100-4,4,230.1

N ☑ **J3360** Injection, diazepam, up to 5 mg
Use this code for Diastat, Dizac, Valium, Zetran.
MED: 100-2,15,50

N ☑ **J3364** Injection, urokinase, 5,000 IU vial
Use this code for Abbokinase Open-Cath.
MED: 100-2,15,50

K ☑ **J3365** Injection, IV, urokinase, 250,000 IU vial
Use this code for Abbokinase.
See code(s): Q0089
MED: 100-2,15,50

N ☑ **J3370** Injection, vancomycin HCl, 500 mg
Use this code for Varocin, Vancoled.
MED: 100-2,15,50; 100-3,280.14

K ☑ **J3396** Injection, verteporfin, 0.1 mg
MED: 100-3,80.2; 100-3,80.3

N ☑ **J3400** Injection, triflupromazine HCl, up to 20 mg
MED: 100-2,15,50

N ☑ **J3410** Injection, hydroxyzine HCl, up to 25 mg
Use this code for Vistaril, Vistaject-25, Hyzine, Hyzine-50.
MED: 100-2,15,50

N ☑ **J3411** Injection, thiamine HCl, 100 mg

N ☑ **J3415** Injection, pyridoxine HCl, 100 mg

N ☑ **J3420** Injection, vitamin B-12 cyanocobalamin, up to 1,000 mcg
Use this code for Sytobex, Redisol, Rubramin PC, Betalin 12, Berubigen, Cobex, Cobal, Crystal B12, Cyano, Cyanocobalamin, Hydroxocobalamin, Hydroxycobal, Nutri-Twelve.
MED: 100-2,15,50; 100-3,150.6

N ☑ **J3430** Injection, phytonadione (vitamin K), per 1 mg
Use this code for AquaMephyton, Konakion, Menadione, Phytonadione.
MED: 100-2,15,50

K ☑ **J3465** Injection, voriconazole, 10 mg
MED: 100-2,15,50

N ☑ **J3470** Injection, hyaluronidase, up to 150 units
Use this code for Wydase.
MED: 100-2,15,50

N **J3471** Injection, hyaluronidase, ovine, preservative free, per 1 USP unit (up to 999 USP units)

K **J3472** Injection, hyaluronidase, ovine, preservative free, per 1000 USP units

● G ☑ **J3473** Injection, hyaluronidase, recombinant, 1 USP unit
Use this code for Hylenex.

N ☑ **J3475** Injection, magnesium sulphate, per 500 mg
Use this code for Mag Sul, Sulfa Mag.
MED: 100-2,15,50

N ☑ **J3480** Injection, potassium chloride, per 2 meq
MED: 100-2,15,50

N ☑ **J3485** Injection, zidovudine, 10 mg
Use this code for Retrovir, Zidovudine.
MED: 100-2,15,50

N ☑ **J3486** Injection, ziprasidone mesylate, 10 mg
Use this code for Geodon.

K **J3487** Injection, zoledronic acid, 1 mg
Use this code for Zometa.

N **J3490** Unclassified drugs
MED: 100-2,15,50

E ☑ **J3520** Edetate disodium, per 150 mg
Use this code for Endrate, Disotate, Meritate. This drug is used in chelation therapy, a treatment for atherosclerosis that is not covered by Medicare.
MED: 100-3,20.21; 100-3,20.22

N **J3530** Nasal vaccine inhalation
MED: 100-2,15,50

E **J3535** Drug administered through a metered dose inhaler
MED: 100-2,15,50

Special Coverage Instructions   Noncovered by Medicare   Carrier Discretion   ☑ Quality Alert   ● New Code   ○ Reinstated Code ▲ Revised Code

   A Age Edit   M Maternity Edit   ♀ Female Only   ♂ Male Only   A - Y APC Status Indicators   *2007 HCPCS*

| E | | J3570 | **Laetrile, amygdalin, vitamin B-17** |

The FDA has found Laetrile to have no safe or effective therapeutic purpose.

MED: 100-3,30.7

| N | | J3590 | **Unclassified biologics** |

MISCELLANEOUS DRUGS AND SOLUTIONS

| N | ☑ | J7030 | **Infusion, normal saline solution, 1,000 cc** |

MED: 100-2,15,50

| N | ☑ | J7040 | **Infusion, normal saline solution, sterile (500 ml = 1 unit)** |

MED: 100-2,15,50

| N | ☑ | J7042 | **5% dextrose/normal saline (500 ml = 1 unit)** |

MED: 100-2,15,50

| N | ☑ | J7050 | **Infusion, normal saline solution, 250 cc** |

MED: 100-2,15,50

| N | ☑ | J7060 | **5% dextrose/water (500 ml = 1 unit)** |

MED: 100-2,15,50

| N | ☑ | J7070 | **Infusion, D-5-W, 1,000 cc** |

MED: 100-2,15,50

| N | ☑ | J7100 | **Infusion, dextran 40, 500 ml** |

Use this code for Gentran, 10% LMD, Rheomacrodex.

MED: 100-2,15,50

| N | ☑ | J7110 | **Infusion, dextran 75, 500 ml** |

Use this code for Gentran 75.

MED: 100-2,15,50

| N | ☑ | J7120 | **Ringer's lactate infusion, up to 1,000 cc** |

MED: 100-2,15,50

| N | ☑ | J7130 | **Hypertonic saline solution, 50 or 100 meq, 20 cc vial** |

MED: 100-2,15,50

● | K | J7187 | **Injection, von Willebrand Factor complex, human, ristocetin cofactor, per IU VWF:RCO**

~~J7188 Injection, Von Willebrand factor complex, human, IU~~
See code(s) J7187

| K | | J7189 | **Factor VIIa (antihemophilic Factor, recombinant), per 1 mcg** |

MED: 100-1,1,10.1; 100-2,6,10; 100-2,15,50; 100-4,3,20.7.3; 100-4,4,230.1

| K | ☑ | J7190 | **Factor VIII (antihemophilic factor, human) per IU** |

Use this code for Monarc-M, Koate-HP, Alphanate, Hemofil-M, Koate-DVI, Kogenate, Monoclate-P.

Medicare jurisdiction: local contractor.

MED: 100-1,1,10.1; 100-2,6,10; 100-2,15,50; 100-4,3,20.7.3; 100-4,4,240; 100-4,17,80.4

| K | ☑ | J7191 | **Factor VIII (antihemophilic factor (porcine)), per IU** |

Use this code for Hyate:C. Medicare jurisdiction: local contractor.

MED: 100-1,1,10.1; 100-2,6,10; 100-2,15,50; 100-4,3,20.7.3; 100-4,4,240; 100-4,17,80.4

| K | ☑ | J7192 | **Factor VIII (antihemophilic factor, recombinant) per IU** |

Use this code for Recombinate, Kogenate, Bioclate, Helixate, Advate rAHF-PFM, Antihemophilic Factor Human Method M Monoclonal Purified, Genarc, Refacto. Medicare jurisdiction: local contractor.

MED: 100-1,1,10.1; 100-2,6,10; 100-2,15,50; 100-4,3,20.7.3; 100-4,4,240; 100-4,17,80.4

| K | ☑ | J7193 | **Factor IX (antihemophilic factor, purified, nonrecombinant) per IU** |

Use this code for AlphaNine SD, Mononine.

MED: 100-1,1,10.1; 100-2,6,10; 100-2,15,50; 100-4,3,20.7.3; 100-4,4,240; 100-4,17,80.4

AHA: 2Q,'02,8

| K | ☑ | J7194 | **Factor IX complex, per IU** |

Use this code for Konyne-80, Profilnine Heat-Treated, Proplex T, Proplex SX-T, Alphanine SD, Bebulin VH, factor IX+ complex, Profilnine SD. Medicare jurisdiction: local contractor.

MED: 100-1,1,10.1; 100-2,6,10; 100-2,15,50; 100-4,3,20.7.3; 100-4,4,240; 100-4,17,80.4

| K | ☑ | J7195 | **Factor IX (antihemophilic factor, recombinant) per IU** |

Use this code for Benefix, Konyne 80, ProplexT.

MED: 100-1,1,10.1; 100-2,6,10; 100-2,15,50; 100-4,3,20.7.3; 100-4,4,240; 100-4,17,80.4

AHA: 2Q,'02,8

| K | ☑ | J7197 | **Antithrombin III (human), per IU** |

Medicare jurisdiction: local contractor. Use this code for Throbate III, ATnativ.

MED: 100-2,15,50

| K | ☑ | J7198 | **Antiinhibitor, per IU** |

Medicare jurisdiction: local contractor. Use this code for Autoplex T, Feiba VH AICC.

| B | | J7199 | **Hemophilia clotting factor, not otherwise classified** |

Medicare jurisdiction: local contractor.

| E | | J7300 | **Intrauterine copper contraceptive** |

Use this code for Paragard T380A.

| E | ☑ | J7302 | **Levonorgestrel-releasing intrauterine contraceptive system, 52 mg**   ♀ |

Use this code for Mirena.

| E | ☑ | J7303 | **Contraceptive supply, hormone containing vaginal ring, each**   ♀ |

Use this code for Nuvaring Vaginal Ring.

| E | ☑ | J7304 | **Contraceptive supply, hormone containing patch, each** |

| E | | J7306 | **Levonorgestrel (contraceptive) implant system, including implants and supplies** |

| K | ☑ | J7308 | **Aminolevulinic acid HCl for topical administration, 20%, single unit dosage form (354 mg)** |

| K | ☑ | J7310 | **Ganciclovir, 4.5 mg, long-acting implant** |

Use this code for Vitrasert.

MED: 100-2,15,50

● | G | J7311 | **Fluocinolone acetonide, intravitreal implant**

Use this code for Retisert.

~~J7317 Sodium hyaluronate, per 20 to 25 mg dose for intra-articular injection~~
See code(s) J7319

● | K | J7319 | **Hyaluronan (sodium hyaluronate) or derivative, intra-articular injection, per injection**

Use this code for hylan G F 20, Hyalgan, Hylan, Provisc, Euflexxa, Supartz, Synvisc.

~~J7320 Hylan G-F 20, 16 mg, for intra-articular injection~~
See code(s) J7319.

| B | ☑ | J7330 | **Autologous cultured chondrocytes, implant** |

Medicare jurisdiction: local contractor. Use this code for Carticel.

Special Coverage Instructions   Noncovered by Medicare   Carrier Discretion   ☑ Quality Alert   ● New Code   ○ Reinstated Code   ▲ Revised Code

2007 HCPCS   ❶-❾ ASC Group   MED: Pub 100/NCD References   ♿ DMEPOS Paid   ⊘ SNF Excluded   J Codes — 87

K ☑ **J7340** Dermal and epidermal, (substitute) tissue of human origin, with or without bioengineered or processed elements, with metabolically active elements, per square centimeter
Use this code for Apligraf, Orcel, TransCyte.

MED: 100-4,4,230.1

K **J7341** Dermal (substitute) tissue of nonhuman origin, with or without other bioengineered or processed elements, with metabolically active elements, per square centimeter

K ☑ **J7342** Dermal (substitute) tissue of human origin, with or without other bioengineered or processed elements, with metabolically active elements, per square centimeter
Use this code for Dermagraft , Dermagraft TC.

MED: 100-4,4,230.1

K **J7343** Dermal and epidermal, (substitute) tissue of non-human origin, with or without other bioengineered or processed elements, without metabolically active elements, per square centimeter
Use this code for Integra.

MED: 100-4,4,230.1

K **J7344** Dermal (substitute) tissue of human origin, with or without other bioengineered or processed elements, without metabolically active elements, per square centimeter

MED: 100-4,4,230.1

● B **J7345** Dermal (substitute) tissue of nonhuman origin, with or without other bioengineered or processed elements, without metabolically active elements, per square centimeter

● K **J7346** Dermal (substitute) tissue of human origin, injectable, with or without other bioengineered or processed elements, but without metabolically active elements, 1 cc

~~J7350~~ ~~Dermal (substitute) tissue of human origin, injectable, with or without other bioengineered or processed elements, but without metabolized active elements, per 10 mg~~
See code(s) J7346

N ☑ **J7500** Azathioprine, oral, 50 mg
Use this code for Azasan, Imuran.

MED: 100-2,15,50.5; 100-4,4,240; 100-4,17,80.3

K ☑ **J7501** Azathioprine, parenteral, 100 mg
Use this code for Imuran.

MED: 100-2,6,10; 100-2,15,50; 100-4,4,230.1; 100-4,4,240; 100-4,17,80.3

K ☑ **J7502** Cyclosporine, oral, 100 mg
Use this code for Neoral, Sandimmune, Gengraf, Sangcya

MED: 100-2,15,50.5; 100-4,4,230.1; 100-4,4,240; 100-4,17,80.3

K ☑ **J7504** Lymphocyte immune globulin, antithymocyte globulin, equine, parenteral, 250 mg
Use this code for Atgam.

MED: 100-2,6,10; 100-2,15,50; 100-3,260.7; 100-4,4,240; 100-4,17,80.3

K ☑ **J7505** Muromonab-CD3, parenteral, 5 mg
Use this code for Orthoclone OKT3.

MED: 100-2,6,10; 100-2,15,50; 100-4,4,240; 100-4,17,80.3

N ☑ **J7506** Prednisone, oral, per 5 mg
Use this code for Deltasone, Liquid Pred Syrup, Levoxyl, Predone, Prednicot, Sterapred.

MED: 100-2,15,50.5; 100-4,4,240; 100-4,17,80.3

K ☑ **J7507** Tacrolimus, oral, per 1 mg
Use this code for Prograf.

MED: 100-2,15,50.5; 100-4,4,240; 100-4,17,80.3

N ☑ **J7509** Methylprednisolone, oral, per 4 mg
Use this code for Medrol, Methylpred.

MED: 100-2,15,50.5; 100-4,4,240; 100-4,17,80.3

N ☑ **J7510** Prednisolone, oral, per 5 mg
Use this code for Delta-Cortef, Cotolone, Pediapred, Prednoral, Prelone.

MED: 100-2,15,50.5; 100-4,4,240; 100-4,17,80.3

K ☑ **J7511** Lymphocyte immune globulin, antithymocyte globulin, rabbit, parenteral, 25 mg
Use this code for Thymoglobulin.

MED: 100-2,6,10; 100-4,4,240; 100-4,17,80.3
AHA: 2Q,'02,8

K ☑ **J7513** Daclizumab, parenteral, 25 mg
Use this code for Zenapax.

MED: 100-2,6,10; 100-2,15,50.5; 100-4,4,240; 100-4,17,80.3

N ☑ **J7515** Cyclosporine, oral, 25 mg
Use this code for Gengraf, Neoral, Sandimmune.

MED: 100-4,4,240; 100-4,17,80.3

N ☑ **J7516** Cyclosporine, parenteral, 250 mg
Use this code for Neoral, Sandimmune.

MED: 100-2,6,10; 100-4,4,240; 100-4,17,80.3

K ☑ **J7517** Mycophenolate mofetil, oral, 250 mg
Use this code for CellCept.

MED: 100-4,4,240; 100-4,17,80.3

K ☑ **J7518** Mycophenolic acid, oral, 180 mg
Use this code for Myfortic Delayed Release.

MED: 100-4,4,240; 100-4,17,80.3.1

K ☑ **J7520** Sirolimus, oral, 1 mg
Use this code for Rapamune.

MED: 100-2,15,50.5; 100-4,4,240; 100-4,17,80.3

K ☑ **J7525** Tacrolimus, parenteral, 5 mg
Use this code for Prograf.

MED: 100-2,6,10; 100-2,15,50.5; 100-4,4,240; 100-4,17,80.3

N **J7599** Immunosuppressive drug, NOC
Determine if an alternative HCPCS Level II or a CPT code better describes the service being reported. This code should be used only if a more specific code is unavailable.

MED: 100-2,6,10; 100-2,15,50.5; 100-4,4,240; 100-4,17,80.3

INHALATION SOLUTIONS

● B **J7607** Levalbuterol, inhalation solution, compounded product, administered through DME, concentrated form, 0.5 mg

B ☑ **J7608** Acetylcysteine, inhalation solution administered through DME, unit dose form, per g
Use this code for Acetadote, Mucomyst, Mucosil.

MED: 100-2,15,110.3

● B **J7609** Albuterol, inhalation solution, compounded product, administered through DME, unit dose, 1 mg

● B **J7610** Albuterol, inhalation solution, compounded product, administered through DME, concentrated form, 1 mg

▲ B ☑ **J7611** Albuterol, inhalation solution, FDA-approved final product, noncompounded, administered through DME, concentrated form, 1 mg
Use this code for Accuneb, Proventil, Respirol, Ventolin.

MED: 100-2,15,110.3

Special Coverage Instructions   Noncovered by Medicare   Carrier Discretion   ☑ Quality Alert   ● New Code   ○ Reinstated Code   ▲ Revised Code

88 — J Codes   A Age Edit   M Maternity Edit   ♀ Female Only   ♂ Male Only   A - Y APC Status Indicators   *2007 HCPCS*

▲ B ☑ **J7612** Levalbuterol, inhalation solution, FDA-approved final product, noncompounded, administered through DME, concentrated form, 0.5 mg
Use this code for Xopenex HFA.
MED: 100-2,15,110.3

▲ B ☑ **J7613** Albuterol, inhalation solution, FDA-approved final product, noncompounded, administered through DME, unit dose, 1 mg
Use this code for Accuneb, Proventil, Respirol, Ventolin.
MED: 100-2,15,110.3

▲ B ☑ **J7614** Levalbuterol, inhalation solution, FDA-approved final product, noncompounded, administered through DME, unit dose, 0.5 mg
Use this code for Xopenex.
MED: 100-2,15,110.3

● B **J7615** Levalbuterol, inhalation solution, compounded product, administered through DME, unit dose, 0.5 mg

▲ B **J7620** Albuterol, up to 2.5 mg and ipratropium bromide, up to 0.5 mg, FDA-approved final product, noncompounded, administered through DME
MED: 100-2,15,110.3

▲ B **J7622** Beclomethasone, inhalation solution, compounded product, administered through DME, unit dose form, per milligram
Use this code for Beclovent, Beconase.

▲ B ☑ **J7624** Betamethasone, inhalation solution, compounded product, administered through DME, unit dose form, per milligram

▲ B ☑ **J7626** Budesonide, inhalation solution, FDA-approved final product, noncompounded, administered through DME, unit dose form, up to 0.5 mg
Use this code for Pulmicort Respules.

▲ B **J7627** Budesonide, inhalation solution, compounded product, administered through DME, unit dose form, up to 0.5 mg

▲ B ☑ **J7628** Bitolterol mesylate, inhalation solution, compounded product, administered through DME, concentrated form, per milligram
Use this code for Tornalate.
MED: 100-2,15,110.3

▲ B ☑ **J7629** Bitolterol mesylate, inhalation solution, compounded product, administered through DME, unit dose form, per milligram
Use this code for Tornalate.
MED: 100-2,15,110.3

B ☑ **J7631** Cromolyn sodium, inhalation solution administered through DME, unit dose form, per 10 mg
Use this code for Intal, Nasalcrom, Gastrocrom.
MED: 100-2,15,110.3

▲ B **J7633** Budesonide, inhalation solution, FDA-approved final product, noncompounded, administered through DME, concentrated form, per 0.25 milligram
Use this code for Pumocort.

● B **J7634** Budesonide, inhalation solution, compounded product, administered through DME, concentrated form, per 0.25 milligram

▲ B ☑ **J7635** Atropine, inhalation solution, compounded product, administered through DME, concentrated form, per milligram
MED: 100-2,15,110.3

▲ B ☑ **J7636** Atropine, inhalation solution, compounded product, administered through DME, unit dose form, per milligram
MED: 100-2,15,110.3

▲ B ☑ **J7637** Dexamethasone, inhalation solution, compounded product, administered through DME, concentrated form, per milligram
MED: 100-2,15,110.3

▲ B ☑ **J7638** Dexamethasone, inhalation solution, compounded product, administered through DME, unit dose form, per milligram
MED: 100-2,15,110.3

B ☑ **J7639** Dornase alpha, inhalation solution administered through DME, unit dose form, per mg
Use this code for Pulmozyme.
MED: 100-2,15,110.3

▲ E **J7640** Formoterol, inhalation solution, compounded product, administered through DME, unit dose form, 12 micrograms

▲ B **J7641** Flunisolide, inhalation solution, compounded product, administered through DME, unit dose, per milligram
Use this code for Aerobid, Flunisolide.

▲ B ☑ **J7642** Glycopyrrolate, inhalation solution, compounded product, administered through DME, concentrated form, per milligram
MED: 100-2,15,110.3

▲ B ☑ **J7643** Glycopyrrolate, inhalation solution, compounded product, administered through DME, unit dose form, per milligram
Use this code for Robinul.
MED: 100-2,15,110.3

▲ B ☑ **J7644** Ipratropium bromide, inhalation solution, FDA-approved final product, noncompounded, administered through DME, unit dose form, per milligram
Use this code for Atrovent.
MED: 100-2,15,110.3

● B **J7645** Ipratropium bromide, inhalation solution, compounded product, administered through DME, unit dose form, per milligram

● B **J7647** Isoetharine HCl, inhalation solution, compounded product, administered through DME, concentrated form, per milligram

▲ B ☑ **J7648** Isoetharine HCl, inhalation solution, FDA-approved final product, noncompounded, administered through DME, concentrated form, per milligram
Use this code for Beta-2.
MED: 100-2,15,110.3

▲ B ☑ **J7649** Isoetharine HCl, inhalation solution, FDA-approved final product, noncompounded, administered through DME, unit dose form, per milligram
MED: 100-2,15,110.3

● B **J7650** Isoetharine HCl, inhalation solution, compounded product, administered through DME, unit dose form, per milligram

● B **J7657** Isoproterenol HCl, inhalation solution, compounded product, administered through DME, concentrated form, per milligram

▲ B ☑ **J7658** Isoproterenol HCl, inhalation solution, FDA-approved final product, noncompounded, administered through DME, concentrated form, per milligram
Use this code for Isuprel HCl, Medihaler-ISO.
MED: 100-2,15,110.3

Special Coverage Instructions | Noncovered by Medicare | Carrier Discretion | ☑ Quality Alert | ● New Code | ○ Reinstated Code | ▲ Revised Code

Chemotherapy Drugs

J7659 — J9001

▲ Ⓑ ☑ **J7659** Isoproterenol HCl, inhalation solution, FDA-approved final product, noncompounded, administered through DME, unit dose form, per milligram
Use this code for Isuprel HCl, Medihaler-ISO.
MED: 100-2,15,110.3

● Ⓑ **J7660** Isoproterenol HCl, inhalation solution, compounded product, administered through DME, unit dose form, per milligram

● Ⓑ **J7667** Metaproterenol sulfate, inhalation solution, compounded product, concentrated form, per 10 milligrams

▲ Ⓑ ☑ **J7668** Metaproterenol sulfate, inhalation solution, FDA-approved final product, noncompounded, administered through DME, concentrated form, per 10 milligrams
Use this code for Alupent, Methaprel.
MED: 100-2,15,110.3

▲ Ⓑ ☑ **J7669** Metaproterenol sulfate, inhalation solution, FDA-approved final product, noncompounded, administered through DME, unit dose form, per 10 milligrams
Use this code for Alupent.
MED: 100-2,15,110.3

● Ⓑ **J7670** Metaproterenol sulfate, inhalation solution, compounded product, administered through DME, unit dose form, per 10 milligrams

Ⓝ ☑ **J7674** Methacholine chloride administered as inhalation solution through a nebulizer, per 1 mg
Use this code for Provocholine Powder.

▲ Ⓑ ☑ **J7680** Terbutaline sulfate, inhalation solution, compounded product, administered through DME, concentrated form, per milligram
Use this code for Brethine, Bricanyl.
MED: 100-2,15,110.3

▲ Ⓑ ☑ **J7681** Terbutaline sulfate, inhalation solution, compounded product, administered through DME, unit dose form, per milligram
Use this code for Brethine, Bricanyl.
MED: 100-2,15,110.3

▲ Ⓑ ☑ **J7682** Tobramycin, inhalation solution, FDA-approved final product, noncompounded, unit dose form, administered through DME, per 300 milligrams
Use this code for Tobi.
MED: 100-2,15,110.3

▲ Ⓑ ☑ **J7683** Triamcinolone, inhalation solution, compounded product, administered through DME, concentrated form, per milligram
Use this code for Azmacort.
MED: 100-2,15,110.3

▲ Ⓑ ☑ **J7684** Triamcinolone, inhalation solution, compounded product, administered through DME, unit dose form, per milligram
Use this code for Azmacort.
MED: 100-2,15,110.3

● Ⓑ **J7685** Tobramycin, inhalation solution, compounded product, administered through DME, unit dose form, per 300 milligrams

Ⓨ **J7699** NOC drugs, inhalation solution administered through DME
MED: 100-2,15,110.3

Ⓝ **J7799** NOC drugs, other than inhalation drugs, administered through DME
MED: 100-2,15,110.3

Ⓑ **J8498** Antiemetic drug, rectal/suppository, not otherwise specified

Ⓔ **J8499** Prescription drug, oral, nonchemotherapeutic, NOS
MED: 100-2,15,50

Ⓖ ☑ **J8501** Aprepitant, oral, 5 mg
Use this code for Emend.
MED: 100-4,4,240; 100-4,17,80.2; 100-4,17,80.2.1; 100-4,17,80.2.4

Ⓚ ☑ **J8510** Bulsulfan; oral, 2 mg
Use this code for Busulfex, Myleran.
MED: 100-2,15,50.5; 100-4,4,240, 100-4,17,00.1.1

Ⓔ **J8515** Cabergoline, oral, 0.25 mg
Use this code for Dostinex.
MED: 100-2,15,50.5; 100-4,4,240

Ⓚ ☑ **J8520** Capecitabine, oral, 150 mg
Use this code for Xeloda.
MED: 100-2,15,50.5; 100-4,4,240; 100-4,17,80.1.1

Ⓑ ☑ **J8521** Capecitabine, oral, 500 mg
Use this code for Xeloda.
MED: 100-2,15,50.5; 100-4,4,240; 100-4,17,80.1.1

Ⓝ ☑ **J8530** Cyclophosphamide, oral, 25 mg
Use this code for Cytoxan.
MED: 100-2,15,50.5; 100-4,4,240; 100-4,17,80.1.1

Ⓝ **J8540** Dexamethasone, oral, 0.25 mg
Use this code for Decadron.

Ⓚ ☑ **J8560** Etoposide, oral, 50 mg
Use this code for VePesid.
MED: 100-2,15,50.5; 100-4,4,230.1; 100-4,4,240; 100-4,17,80.1.1

Ⓔ ☑ **J8565** Gefitinib, oral, 250 mg
Use this code for Iressa.
MED: 100-4,4,240; 100-4,17,80.1.1

Ⓝ **J8597** Antiemetic drug, oral, not otherwise specified

Ⓝ ☑ **J8600** Melphalan, oral 2 mg
Use this code for Alkeran.
MED: 100-2,15,50.5; 100-4,4,240; 100-4,17,80.1.1

Ⓝ ☑ **J8610** Methotrexate, oral, 2.5 mg
Use this code for Rheumatrex Dose Pack.
MED: 100-2,15,50.5; 100-4,4,240; 100-4,17,80.1.1

● Ⓚ ☑ **J8650** Nabilone, oral, 1 mg
Use this code for Cesamet.

Ⓚ ☑ **J8700** Temozolomide, oral, 5 mg
Use this code for Temodar.
MED: 100-2,15,50.5; 100-4,4,240

Ⓑ **J8999** Prescription drug, oral, chemotherapeutic, NOS
Determine if an alternative HCPCS Level II or a CPT code better describes the service being reported. This code should be used only if a more specific code is unavailable.
MED: 100-2,15,50.5; 100-4,4,240; 100-4,17,80.1.1; 100-4,17,80.1.2

CHEMOTHERAPY DRUGS J9000-J9999

These codes cover the cost of the chemotherapy drug only, not the administration. See also J8999.

Ⓚ ☑ **J9000** Doxorubicin HCl, 10 mg   ⊘
Use this code for Adriamycin PFS, Adriamycin RDF, Rubex.
MED: 100-2,15,50; 100-4,4,230.1; 100-4,17,80.2

Ⓚ ☑ **J9001** Doxorubicin HCl, all lipid formulations, 10 mg   ⊘
Use this code for Doxil.
MED: 100-2,15,50; 100-4,17,80.2

Special Coverage Instructions   Noncovered by Medicare   Carrier Discretion   ☑ Quality Alert   ● New Code   ○ Reinstated Code   ▲ Revised Code

90 — J Codes   Ⓐ Age Edit   Ⓜ Maternity Edit   ♀ Female Only   ♂ Male Only   Ⓐ - Ⓨ APC Status Indicators   2007 HCPCS

K	**J9010** Alemtuzumab, 10 mg	⊘
	Use this code for Campath.	
K ☑	**J9015** Aldesleukin, per single use vial	⊘
	Use this code for Proleukin, IL-2, Interleukin.	
	MED: 100-2,15,50	
K ☑	**J9017** Arsenic trioxide, 1 mg	⊘
	Use this code for Trisenox.	
	AHA: 2Q,'02,8	
K ☑	**J9020** Asparaginase, 10,000 units	⊘
	Use this code for Elspar.	
	MED: 100-2,15,50	
K	**J9025** Injection, azacitidine, 1 mg	⊘
	Use this code for Vidaza.	
	MED: 100-4,4,230.1	
G	**J9027** Injection, clofarabine, 1 mg	⊘
	Use this code for Clolar.	
	MED: 100-4,4,230.1	
K ☑	**J9031** BCG live (intravesical), per instillation	
	Use this code for Tice BCG, PACIS BCG, TheraCys.	
	MED: 100-2,15,50	
K ☑	**J9035** Injection, bevacizumab, 10 mg	⊘
	Use this code for Avastin, Imuron.	
K ☑	**J9040** Bleomycin sulfate, 15 units	⊘
	Use this code for Blenoxane.	
	MED: 100-2,15,50; 100-4,4,230.1	
K ☑	**J9041** Injection, bortezomib, 0.1 mg	⊘
	Use this code for Velcade.	
K ☑	**J9045** Carboplatin, 50 mg	⊘
	Use this code for Paraplatin, Platinol AQ.	
	MED: 100-2,15,50	
K ☑	**J9050** Carmustine, 100 mg	⊘
	Use this code for BiCNU.	
	MED: 100-2,15,50; 100-4,4,230.1; 100-4,17,80.2	
K ☑	**J9055** Injection, cetuximab, 10 mg	⊘
	Use this code for Erbitux.	
N ☑	**J9060** Cisplatin, powder or solution, per 10 mg	⊘
	Use this code for Plantinol AQ.	
	MED: 100-2,15,50; 100-4,4,230.1; 100-4,17,80.2	
B ☑	**J9062** Cisplatin, 50 mg	⊘
	Use this code for Plantinol AQ.	
	MED: 100-2,15,50; 100-4,17,80.2	
K ☑	**J9065** Injection, cladribine, per 1 mg	⊘
	Use this code for Leustatin.	
	MED: 100-2,15,50; 100-4,4,230.1	
N ☑	**J9070** Cyclophosphamide, 100 mg	⊘
	Use this code for Endoxan-Asta.	
	MED: 100-2,15,50; 100-4,4,230.1; 100-4,17,80.2	
B ☑	**J9080** Cyclophosphamide, 200 mg	⊘
	Use this code for Cytoxan, Neosar.	
	MED: 100-2,15,50; 100-4,17,80.2	
B ☑	**J9090** Cyclophosphamide, 500 mg	⊘
	Use this code for Cytoxan, Neosar.	
	MED: 100-2,15,50; 100-4,17,80.2	
B ☑	**J9091** Cyclophosphamide, 1 g	⊘
	Use this code for Cytoxan, Neosar.	
	MED: 100-2,15,50; 100-4,17,80.2	

B ☑	**J9092** Cyclophosphamide, 2 g	⊘
	Use this code for Cytoxan, Neosar.	
	MED: 100-2,15,50; 100-4,17,80.2	
K ☑	**J9093** Cyclophosphamide, lyophilized, 100 mg	⊘
	Use this code for Cytoxan Lyophilized.	
	MED: 100-2,15,50; 100-4,4,230.1; 100-4,17,80.2	
B ☑	**J9094** Cyclophosphamide, lyophilized, 200 mg	⊘
	Use this code for Cytoxan Lyophilized.	
	MED: 100-2,15,50; 100-4,17,80.2	
B ☑	**J9095** Cyclophosphamide, lyophilized, 500 mg	⊘
	Use this code for Cytoxan Lyophilized.	
	MED: 100-2,15,50; 100-4,17,80.2	
B ☑	**J9096** Cyclophosphamide, lyophilized, 1 g	⊘
	Use this code for Cytoxan Lyophilized.	
	MED: 100-2,15,50; 100-4,17,80.2	
B ☑	**J9097** Cyclophosphamide, lyophilized, 2 g	⊘
	Use this code for Cytoxan Lyophilized.	
	MED: 100-2,15,50; 100-4,17,80.2	
K ☑	**J9098** Cytarabine liposome, 10 mg	⊘
	Use this code for Depocyt.	
N ☑	**J9100** Cytarabine, 100 mg	⊘
	Use this code for Cytosar-U, Ara-C, Tarabin CFS.	
	MED: 100-2,15,50; 100-4,4,230.1	
B ☑	**J9110** Cytarabine, 500 mg	⊘
	Use this code for Cytosar-U.	
	MED: 100-2,15,50	
K ☑	**J9120** Dactinomycin, 0.5 mg	⊘
	Use this code for Cosmegen.	
	MED: 100-2,15,50	
K ☑	**J9130** Dacarbazine, 100 mg	⊘
	Use this code for DTIC-Dome.	
	MED: 100-2,15,50; 100-4,4,230.1; 100-4,17,80.2	
B ☑	**J9140** Dacarbazine, 200 mg	⊘
	Use this code for DTIC-Dome.	
	MED: 100-2,15,50; 100-4,17,80.2	
K ☑	**J9150** Daunorubicin HCl, 10 mg	⊘
	Use this code for Cerubidine.	
	MED: 100-2,15,50; 100-4,4,230.1	
K ☑	**J9151** Daunorubicin citrate, liposomal formulation, 10 mg	⊘
	Use this code for Daunoxome.	
	MED: 100-2,15,50	
K ☑	**J9160** Denileukin diftitox, 300 mcg	⊘
	Use this code for Ontak.	
N ☑	**J9165** Diethylstilbestrol diphosphate, 250 mg	⊘
	Use this code for Stilphostrol.	
	MED: 100-2,15,50; 100-4,4,230.1	
K ☑	**J9170** Docetaxel, 20 mg	⊘
	Use this code for Taxotere.	
	MED: 100-2,15,50	
N	**J9175** Injection, Elliotts B Solution, 1 ml	
	MED: 100-2,15,50; 100-4,4,230.1	
K ☑	**J9178** Injection, epirubicin HCl, 2 mg	⊘
	Use this code for Ellence.	
	MED: 100-4,17,80.2	
N ☑	**J9181** Etoposide, 10 mg	⊘
	Use this code for VePesid, Toposar.	
	MED: 100-2,15,50; 100-4,4,230.1	

Special Coverage Instructions   Noncovered by Medicare   Carrier Discretion   ☑ Quality Alert   ● New Code   ○ Reinstated Code   ▲ Revised Code

2007 HCPCS   **1**-**9** ASC Group   MED: Pub 100/NCD References   ᠔ DMEPOS Paid   ⊘ SNF Excluded   **J Codes — 91**

Chemotherapy Drugs

J9182 — J9320

B ☑ **J9182** Etoposide, 100 mg ⊘
Use this code for VePesid, Toposar.
MED: 100-2,15,50

K ☑ **J9185** Fludarabine phosphate, 50 mg ⊘
Use this code for Fludara.
MED: 100-2,15,50

N ☑ **J9190** Fluorouracil, 500 mg ⊘
Use this code for Adrucil.
MED: 100-2,15,50

K ☑ **J9200** Floxuridine, 500 mg ⊘
Use this code for FUDR.
MED: 100-2,15,50; 100-4,4,230.1

K ☑ **J9201** Gemcitabine HCl, 200 mg ⊘
Use this code for Gemzar.
MED: 100-2,15,50

K ☑ **J9202** Goserelin acetate implant, per 3.6 mg
Use this code for Zoladex.
MED: 100-2,15,50

K ☑ **J9206** Irinotecan, 20 mg ⊘
Use this code for Camptosar.
MED: 100-2,15,50

K ☑ **J9208** Ifosfamide, per 1 g ⊘
Use this code for IFEX, Mitoxana.
MED: 100-2,15,50; 100-4,4,230.1

K ☑ **J9209** Mesna, 200 mg
Use this code for Mesnex.
MED: 100-2,15,50; 100-4,4,230.1

K ☑ **J9211** Idarubicin HCl, 5 mg ⊘
Use this code for Idamycin.
MED: 100-2,15,50; 100-4,4,230.1

K ☑ **J9212** Injection, interferon alfacon-1, recombinant, 1 mcg
Use this code for Infergen.
MED: 100-2,15,50

K ☑ **J9213** Interferon alfa-2A, recombinant, 3 million units
Use this code for Roferon-A.
MED: 100-2,15,50

K ☑ **J9214** Interferon alfa-2B, recombinant, 1 million units
Use this code for Intron A, Rebetron Kit.
MED: 100-2,15,50

K ☑ **J9215** Interferon alfa-N3, (human leukocyte derived), 250,000 IU
Use this code for Alferon N.
MED: 100-2,15,50

K ☑ **J9216** Interferon gamma-1B, 3 million units
Use this code for Actimmune.
MED: 100-2,15,50

K ☑ **J9217** Leuprolide acetate (for depot suspension), 7.5 mg
Use this code for Lupron Depot, Eligard.
MED: 100-2,15,50

K ☑ **J9218** Leuprolide acetate, per 1 mg
Use this code for Lupron, Eligard.
MED: 100-2,15,50; 100-4,4,230.1

K ☑ **J9219** Leuprolide acetate implant, 65 mg
Use this code for Lupron Implant.
MED: 100-2,15,50
AHA: 4Q,'01,5

K **J9225** Histrelin implant, 50 mg ⊘
Use this code for Vantas.
MED: 100-2,15,50

K ☑ **J9230** Mechlorethamine HCl, (nitrogen mustard), 10 mg ⊘
Use this code for Mustargen.
MED: 100-2,15,50; 100-4,17,80.2

K ☑ **J9245** Injection, melphalan HCl, 50 mg ⊘
Use this code for Alkeran, L-phenylalanine mustard.
MED: 100-2,15,50

N ☑ **J9250** Methotrexate sodium, 5 mg ⊘
Use this code for Folex, Folex PFS, Methotrexate LPF.
MED: 100-2,15,50

B ☑ **J9260** Methotrexate sodium, 50 mg ⊘
Use this code for Folex, Folex PFS, Methotrexate LPF.
MED: 100-2,15,50

● K **J9261** Injection, nelarabine, 50 mg
Use this code for Arranon

K ☑ **J9263** Injection, oxaliplatin, 0.5 mg ⊘
Use this code for Eloxatin.
MED: 100-4,4,230.1

G **J9264** Injection, paclitaxel protein-bound particles, 1 mg ⊘
Use this code for Abraxane.
MED: 100-4,4,230.1

K ☑ **J9265** Paclitaxel, 30 mg ⊘
Use this code for Taxol, Nov-Onxol.
MED: 100-2,15,50; 100-4,4,230.1

K ☑ **J9266** Pegaspargase, per single dose vial ⊘
Use this code for Oncaspar.
MED: 100-2,15,50
AHA: 2Q,'02,8

K ☑ **J9268** Pentostatin, per 10 mg ⊘
Use this code for Nipent.
MED: 100-2,15,50

K ☑ **J9270** Plicamycin, 2.5 mg ⊘
Use this code for Mithacin.
MED: 100-2,15,50

K ☑ **J9280** Mitomycin, 5 mg ⊘
Use this code for Mutamycin.
MED: 100-2,15,50; 100-4,4,230.1

B ☑ **J9290** Mitomycin, 20 mg ⊘
Use this code for Mutamycin.
MED: 100-2,15,50

B ☑ **J9291** Mitomycin, 40 mg ⊘
Use this code for Mutamycin.
MED: 100-2,15,50

K ☑ **J9293** Injection, mitoxantrone HCl, per 5 mg ⊘
Use this code for Navantrone.
MED: 100-2,15,50

K **J9300** Gemtuzumab ozogamicin, 5 mg ⊘
Use this code for Mylotarg.
AHA: 2Q,'02,8

K ☑ **J9305** Injection, pemetrexed, 10 mg ⊘
Use this code for Alimta.

K ☑ **J9310** Rituximab, 100 mg ⊘
Use this code for RituXan.
MED: 100-2,15,50

K ☑ **J9320** Streptozocin, 1 g ⊘
Use this code for Zanosar.
MED: 100-2,15,50; 100-4,17,80.2

Special Coverage Instructions   Noncovered by Medicare   Carrier Discretion   ☑ Quality Alert   ● New Code   ○ Reinstated Code   ▲ Revised Code

   A Age Edit   M Maternity Edit   ♀ Female Only   ♂ Male Only   A - Ⓩ APC Status Indicators   *2007 HCPCS*

K ☑ **J9340** Thiotepa, 15 mg ⊘
Use this code for Thioplex.
MED: 100-2,15,50; 100-4,4,230.1

K ☑ **J9350** Topotecan, 4 mg ⊘
Use this code for Hycamtin.
MED: 100-2,15,50

K ☑ **J9355** Trastuzumab, 10 mg ⊘
Use this code for Herceptin.

K ☑ **J9357** Valrubicin, intravesical, 200 mg ⊘
Use this code for Valstar.
MED: 100-2,15,50

N ☑ **J9360** Vinblastine sulfate, 1 mg ⊘
Use this code for Velban.
MED: 100-2,15,50

N ☑ **J9370** Vincristine sulfate, 1 mg ⊘
Use this code for Oncovin, Vincasar PFS.
MED: 100-2,15,50

B ☑ **J9375** Vincristine sulfate, 2 mg ⊘
Use this code for Oncovin, Vincasar PFS.
MED: 100-2,15,50

B ☑ **J9380** Vincristine sulfate, 5 mg ⊘
Use this code for Oncovin.
MED: 100-2,15,50

K ☑ **J9390** Vinorelbine tartrate, per 10 mg ⊘
Use this code for Navelbine.
MED: 100-2,15,50; 100-4,4,230.1

K ☑ **J9395** Injection, fulvestrant, 25 mg ⊘
Use this code for Fastodex.

K ☑ **J9600** Porfimer sodium, 75 mg ⊘
Use this code for Photofrin.
MED: 100-2,15,50

N **J9999** NOC, antineoplastic drug
Determine if an alternative HCPCS Level II or a CPT code better describes the service being reported. This code should be used only if a more specific code is unavailable.
MED: 100-2,15,50; 100-3,110.2

Special Coverage Instructions | Noncovered by Medicare | Carrier Discretion | ☑ Quality Alert | ● New Code ○ Reinstated Code ▲ Revised Code

2007 HCPCS | **1**-**9** ASC Group | **MED:** Pub 100/NCD References | ᕹ DMEPOS Paid | ⊘ SNF Excluded | J Codes — 93

TEMPORARY CODES K0000-K9999

The K codes were established for use by the DME Medicare Administrative Contractors (DME MACs). The K codes are developed when the currently existing permanent national codes for supplies and certain product categories do not include the codes needed to implement a DME MAC medical review policy.

K CODES ASSIGNED TO DURABLE MEDICAL EQUIPMENT ADMINISTRATIVE CONTRACTORS (DME MACS)

WHEELCHAIR AND WHEELCHAIR ACCESSORIES

☑		K0001	Standard wheelchair	⊘ ᕃ
☑		K0002	Standard hemi (low seat) wheelchair	⊘ ᕃ
☑		K0003	Lightweight wheelchair	⊘ ᕃ
☑		K0004	High strength, lightweight wheelchair	⊘ ᕃ
☑		K0005	Ultralightweight wheelchair	⊘ ᕃ
☑		K0006	Heavy-duty wheelchair	⊘ ᕃ
☑		K0007	Extra heavy-duty wheelchair	⊘ ᕃ
☑		K0009	Other manual wheelchair/base	⊘
☑		K0010	Standard-weight frame motorized/power wheelchair	⊘ ᕃ
☑		K0011	Standard-weight frame motorized/power wheelchair with programmable control parameters for speed adjustment, tremor dampening, acceleration control and braking	⊘ ᕃ
☑		K0012	Lightweight portable motorized/power wheelchair	⊘ ᕃ
☑		K0014	Other motorized/power wheelchair base	⊘
☑	☑	K0015	Detachable, nonadjustable height armrest, each	⊘ ᕃ
☑	☑	K0017	Detachable, adjustable height armrest, base, each	⊘ ᕃ
☑	☑	K0018	Detachable, adjustable height armrest, upper portion, each	⊘ ᕃ
☑	☑	K0019	Arm pad, each	⊘ ᕃ
☑	☑	K0020	Fixed, adjustable height armrest, pair	⊘ ᕃ
☑	☑	K0037	High mount flip-up footrest, each	⊘ ᕃ
☑	☑	K0038	Leg strap, each	⊘ ᕃ
☑	☑	K0039	Leg strap, H style, each	⊘ ᕃ
☑	☑	K0040	Adjustable angle footplate, each	⊘ ᕃ
☑	☑	K0041	Large size footplate, each	⊘ ᕃ
☑	☑	K0042	Standard size footplate, each	⊘ ᕃ
☑	☑	K0043	Footrest, lower extension tube, each	⊘ ᕃ
☑	☑	K0044	Footrest, upper hanger bracket, each	⊘ ᕃ
☑		K0045	Footrest, complete assembly	⊘ ᕃ
☑	☑	K0046	Elevating legrest, lower extension tube, each	⊘ ᕃ
☑	☑	K0047	Elevating legrest, upper hanger bracket, each	⊘ ᕃ
☑		K0050	Ratchet assembly	⊘ ᕃ
☑	☑	K0051	Cam release assembly, footrest or legrest, each	⊘ ᕃ
☑	☑	K0052	Swingaway, detachable footrests, each	⊘ ᕃ
☑	☑	K0053	Elevating footrests, articulating (telescoping), each	⊘ ᕃ
☑	☑	K0056	Seat height less than 17 in. or equal to or greater than 21 in. for a high strength, lightweight, or ultralightweight wheelchair	⊘ ᕃ

☑	☑	K0065	Spoke protectors, each	⊘ ᕃ
☑	☑	K0069	Rear wheel assembly, complete, with solid tire, spokes or molded, each	⊘ ᕃ
☑	☑	K0070	Rear wheel assembly, complete with pneumatic tire, spokes or molded, each	⊘ ᕃ
☑	☑	K0071	Front caster assembly, complete, with pneumatic tire, each	⊘ ᕃ
☑	☑	K0072	Front caster assembly, complete, with semipneumatic tire, each	⊘ ᕃ
☑	☑	K0073	Caster pin lock, each	⊘ ᕃ
☑	☑	K0077	Front caster assembly, complete, with solid tire, each	⊘ ᕃ
		~~K0090~~	~~Rear wheel tire for power wheelchair, any size, each~~	
		~~K0091~~	~~Rear wheel tire tube other than zero pressure for power wheelchair, any size, each~~	
		~~K0092~~	~~Rear wheel assembly for power wheelchair, complete, each~~	
		~~K0093~~	~~Rear wheel zero pressure tire tube (flat free insert) for power wheelchair, any size, each~~	
		~~K0094~~	~~Wheel tire for power base, any size, each~~	
		~~K0095~~	~~Wheel tire tube other than zero pressure for each base, any size, each~~	
		~~K0096~~	~~Wheel assembly for power base, complete, each~~	
		~~K0097~~	~~Wheel zero-pressure tire tube (flat free insert) for power base, any size, each~~	
☑		K0098	Drive belt for power wheelchair	⊘ ᕃ
		~~K0099~~	~~Front caster for power wheelchair~~	
☑	☑	K0105	IV hanger, each	⊘ ᕃ
☑		K0108	Wheelchair component or accessory, not otherwise specified	⊘
☑		K0195	Elevating legrest, pair (for use with capped rental wheelchair base)	⊘ ᕃ
			MED: 100-3,230.10	
☑		K0455	Infusion pump used for uninterrupted parenteral administration of medication, (e.g., epoprostenol or treprostinol)	⊘ ᕃ
			MED: 100-3,280.14	
☑		K0462	Temporary replacement for patient owned equipment being repaired, any type	⊘
			MED: 100-4,20,40.1	
☑	☑	K0552	Supplies for external drug infusion pump, syringe type cartridge, sterile, each	⊘ ᕃ
			MED: 100-3,280.14	
☑	☑	K0601	Replacement battery for external infusion pump owned by patient, silver oxide, 1.5 volt, each	⊘ ᕃ
			AHA: 2Q,'03,7	
☑	☑	K0602	Replacement battery for external infusion pump owned by patient, silver oxide, 3 volt, each	⊘ ᕃ
			AHA: 2Q,'03,7	
☑	☑	K0603	Replacement battery for external infusion pump owned by patient, alkaline, 1.5 volt, each	⊘ ᕃ
			AHA: 2Q,'03,7	
☑	☑	K0604	Replacement battery for external infusion pump owned by patient, lithium, 3.6 volt, each	⊘ ᕃ
			AHA: 2Q,'03,7	
☑	☑	K0605	Replacement battery for external infusion pump owned by patient, lithium, 4.5 volt, each	⊘ ᕃ
			AHA: 2Q,'03,7	

Special Coverage Instructions	Noncovered by Medicare	Carrier Discretion	☑ Quality Alert ● New Code ○ Reinstated Code ▲ Revised Code

☑ **K0606** Automatic external defibrillator, with integrated electrocardiogram analysis, garment type ⊘ ᶧ
AHA: 4Q,'03,4

☑ ☑ **K0607** Replacement battery for automated external defibrillator, garment type only, each ⊘ ᶧ
AHA: 4Q,'03,4

☑ ☑ **K0608** Replacement garment for use with automated external defibrillator, each ⊘ ᶧ
AHA: 4Q,'03,4

☑ ☑ **K0609** Replacement electrodes for use with automated external defibrillator, garment type only, each ⊘ ᶧ
AHA: 4Q,'03,4

☑ **K0669** Wheelchair accessory, wheelchair seat or back cushion, does not meet specific code criteria or no written coding verification from SADMERC

☑ **K0730** Controlled dose inhalation drug delivery system

● ☑ **K0733** Power wheelchair accessory, 12 to 24 amp hour sealed lead acid battery, each (e.g. gel cell, absorbed glassmat) ᶧ

● ☑ **K0734** Skin protection wheelchair seat cushion, adjustable, width less than 22 inches, any depth

● ☑ **K0735** Skin protection wheelchair seat cushion, adjustable, width 22 inches or greater, any depth

● ☑ **K0736** Skin protection and positioning wheelchair seat cushion, adjustable, width less than 22 inches, any depth

● ☑ **K0737** Skin protection and positioning wheelchair seat cushion, adjustable, width 22 inches or greater, any depth

● ☑ **K0738** Portable gaseous oxygen system, rental; home compressor used to fill portable oxygen cylinders; includes portable containers, regulator, flowmeter, humidifier, cannula or mask, and tubing

● ☑ **K0800** Power operated vehicle, group 1 standard, patient weight capacity up to and including 300 pounds ᶧ

● ☑ **K0801** Power operated vehicle, group 1 heavy duty, patient weight capacity 301 to 450 pounds ᶧ

● ☑ **K0802** Power operated vehicle, group 1 very heavy duty, patient weight capacity 451 to 600 pounds ᶧ

● ☑ **K0806** Power operated vehicle, group 2 standard, patient weight capacity up to and including 300 pounds ᶧ

● ☑ **K0807** Power operated vehicle, group 2 heavy duty, patient weight capacity 301 to 450 pounds ᶧ

● ☑ **K0808** Power operated vehicle, group 2 very heavy duty, patient weight capacity 451 to 600 pounds ᶧ

● ☑ **K0812** Power operated vehicle, not otherwise classified ᶧ

● ☑ **K0813** Power wheelchair, group 1 standard, portable, sling/solid seat and back, patient weight capacity up to and including 300 pounds ᶧ

● ☑ **K0814** Power wheelchair, group 1 standard, portable, captain's chair, patient weight capacity up to and including 300 pounds ᶧ

● ☑ **K0815** Power wheelchair, group 1 standard, sling/solid seat and back, patient weight capacity up to and including 300 pounds ᶧ

● ☑ **K0816** Power wheelchair, group 1 standard, captain's chair, patient weight capacity up to and including 300 pounds ᶧ

● ☑ **K0820** Power wheelchair, group 2 standard, portable, sling/solid seat/back, patient weight capacity up to and including 300 pounds ᶧ

● ☑ **K0821** Power wheelchair, group 2 standard, portable, captain's chair, patient weight capacity up to and including 300 pounds ᶧ

● ☑ **K0822** Power wheelchair, group 2 standard, sling/solid seat/back, patient weight capacity up to and including 300 pounds ᶧ

● ☑ **K0823** Power wheelchair, group 2 standard, captain's chair, patient weight capacity up to and including 300 pounds ᶧ

● ☑ **K0824** Power wheelchair, group 2 heavy duty, sling/solid seat/back, patient weight capacity 301 to 450 pounds ᶧ

● ☑ **K0825** Power wheelchair, group 2 heavy duty, captain's chair, patient weight capacity 301 to 450 pounds ᶧ

● ☑ **K0826** Power wheelchair, group 2 very heavy duty, sling/solid seat/back, patient weight capacity 451 to 600 pounds ᶧ

● ☑ **K0827** Power wheelchair, group 2 very heavy duty, captain's chair, patient weight capacity 451 to 600 pounds ᶧ

● ☑ **K0828** Power wheelchair, group 2 extra heavy duty, sling/solid seat/back, patient weight capacity 601 pounds or more ᶧ

● ☑ **K0829** Power wheelchair, group 2 extra heavy duty, captain's chair, patient weight capacity 601 pounds or more ᶧ

● ☑ **K0830** Power wheelchair, group 2 standard, seat elevator, sling/solid seat/back, patient weight capacity up to and including 300 pounds ᶧ

● ☑ **K0831** Power wheelchair, group 2 standard, seat elevator, captain's chair, patient weight capacity up to and including 300 pounds ᶧ

● ☑ **K0835** Power wheelchair, group 2 standard, single power option, sling/solid seat/back, patient weight capacity up to and including 300 pounds ᶧ

● ☑ **K0836** Power wheelchair, group 2 standard, single power option, captain's chair, patient weight capacity up to and including 300 pounds ᶧ

● ☑ **K0837** Power wheelchair, group 2 heavy duty, single power option, sling/solid seat/back, patient weight capacity 301 to 450 pounds ᶧ

● ☑ **K0838** Power wheelchair, group 2 heavy duty, single power option, captain's chair, patient weight capacity 301 to 450 pounds ᶧ

● ☑ **K0839** Power wheelchair, group 2 very heavy duty, single power option, sling/solid seat/back, patient weight capacity 451 to 600 pounds ᶧ

● ☑ **K0840** Power wheelchair, group 2 extra heavy duty, single power option, sling/solid seat/back, patient weight capacity 601 pounds or more ᶧ

● ☑ **K0841** Power wheelchair, group 2 standard, multiple power option, sling/solid seat/back, patient weight capacity up to and including 300 pounds ᶧ

● ☑ **K0842** Power wheelchair, group 2 standard, multiple power option, captain's chair, patient weight capacity up to and including 300 pounds ᶧ

● ☑ **K0843** Power wheelchair, group 2 heavy duty, multiple power option, sling/solid seat/back, patient weight capacity 301 to 450 pounds ᶧ

● ☑ **K0848** Power wheelchair, group 3 standard, sling/solid seat/back, patient weight capacity up to and including 300 pounds ᶧ

Special Coverage Instructions   Noncovered by Medicare   Carrier Discretion   ☑ Quality Alert   ● New Code   ○ Reinstated Code   ▲ Revised Code

96 — K Codes   Ⓐ Age Edit   Ⓜ Maternity Edit   ♀ Female Only   ♂ Male Only   Ⓐ - Ⓨ APC Status Indicators   *2007 HCPCS*

● ☑ K0849 Power wheelchair, group 3 standard, captain's chair, patient weight capacity up to and including 300 pounds &

● ☑ K0850 Power wheelchair, group 3 heavy duty, sling/solid seat/back, patient weight capacity 301 to 450 pounds &

● ☑ K0851 Power wheelchair, group 3 heavy duty, captain's chair, patient weight capacity 301 to 450 pounds &

● ☑ K0852 Power wheelchair, group 3 very heavy duty, sling/solid seat/back, patient weight capacity 451 to 600 pounds &

● ☑ K0853 Power wheelchair, group 3 very heavy duty, captain's chair, patient weight capacity, 451 to 600 pounds &

● ☑ K0854 Power wheelchair, group 3 extra heavy duty, sling/solid seat/back, patient weight capacity 601 pounds or more &

● ☑ K0855 Power wheelchair, group 3 extra heavy duty, captain's chair, patient weight 601 pounds or more &

● ☑ K0856 Power wheelchair, group 3 standard, single power option, sling/solid seat/back, patient weight capacity up to and including 300 pounds &

● ☑ K0857 Power wheelchair, group 3 standard, single power option, captain's chair, patient weight capacity up to and including 300 pounds &

● ☑ K0858 Power wheelchair, group 3 heavy duty, single power option, sling/solid seat/back, patient weight capacity 301 to 450 pounds &

● ☑ K0859 Power wheelchair, group 3 heavy duty, single power option, captain's chair, patient weight capacity 301 to 450 pounds &

● ☑ K0860 Power wheelchair, group 3 very heavy duty, single power option, sling/solid seat/back, patient weight capacity 451 to 600 pounds &

● ☑ K0861 Power wheelchair, group 3 standard, multiple power option, sling/solid seat/back, patient weight capacity up to and including 300 pounds &

● ☑ K0862 Power wheelchair, group 3 heavy duty, multiple power option, sling/solid seat/back, patient weight capacity 301 to 450 pounds &

● ☑ K0863 Power wheelchair, group 3 very heavy duty, multiple power option, sling/solid seat/back, patient weight capacity 451 to 600 pounds &

● ☑ K0864 Power wheelchair, group 3 extra heavy duty, multiple power option, sling/solid seat/back, patient weight capacity 601 pounds or more &

● ☑ K0868 Power wheelchair, group 4 standard, sling/solid seat/back, patient weight capacity up to and including 300 pounds &

● ☑ K0869 Power wheelchair, group 4 standard, captain's chair, patient weight capacity up to and including 300 pounds &

● ☑ K0870 Power wheelchair, group 4 heavy duty, sling/solid seat/back, patient weight capacity 301 to 450 pounds &

● ☑ K0871 Power wheelchair, group 4 very heavy duty, sling/solid seat/back, patient weight capacity 451 to 600 pounds &

● ☑ K0877 Power wheelchair, group 4 standard, single power option, sling/solid seat/back, patient weight capacity up to and including 300 pounds &

● ☑ K0878 Power wheelchair, group 4 standard, single power option, captain's chair, patient weight capacity up to and including 300 pounds &

● ☑ K0879 Power wheelchair, group 4 heavy duty, single power option, sling/solid seat/back, patient weight capacity 301 to 450 pounds &

● ☑ K0880 Power wheelchair, group 4 very heavy duty, single power option, sling/solid seat/back, patient weight 451 to 600 pounds &

● ☑ K0884 Power wheelchair, group 4 standard multiple power option, sling/solid seat/back, patient weight capacity up to and including 300 pounds &

● ☑ K0885 Power wheelchair, group 4 standard, multiple power option, captain's chair, weight capacity up to and including 300 pounds &

● ☑ K0886 Power wheelchair, group 4 heavy duty, multiple power option, sling/solid seat/back, patient weight capacity 301 to 450 pounds &

● ☑ K0890 Power wheelchair, group 5 pediatric, single power option, sling/solid seat/back, patient weight capacity up to and including 125 pounds &

● ☑ K0891 Power wheelchair, group 5 pediatric, multiple power option, sling/solid seat/back, patient weight capacity up to and including 125 pounds &

● ☑ K0898 Power wheelchair, not otherwise classified &

● ☑ K0899 Power mobility device, not coded by SADMERC or does not meet criteria &

Special Coverage Instructions   Noncovered by Medicare   Carrier Discretion   ☑ Quality Alert   ● New Code   ○ Reinstated Code   ▲ Revised Code

Orthotic Procedures

L0100 — L0462

ORTHOTIC PROCEDURES AND DEVICES L0000-L4999

L codes include orthotic and prosthetic procedures and devices, as well as scoliosis equipment, orthopedic shoes, and prosthetic implants.

ORTHOTIC DEVICES - SPINAL

CERVICAL

Medicare claims for L codes fall under the jurisdiction of the DME Medicare Administrative Contractors (DME MAC), unless otherwise noted.

L0100 ~~Cranial orthosis (helmet), with or without soft interface, molded to patient model~~
See code(s) A8002, A8003.

L0110 ~~Cranial orthosis (helmet), with or without soft interface, nonmolded~~
See code(s) A8000, A8001.

Ⓐ L0112 Cranial cervical orthosis, congenital torticollis type, with or without soft interface material, adjustable range of motion joint, custom fabricated

Ⓐ L0120 Cervical, flexible, nonadjustable (foam collar)

Ⓐ L0130 Cervical, flexible, thermoplastic collar, molded to patient

Ⓐ L0140 Cervical, semi-rigid, adjustable (plastic collar)

Ⓐ L0150 Cervical, semi-rigid, adjustable molded chin cup (plastic collar with mandibular/occipital piece)

Ⓐ L0160 Cervical, semi-rigid, wire frame occipital/mandibular support

Ⓐ L0170 Cervical, collar, molded to patient model

Ⓐ ☑ L0172 Cervical, collar, semi-rigid thermoplastic foam, two piece

Ⓐ ☑ L0174 Cervical, collar, semi-rigid, thermoplastic foam, two piece with thoracic extension

MULTIPLE POST COLLAR

Ⓐ L0180 Cervical, multiple post collar, occipital/mandibular supports, adjustable

Ⓐ L0190 Cervical, multiple post collar, occipital/mandibular supports, adjustable cervical bars (SOMI, Guilford, Taylor types)

Ⓐ L0200 Cervical, multiple post collar, occipital/mandibular supports, adjustable cervical bars, and thoracic extension

THORACIC

Ⓐ L0210 Thoracic, rib belt

Ⓐ L0220 Thoracic, rib belt, custom fabricated

Ⓐ L0430 Spinal orthosis, anterior-posterior-lateral control, with interface material, custom fitted (DeWall Posture Protector only)

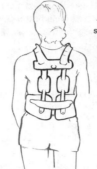
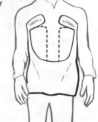

TLSO brace with adjustable straps and pads (L0450). The model at right and similar devices such as the Boston brace are molded polymer over foam and may be bivalve (front and back components)

Thoracic lumbar sacral orthosis (TLSO)

Ⓐ L0450 TLSO, flexible, provides trunk support, upper thoracic region, produces intracavitary pressure to reduce load on the intervertebral disks with rigid stays or panel(s), includes shoulder straps and closures, prefabricated, includes fitting and adjustment

Ⓐ L0452 TLSO, flexible, provides trunk support, upper thoracic region, produces intracavitary pressure to reduce load on the intervertebral disks with rigid stays or panel(s), includes shoulder straps and closures, custom fabricated

Ⓐ L0454 TLSO flexible, provides trunk support, extends from sacrococcygeal junction to above T-9 vertebra, restricts gross trunk motion in the sagittal plane, produces intracavitary pressure to reduce load on the intervertebral disks with rigid stays or panel(s), includes shoulder straps and closures, prefabricated, includes fitting and adjustment

Ⓐ L0456 TLSO, flexible, provides trunk support, thoracic region, rigid posterior panel and soft anterior apron, extends from the sacrococcygeal junction and terminates just inferior to the scapular spine, restricts gross trunk motion in the sagittal plane, produces intracavitary pressure to reduce load on the intervertebral disks, includes straps and closures, prefabricated, includes fitting and adjustment

Ⓐ L0458 TLSO, triplanar control, modular segmented spinal system, two rigid plastic shells, posterior extends from the sacrococcygeal junction and terminates just inferior to the scapular spine, anterior extends from the symphysis pubis to the xiphoid, soft liner, restricts gross trunk motion in the sagittal, coronal, and transverse planes, lateral strength is provided by overlapping plastic and stabilizing closures, includes straps and closures, prefabricated, includes fitting and adjustment

Ⓐ L0460 TLSO, triplanar control, modular segmented spinal system, two rigid plastic shells, posterior extends from the sacrococcygeal junction and terminates just inferior to the scapular spine, anterior extends from the symphysis pubis to the sternal notch, soft liner, restricts gross trunk motion in the sagittal, coronal, and transverse planes, lateral strength is provided by overlapping plastic and stabilizing closures, includes straps and closures, prefabricated, includes fitting and adjustment ♿

Ⓐ L0462 TLSO, triplanar control, modular segmented spinal system, three rigid plastic shells, posterior extends from the sacrococcygeal junction and terminates just inferior to the scapular spine, anterior extends from the symphysis pubis to the sternal notch, soft liner, restricts gross trunk motion in the sagittal, coronal, and transverse planes, lateral strength is provided by overlapping plastic and stabilizing closures, includes straps and closures, prefabricated, includes fitting and adjustment ♿

Special Coverage Instructions | Noncovered by Medicare | Carrier Discretion | ☑ Quality Alert | ● New Code | ○ Reinstated Code | ▲ Revised Code

98 — L Codes | Ⓐ Age Edit | Ⓜ Maternity Edit | ♀ Female Only | ♂ Male Only | Ⓐ - Ⓨ APC Status Indicators | *2007 HCPCS*

A L0464 TLSO, triplanar control, modular segmented spinal system, four rigid plastic shells, posterior extends from sacrococcygeal junction and terminates just inferior to scapular spine, anterior extends from symphysis pubis to the sternal notch, soft liner, restricts gross trunk motion in sagittal, coronal, and transverse planes, lateral strength is provided by overlapping plastic and stabilizing closures, includes straps and closures, prefabricated, includes fitting and adjustment

A L0466 TLSO, sagittal control, rigid posterior frame and flexible soft anterior apron with straps, closures and padding, restricts gross trunk motion in sagittal plane, produces intracavitary pressure to reduce load on intervertebral disks, includes fitting and shaping the frame, prefabricated, includes fitting and adjustment

A L0468 TLSO, sagittal-coronal control, rigid posterior frame and flexible soft anterior apron with straps, closures and padding, extends from sacrococcygeal junction over scapulae, lateral strength provided by pelvic, thoracic, and lateral frame pieces, restricts gross trunk motion in sagittal, and coronal planes, produces intracavitary pressure to reduce load on intervertebral disks, includes fitting and shaping the frame, prefabricated, includes fitting and adjustment

A L0470 TLSO, triplanar control, rigid posterior frame and flexible soft anterior apron with straps, closures and padding, extends from sacrococcygeal junction to scapula, lateral strength provided by pelvic, thoracic, and lateral frame pieces, rotational strength provided by subclavicular extensions, restricts gross trunk motion in sagittal, coronal, and transverse planes, produces intracavitary pressure to reduce load on the intervertebral disks, includes fitting and shaping the frame, prefabricated, includes fitting and adjustment

A L0472 TLSO, triplanar control, hyperextension, rigid anterior and lateral frame extends from symphysis pubis to sternal notch with two anterior components (one pubic and one sternal), posterior and lateral pads with straps and closures, limits spinal flexion, restricts gross trunk motion in sagittal, coronal, and transverse planes, includes fitting and shaping the frame, prefabricated, includes fitting and adjustment

A L0480 TLSO, triplanar control, one piece rigid plastic shell without interface liner, with multiple straps and closures, posterior extends from sacrococcygeal junction and terminates just inferior to scapular spine, anterior extends from symphysis pubis to sternal notch, anterior or posterior opening, restricts gross trunk motion in sagittal, coronal, and transverse planes, includes a carved plaster or CAD-CAM model, custom fabricated

A L0482 TLSO, triplanar control, one piece rigid plastic shell with interface liner, multiple straps and closures, posterior extends from sacrococcygeal junction and terminates just inferior to scapular spine, anterior extends from symphysis pubis to sternal notch, anterior or posterior opening, restricts gross trunk motion in sagittal, coronal, and transverse planes, includes a carved plaster or CAD-CAM model, custom fabricated

A L0484 TLSO, triplanar control, two piece rigid plastic shell without interface liner, with multiple straps and closures, posterior extends from sacrococcygeal junction and terminates just inferior to scapular spine, anterior extends from symphysis pubis to sternal notch, lateral strength is enhanced by overlapping plastic, restricts gross trunk motion in the sagittal, coronal, and transverse planes, includes a carved plaster or CAD-CAM model, custom fabricated

A L0486 TLSO, triplanar control, two piece rigid plastic shell with interface liner, multiple straps and closures, posterior extends from sacrococcygeal junction and terminates just inferior to scapular spine, anterior extends from symphysis pubis to sternal notch, lateral strength is enhanced by overlapping plastic, restricts gross trunk motion in the sagittal, coronal, and transverse planes, includes a carved plaster or CAD-CAM model, custom fabricated

A L0488 TLSO, triplanar control, one piece rigid plastic shell with interface liner, multiple straps and closures, posterior extends from sacrococcygeal junction and terminates just inferior to scapular spine, anterior extends from symphysis pubis to sternal notch, anterior or posterior opening, restricts gross trunk motion in sagittal, coronal, and transverse planes, prefabricated, includes fitting and adjustment

A L0490 TLSO, sagittal-coronal control, one piece rigid plastic shell, with overlapping reinforced anterior, with multiple straps and closures, posterior extends from sacrococcygeal junction and terminates at or before the T-9 vertebra, anterior extends from symphysis pubis to xiphoid, anterior opening, restricts gross trunk motion in sagittal and coronal planes, prefabricated, includes fitting and adjustment

A L0491 TLSO, sagittal-coronal control, modular segmented spinal sytem, two rigid plastic shells, posterior extends from the sacrococcygeal junction and terminates just inferior to the scapular spine, anterior extends from the symphysis pubis to the xiphoid, soft liner, restricts gross trunk motion in the sagittal and coronal planes, lateral strength is provided by overlapping plastic and stabilizing closures, includes straps and closures, prefabricated, includes fitting and adjustment

A L0492 TLSO, sagittal-coronal control, modular segmented spinal system, three rigid plastic shells, posterior extends from the sacrococcygeal junction and terminates just inferior to the scapular spine, anterior extends from the symphysis pubis to the xiphoid, soft liner, restricts gross trunk motion in the sagittal and coronal planes, lateral strength is provided by overlapping plastic and stabilizing closures, includes straps and closures, prefabricated, includes fitting and adjustment

CERVICAL-THORACIC-LUMBAR-SACRAL ORTHOSIS (CTLSO)

A L0621 Sacroiliac orthosis, flexible, provides pelvic-sacral support, reduces motion about the sacroiliac joint, includes straps, closures, may include pendulous abdomen design, prefabricated, includes fitting and adjustment

A L0622 Sacroiliac orthosis, flexible, provides pelvic-sacral support, reduces motion about the sacroiliac joint, includes straps, closures, may include pendulous abdomen design, custom fabricated

Ⓐ **L0623** Sacroiliac orthosis, provides pelvic-sacral support, with rigid or semi-rigid panels over the sacrum and abdomen, reduces motion about the sacroiliac joint, includes straps, closures, may include pendulous abdomen design, prefabricated, includes fitting and adjustment

Ⓐ **L0624** Sacroiliac orthosis, provides pelvic-sacral support, with rigid or semi-rigid panels placed over the sacrum and abdomen, reduces motion about the sacroiliac joint, includes straps, closures, may include pendulous abdomen design, custom fabricated

Ⓐ **L0625** Lumbar orthosis, flexible, provides lumbar support, posterior extends from L-1 to below L-5 vertebra, produces intracavitary pressure to reduce load on the intervertebral discs, includes straps, closures, may include pendulous abdomen design, shoulder straps, stays, prefabricated, includes fitting and adjustment

Ⓐ **L0626** Lumbar orthosis, sagittal control, with rigid posterior panel(s), posterior extends from L-1 to below L-5 vertebra, produces intracavitary pressure to reduce load on the intervertebral discs, includes straps, closures, may include padding, stays, shoulder straps, pendulous abdomen design, prefabricated, includes fitting and adjustment

Ⓐ **L0627** Lumbar orthosis, sagittal control, with rigid anterior and posterior panels, posterior extends from L-1 to below L-5 vertebra, produces intracavitary pressure to reduce load on the intervertebral discs, includes straps, closures, may include padding, shoulder straps, pendulous abdomen design, prefabricated, includes fitting and adjustment

Ⓐ **L0628** Lumbar-sacral orthosis, flexible, provides lumbo-sacral support, posterior extends from sacrococcygeal junction to T-9 vertebra, produces intracavitary pressure to reduce load on the intervertebral discs, includes straps, closures, may include stays, shoulder straps, pendulous abdomen design, prefabricated, includes fitting and adjustment

Ⓐ **L0629** Lumbar-sacral orthosis, flexible, provides lumbo-sacral support, posterior extends from sacrococcygeal junction to T-9 vertebra, produces intracavitary pressure to reduce load on the intervertebral discs, includes straps, closures, may include stays, shoulder straps, pendulous abdomen design, custom fabricated

Ⓐ **L0630** Lumbar-sacral orthosis, sagittal control, with rigid posterior panel(s), posterior extends from sacrococcygeal junction to T-9 vertebra, produces intracavitary pressure to reduce load on the intervertebral discs, includes straps, closures, may include padding, stays, shoulder straps, pendulous abdomen design, prefabricated, includes fitting and adjustment

▲ Ⓐ **L0631** Lumbar-sacral orthosis, sagittal control, with rigid anterior and posterior panels, posterior extends from sacrococcygeal junction to T-9 vertebra, produces intracavitary pressure to reduce load on the intervertebral discs, includes straps, closures, may include padding, shoulder straps, pendulous abdomen design, prefabricated, includes fitting and adjustment

Ⓐ **L0632** LSO, sagittal control, with rigid anterior and posterior panels, posterior extends from sacrococcygeal junction to T-9 vertebra, produces intracavitary pressure to reduce load on the intervertebral discs, includes straps, closures, may include padding, shoulder straps, pendulous abdomen design, custom fabricated

Ⓐ **L0633** LSO, sagittal-coronal control, with rigid posterior frame/panel(s), posterior extends from sacrococcygeal junction to T-9 vertebra, lateral strength provided by rigid lateral frame/panels, produces intracavitary pressure to reduce load on intervertebral discs, includes straps, closures, may include padding, stays, shoulder straps, pendulous abdomen design, prefabricated, includes fitting and adjustment

Ⓐ **L0634** LSO, sagittal-coronal control, with rigid posterior frame/panel(s), posterior extends from sacrococcygeal junction to T-9 vertebra, lateral strength provided by rigid lateral frame/panel(s), produces intracavitary pressure to reduce load on intervertebral discs, includes straps, closures, may include padding, stays, shoulder straps, pendulous abdomen design, custom fabricated

Ⓐ **L0635** LSO, sagittal-coronal control, lumbar flexion, rigid posterior frame/panel(s), lateral articulating design to flex the lumbar spine, posterior extends from sacrococcygeal junction to T-9 vertebra, lateral strength provided by rigid lateral frame/panel(s), produces intracavitary pressure to reduce load on intervertebral discs, includes straps, closures, may include padding, anterior panel, pendulous abdomen design, prefabricated, includes fitting and adjustment

Ⓐ **L0636** LSO, sagittal-coronal control, lumbar flexion, rigid posterior frame/panels, lateral articulating design to flex the lumbar spine, posterior extends from sacrococcygeal junction to T-9 vertebra, lateral strength provided by rigid lateral frame/panels, produces intracavitary pressure to reduce load on intervertebral discs, includes straps, closures, may include padding, anterior panel, pendulous abdomen design, custom fabricated

Ⓐ **L0637** LSO, sagittal-coronal control, with rigid anterior and posterior frame/panels, posterior extends from sacrococcygeal junction to T-9 vertebra, lateral strength provided by rigid lateral frame/panels, produces intracavitary pressure to reduce load on intervertebral discs, includes straps, closures, may include padding, shoulder straps, pendulous abdomen design, prefabricated, includes fitting and adjustment

Ⓐ **L0638** LSO, sagittal-coronal control, with rigid anterior and posterior frame/panels, posterior extends from sacrococcygeal junction to T-9 vertebra, lateral strength provided by rigid lateral frame/panels, produces intracavitary pressure to reduce load on intervertebral discs, includes straps, closures, may include padding, shoulder straps, pendulous abdomen design, custom fabricated

Ⓐ **L0639** LSO, sagittal-coronal control, rigid shell(s)/panel(s), posterior extends from sacrococcygeal junction to T-9 vertebra, anterior extends from symphysis pubis to xyphoid, produces intracavitary pressure to reduce load on the intervertebral discs, overall strength is provided by overlapping rigid material and stabilizing closures, includes straps, closures, may include soft interface, pendulous abdomen design, prefabricated, includes fitting and adjustment

Ⓐ **L0640** LSO, sagittal-coronal control, rigid shell(s)/panel(s), posterior extends from sacrococcygeal junction to T-9 vertebra, anterior extends from symphysis pubis to xyphoid, produces intracavitary pressure to reduce load on the intervertebral discs, overall strength is provided by overlapping rigid material and stabilizing closures, includes straps, closures, may include soft interface, pendulous abdomen design, custom fabricated

Special Coverage Instructions · Noncovered by Medicare · Carrier Discretion · ☑ Quality Alert · ● New Code · ○ Reinstated Code · ▲ Revised Code

100 — L Codes · Ⓐ Age Edit · Ⓜ Maternity Edit · ♀ Female Only · ♂ Male Only · Ⓐ - ☑ APC Status Indicators · *2007 HCPCS*

ANTERIOR-POSTERIOR-LATERAL CONTROL

Ⓐ **L0700** CTLSO, anterior-posterior-lateral control, molded to patient model (Minerva type) ⓑ

Ⓐ **L0710** CTLSO, anterior-posterior-lateral control, molded to patient model, with interface material (Minerva type) ⓑ

HALO PROCEDURE

Ⓐ **L0810** Halo procedure, cervical halo incorporated into jacket vest ⓑ

Ⓐ **L0820** Halo procedure, cervical halo incorporated into plaster body jacket ⓑ

Ⓐ **L0830** Halo procedure, cervical halo incorporated into Milwaukee type orthosis ⓑ

Ⓐ **L0859** Addition to halo procedure, magnetic resonance image compatible systems, rings and pins, any material

Ⓐ **L0861** Addition to halo procedure, replacement liner/interface material ⓑ

Ⓐ **L0960** Torso support, postsurgical support, pads for postsurgical support ⓑ

ADDITIONS TO SPINAL ORTHOSIS

Ⓐ **L0970** TLSO, corset front ⓑ

Ⓐ **L0972** LSO, corset front ⓑ

Ⓐ **L0974** TLSO, full corset ⓑ

Ⓐ **L0976** LSO, full corset ⓑ

Ⓐ **L0978** Axillary crutch extension ⓑ

Ⓐ ☑ **L0980** Peroneal straps, pair ⓑ

Ⓐ ☑ **L0982** Stocking supporter grips, set of four (4) ⓑ

Ⓐ ☑ **L0984** Protective body sock, each ⓑ

Ⓐ **L0999** Addition to spinal orthosis, NOS
Determine if an alternative HCPCS Level II or a CPT code better describes the service being reported. This code should be used only if a more specific code is unavailable.

ORTHOTIC DEVICES - SCOLIOSIS PROCEDURES

The orthotic care of scoliosis differs from other orthotic care in that the treatment is more dynamic in nature and uses continual modification of the orthosis to the patient's changing condition. This coding structure uses the proper names - or eponyms - of the procedures because they have historic and universal acceptance in the profession. It should be recognized that variations to the basic procedures described by the founders/developers are accepted in various medical and orthotic practices throughout the country. All procedures include model of patient when indicated.

CERVICAL-THORACIC-LUMBAR-SACRAL ORTHOSIS (CTLSO)

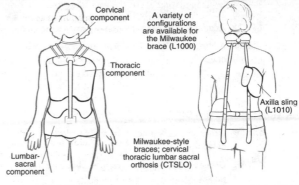

Cervical component

A variety of configurations are available for the Milwaukee brace (L1000)

Thoracic component

Axilla sling (L1010)

Lumbar-sacral component

Milwaukee-style braces; cervical thoracic lumbar sacral orthosis (CTLSO)

Ⓐ **L1000** CTLSO (Milwaukee), inclusive of furnishing initial orthosis, including model ⓑ

● Ⓐ **L1001** Cervical thoracic lumbar sacral orthosis, immobilizer, infant size, prefabricated, includes fitting and adjustment Ⓐ

Ⓐ **L1005** Tension based scoliosis orthosis and accessory pads, includes fitting and adjustment ⓑ

Ⓐ **L1010** Addition to CTLSO or scoliosis orthosis, axilla sling ⓑ

Ⓐ **L1020** Addition to CTLSO or scoliosis orthosis, kyphosis pad ⓑ

Ⓐ **L1025** Addition to CTLSO or scoliosis orthosis, kyphosis pad, floating ⓑ

Ⓐ **L1030** Addition to CTLSO or scoliosis orthosis, lumbar bolster pad ⓑ

Ⓐ **L1040** Addition to CTLSO or scoliosis orthosis, lumbar or lumbar rib pad ⓑ

Ⓐ **L1050** Addition to CTLSO or scoliosis orthosis, sternal pad ⓑ

Ⓐ **L1060** Addition to CTLSO or scoliosis orthosis, thoracic pad ⓑ

Ⓐ **L1070** Addition to CTLSO or scoliosis orthosis, trapezius sling ⓑ

Ⓐ **L1080** Addition to CTLSO or scoliosis orthosis, outrigger ⓑ

Ⓐ **L1085** Addition to CTLSO or scoliosis orthosis, outrigger, bilateral with vertical extensions ⓑ

Ⓐ **L1090** Addition to CTLSO or scoliosis orthosis, lumbar sling ⓑ

Ⓐ **L1100** Addition to CTLSO or scoliosis orthosis, ring flange, plastic or leather ⓑ

Ⓐ **L1110** Addition to CTLSO or scoliosis orthosis, ring flange, plastic or leather, molded to patient model ⓑ

Ⓐ ☑ **L1120** Addition to CTLSO, scoliosis orthosis, cover for upright, each ⓑ

THORACIC-LUMBAR-SACRAL ORTHOSIS (TLSO) (LOW PROFILE)

Ⓐ **L1200** TLSO, inclusive of furnishing initial orthosis only ⓑ

Ⓐ **L1210** Addition to TLSO, (low profile), lateral thoracic extension ⓑ

Ⓐ **L1220** Addition to TLSO, (low profile), anterior thoracic extension ⓑ

Ⓐ **L1230** Addition to TLSO, (low profile), Milwaukee type superstructure ⓑ

Ⓐ **L1240** Addition to TLSO, (low profile), lumbar derotation pad ⓑ

Special Coverage Instructions   Noncovered by Medicare   Carrier Discretion   ☑ Quality Alert   ● New Code   ○ Reinstated Code   ▲ Revised Code

2007 HCPCS   **1**-**9** ASC Group   **MED:** Pub 100/NCD References   ⓑ DMEPOS Paid   ⊘ SNF Excluded   **L Codes — 101**

Orthotic Procedures

L1250 — L1845

Ⓐ **L1250** Addition to TLSO, (low profile), anterior asis pad �

Ⓐ **L1260** Addition to TLSO, (low profile), anterior thoracic derotation pad ㄱ

Ⓐ **L1270** Addition to TLSO, (low profile), abdominal pad ㄱ

Ⓐ ☑ **L1280** Addition to TLSO, (low profile), rib gusset (elastic), each

Ⓐ **L1290** Addition to TLSO, (low profile), lateral trochanteric pad ㄱ

OTHER SCOLIOSIS PROCEDURES

Ⓐ **L1300** Other scoliosis procedure, body jacket molded to patient model

Ⓐ **L1310** Other scoliosis procedure, postoperative body jacket ㄱ

Ⓐ **L1499** Spinal orthosis, not otherwise specified
Determine if an alternative HCPCS Level II or a CPT code better describes the service being reported. This code should be used only if a more specific code is unavailable.

THORACIC-HIP-KNEE-ANKLE ORTHOSIS (THKAO)

Ⓐ **L1500** THKAO, mobility frame (Newington, Parapodium types) ㄱ

Ⓐ **L1510** THKAO, standing frame, with or without tray and accessories ㄱ

Ⓐ **L1520** THKAO, swivel walker ㄱ

ORTHOTIC DEVICES - LOWER LIMB

The procedures in L1600-L2999 are considered as "base" or "basic procedures" and may be modified by listing procedure from the "additions" sections and adding them to the base procedures.

HIP ORTHOSIS (HO) - FLEXIBLE

Ⓐ **L1600** HO, abduction control of hip joints, flexible, Frejka type with cover, prefabricated, includes fitting and adjustment ㄱ

Ⓐ **L1610** HO, abduction control of hip joints, flexible, (Frejka cover only), prefabricated, includes fitting and adjustment ㄱ

Ⓐ **L1620** HO, abduction control of hip joints, flexible, (Pavlik harness), prefabricated, includes fitting and adjustment ㄱ

Ⓐ **L1630** HO, abduction control of hip joints, semi-flexible (Von Rosen type), custom fabricated ㄱ

Ⓐ **L1640** HO, abduction control of hip joints, static, pelvic band or spreader bar, thigh cuffs, custom fabricated ㄱ

Ⓐ **L1650** HO, abduction control of hip joints, static, adjustable (Ilfled type), prefabricated, includes fitting and adjustment ㄱ

Ⓐ **L1652** Hip orthosis, bilateral thigh cuffs with adjustable abductor spreader bar, adult size, prefabricated, includes fitting and adjustment, any type ㄱ

Ⓐ **L1660** HO, abduction control of hip joints, static, plastic, prefabricated, includes fitting and adjustment ㄱ

Ⓐ **L1680** HO, abduction control of hip joints, dynamic, pelvic control, adjustable hip motion control, thigh cuffs (Rancho hip action type), custom fabricated ㄱ

Ⓐ **L1685** HO, abduction control of hip joint, postoperative hip abduction type, custom fabricated ㄱ

Ⓐ **L1686** HO, abduction control of hip joint, postoperative hip abduction type, prefabricated, includes fitting and adjustments

Ⓐ **L1690** Combination, bilateral, lumbo-sacral, hip, femur orthosis providing adduction and internal rotation control, prefabricated, includes fitting and adjustment ㄱ

LEGG PERTHES

Ⓐ **L1700** Legg Perthes orthosis, (Toronto type), custom fabricated ㄱ

Ⓐ **L1710** Legg Perthes orthosis, (Newington type), custom fabricated ㄱ

Ⓐ **L1720** Legg Perthes orthosis, trilateral, (Tachdijan type), custom fabricated ㄱ

Ⓐ **L1730** Legg Perthes orthosis, (Scottish Rite type), custom fabricated ㄱ

Ⓐ **L1755** Legg Perthes orthosis, (Patten bottom type), custom fabricated ㄱ

KNEE ORTHOSIS (KO)

Ⓐ **L1800** KO, elastic with stays, prefabricated, includes fitting and adjustment ㄱ

Ⓐ **L1810** KO, elastic with joints, prefabricated, includes fitting and adjustment ㄱ

Ⓐ **L1815** KO, elastic or other elastic type material with condylar pad(s), prefabricated, includes fitting and adjustment ㄱ

Ⓐ **L1820** Knee orthosis, elastic with condylar pads and joints, with or without patellar control, prefabricated, includes fitting and adjustment ㄱ

Ⓐ **L1825** KO, elastic knee cap, prefabricated, includes fitting and adjustment ㄱ

Ⓐ **L1830** KO, immobilizer, canvas longitudinal, prefabricated, includes fitting and adjustment ㄱ

Ⓐ **L1831** Knee orthosis, locking knee joint(s), positional orthosis, prefabricated, includes fitting and adjustment ㄱ

Ⓐ **L1832** Knee orthosis, adjustable knee joints (unicentric or polycentric), positional orthosis, rigid support, prefabricated, includes fitting and adjustment ㄱ

Ⓐ **L1834** KO, without knee joint, rigid, custom fabricated ㄱ

Ⓐ **L1836** Knee orthosis, rigid, without joint(s), includes soft interface material, prefabricated, includes fitting and adjustment ㄱ

Ⓐ **L1840** KO, derotation, medial-lateral, anterior cruciate ligament, custom fabricated ㄱ

Ⓐ **L1843** Knee orthosis, single upright, thigh and calf, with adjustable flexion and extension joint (unicentric or polycentric), medial-lateral and rotation control, with or without varus/valgus adjustment, prefabricated, includes fitting and adjustment ㄱ

Ⓐ **L1844** Knee orthosis, single upright, thigh and calf, with adjustable flexion and extension joint (unicentric or polycentric), medial-lateral and rotation control, with or without varus/valgus adjustment, custom fabricated ㄱ

Ⓐ **L1845** Knee orthosis, double upright, thigh and calf, with adjustable flexion and extension joint (unicentric or polycentric), medial-lateral and rotation control, with or without varus/valgus adjustment, prefabricated, includes fitting and adjustment ㄱ

Special Coverage Instructions   Noncovered by Medicare   Carrier Discretion   ☑ Quality Alert   ● New Code   ○ Reinstated Code   ▲ Revised Code

102 — L Codes   Ⓐ Age Edit   Ⓜ Maternity Edit   ♀ Female Only   ♂ Male Only   Ⓐ - ☑ APC Status Indicators   *2007 HCPCS*

Ⓐ **L1846** Knee orthosis, double upright, thigh and calf, with adjustable flexion and extension joint (unicentric or polycentric), medial-lateral and rotation control, with or without varus/valgus adjustment, custom fabricated ⅄

Ⓐ **L1847** KO, double upright with adjustable joint, with inflatable air support chamber(s), prefabricated, includes fitting and adjustment ⅄

Ⓐ **L1850** KO, Swedish type, prefabricated, includes fitting and adjustment ⅄

Ⓐ **L1855** KO, molded plastic, thigh and calf sections, with double upright knee joints, custom fabricated ⅄

Ⓐ **L1858** KO, molded plastic, polycentric knee joints, pneumatic knee pads (CTI), custom fabricated ⅄

Ⓐ **L1860** KO, modification of supracondylar prosthetic socket, custom fabricated (SK) ⅄

Ⓐ **L1870** KO, double upright, thigh and calf lacers, with knee joints, custom fabricated ⅄

Ⓐ **L1880** KO, double upright, nonmolded thigh and calf cuffs/lacers with knee joints, custom fabricated ⅄

ANKLE-FOOT ORTHOSIS (AFO)

Ⓐ **L1900** AFO, spring wire, dorsiflexion assist calf band, custom fabricated ⅄

Ⓐ **L1901** Ankle orthosis, elastic, prefabricated, includes fitting and adjustment (e.g., neoprene, Lycra) ⅄

Ⓐ **L1902** AFO, ankle gauntlet, prefabricated, includes fitting and adjustment ⅄

Ⓐ **L1904** AFO, molded ankle gauntlet, custom fabricated ⅄

Ⓐ **L1906** AFO, multiligamentus ankle support, prefabricated, includes fitting and adjustment ⅄

Ⓐ **L1907** AFO, supramalleolar with straps, with or without interface/pads, custom fabricated ⅄

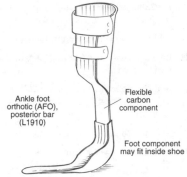

Ankle foot orthotic (AFO), posterior bar (L1910)

Flexible carbon component

Foot component may fit inside shoe

Ⓐ **L1910** AFO, posterior, single bar, clasp attachment to shoe counter, prefabricated, includes fitting and adjustment ⅄

Ⓐ **L1920** AFO, single upright with static or adjustable stop (Phelps or Perlstein type), custom fabricated ⅄

Ⓐ **L1930** AFO, plastic or other material, prefabricated, includes fitting and adjustment ⅄

Ⓐ **L1932** AFO, rigid anterior tibial section, total carbon fiber or equal material, prefabricated, includes fitting and adjustment ⅄

Ⓐ **L1940** AFO, plastic or other material, custom-fabricated ⅄

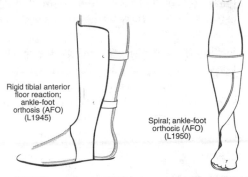

Rigid tibial anterior floor reaction; ankle-foot orthosis (AFO) (L1945)

Spiral; ankle-foot orthosis (AFO) (L1950)

Ⓐ **L1945** AFO, molded to patient model, plastic, rigid anterior tibial section (floor reaction), custom fabricated ⅄

Ⓐ **L1950** Ankle foot orthosis, spiral, (Institute of Rehabilitative Medicine type), plastic, custom-fabricated ⅄

Ⓐ **L1951** Ankle foot orthosis, spiral, (Institute of Rehabilitative Medicine type), plastic or other material, prefabricated, includes fitting and adjustment ⅄

Ⓐ **L1960** AFO, posterior solid ankle, plastic, custom fabricated ⅄

Ⓐ **L1970** AFO, plastic, with ankle joint, custom fabricated ⅄

Ⓐ **L1971** Ankle foot orthosis, plastic or other material with ankle joint, prefabricated, includes fitting and adjustment ⅄

Ⓐ **L1980** AFO, single upright free plantar dorsiflexion, solid stirrup, calf band/cuff (single bar BK orthosis), custom fabricated ⅄

Ⓐ **L1990** AFO, double upright free plantar dorsiflexion, solid stirrup, calf band/cuff (double bar BK orthosis), custom fabricated ⅄

KNEE-ANKLE-FOOT ORTHOSIS (KAFO) - OR ANY COMBINATION

Ⓐ **L2000** KAFO, single upright, free knee, free ankle, solid stirrup, thigh and calf bands/cuffs (single bar AK orthosis), custom fabricated ⅄

Ⓐ **L2005** Knee ankle foot orthosis, any material, single or double upright, stance control, automatic lock and swing phase release, mechanical activation, includes ankle joint, any type, custom fabricated

Ⓐ **L2010** KAFO, single upright, free ankle, solid stirrup, thigh and calf bands/cuffs (single bar AK orthosis), without knee joint, custom fabricated ⅄

Ⓐ **L2020** KAFO, double upright, free knee, free ankle, solid stirrup, thigh and calf bands/cuffs (double bar AK orthosis), custom fabricated ⅄

Ⓐ **L2030** KAFO, double upright, free ankle, solid stirrup, thigh and calf bands/cuffs, (double bar AK orthosis), without knee joint, custom fabricated ⅄

Ⓐ **L2034** Knee ankle foot orthosis, full plastic, single upright, with or without free motion knee, medial lateral rotation control, with or without free motion ankle, custom fabricated

Ⓐ **L2035** Knee ankle foot orthosis, full plastic, static (pediatric size), without free motion ankle, prefabricated, includes fitting and adjustment ⅄

Ⓐ **L2036** Knee ankle foot orthosis, full plastic, double upright, with or without free motion knee, with or without free motion ankle, custom fabricated ⅄

Ⓐ **L2037** Knee ankle foot orthosis, full plastic, single upright, with or without free motion knee, with or without free motion ankle, custom fabricated ⅄

Special Coverage Instructions   Noncovered by Medicare   Carrier Discretion   ☑ Quality Alert   ● New Code   ○ Reinstated Code   ▲ Revised Code

2007 HCPCS   🔟-🌀 ASC Group   **MED:** Pub 100/NCD References   ⅄ DMEPOS Paid   ⊘ SNF Excluded   **L Codes — 103**

Orthotic Procedures

L2038 — L2397

[A] L2038 Knee ankle foot orthosis, full plastic, with or without free motion knee, multi-axis ankle, custom fabricated &

TORSION CONTROL: HIP-KNEE-ANKLE-FOOT ORTHOSIS (HKAFO)

[A] L2040 HKAFO, torsion control, bilateral rotation straps, pelvic band/belt, custom fabricated &

[A] L2050 HKAFO, torsion control, bilateral torsion cables, hip joint, pelvic band/belt, custom fabricated &

[A] L2060 HKAFO, torsion control, bilateral torsion cables, ball bearing hip joint, pelvic band/ belt, custom fabricated &

[A] L2070 HKAFO, torsion control, unilateral rotation straps, pelvic band/belt, custom fabricated &

[A] L2080 HKAFO, torsion control, unilateral torsion cable, hip joint, pelvic band/belt, custom fabricated &

[A] L2090 HKAFO, torsion control, unilateral torsion cable, ball bearing hip joint, pelvic band/belt, custom fabricated &

[A] L2106 AFO, fracture orthosis, tibial fracture cast orthosis, thermoplastic type casting material, custom fabricated &

[A] L2108 AFO, fracture orthosis, tibial fracture cast orthosis, custom fabricated &

[A] L2112 AFO, fracture orthosis, tibial fracture orthosis, soft, prefabricated, includes fitting and adjustment &

[A] L2114 AFO, fracture orthosis, tibial fracture orthosis, semi-rigid, prefabricated, includes fitting and adjustment &

[A] L2116 AFO, fracture orthosis, tibial fracture orthosis, rigid, prefabricated, includes fitting and adjustment &

[A] L2126 KAFO, fracture orthosis, femoral fracture cast orthosis, thermoplastic type casting material, custom fabricated &

[A] L2128 KAFO, fracture orthosis, femoral fracture cast orthosis, custom fabricated &

[A] L2132 KAFO, fracture orthosis, femoral fracture cast orthosis, soft, prefabricated, includes fitting and adjustment &

[A] L2134 KAFO, fracture orthosis, femoral fracture cast orthosis, semi-rigid, prefabricated, includes fitting and adjustment &

[A] L2136 KAFO, fracture orthosis, femoral fracture cast orthosis, rigid, prefabricated, includes fitting and adjustment &

ADDITIONS TO FRACTURE ORTHOSIS

[A] L2180 Addition to lower extremity fracture orthosis, plastic shoe insert with ankle joints &

[A] L2182 Addition to lower extremity fracture orthosis, drop lock knee joint &

[A] L2184 Addition to lower extremity fracture orthosis, limited motion knee joint &

[A] L2186 Addition to lower extremity fracture orthosis, adjustable motion knee joint, Lerman type &

[A] L2188 Addition to lower extremity fracture orthosis, quadrilateral brim &

[A] L2190 Addition to lower extremity fracture orthosis, waist belt &

[A] L2192 Addition to lower extremity fracture orthosis, hip joint, pelvic band, thigh flange, and pelvic belt &

ADDITIONS TO LOWER EXTREMITY ORTHOSIS: SHOE-ANKLE-SHIN-KNEE

[A] [✓] L2200 Addition to lower extremity, limited ankle motion, each joint &

[A] [✓] L2210 Addition to lower extremity, dorsiflexion assist (plantar flexion resist), each joint &

[A] [✓] L2220 Addition to lower extremity, dorsiflexion and plantar flexion assist/resist, each joint &

[A] L2230 Addition to lower extremity, split flat caliper stirrups and plate attachment &

[A] L2232 Addition to lower extremity orthosis, rocker bottom for total contact ankle foot orthosis, for custom fabricated orthosis only

[A] L2240 Addition to lower extremity, round caliper and plate attachment &

[A] L2250 Addition to lower extremity, foot plate, molded to patient model, stirrup attachment &

[A] L2260 Addition to lower extremity, reinforced solid stirrup (Scott-Craig type) &

[A] L2265 Addition to lower extremity, long tongue stirrup &

[A] L2270 Addition to lower extremity, varus/valgus correction (T) strap, padded/lined or malleolus pad &

[A] L2275 Addition to lower extremity, varus/valgus correction, plastic modification, padded/lined &

[A] L2280 Addition to lower extremity, molded inner boot &

[A] L2300 Addition to lower extremity, abduction bar (bilateral hip involvement), jointed, adjustable &

[A] L2310 Addition to lower extremity, abduction bar, straight &

[A] L2320 Addition to lower extremity, nonmolded lacer, for custom fabricated orthosis only &

[A] L2330 Addition to lower extremity, lacer molded to patient model, for custom fabricated orthosis only &

[A] L2335 Addition to lower extremity, anterior swing band &

[A] L2340 Addition to lower extremity, pretibial shell, molded to patient model &

[A] L2350 Addition to lower extremity, prosthetic type, (BK) socket, molded to patient model, (used for PTB, AFO orthoses) &

[A] L2360 Addition to lower extremity, extended steel shank &

[A] L2370 Addition to lower extremity, Patten bottom &

[A] L2375 Addition to lower extremity, torsion control, ankle joint and half solid stirrup &

[A] [✓] L2380 Addition to lower extremity, torsion control, straight knee joint, each joint &

[A] [✓] L2385 Addition to lower extremity, straight knee joint, heavy duty, each joint &

[A] L2387 Addition to lower extremity, polycentric knee joint, for custom fabricated knee ankle foot orthosis, each joint &

[A] [✓] L2390 Addition to lower extremity, offset knee joint, each joint &

[A] [✓] L2395 Addition to lower extremity, offset knee joint, heavy duty, each joint &

[A] L2397 Addition to lower extremity orthosis, suspension sleeve &

| Special Coverage Instructions | Noncovered by Medicare | Carrier Discretion | ☑ Quality Alert | ● New Code | ○ Reinstated Code | ▲ Revised Code |

104 — L Codes   [A] Age Edit   [M] Maternity Edit   ♀ Female Only   ♂ Male Only   [A] - [Y] APC Status Indicators   *2007 HCPCS*

ADDITIONS TO STRAIGHT KNEE OR OFFSET KNEE JOINTS

- [A] ☑ **L2405** Addition to knee joint, drop lock, each &
- [A] ☑ **L2415** Addition to knee lock with integrated release mechanism (bail, cable, or equal), any material, each joint &
- [A] ☑ **L2425** Addition to knee joint, disc or dial lock for adjustable knee flexion, each joint &
- [A] ☑ **L2430** Addition to knee joint, ratchet lock for active and progressive knee extension, each joint &
- [A] **L2492** Addition to knee joint, lift loop for drop lock ring &

ADDITIONS: THIGH/WEIGHT BEARING - GLUTEAL/ISCHIAL WEIGHT BEARING

- [A] **L2500** Addition to lower extremity, thigh/weight bearing, gluteal/ischial weight bearing, ring &
- [A] **L2510** Addition to lower extremity, thigh/weight bearing, quadri-lateral brim, molded to patient model &
- [A] **L2520** Addition to lower extremity, thigh/weight bearing, quadri-lateral brim, custom fitted &
- [A] **L2525** Addition to lower extremity, thigh/weight bearing, ischial containment/narrow M–L brim molded to patient model &
- [A] **L2526** Addition to lower extremity, thigh/weight bearing, ischial containment/narrow M–L brim, custom fitted &
- [A] **L2530** Addition to lower extremity, thigh/weight bearing, lacer, nonmolded &
- [A] **L2540** Addition to lower extremity, thigh/weight bearing, lacer, molded to patient model &
- [A] **L2550** Addition to lower extremity, thigh/weight bearing, high roll cuff &

ADDITIONS: PELVIC AND THORACIC CONTROL

- [A] ☑ **L2570** Addition to lower extremity, pelvic control, hip joint, Clevis type, two position joint, each &
- [A] **L2580** Addition to lower extremity, pelvic control, pelvic sling &
- [A] ☑ **L2600** Addition to lower extremity, pelvic control, hip joint, Clevis type, or thrust bearing, free, each &
- [A] ☑ **L2610** Addition to lower extremity, pelvic control, hip joint, Clevis or thrust bearing, lock, each &
- [A] ☑ **L2620** Addition to lower extremity, pelvic control, hip joint, heavy-duty, each &
- [A] ☑ **L2622** Addition to lower extremity, pelvic control, hip joint, adjustable flexion, each &
- [A] ☑ **L2624** Addition to lower extremity, pelvic control, hip joint, adjustable flexion, extension, abduction control, each &
- [A] **L2627** Addition to lower extremity, pelvic control, plastic, molded to patient model, reciprocating hip joint and cables &
- [A] **L2628** Addition to lower extremity, pelvic control, metal frame, reciprocating hip joint and cables &
- [A] **L2630** Addition to lower extremity, pelvic control, band and belt, unilateral &
- [A] **L2640** Addition to lower extremity, pelvic control, band and belt, bilateral &
- [A] ☑ **L2650** Addition to lower extremity, pelvic and thoracic control, gluteal pad, each &

- [A] **L2660** Addition to lower extremity, thoracic control, thoracic band &
- [A] **L2670** Addition to lower extremity, thoracic control, paraspinal uprights &
- [A] **L2680** Addition to lower extremity, thoracic control, lateral support uprights &

ADDITIONS: GENERAL

- [A] ☑ **L2750** Addition to lower extremity orthosis, plating chrome or nickel, per bar &
- [A] **L2755** Addition to lower extremity orthosis, high strength, lightweight material, all hybrid lamination/prepreg composite, per segment, for custom fabricated orthosis only &
- [A] **L2760** Addition to lower extremity orthosis, extension, per extension, per bar (for lineal adjustment for growth) &
- [A] ☑ **L2768** Orthotic side bar disconnect device, per bar &
- [A] ☑ **L2770** Addition to lower extremity orthosis, any material, per bar or joint &
- [A] ☑ **L2780** Addition to lower extremity orthosis, noncorrosive finish, per bar &
- [A] ☑ **L2785** Addition to lower extremity orthosis, drop lock retainer, each &
- [A] **L2795** Addition to lower extremity orthosis, knee control, full kneecap &
- [A] **L2800** Addition to lower extremity orthosis, knee control, knee cap, medial or lateral pull, for use with custom fabricated orthosis only &
- [A] **L2810** Addition to lower extremity orthosis, knee control, condylar pad &
- [A] **L2820** Addition to lower extremity orthosis, soft interface for molded plastic, below knee section &
- [A] **L2830** Addition to lower extremity orthosis, soft interface for molded plastic, above knee section &
- [A] ☑ **L2840** Addition to lower extremity orthosis, tibial length sock, fracture or equal, each &
- [A] ☑ **L2850** Addition to lower extremity orthosis, femoral length sock, fracture or equal, each &
- [A] ☑ **L2860** Addition to lower extremity joint, knee or ankle, concentric adjustable torsion style mechanism, each
- [A] **L2999** Lower extremity orthoses, NOS
  Determine if an alternative HCPCS Level II or a CPT code better describes the service being reported. This code should be used only if a more specific code is unavailable.

ORTHOPEDIC SHOES

INSERTS

- [A] ☑ **L3000** Foot insert, removable, molded to patient model, UCB type, Berkeley shell, each
  MED: 100-2,15,290
- [A] ☑ **L3001** Foot insert, removable, molded to patient model, Spenco, each
  MED: 100-2,15,290
- [A] ☑ **L3002** Foot insert, removable, molded to patient model, Plastazote or equal, each
  MED: 100-2,15,290

Special Coverage Instructions   Noncovered by Medicare   Carrier Discretion   ☑ Quality Alert   ● New Code   ○ Reinstated Code   ▲ Revised Code

2007 HCPCS   **1**-**9** ASC Group   **MED:** Pub 100/NCD References   & DMEPOS Paid   ⊘ SNF Excluded   **L Codes — 105**

Orthotic Procedures

L3003 — L3252

Ⓐ ☑ **L3003** Foot insert, removable, molded to patient model, silicone gel, each
MED: 100-2,15,290

Ⓐ ☑ **L3010** Foot insert, removable, molded to patient model, longitudinal arch support, each
MED: 100-2,15,290

Ⓐ ☑ **L3020** Foot insert, removable, molded to patient model, longitudinal/metatarsal support, each
MED: 100-2,15,290

Ⓐ ☑ **L3030** Foot insert, removable, formed to patient foot, each
MED: 100-2,15,290

Ⓐ ☑ **L3031** Foot, insert/plate, removable, addition to lower extremity orthosis, high strength, lightweight material, all hybrid lamination/prepreg composite, each

ARCH SUPPORT, REMOVABLE, PREMOLDED

Ⓐ ☑ **L3040** Foot, arch support, removable, premolded, longitudinal, each
MED: 100-2,15,290

Ⓐ ☑ **L3050** Foot, arch support, removable, premolded, metatarsal, each
MED: 100-2,15,290

Ⓐ ☑ **L3060** Foot, arch support, removable, premolded, longitudinal/metatarsal, each
MED: 100-2,15,290

ARCH SUPPORT, NONREMOVABLE, ATTACHED TO SHOE

Ⓐ ☑ **L3070** Foot, arch support, nonremovable, attached to shoe, longitudinal, each
MED: 100-2,15,290

Ⓐ ☑ **L3080** Foot, arch support, nonremovable, attached to shoe, metatarsal, each
MED: 100-2,15,290

Ⓐ ☑ **L3090** Foot, arch support, nonremovable, attached to shoe, longitudinal/metatarsal, each
MED: 100-2,15,290

Ⓐ **L3100** Hallus-valgus night dynamic splint
MED: 100-2,15,290; 100-4,4,240

ABDUCTION AND ROTATION BARS

A Denis-Browne style splint is a bar that can be applied by strapping or mounted on a shoe. This type of splint generally corrects congenital conditions such as genu varus

Denis-Browne splint

The angle may be adjusted on a plate on the sole of the shoe

Ⓐ **L3140** Foot, abduction rotation bar, including shoes
MED: 100-2,15,290

Ⓐ **L3150** Foot, abduction rotation bar, without shoes
MED: 100-2,15,290

Ⓐ **L3160** Foot, adjustable shoe-styled positioning device

Ⓐ **L3170** Foot, plastic, silicone or equal, heel stabilizer, each
MED: 100-2,15,290

ORTHOPEDIC FOOTWEAR

Ⓐ **L3201** Orthopedic shoe, Oxford with supinator or pronator, infant   Ⓐ
MED: 100-2,15,290

Ⓐ **L3202** Orthopedic shoe, Oxford with supinator or pronator, child   Ⓐ
MED: 100-2,15,290

Ⓐ **L3203** Orthopedic shoe, Oxford with supinator or pronator, junior   Ⓐ
MED: 100-2,15,290

Ⓐ **L3204** Orthopedic shoe, hightop with supinator or pronator, infant   Ⓐ
MED: 100-2,15,290

Ⓐ **L3206** Orthopedic shoe, hightop with supinator or pronator, child   Ⓐ
MED: 100-2,15,290

Ⓐ **L3207** Orthopedic shoe, hightop with supinator or pronator, junior   Ⓐ
MED: 100-2,15,290

Ⓐ ☑ **L3208** Surgical boot, each, infant   Ⓐ
MED: 100-2,15,100

Ⓐ ☑ **L3209** Surgical boot, each, child   Ⓐ
MED: 100-2,15,100

Ⓐ ☑ **L3211** Surgical boot, each, junior   Ⓐ
MED: 100-2,15,100

Ⓐ ☑ **L3212** Benesch boot, pair, infant   Ⓐ
MED: 100-2,15,100

Ⓐ ☑ **L3213** Benesch boot, pair, child   Ⓐ
MED: 100-2,15,100

Ⓐ ☑ **L3214** Benesch boot, pair, junior   Ⓐ
MED: 100-2,15,100

Ⓐ **L3215** Orthopedic footwear, ladies shoe, oxford, each   Ⓐ ♀

Ⓐ **L3216** Orthopedic footwear, ladies shoe, depth inlay, each   Ⓐ ♀

Ⓐ **L3217** Orthopedic footwear, ladies shoe, hightop, depth inlay, each   Ⓐ ♀

Ⓐ **L3219** Orthopedic footwear, mens shoe, oxford, each   Ⓐ ♂

Ⓐ **L3221** Orthopedic footwear, mens shoe, depth inlay, each   Ⓐ ♂

Ⓐ **L3222** Orthopedic footwear, mens shoe, hightop, depth inlay, each   Ⓐ ♂

Ⓐ **L3224** Orthopedic footwear, woman's shoe, Oxford, used as an integral part of a brace (orthosis)   ♀ ♿
MED: 100-2,15,290

Ⓐ **L3225** Orthopedic footwear, man's shoe, Oxford, used as an integral part of a brace (orthosis)   ♂ ♿
MED: 100-2,15,290

Ⓐ **L3230** Orthopedic footwear, custom shoe, depth inlay, each
MED: 100-2,15,290

Ⓐ ☑ **L3250** Orthopedic footwear, custom molded shoe, removable inner mold, prosthetic shoe, each
MED: 100-2,15,290

Ⓐ ☑ **L3251** Foot, shoe molded to patient model, silicone shoe, each
MED: 100-2,15,290

Ⓐ ☑ **L3252** Foot, shoe molded to patient model, Plastazote (or similar), custom fabricated, each
MED: 100-2,15,290

Special Coverage Instructions   Noncovered by Medicare   Carrier Discretion   ☑ Quality Alert   ● New Code   ○ Reinstated Code   ▲ Revised Code

106 — L Codes   Ⓐ Age Edit   Ⓜ Maternity Edit   ♀ Female Only   ♂ Male Only   Ⓐ - ☑ APC Status Indicators   2007 HCPCS

Ⓐ ☑ **L3253** Foot, molded shoe Plastazote (or similar), custom fitted, each
MED: 100-2,15,290

Ⓐ **L3254** Nonstandard size or width
MED: 100-2,15,290

Ⓐ **L3255** Nonstandard size or length
MED: 100-2,15,290

Ⓐ **L3257** Orthopedic footwear, additional charge for split size
MED: 100-2,15,290

Ⓔ ☑ **L3260** Surgical boot / shoe, each
MED: 100-2,15,100

Ⓐ ☑ **L3265** Plastazote sandal, each

SHOE MODIFICATION - LIFTS

Ⓐ ☑ **L3300** Lift, elevation, heel, tapered to metatarsals, per in.
MED: 100-2,15,290

Ⓐ ☑ **L3310** Lift, elevation, heel and sole, neoprene, per in.
MED: 100-2,15,290

Ⓐ ☑ **L3320** Lift, elevation, heel and sole, cork, per in.
MED: 100-2,15,290

Ⓐ **L3330** Lift, elevation, metal extension (skate)
MED: 100-2,15,290

Ⓐ ☑ **L3332** Lift, elevation, inside shoe, tapered, up to one-half in.
MED: 100-2,15,290

Ⓐ ☑ **L3334** Lift, elevation, heel, per in.
MED: 100-2,15,290

SHOE MODIFICATION - WEDGES

Ⓐ **L3340** Heel wedge, SACH
MED: 100-2,15,290

Ⓐ **L3350** Heel wedge
MED: 100-2,15,290

Ⓐ **L3360** Sole wedge, outside sole
MED: 100-2,15,290

Ⓐ **L3370** Sole wedge, between sole
MED: 100-2,15,290

Ⓐ **L3380** Clubfoot wedge
MED: 100-2,15,290

Ⓐ **L3390** Outflare wedge
MED: 100-2,15,290

Ⓐ **L3400** Metatarsal bar wedge, rocker
MED: 100-2,15,290

Ⓐ **L3410** Metatarsal bar wedge, between sole
MED: 100-2,15,290

Ⓐ **L3420** Full sole and heel wedge, between sole
MED: 100-2,15,290

SHOE MODIFICATIONS - HEELS

Ⓐ **L3430** Heel, counter, plastic reinforced
MED: 100-2,15,290

Ⓐ **L3440** Heel, counter, leather reinforced
MED: 100-2,15,290

Ⓐ **L3450** Heel, SACH cushion type
MED: 100-2,15,290

Ⓐ **L3455** Heel, new leather, standard
MED: 100-2,15,290

Ⓐ **L3460** Heel, new rubber, standard
MED: 100-2,15,290

Ⓐ **L3465** Heel, Thomas with wedge
MED: 100-2,15,290

Ⓐ **L3470** Heel, Thomas extended to ball
MED: 100-2,15,290

Ⓐ **L3480** Heel, pad and depression for spur
MED: 100-2,15,290

Ⓐ **L3485** Heel, pad, removable for spur
MED: 100-2,15,290

MISCELLANEOUS SHOE ADDITIONS

Ⓐ **L3500** Orthopedic shoe addition, insole, leather
MED: 100-2,15,290

Ⓐ **L3510** Orthopedic shoe addition, insole, rubber
MED: 100-2,15,290

Ⓐ **L3520** Orthopedic shoe addition, insole, felt covered with leather
MED: 100-2,15,290

Ⓐ **L3530** Orthopedic shoe addition, sole, half
MED: 100-2,15,290

Ⓐ **L3540** Orthopedic shoe addition, sole, full
MED: 100-2,15,290

Ⓐ **L3550** Orthopedic shoe addition, toe tap, standard
MED: 100-2,15,290

Ⓐ **L3560** Orthopedic shoe addition, toe tap, horseshoe
MED: 100-2,15,290

Ⓐ **L3570** Orthopedic shoe addition, special extension to instep (leather with eyelets)
MED: 100-2,15,290

Ⓐ **L3580** Orthopedic shoe addition, convert instep to Velcro closure
MED: 100-2,15,290

Ⓐ **L3590** Orthopedic shoe addition, convert firm shoe counter to soft counter
MED: 100-2,15,290

Ⓐ **L3595** Orthopedic shoe addition, March bar
MED: 100-2,15,290

TRANSFER OR REPLACEMENT

Ⓐ **L3600** Transfer of an orthosis from one shoe to another, caliper plate, existing
MED: 100-2,15,290

Ⓐ **L3610** Transfer of an orthosis from one shoe to another, caliper plate, new
MED: 100-2,15,290

Ⓐ **L3620** Transfer of an orthosis from one shoe to another, solid stirrup, existing
MED: 100-2,15,290

Ⓐ **L3630** Transfer of an orthosis from one shoe to another, solid stirrup, new
MED: 100-2,15,290

Ⓐ **L3640** Transfer of an orthosis from one shoe to another, Dennis Browne splint (Riveton), both shoes
MED: 100-2,15,290

Ⓐ **L3649** Orthopedic shoe, modification, addition or transfer, NOS
Determine if an alternative HCPCS Level II or a CPT code better describes the service being reported. This code should be used only if a more specific code is unavailable.
MED: 100-2,15,290

Special Coverage Instructions   Noncovered by Medicare   Carrier Discretion   ☑ Quality Alert   ● New Code   ○ Reinstated Code   ▲ Revised Code

Orthotic Procedures

L3650 — L3900

ORTHOTIC DEVICES - UPPER LIMB

The procedures in this section are considered as "base" or "basic procedures" and may be modified by listing procedures from the "additions" sections and adding them to the base procedure.

SHOULDER ORTHOSIS (SO)

[A] **L3650** SO, figure of eight design abduction restrainer, prefabricated, includes fitting and adjustment   占

[A] **L3651** SO, single shoulder, elastic, prefabricated, includes fitting and adjustment (e.g., neoprene, Lycra)   占

[A] **L3652** SO, double shoulder, elastic, prefabricated, includes fitting and adjustment (e.g., neoprene, Lycra)   占

[A] **L3660** SO, figure of eight design abduction restrainer, canvas and webbing, prefabricated, includes fitting and adjustment   占

[A] **L3670** SO, acromio/clavicular (canvas and webbing type), prefabricated, includes fitting and adjustment   占

[A] **L3671** Shoulder orthosis, shoulder cap design, without joints, may include soft interface, straps, custom fabricated, includes fitting and adjustment

[A] **L3672** Shoulder orthosis, abduction positioning (airplane design), thoracic component and support bar, without joints, may include soft interface, straps, custom fabricated, includes fitting and adjustment

[A] **L3673** Shoulder orthosis, abduction positioning (airplane design), thoracic component and support bar, includes nontorsion joint/turnbuckle, may include soft interface, straps, custom fabricated, includes fitting and adjustment

[A] **L3675** SO, vest type abduction restrainer, canvas webbing type, or equal, prefabricated, includes fitting and adjustment   占

[E] **L3677** Shoulder orthosis, hard plastic, shoulder stabilizer, prefabricated, includes fitting and adjustment
MED: 100-2,15,120

ELBOW ORTHOSIS (EO)

[A] **L3700** EO, elastic with stays, prefabricated, includes fitting and adjustment   占

[A] **L3701** EO, elastic, prefabricated, includes fitting and adjustment (e.g., neoprene, Lycra)   占

[A] **L3702** Elbow orthosis, without joints, may include soft interface, straps, custom fabricated, includes fitting and adjustment

[A] **L3710** EO, elastic with metal joints, prefabricated, includes fitting and adjustment   占

[A] **L3720** EO, double upright with forearm/arm cuffs, free motion, custom fabricated   占

[A] **L3730** EO, double upright with forearm/arm cuffs, extension/flexion assist, custom fabricated   占

[A] **L3740** EO, double upright with forearm/arm cuffs, adjustable position lock with active control, custom fabricated   占

[A] **L3760** Elbow orthosis, with adjustable position locking joint(s), prefabricated, includes fitting and adjustments, any type   占

[A] **L3762** Elbow orthosis, rigid, without joints, includes soft interface material, prefabricated, includes fitting and adjustment   占

[A] **L3763** Elbow wrist hand orthosis, rigid, without joints, may include soft interface, straps, custom fabricated, includes fitting and adjustment

[A] **L3764** Elbow wrist hand orthosis, includes one or more nontorsion joints, elastic bands, turnbuckles, may include soft interface, straps, custom fabricated, includes fitting and adjustment

[A] **L3765** Elbow wrist hand finger orthosis, rigid, without joints, may include soft interface, straps, custom fabricated, includes fitting and adjustment

[A] **L3766** Elbow wrist hand finger orthosis, includes one or more nontorsion joints, elastic bands, turnbuckles, may include soft interface, straps, custom fabricated, includes fitting and adjustment

WRIST-HAND-FINGER ORTHOSIS (WHFO)

[A] **L3800** WHFO, short opponens, no attachments, custom fabricated   占

[A] **L3805** WHFO, long opponens, no attachment, custom fabricated   占

● [A] **L3806** Wrist hand finger orthosis, includes one or more nontorsion joint(s), elastic bands, turnbuckles, may include soft interface material, straps, custom fabricated, includes fitting and adjustment

[A] **L3807** WHFO, without joint(s), prefabricated, includes fitting and adjustments, any type   占

● [A] **L3808** Wrist hand finger orthosis, rigid without joints, may include soft interface material; straps, custom fabricated, includes fitting and adjustment

ADDITIONS

[A] **L3810** WHFO, addition to short and long opponens, thumb abduction (C) bar   占

[A] **L3815** WHFO, addition to short and long opponens, second M.P. abduction assist   占

[A] **L3820** WHFO, addition to short and long opponens, I.P. extension assist, with M.P. extension stop   占

[A] **L3825** WHFO, addition to short and long opponens, M.P. extension stop   占

[A] **L3830** WHFO, addition to short and long opponens, M.P. extension assist   占

[A] **L3835** WHFO, addition to short and long opponens, M.P. spring extension assist   占

[A] **L3840** WHFO, addition to short and long opponens, spring swivel thumb   占

[A] **L3845** WHFO, addition to short and long opponens, thumb I.P. extension assist, with M.P. stop   占

[A] **L3850** WHFO, addition to short and long opponens, action wrist, with dorsiflexion assist   占

[A] **L3855** WHFO, addition to short and long opponens, adjustable M.P. flexion control   占

[A] **L3860** WHFO, addition to short and long opponens, adjustable M.P. flexion control and I.P.   占

[B] **L3890** Addition to upper extremity joint, wrist or elbow, concentric adjustable torsion style mechanism, each

DYNAMIC FLEXOR HINGE, RECIPROCAL WRIST EXTENSION/FLEXION, FINGER FLEXION/EXTENSION

[A] **L3900** WHFO, dynamic flexor hinge, reciprocal wrist extension/flexion, finger flexion/extension, wrist or finger driven, custom fabricated   占

Special Coverage Instructions   Noncovered by Medicare   Carrier Discretion   ☑ Quality Alert   ● New Code   ○ Reinstated Code   ▲ Revised Code

108 — L Codes   [A] Age Edit   [M] Maternity Edit   ♀ Female Only   ♂ Male Only   [A] - [Y] APC Status Indicators   *2007 HCPCS*

Ⓐ	L3901	WHFO, dynamic flexor hinge, reciprocal wrist extension/flexion, finger flexion/extension, cable driven, custom fabricated ╘

EXTERNAL POWER

	~~L3902~~	~~WHFO, external powered, compressed gas, custom fabricated~~ See code(s) L6624.
Ⓐ	L3904	WHFO, external powered, electric, custom fabricated ╘

OTHER WHFOS - CUSTOM FITTED

Ⓐ	L3905	Wrist hand orthosis, includes one or more nontorsion joints, elastic bands, turnbuckles, may include soft interface, straps, custom fabricated, includes fitting and adjustment
Ⓐ	L3906	Wrist hand orthosis, without joints, may include soft interface, straps, custom fabricated, includes fitting and adjustment ╘
Ⓐ	L3907	WHFO, wrist gauntlet with thumb spica, molded to patient model, custom fabricated ╘
Ⓐ	L3908	WHO, wrist extension control cock-up, nonmolded, prefabricated, includes fitting and adjustment
Ⓐ	L3909	WO, elastic, prefabricated, includes fitting and adjustment (e.g., neoprene, Lycra) ╘
Ⓐ	L3910	WHFO, Swanson design, prefabricated, includes fitting and adjustment ╘
Ⓐ	L3911	WHFO, elastic, prefabricated, includes fitting and adjustment (e.g., neoprene, Lycra) ╘
Ⓐ	L3912	HFO, flexion glove with elastic finger control, prefabricated, includes fitting and adjustment ╘
Ⓐ	L3913	Hand finger orthosis, without joints, may include soft interface, straps, custom fabricated, includes fitting and adjustment
	~~L3914~~	~~WHO, wrist extension cock-up, prefabricated, includes fitting and adjustment~~ See code(s) L3908.
● Ⓐ	L3915	Wrist hand orthosis, includes one or more nontorsion joint(s), elastic bands, turnbuckles, may include soft interface, straps, prefabricated, includes fitting and adjustment
Ⓐ	L3916	WHFO, wrist extension cock-up, with outrigger, prefabricated, includes fitting and adjustment ╘
Ⓐ	L3917	Hand orthosis, metacarpal fracture orthosis, prefabricated, includes fitting and adjustment ╘
Ⓐ	L3918	HFO, knuckle bender, prefabricated, includes fitting and adjustment ╘
Ⓐ	L3919	Hand orthosis, without joints, may include soft interface, straps, custom fabricated, includes fitting and adjustment
Ⓐ	L3920	HFO, knuckle bender, with outrigger, prefabricated, includes fitting and adjustment
Ⓐ	L3921	Hand finger orthosis, includes one or more nontorsion joints, elastic bands, turnbuckles, may include soft interface, straps, custom fabricated, includes fitting and adjustment
Ⓐ	L3922	HFO, knuckle bender, two segment to flex joints, prefabricated, includes fitting and adjustment ╘
Ⓐ	L3923	Hand finger orthosis, without joints, may include soft interface, straps, custom fabricated, includes fitting and adjustment ╘

Ⓐ	L3924	WHFO, Oppenheimer, prefabricated, includes fitting and adjustment ╘
Ⓐ	L3926	WHFO, Thomas suspension, prefabricated, includes fitting and adjustment ╘
Ⓐ	L3928	HFO, finger extension, with clock spring, prefabricated, includes fitting and adjustment ╘
Ⓐ	L3930	WHFO, finger extension, with wrist support, prefabricated, includes fitting and adjustment ╘
Ⓐ	L3932	FO, safety pin, spring wire, prefabricated, includes fitting and adjustment ╘
Ⓐ	L3933	Finger orthosis, without joints, may include soft interface, custom fabricated, includes fitting and adjustment
Ⓐ	L3934	FO, safety pin, modified, prefabricated, includes fitting and adjustment ╘
Ⓐ	L3935	Finger orthosis, nontorsion joint, may include soft interface, custom fabricated, includes fitting and adjustment
Ⓐ	L3936	WHFO, Palmer, prefabricated, includes fitting and adjustment ╘
Ⓐ	L3938	WHFO, dorsal wrist, prefabricated, includes fitting and adjustment ╘
Ⓐ	L3940	WHFO, dorsal wrist, with outrigger attachment, prefabricated, includes fitting and adjustment ╘
Ⓐ	L3942	HFO, reverse knuckle bender, prefabricated, includes fitting and adjustment ╘
Ⓐ	L3944	HFO, reverse knuckle bender, with outrigger, prefabricated, includes fitting and adjustment ╘
Ⓐ	L3946	HFO, composite elastic, prefabricated, includes fitting and adjustment ╘
Ⓐ	L3948	FO, finger knuckle bender, prefabricated, includes fitting and adjustment ╘
Ⓐ	L3950	WHFO, combination Oppenheimer, with knuckle bender and two attachments, prefabricated, includes fitting and adjustment ╘
Ⓐ	L3952	WHFO, combination Oppenheimer, with reverse knuckle and two attachments, prefabricated, includes fitting and adjustment ╘
Ⓐ	L3954	HFO, spreading hand, prefabricated, includes fitting and adjustment ╘
Ⓐ ☑	L3956	Addition of joint to upper extremity orthosis, any material; per joint ╘

SHOULDER-ELBOW-WRIST-HAND ORTHOSIS (SEWHO)

ABDUCTION POSITION, CUSTOM FITTED

Ⓐ	L3960	SEWHO, abduction positioning, airplane design, prefabricated, includes fitting and adjustment ╘
Ⓐ	L3961	Shoulder elbow wrist hand orthosis, shoulder cap design, without joints, may include soft interface, straps, custom fabricated, includes fitting and adjustment
Ⓐ	L3962	SEWHO, abduction positioning, Erb's palsy design, prefabricated, includes fitting and adjustment ╘
Ⓨ	L3964	SEO, mobile arm support attached to wheelchair, balanced, adjustable, prefabricated, includes fitting and adjustment ╘
Ⓨ	L3965	SEO, mobile arm support attached to wheelchair, balanced, adjustable Rancho type, prefabricated, includes fitting and adjustment ╘

Special Coverage Instructions | Noncovered by Medicare | Carrier Discretion | ☑ Quality Alert | ● New Code | ○ Reinstated Code | ▲ Revised Code

2007 HCPCS | 1-9 ASC Group | MED: Pub 100/NCD References | ╘ DMEPOS Paid | ⊘ SNF Excluded | L Codes — 109

Orthotic Procedures

L3966 — L4394

Y   **L3966** SEO, mobile arm support attached to wheelchair, balanced, reclining, prefabricated, includes fitting and adjustment

A   **L3967** Shoulder elbow wrist hand orthosis, abduction positioning (airplane design), thoracic component and support bar, without joints, may include soft interface, straps, custom fabricated, includes fitting and adjustment

Y   **L3968** SEO, mobile arm support attached to wheelchair, balanced, friction arm support (friction dampening to proximal and distal joints), prefabricated, includes fitting and adjustment

Y   **L3969** SEO, mobile arm support, monosuspension arm and hand support, overhead elbow forearm hand sling support, yoke type arm suspension support, prefabricated, includes fitting and adjustment

ADDITIONS TO MOBILE ARM SUPPORTS

Y   **L3970** SEO, addition to mobile arm support, elevating proximal arm

A   **L3971** Shoulder elbow wrist hand orthosis, shoulder cap design, includes one or more nontorsion joints, elastic bands, turnbuckles, may include soft interface, straps, custom fabricated, includes fitting and adjustment

Y   **L3972** SEO, addition to mobile arm support, offset or lateral rocker arm with elastic balance control

A   **L3973** Shoulder elbow wrist hand orthosis, abduction positioning (airplane design), thoracic component and support bar, includes one or more nontorsion joints, elastic bands, turnbuckles, may include soft interface, straps, custom fabricated, includes fitting and adjustment

Y   **L3974** SEO, addition to mobile arm support, supinator

A   **L3975** Shoulder elbow wrist hand finger orthosis, shoulder cap design, without joints, may include soft interface, straps, custom fabricated, includes fitting and adjustment

A   **L3976** Shoulder elbow wrist hand finger orthosis, abduction positioning (airplane design), thoracic component and support bar, without joints, may include soft interface, straps, custom fabricated, includes fitting and adjustment

A   **L3977** Shoulder elbow wrist hand finger orthosis, shoulder cap design, includes one or more nontorsion joints, elastic bands, turnbuckles, may include soft interface, straps, custom fabricated, includes fitting and adjustment

A   **L3978** Shoulder elbow wrist hand finger orthosis, abduction positioning (airplane design), thoracic component and support bar, includes one or more nontorsion joints, elastic bands, turnbuckles, may include soft interface, straps, custom fabricated, includes fitting and adjustment

FRACTURE ORTHOSIS

A   **L3980** Upper extremity fracture orthosis, humeral, prefabricated, includes fitting and adjustment

A   **L3982** Upper extremity fracture orthosis, radius/ulnar, prefabricated, includes fitting and adjustment

A   **L3984** Upper extremity fracture orthosis, wrist, prefabricated, includes fitting and adjustment

A   **L3985** Upper extremity fracture orthosis, forearm, hand with wrist hinge, custom fabricated

A   **L3986** Upper extremity fracture orthosis, combination of humeral, radius/ulnar, wrist (example: Colles' fracture), custom fabricated

A   **L3995** Addition to upper extremity orthosis, sock, fracture or equal, each

A   **L3999** Upper limb orthosis, NOS

SPECIFIC REPAIR

A   **L4000** Replace girdle for spinal orthosis (CTLSO or SO)

A   **L4002** Replacement strap, any orthosis, includes all components, any length, any type

A   **L4010** Replace trilateral socket brim

A   **L4020** Replace quadrilateral socket brim, molded to patient model

A   **L4030** Replace quadrilateral socket brim, custom fitted

A   **L4040** Replace molded thigh lacer, for custom fabricated orthosis only

A   **L4045** Replace nonmolded thigh lacer, for custom fabricated orthosis only

A   **L4050** Replace molded calf lacer, for custom fabricated orthosis only

A   **L4055** Replace nonmolded calf lacer, for custom fabricated orthosis only

A   **L4060** Replace high roll cuff

A   **L4070** Replace proximal and distal upright for KAFO

A   **L4080** Replace metal bands KAFO, proximal thigh

A   **L4090** Replace metal bands KAFO-AFO, calf or distal thigh

A   **L4100** Replace leather cuff KAFO, proximal thigh

A   **L4110** Replace leather cuff KAFO-AFO, calf or distal thigh

A   **L4130** Replace pretibial shell

REPAIRS

A ☑   **L4205** Repair of orthotic device, labor component, per 15 minutes
     MED: 100-2,15,110.2

A   **L4210** Repair of orthotic device, repair or replace minor parts
     MED: 100-2,15,110.2; 100-2,15,120

A   **L4350** Ankle control orthosis, stirrup style, rigid, includes any type interface (e.g., pneumatic, gel), prefabricated, includes fitting and adjustment

A   **L4360** Walking boot, pneumatic, with or without joints, with or without interface material, prefabricated, includes fitting and adjustment

A   **L4370** Pneumatic full leg splint, prefabricated, includes fitting and adjustment
     MED: 100-4,4,240

A   **L4380** Pneumatic knee splint, prefabricated, includes fitting and adjustment
     MED: 100-4,4,240

A   **L4386** Walking boot, nonpneumatic, with or without joints, with or without interface material, prefabricated, includes fitting and adjustment

A   **L4392** Replacement soft interface material, static AFO

A   **L4394** Replace soft interface material, foot drop splint

---

Special Coverage Instructions   Noncovered by Medicare   Carrier Discretion   ☑ Quality Alert   ● New Code   ○ Reinstated Code   ▲ Revised Code

110 — L Codes   A Age Edit   M Maternity Edit   ♀ Female Only   ♂ Male Only   A - Y APC Status Indicators   *2007 HCPCS*

[A] **L4396** Static ankle foot orthosis, including soft interface material, adjustable for fit, for positioning, pressure reduction, may be used for minimal ambulation, prefabricated, includes fitting and adjustment &

[A] **L4398** Foot drop splint, recumbent positioning device, prefabricated, includes fitting and adjustment &
MED: 100-4,4,240

PROSTHETIC PROCEDURES L5000-L9999

LOWER LIMB

The procedures in this section are considered as "base" or "basic procedures" and may be modified by listing items/procedures or special materials from the "additions" sections and adding them to the base procedure.

PARTIAL FOOT

[A] **L5000** Partial foot, shoe insert with longitudinal arch, toe filler
MED: 100-2,15,290; 100-4,3,10.4

[A] **L5010** Partial foot, molded socket, ankle height, with toe filler
MED: 100-2,15,290; 100-4,3,10.4

[A] **L5020** Partial foot, molded socket, tibial tubercle height, with toe filler
MED: 100-2,15,290; 100-4,3,10.4

ANKLE

[A] **L5050** Ankle, Symes, molded socket, SACH foot ⊘&
MED: 100-4,3,10.4

[A] **L5060** Ankle, Symes, metal frame, molded leather socket, articulated ankle/foot ⊘&
MED: 100-4,3,10.4

BELOW KNEE

[A] **L5100** Below knee, molded socket, shin, SACH foot ⊘&
MED: 100-4,3,10.4

[A] **L5105** Below knee, plastic socket, joints and thigh lacer, SACH foot ⊘&
MED: 100-4,3,10.4

KNEE DISARTICULATION

[A] **L5150** Knee disarticulation (or through knee), molded socket, external knee joints, shin, SACH foot ⊘&
MED: 100-4,3,10.4

[A] **L5160** Knee disarticulation (or through knee), molded socket, bent knee configuration, external knee joints, shin, SACH foot ⊘&
MED: 100-4,3,10.4

ABOVE KNEE

[A] **L5200** Above knee, molded socket, single axis constant friction knee, shin, SACH foot ⊘&
MED: 100-4,3,10.4

[A] ☑ **L5210** Above knee, short prosthesis, no knee joint (stubbies), with foot blocks, no ankle joints, each ⊘&
MED: 100-4,3,10.4

[A] ☑ **L5220** Above knee, short prosthesis, no knee joint (stubbies), with articulated ankle/foot, dynamically aligned, each ⊘&
MED: 100-4,3,10.4

[A] **L5230** Above knee, for proximal femoral focal deficiency, constant friction knee, shin, sach foot ⊘&
MED: 100-4,3,10.4

HIP DISARTICULATION

[A] **L5250** Hip disarticulation, Canadian type; molded socket, hip joint, single axis constant friction knee, shin, SACH foot ⊘&
MED: 100-4,3,10.4

[A] **L5270** Hip disarticulation, tilt table type; molded socket, locking hip joint, single axis constant friction knee, shin, SACH foot ⊘&
MED: 100-4,3,10.4

HEMIPELVECTOMY

[A] **L5280** Hemipelvectomy, Canadian type; molded socket, hip joint, single axis constant friction knee, shin, SACH foot ⊘&
MED: 100-4,3,10.4

[A] **L5301** Below knee, molded socket, shin, SACH foot, endoskeletal system ⊘&
MED: 100-4,3,10.4

[A] **L5311** Knee disarticulation (or through knee), molded socket, external knee joints, shin, SACH foot, endoskeletal system ⊘&
MED: 100-4,3,10.4

[A] **L5321** Above knee, molded socket, open end, SACH foot, endoskeletal system, single axis knee ⊘&
MED: 100-4,3,10.4

[A] **L5331** Hip disarticulation, Canadian type, molded socket, endoskeletal system, hip joint, single axis knee, SACH foot ⊘&
MED: 100-4,3,10.4

[A] **L5341** Hemipelvectomy, Canadian type, molded socket, endoskeletal system, hip joint, single axis knee, SACH foot ⊘&
MED: 100-4,3,10.4

IMMEDIATE POSTSURGICAL OR EARLY FITTING PROCEDURES

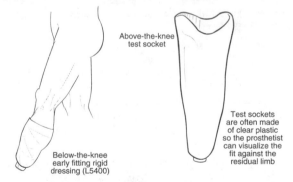

Above-the-knee test socket

Test sockets are often made of clear plastic so the prosthetist can visualize the fit against the residual limb

Below-the-knee early fitting rigid dressing (L5400)

[A] ☑ **L5400** Immediate postsurgical or early fitting, application of initial rigid dressing, including fitting, alignment, suspension, and one cast change, below knee

[A] ☑ **L5410** Immediate postsurgical or early fitting, application of initial rigid dressing, including fitting, alignment and suspension, below knee, each additional cast change and realignment ⊘&

[A] ☑ **L5420** Immediate postsurgical or early fitting, application of initial rigid dressing, including fitting, alignment and suspension and one cast change AK or knee disarticulation ⊘&

[A] ☑ **L5430** Immediate postsurgical or early fitting, application of initial rigid dressing, including fitting, alignment and suspension, AK or knee disarticulation, each additional cast change and realignment ⊘&

| Special Coverage Instructions | Noncovered by Medicare | Carrier Discretion | ☑ Quality Alert | ● New Code | ○ Reinstated Code | ▲ Revised Code |

2007 HCPCS   **1**-**9** ASC Group   **MED:** Pub 100/NCD References   & DMEPOS Paid   ⊘ SNF Excluded   **L Codes — 111**

[A] **L5450** Immediate postsurgical or early fitting, application of nonweight bearing rigid dressing, below knee ⊘ ᴋ

[A] **L5460** Immediate postsurgical or early fitting, application of nonweight bearing rigid dressing, above knee ⊘ ᴋ

INITIAL PROSTHESIS

[A] **L5500** Initial, below knee PTB type socket, nonalignable system, pylon, no cover, SACH foot, plaster socket, direct formed ⊘ ᴋ

MED: 100-2,1,40; 100-4,3,10.4

[A] **L5505** Initial, above knee — knee disarticulation, ischial level socket, nonalignable system, pylon, no cover, SACH foot plaster socket, direct formed ⊘ ᴋ

MED: 100-2,1,40; 100-4,3,10.4

PREPARATORY PROSTHESIS

[A] **L5510** Preparatory, below knee PTB type socket, nonalignable system, pylon, no cover, SACH foot, plaster socket, molded to model ⊘ ᴋ

[A] **L5520** Preparatory, below knee PTB type socket, nonalignable system, pylon, no cover, SACH foot, thermoplastic or equal, direct formed ⊘ ᴋ

[A] **L5530** Preparatory, below knee PTB type socket, nonalignable system, pylon, no cover, SACH foot, thermoplastic or equal, molded to model ⊘ ᴋ

[A] **L5535** Preparatory, below knee PTB type socket, nonalignable system, pylon, no cover, SACH foot, prefabricated, adjustable open end socket ⊘ ᴋ

[A] **L5540** Preparatory, below knee PTB type socket, nonalignable system, pylon, no cover, SACH foot, laminated socket, molded to model ⊘ ᴋ

[A] **L5560** Preparatory, above knee — knee disarticulation, ischial level socket, nonalignable system, pylon, no cover, SACH foot, plaster socket, molded to model ⊘ ᴋ

[A] **L5570** Preparatory, above knee — knee disarticulation, ischial level socket, nonalignable system, pylon, no cover, SACH foot, thermoplastic or equal, direct formed ⊘ ᴋ

[A] **L5580** Preparatory, above knee — knee disarticulation, ischial level socket, nonalignable system, pylon, no cover, SACH foot, thermoplastic or equal, molded to model ⊘ ᴋ

[A] **L5585** Preparatory, above knee — knee disarticulation, ischial level socket, nonalignable system, pylon, no cover, SACH foot, prefabricated adjustable open end socket ⊘ ᴋ

[A] **L5590** Preparatory, above knee — knee disarticulation, ischial level socket, nonalignable system, pylon, no cover, SACH foot, laminated socket, molded to model ⊘ ᴋ

[A] **L5595** Preparatory, hip disarticulation — hemipelvectomy, pylon, no cover, SACH foot, thermoplastic or equal, molded to patient model ⊘ ᴋ

[A] **L5600** Preparatory, hip disarticulation — hemipelvectomy, pylon, no cover, SACH foot, laminated socket, molded to patient model ⊘ ᴋ

ADDITIONS: LOWER EXTREMITY

[A] **L5610** Addition to lower extremity, endoskeletal system, above knee, hydracadence system ⊘ ᴋ

[A] **L5611** Addition to lower extremity, endoskeletal system, above knee — knee disarticulation, 4-bar linkage, with friction swing phase control ⊘ ᴋ

[A] **L5613** Addition to lower extremity, endoskeletal system, above knee — knee disarticulation, 4-bar linkage, with hydraulic swing phase control ⊘ ᴋ

[A] **L5614** Addition to lower extremity, endoskeletal system, above knee — knee disarticulation, 4-bar linkage, with pneumatic swing phase control ⊘ ᴋ

[A] **L5616** Addition to lower extremity, endoskeletal system, above knee, universal multiplex system, friction swing phase control ⊘ ᴋ

[A] ☑ **L5617** Addition to lower extremity, quick change self-aligning unit, above or below knee, each ⊘ ᴋ

ADDITIONS: TEST SOCKETS

[A] **L5618** Addition to lower extremity, test socket, Symes ⊘ ᴋ

[A] **L5620** Addition to lower extremity, test socket, below knee ⊘ ᴋ

[A] **L5622** Addition to lower extremity, test socket, knee disarticulation ⊘ ᴋ

[A] **L5624** Addition to lower extremity, test socket, above knee ⊘ ᴋ

[A] **L5626** Addition to lower extremity, test socket, hip disarticulation ⊘ ᴋ

[A] **L5628** Addition to lower extremity, test socket, hemipelvectomy ⊘ ᴋ

[A] **L5629** Addition to lower extremity, below knee, acrylic socket ⊘ ᴋ

ADDITIONS: SOCKET VARIATIONS

[A] **L5630** Addition to lower extremity, Symes type, expandable wall socket ⊘ ᴋ

[A] **L5631** Addition to lower extremity, above knee or knee disarticulation, acrylic socket ⊘ ᴋ

[A] **L5632** Addition to lower extremity, Symes type, PTB brim design socket ⊘ ᴋ

[A] **L5634** Addition to lower extremity, Symes type, posterior opening (Canadian) socket ⊘ ᴋ

[A] **L5636** Addition to lower extremity, Symes type, medial opening socket ⊘ ᴋ

[A] **L5637** Addition to lower extremity, below knee, total contact ⊘ ᴋ

[A] **L5638** Addition to lower extremity, below knee, leather socket ⊘ ᴋ

[A] **L5639** Addition to lower extremity, below knee, wood socket ⊘ ᴋ

[A] **L5640** Addition to lower extremity, knee disarticulation, leather socket ⊘ ᴋ

[A] **L5642** Addition to lower extremity, above knee, leather socket ⊘ ᴋ

[A] **L5643** Addition to lower extremity, hip disarticulation, flexible inner socket, external frame ⊘ ᴋ

[A] **L5644** Addition to lower extremity, above knee, wood socket ⊘ ᴋ

[A] **L5645** Addition to lower extremity, below knee, flexible inner socket, external frame ⊘ ᴋ

[A] **L5646** Addition to lower extremity, below knee, air, fluid, gel or equal, cushion socket ⊘ ᴋ

[A] **L5647** Addition to lower extremity, below knee, suction socket ⊘ ᴋ

[A] **L5648** Addition to lower extremity, above knee, air, fluid, gel or equal, cushion socket ⊘ ᴋ

Special Coverage Instructions   Noncovered by Medicare   Carrier Discretion   ☑ Quality Alert   ● New Code   ○ Reinstated Code   ▲ Revised Code

112 — L Codes   [A] Age Edit   [M] Maternity Edit   ♀ Female Only   ♂ Male Only   [A] - [Y] APC Status Indicators   *2007 HCPCS*

[A]	L5649	Addition to lower extremity, ischial containment/narrow M-L socket	⊘ ♿
[A]	L5650	Addition to lower extremity, total contact, above knee or knee disarticulation socket	⊘ ♿
[A]	L5651	Addition to lower extremity, above knee, flexible inner socket, external frame	⊘ ♿
[A]	L5652	Addition to lower extremity, suction suspension, above knee or knee disarticulation socket	⊘ ♿
[A]	L5653	Addition to lower extremity, knee disarticulation, expandable wall socket	⊘ ♿

ADDITIONS: SOCKET INSERT AND SUSPENSION

[A]	L5654	Addition to lower extremity, socket insert, Symes (Kemblo, Pelite, Aliplast, Plastazote or equal)	⊘ ♿
[A]	L5655	Addition to lower extremity, socket insert, below knee (Kemblo, Pelite, Aliplast, Plastazote or equal)	⊘ ♿
[A]	L5656	Addition to lower extremity, socket insert, knee disarticulation (Kemblo, Pelite, Aliplast, Plastazote or equal)	⊘ ♿
[A]	L5658	Addition to lower extremity, socket insert, above knee (Kemblo, Pelite, Aliplast, Plastazote or equal)	⊘ ♿
[A]	L5661	Addition to lower extremity, socket insert, multidurometer, Symes	⊘ ♿
[A]	L5665	Addition to lower extremity, socket insert, multidurometer, below knee	⊘ ♿
[A]	L5666	Addition to lower extremity, below knee, cuff suspension	⊘ ♿
[A]	L5668	Addition to lower extremity, below knee, molded distal cushion	⊘ ♿

As the suspension sleeve is donned, air is driven out through a valve

The valve is closed upon donning and a suction fit is formed around the residual limb

Residual limb

Sealing membrane

Sleeve

Open valve

Closed valve

[A]	L5670	Addition to lower extremity, below knee, molded supracondylar suspension (PTS or similar)	⊘ ♿
[A]	L5671	Addition to lower extremity, below knee/above knee suspension locking mechanism (shuttle, lanyard or equal), excludes socket insert	⊘ ♿
[A]	L5672	Addition to lower extremity, below knee, removable medial brim suspension	⊘ ♿
[A]	L5673	Addition to lower extremity, below knee/above knee, custom fabricated from existing mold or prefabricated, socket insert, silicone gel, elastomeric or equal, for use with locking mechanism	⊘ ♿
[A] ☑	L5676	Addition to lower extremity, below knee, knee joints, single axis, pair	⊘ ♿
[A] ☑	L5677	Addition to lower extremity, below knee, knee joints, polycentric, pair	⊘ ♿
[A] ☑	L5678	Addition to lower extremity, below knee joint covers, pair	⊘ ♿

[A]	L5679	Addition to lower extremity, below knee/above knee, custom fabricated from existing mold or prefabricated, socket insert, silicone gel, elastomeric or equal, not for use with locking mechanism	⊘ ♿
[A]	L5680	Addition to lower extremity, below knee, thigh lacer, nonmolded	⊘ ♿
[A]	L5681	Addition to lower extremity, below knee/above knee, custom fabricated socket insert for congenital or atypical traumatic amputee, silicone gel, elastomeric or equal, for use with or without locking mechanism, initial only (for other than initial, use code L5673 or L5679)	⊘ ♿
[A]	L5682	Addition to lower extremity, below knee, thigh lacer, gluteal/ischial, molded	⊘ ♿
[A]	L5683	Addition to lower extremity, below knee/above knee, custom fabricated socket insert for other than congenital or atypical traumatic amputee, silicone gel, elastomeric or equal, for use with or without locking mechanism, initial only (for other than initial, use code L5673 or L5679)	⊘ ♿
[A]	L5684	Addition to lower extremity, below knee, fork strap	⊘ ♿
[A]	L5685	Addition to lower extremity prosthesis, below knee, suspension/sealing sleeve, with or without valve, any material, each	⊘
[A]	L5686	Addition to lower extremity, below knee, back check (extension control)	⊘ ♿
[A]	L5688	Addition to lower extremity, below knee, waist belt, webbing	⊘ ♿
[A]	L5690	Addition to lower extremity, below knee, waist belt, padded and lined	⊘ ♿
[A]	L5692	Addition to lower extremity, above knee, pelvic control belt, light	⊘ ♿
[A]	L5694	Addition to lower extremity, above knee, pelvic control belt, padded and lined	⊘ ♿
[A] ☑	L5695	Addition to lower extremity, above knee, pelvic control, sleeve suspension, neoprene or equal, each	⊘
[A]	L5696	Addition to lower extremity, above knee or knee disarticulation, pelvic joint	⊘
[A]	L5697	Addition to lower extremity, above knee or knee disarticulation, pelvic band	⊘
[A]	L5698	Addition to lower extremity, above knee or knee disarticulation, Silesian bandage	⊘
[A]	L5699	All lower extremity prostheses, shoulder harness	⊘

REPLACEMENTS

[A]	L5700	Replacement, socket, below knee, molded to patient model	⊘
[A]	L5701	Replacement, socket, above knee/knee disarticulation, including attachment plate, molded to patient model	⊘
[A]	L5702	Replacement, socket, hip disarticulation, including hip joint, molded to patient model	⊘
[A]	L5703	Ankle, Symes, molded to patient model, socket without solid ankle cushion heel (SACH) foot, replacement only	⊘
[A]	L5704	Custom shaped protective cover, below knee	⊘
[A]	L5705	Custom shaped protective cover, above knee	⊘
[A]	L5706	Custom shaped protective cover, knee disarticulation	⊘

Special Coverage Instructions   Noncovered by Medicare   Carrier Discretion   ☑ Quality Alert   ● New Code   ○ Reinstated Code   ▲ Revised Code

2007 HCPCS   **1-9** ASC Group   **MED:** Pub 100/NCD References   ♿ DMEPOS Paid   ⊘ SNF Excluded   **L Codes — 113**

[A] **L5707** Custom shaped protective cover, hip disarticulation ⊘

ADDITIONS: EXOSKELETAL KNEE-SHIN SYSTEM

[A] **L5710** Addition, exoskeletal knee-shin system, single axis, manual lock ⊘

[A] **L5711** Addition, exoskeletal knee-shin system, single axis, manual lock, ultra-light material ⊘

[A] **L5712** Addition, exoskeletal knee-shin system, single axis, friction swing and stance phase control (safety knee) ⊘

[A] **L5714** Addition, exoskeletal knee-shin system, single axis, variable friction swing phase control ⊘

[A] **L5716** Addition, exoskeletal knee-shin system, polycentric, mechanical stance phase lock ⊘

[A] **L5718** Addition, exoskeletal knee-shin system, polycentric, friction swing and stance phase control ⊘

[A] **L5722** Addition, exoskeletal knee-shin system, single axis, pneumatic swing, friction stance phase control ⊘

[A] **L5724** Addition, exoskeletal knee-shin system, single axis, fluid swing phase control ⊘

[A] **L5726** Addition, exoskeletal knee-shin system, single axis, external joints, fluid swing phase control ⊘

[A] **L5728** Addition, exoskeletal knee-shin system, single axis, fluid swing and stance phase control ⊘

[A] **L5780** Addition, exoskeletal knee-shin system, single axis, pneumatic/hydra pneumatic swing phase control ⊘

[A] **L5781** Addition to lower limb prosthesis, vacuum pump, residual limb volume management and moisture evacuation system ⊘

[A] **L5782** Addition to lower limb prosthesis, vacuum pump, residual limb volume management and moisture evacuation system, heavy duty ⊘

COMPONENT MODIFICATION

[A] **L5785** Addition, exoskeletal system, below knee, ultra-light material (titanium, carbon fiber or equal) ⊘

[A] **L5790** Addition, exoskeletal system, above knee, ultra-light material (titanium, carbon fiber or equal) ⊘

[A] **L5795** Addition, exoskeletal system, hip disarticulation, ultra-light material (titanium, carbon fiber or equal) ⊘

ADDITIONS: ENDOSKELETAL KNEE-SHIN SYSTEM

[A] **L5810** Addition, endoskeletal knee-shin system, single axis, manual lock ⊘

[A] **L5811** Addition, endoskeletal knee-shin system, single axis, manual lock, ultra-light material ⊘

[A] **L5812** Addition, endoskeletal knee-shin system, single axis, friction swing and stance phase control (safety knee) ⊘

[A] **L5814** Addition, endoskeletal knee-shin system, polycentric, hydraulic swing phase control, mechanical stance phase lock ⊘

[A] **L5816** Addition, endoskeletal knee-shin system, polycentric, mechanical stance phase lock ⊘

[A] **L5818** Addition, endoskeletal knee-shin system, polycentric, friction swing and stance phase control ⊘

[A] **L5822** Addition, endoskeletal knee-shin system, single axis, pneumatic swing, friction stance phase control ⊘

[A] **L5824** Addition, endoskeletal knee-shin system, single axis, fluid swing phase control ⊘

[A] **L5826** Addition, endoskeletal knee-shin system, single axis, hydraulic swing phase control, with miniature high activity frame ⊘

[A] **L5828** Addition, endoskeletal knee-shin system, single axis, fluid swing and stance phase control ⊘

[A] **L5830** Addition, endoskeletal knee-shin system, single axis, pneumatic/swing phase control ⊘

[A] **L5840** Addition, endoskeletal knee-shin system, 4-bar linkage or multiaxial, pneumatic swing phase control ⊘

[A] **L5845** Addition, endoskeletal knee-shin system, stance flexion feature, adjustable ⊘

▲ [A] **L5848** Addition to endoskeletal knee-shin system, fluid stance extension, dampening feature, with or without adjustability ⊘

[A] **L5850** Addition, endoskeletal system, above knee or hip disarticulation, knee extension assist ⊘

[A] **L5855** Addition, endoskeletal system, hip disarticulation, mechanical hip extension assist ⊘

[A] **L5856** Addition to lower extremity prosthesis, endoskeletal knee-shin system, microprocessor control feature, swing and stance phase, includes electronic sensor(s), any type ⊘

[A] **L5857** Addition to lower extremity prosthesis, endoskeletal knee-shin system, microprocessor control feature, swing phase only, includes electronic sensor(s), any type ⊘

[A] **L5858** Addition to lower extremity prosthesis, endoskeletal knee shin system, microprocessor control feature, stance phase only, includes electronic sensor(s), any type ⊘

[A] **L5910** Addition, endoskeletal system, below knee, alignable system ⊘

[A] **L5920** Addition, endoskeletal system, above knee or hip disarticulation, alignable system ⊘

[A] **L5925** Addition, endoskeletal system, above knee, knee disarticulation or hip disarticulation, manual lock ⊘

[A] **L5930** Addition, endoskeletal system, high activity knee control frame ⊘

[A] **L5940** Addition, endoskeletal system, below knee, ultra-light material (titanium, carbon fiber or equal) ⊘

[A] **L5950** Addition, endoskeletal system, above knee, ultra-light material (titanium, carbon fiber or equal) ⊘

[A] **L5960** Addition, endoskeletal system, hip disarticulation, ultra-light material (titanium, carbon fiber or equal) ⊘

[A] **L5962** Addition, endoskeletal system, below knee, flexible protective outer surface covering system ⊘

[A] **L5964** Addition, endoskeletal system, above knee, flexible protective outer surface covering system ⊘

[A] **L5966** Addition, endoskeletal system, hip disarticulation, flexible protective outer surface covering system ⊘

[A] **L5968** Addition to lower limb prosthesis, multiaxial ankle with swing phase active dorsiflexion feature ⊘

[A] **L5970** All lower extremity prostheses, foot, external keel, SACH foot ⊘

[A] **L5971** All lower extremity prosthesis, solid ankle cushion heel (SACH) foot, replacement only ⊘

Special Coverage Instructions   Noncovered by Medicare   Carrier Discretion   ☑ Quality Alert   ● New Code   ○ Reinstated Code   ▲ Revised Code

[A] **L5972** All lower extremity prostheses, flexible keel foot (SAFE, STEN, Bock Dynamic or equal) ⊘

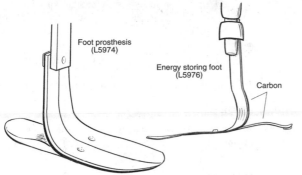

Foot prosthesis
(L5974)

Energy storing foot
(L5976)

Carbon

[A] **L5974** All lower extremity prostheses, foot, single axis ankle/foot ⊘

[A] **L5975** All lower extremity prosthesis, combination single axis ankle and flexible keel foot ⊘

[A] **L5976** All lower extremity prostheses, energy storing foot (Seattle Carbon Copy II or equal) ⊘

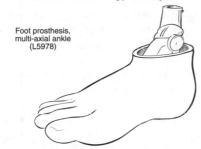

Foot prosthesis,
multi-axial ankle
(L5978)

[A] **L5978** All lower extremity prostheses, foot, multiaxial ankle/foot ⊘

[A] **L5979** All lower extremity prostheses, multiaxial ankle, dynamic response foot, one piece system ⊘

[A] **L5980** All lower extremity prostheses, flex-foot system ⊘

[A] **L5981** All lower extremity prostheses, flex-walk system or equal ⊘

[A] **L5982** All exoskeletal lower extremity prostheses, axial rotation unit ⊘

[A] **L5984** All endoskeletal lower extremity prosthesis, axial rotation unit, with or without adjustability ⊘

[A] **L5985** All endoskeletal lower extremity prostheses, dynamic prosthetic pylon ⊘

[A] **L5986** All lower extremity prostheses, multiaxial rotation unit (MCP or equal) ⊘

[A] **L5987** All lower extremity prosthesis, shank foot system with vertical loading pylon ⊘

[A] **L5988** Addition to lower limb prosthesis, vertical shock reducing pylon feature ⊘

[A] **L5990** Addition to lower extremity prosthesis, user adjustable heel height ⊘

● [A] **L5993** Addition to lower extremity prosthesis, heavy duty feature, foot only, (for patient weight greater than 300 lbs) ⊘

● [A] **L5994** Addition to lower extremity prosthesis, heavy duty feature, knee only, (for patient weight greater than 300 lbs) ⊘

▲ [A] **L5995** Addition to lower extremity prosthesis, heavy duty feature, other than foot or knee, (for patient weight greater than 300 lbs) ⊘

[A] **L5999** Lower extremity prosthesis, not otherwise specified Determine if an alternative HCPCS Level II or a CPT code better describes the service being reported. This code should be used only if a more specific code is unavailable.

UPPER LIMB

The procedures in L6000-L6590 are considered as "base" or "basic procedures" and may be modified by listing procedures from the "addition" sections. The base procedures include only standard friction wrist and control cable system unless otherwise specified.

PARTIAL HAND

[A] **L6000** Partial hand, Robin-Aids, thumb remaining (or equal)

[A] **L6010** Partial hand, Robin-Aids, little and/or ring finger remaining (or equal)

[A] **L6020** Partial hand, Robin-Aids, no finger remaining (or equal)

[A] **L6025** Transcarpal/metacarpal or partial hand disarticulation prosthesis, external power, self-suspended, inner socket with removable forearm section, electrodes and cables, two batteries, charger, myoelectric control of terminal device

WRIST DISARTICULATION

[A] **L6050** Wrist disarticulation, molded socket, flexible elbow hinges, triceps pad ⊘

[A] **L6055** Wrist disarticulation, molded socket with expandable interface, flexible elbow hinges, triceps pad ⊘

BELOW ELBOW

[A] **L6100** Below elbow, molded socket, flexible elbow hinge, triceps pad ⊘

[A] **L6110** Below elbow, molded socket (Muenster or Northwestern suspension types) ⊘

[A] **L6120** Below elbow, molded double wall split socket, step-up hinges, half cuff ⊘

[A] **L6130** Below elbow, molded double wall split socket, stump activated locking hinge, half cuff ⊘

ELBOW DISARTICULATION

[A] **L6200** Elbow disarticulation, molded socket, outside locking hinge, forearm ⊘

[A] **L6205** Elbow disarticulation, molded socket with expandable interface, outside locking hinges, forearm ⊘ �

ABOVE ELBOW

[A] **L6250** Above elbow, molded double wall socket, internal locking elbow, forearm ⊘ 㓱

SHOULDER DISARTICULATION

[A] **L6300** Shoulder disarticulation, molded socket, shoulder bulkhead, humeral section, internal locking elbow, forearm ⊘ 㓱

[A] **L6310** Shoulder disarticulation, passive restoration (complete prosthesis) ⊘ 㓱

[A] **L6320** Shoulder disarticulation, passive restoration (shoulder cap only) ⊘ 㓱

INTERSCAPULAR THORACIC

[A] **L6350** Interscapular thoracic, molded socket, shoulder bulkhead, humeral section, internal locking elbow, forearm ⊘ 㓱

Special Coverage Instructions   Noncovered by Medicare   Carrier Discretion   ☑ Quality Alert   ● New Code   ○ Reinstated Code   ▲ Revised Code

2007 HCPCS   **1-9** ASC Group   **MED:** Pub 100/NCD References   㓱 DMEPOS Paid   ⊘ SNF Excluded   **L Codes — 115**

Prosthetic Procedures

L6360 — L6642

[A] **L6360** Interscapular thoracic, passive restoration (complete prosthesis) ⊘ ö

[A] **L6370** Interscapular thoracic, passive restoration (shoulder cap only) ⊘ ö

IMMEDIATE AND EARLY POSTSURGICAL PROCEDURES

[A] **L6380** Immediate postsurgical or early fitting, application of initial rigid dressing, including fitting alignment and suspension of components, and one cast change, wrist disarticulation or below elbow ö

[A] ☑ **L6382** Immediate postsurgical or early fitting, application of initial rigid dressing including fitting alignment and suspension of components, and one cast change, elbow disarticulation or above elbow ö

[A] ☑ **L6384** Immediate postsurgical or early fitting, application of initial rigid dressing including fitting alignment and suspension of components, and one cast change, shoulder disarticulation or interscapular thoracic ö

[A] ☑ **L6386** Immediate postsurgical or early fitting, each additional cast change and realignment ö

[A] **L6388** Immediate postsurgical or early fitting, application of rigid dressing only ö

ENDOSKELETAL: BELOW ELBOW

[A] **L6400** Below elbow, molded socket, endoskeletal system, including soft prosthetic tissue shaping ⊘ ö

ENDOSKELETAL: ELBOW DISARTICULATION

[A] **L6450** Elbow disarticulation, molded socket, endoskeletal system, including soft prosthetic tissue shaping ⊘ ö

ENDOSKELETAL: ABOVE ELBOW

[A] **L6500** Above elbow, molded socket, endoskeletal system, including soft prosthetic tissue shaping ⊘ ö

ENDOSKELETAL: SHOULDER DISARTICULATION

[A] **L6550** Shoulder disarticulation, molded socket, endoskeletal system, including soft prosthetic tissue shaping ⊘ ö

ENDOSKELETAL: INTERSCAPULAR THORACIC

[A] **L6570** Interscapular thoracic, molded socket, endoskeletal system, including soft prosthetic tissue shaping ⊘ ö

[A] **L6580** Preparatory, wrist disarticulation or below elbow, single wall plastic socket, friction wrist, flexible elbow hinges, figure of eight harness, humeral cuff, Bowden cable control, USMC or equal pylon, no cover, molded to patient model ⊘ ö

[A] **L6582** Preparatory, wrist disarticulation or below elbow, single wall socket, friction wrist, flexible elbow hinges, figure of eight harness, humeral cuff, Bowden cable control, USMC or equal pylon, no cover, direct formed ⊘ ö

[A] **L6584** Preparatory, elbow disarticulation or above elbow, single wall plastic socket, friction wrist, locking elbow, figure of eight harness, fair lead cable control, USMC or equal pylon, no cover, molded to patient model ⊘ ö

[A] **L6586** Preparatory, elbow disarticulation or above elbow, single wall socket, friction wrist, locking elbow, figure of eight harness, fair lead cable control, USMC or equal pylon, no cover, direct formed ⊘ ö

[A] **L6588** Preparatory, shoulder disarticulation or interscapular thoracic, single wall plastic socket, shoulder joint, locking elbow, friction wrist, chest strap, fair lead cable control, USMC or equal pylon, no cover, molded to patient model ⊘ ö

[A] **L6590** Preparatory, shoulder disarticulation or interscapular thoracic, single wall socket, shoulder joint, locking elbow, friction wrist, chest strap, fair lead cable control, USMC or equal pylon, no cover, direct formed ⊘ ö

ADDITIONS: UPPER LIMB

The following procedures/modifications/components may be added to other base procedures. The items in this section should reflect the additional complexity of each modification procedure, in addition to the base procedure, at the time of the original order.

[A] ☑ **L6600** Upper extremity additions, polycentric hinge, pair ⊘ ö

[A] ☑ **L6605** Upper extremity additions, single pivot hinge, pair ⊘ ö

[A] ☑ **L6610** Upper extremity additions, flexible metal hinge, pair ⊘ ö

● [A] **L6611** Addition to upper extremity prosthesis, external powered, additional switch, any type

[A] **L6615** Upper extremity addition, disconnect locking wrist unit ⊘ ö

[A] ☑ **L6616** Upper extremity addition, additional disconnect insert for locking wrist unit, each ⊘ ö

[A] **L6620** Upper extremity addition, flexion/extension wrist unit, with or without friction ⊘ ö

[A] **L6621** Upper extremity prosthesis addition, flexion/extension wrist with or without friction, for use with external powered terminal device ⊘

[A] **L6623** Upper extremity addition, spring assisted rotational wrist unit with latch release ⊘ ö

● [A] **L6624** Upper extremity addition, flexion/extension and rotation wrist unit

[A] **L6625** Upper extremity addition, rotation wrist unit with cable lock ⊘ ö

[A] **L6628** Upper extremity addition, quick disconnect hook adapter, Otto Bock or equal ⊘ ö

[A] **L6629** Upper extremity addition, quick disconnect lamination collar with coupling piece, Otto Bock or equal ⊘ ö

[A] **L6630** Upper extremity addition, stainless steel, any wrist ⊘ ö

[A] ☑ **L6632** Upper extremity addition, latex suspension sleeve, each ⊘ ö

[A] **L6635** Upper extremity addition, lift assist for elbow ⊘ ö

[A] **L6637** Upper extremity addition, nudge control elbow lock ⊘ ö

[A] **L6638** Upper extremity addition to prosthesis, electric locking feature, only for use with manually powered elbow ⊘ ö

● [A] **L6639** Upper extremity addition, heavy duty feature, any elbow

[A] ☑ **L6640** Upper extremity additions, shoulder abduction joint, pair ⊘ ö

[A] **L6641** Upper extremity addition, excursion amplifier, pulley type ⊘ ö

[A] **L6642** Upper extremity addition, excursion amplifier, lever type ⊘ ö

Special Coverage Instructions   Noncovered by Medicare   Carrier Discretion   ☑ Quality Alert   ● New Code   ○ Reinstated Code   ▲ Revised Code

116 — L Codes   [A] Age Edit   [M] Maternity Edit   ♀ Female Only   ♂ Male Only   [A] - [V] APC Status Indicators   *2007 HCPCS*

Ⓐ ☑ L6645 Upper extremity addition, shoulder flexion-abduction joint, each ⃠ ᕷ

Ⓐ L6646 Upper extremity addition, shoulder joint, multipositional locking, flexion, adjustable abduction friction control, for use with body powered or external powered system ⃠ ᕷ

Ⓐ L6647 Upper extremity addition, shoulder lock mechanism, body powered actuator ⃠ ᕷ

Ⓐ L6648 Upper extremity addition, shoulder lock mechanism, external powered actuator ⃠ ᕷ

Ⓐ ☑ L6650 Upper extremity addition, shoulder universal joint, each ⃠ ᕷ

Ⓐ L6655 Upper extremity addition, standard control cable, extra ⃠ ᕷ

Ⓐ L6660 Upper extremity addition, heavy duty control cable ⃠ ᕷ

Ⓐ L6665 Upper extremity addition, Teflon, or equal, cable lining ⃠ ᕷ

Ⓐ L6670 Upper extremity addition, hook to hand, cable adapter ⃠ ᕷ

Ⓐ L6672 Upper extremity addition, harness, chest or shoulder, saddle type ⃠ ᕷ

Ⓐ L6675 Upper extremity addition, harness, (e.g., figure of eight type), single cable design ⃠ ᕷ

Ⓐ L6676 Upper extremity addition, harness, (e.g., figure of eight type), dual cable design ⃠ ᕷ

Ⓐ L6677 Upper extremity addition, harness, triple control, simultaneous operation of terminal device and elbow ⃠

Ⓐ L6680 Upper extremity addition, test socket, wrist disarticulation or below elbow ⃠ ᕷ

Ⓐ L6682 Upper extremity addition, test socket, elbow disarticulation or above elbow ⃠ ᕷ

Ⓐ L6684 Upper extremity addition, test socket, shoulder disarticulation or interscapular thoracic ⃠ ᕷ

Ⓐ L6686 Upper extremity addition, suction socket ⃠ ᕷ

Ⓐ L6687 Upper extremity addition, frame type socket, below elbow or wrist disarticulation ⃠ ᕷ

Ⓐ L6688 Upper extremity addition, frame type socket, above elbow or elbow disarticulation ⃠ ᕷ

Ⓐ L6689 Upper extremity addition, frame type socket, shoulder disarticulation ⃠ ᕷ

Ⓐ L6690 Upper extremity addition, frame type socket, interscapular-thoracic ⃠ ᕷ

Ⓐ ☑ L6691 Upper extremity addition, removable insert, each ⃠ ᕷ

Ⓐ ☑ L6692 Upper extremity addition, silicone gel insert or equal, each ⃠ ᕷ

Ⓐ L6693 Upper extremity addition, locking elbow, forearm counterbalance ⃠ ᕷ

Ⓐ L6694 Addition to upper extremity prosthesis, below elbow/above elbow, custom fabricated from existing mold or prefabricated, socket insert, silicone gel, elastomeric or equal, for use with locking mechanism ⃠

Ⓐ L6695 Addition to upper extremity prosthesis, below elbow/above elbow, custom fabricated from existing mold or prefabricated, socket insert, silicone gel, elastomeric or equal, not for use with locking mechanism ⃠

Ⓐ L6696 Addition to upper extremity prosthesis, below elbow/above elbow, custom fabricated socket insert for congenital or atypical traumatic amputee, silicone gel, elastomeric or equal, for use with or without locking mechanism, initial only (for other than initial, use code L6694 or L6695) ⃠

Ⓐ L6697 Addition to upper extremity prosthesis, below elbow/above elbow, custom fabricated socket insert for other than congenital or atypical traumatic amputee, silicone gel, elastomeric or equal, for use with or without locking mechanism, initial only (for other than initial, use code L6694 or L6695) ⃠

Ⓐ L6698 Addition to upper extremity prosthesis, below elbow/above elbow, lock mechanism, excludes socket insert ⃠

TERMINAL DEVICES

HOOKS

L6700 Terminal device, hook, Dorrance or equal, model #3
See code(s) L6706, L6707.

● Ⓐ L6703 Terminal device, passive hand/mitt, any material, any size

● Ⓐ L6704 Terminal device, sport/recreational/work attachment, any material, any size

L6705 Terminal device, hook, Dorrance or equal, model #5
See code(s) L6706, L6707.

● Ⓐ L6706 Terminal device, hook, mechanical, voluntary opening, any material, any size, lined or unlined

● Ⓐ L6707 Terminal device, hook, mechanical, voluntary closing, any material, any size, lined or unlined

● Ⓐ L6708 Terminal device, hand, mechanical, voluntary opening, any material, any size

● Ⓐ L6709 Terminal device, hand, mechanical, voluntary closing, any material, any size

L6710 Terminal device, hook, Dorrance or equal, model #5X
See code(s) L6706, L6707.

L6715 Terminal device, hook, Dorrance or equal, model #5XA
See code(s) L6706, L6707.

L6720 Terminal device, hook, Dorrance or equal, model #6
See code(s) L6706, L6707.

L6725 Terminal device, hook, Dorrance or equal, model #7
See code(s) L6706, L6707.

L6730 Terminal device, hook, Dorrance or equal, model #7LO
See code(s) L6706, L6707.

L6735 Terminal device, hook, Dorrance or equal, model #8
See code(s) L6706, L6707.

L6740 Terminal device, hook, Dorrance or equal, model #8X
See code(s) L6706, L6707.

L6745 Terminal device, hook, Dorrance or equal, model #88X
See code(s) L6706, L6707.

L6750 Terminal device, hook, Dorrance or equal, model #10P
See code(s) L6706, L6707.

Special Coverage Instructions   Noncovered by Medicare   Carrier Discretion   ☑ Quality Alert   ● New Code   ○ Reinstated Code   ▲ Revised Code

Prosthetic Procedures

L6755 — L6925

~~L6755~~ ~~Terminal device, hook, Dorrance or equal, model #10X~~
See code(s) L6706, L6707.

~~L6765~~ ~~Terminal device, hook, Dorrance or equal, model #12P~~
See code(s) L6706, L6707.

~~L6770~~ ~~Terminal device, hook, Dorrance or equal, model #99X~~
See code(s) L6706, L6707.

~~L6775~~ ~~Terminal device, hook, Dorrance or equal, model #555~~
See code(s) L6706, L6707.

~~L6780~~ ~~Terminal device, hook, Dorrance or equal, model #SS555~~
See code(s) L6706, L6707.

~~L6790~~ ~~Terminal device, hook, Accu hook or equal~~
See code(s) L6706, L6707.

~~L6795~~ ~~Terminal device, hook, 2 load or equal~~
See code(s) L6706, L6707.

~~L6800~~ ~~Terminal device, hook, APRL VC or equal~~
See code(s) L6706, L6707.

▲ Ⓐ **L6805** Addition to terminal device, modifier wrist unit ⊘ �
MED: 100-2,15,120; 100-4,3,10.4

~~L6806~~ ~~Terminal device, hook, TRS Grip, Grip III, VC, or equal~~
See code(s) L6706, L6707.

~~L6807~~ ~~Terminal device, hook, Grip I, Grip II, VC, or equal~~
See code(s) L6706, L6707.

~~L6808~~ ~~Terminal device, hook, TRS Adept, infant or child, VC, or equal~~
See code(s) L6706, L6707.

~~L6809~~ ~~Terminal device, hook, TRS Super Sport, passive~~
See code(s) L6704.

▲ Ⓐ **L6810** Addition to terminal device, precision pinch device ⊘ ዻ
MED: 100-2,15,120; 100-4,3,10.4

HANDS

~~L6825~~ ~~Terminal device, hand, Dorrance, VO~~
See code(s) L6708, L6709.

~~L6830~~ ~~Terminal device, hand, APRL, VC~~
See code(s) L6708, L6709.

~~L6835~~ ~~Terminal device, hand, Sierra, VO~~
See code(s) L6708, L6709.

~~L6840~~ ~~Terminal device, hand, Becker Imperial~~
See code(s) L6708, L6709.

~~L6845~~ ~~Terminal device, hand, Becker Lock Grip~~
See code(s) L6708, L6709.

~~L6850~~ ~~Terminal device, hand, Becker Plylite~~
See code(s) L6708, L6709.

~~L6855~~ ~~Terminal device, hand, Robin-Aids, VO~~
See code(s) L6708, L6709.

~~L6860~~ ~~Terminal device, hand, Robin-Aids, VO soft~~
See code(s) L6708, L6709.

~~L6865~~ ~~Terminal device, hand, passive hand~~
See code(s) L6703.

~~L6867~~ ~~Terminal device, hand, Detroit infant hand (mechanical)~~
See code(s) L6708, L6709

~~L6868~~ ~~Terminal device, hand, passive infant hand, Steeper, Hosmer or equal~~
See code(s) L6703.

~~L6870~~ ~~Terminal device, hand, child mitt~~
See code(s) L6703.

~~L6872~~ ~~Terminal device, hand, NYU child hand~~
See code(s) L6708, L6709.

~~L6873~~ ~~Terminal device, hand, mechanical infant hand, Steeper or equal~~
See code(s) L6708, L6709

~~L6875~~ ~~Terminal device, hand, Bock, VC~~
See code(s) L6708, L6709.

~~L6880~~ ~~Terminal device, hand, Bock, VO~~
See code(s) L6708, L6709.

▲ Ⓐ **L6881** Automatic grasp feature, addition to upper limb electric prosthetic terminal device ⊘ ዻ

Ⓐ **L6882** Microprocessor control feature, addition to upper limb prosthetic terminal device ⊘ ዻ
MED: 100-2,15,120; 100-4,3,10.4

Ⓐ **L6883** Replacement socket, below elbow/wrist disarticulation, molded to patient model, for use with or without external power

▲ Ⓐ **L6884** Replacement socket, above elbow/elbow disarticulation, molded to patient model, for use with or without external power

Ⓐ **L6885** Replacement socket, shoulder disarticulation/interscapular thoracic, molded to patient model, for use with or without external power

GLOVES FOR ABOVE HANDS

Ⓐ **L6890** Addition to upper extremity prosthesis, glove for terminal device, any material, prefabricated, includes fitting and adjustment ዻ

Ⓐ **L6895** Addition to upper extremity prosthesis, glove for terminal device, any material, custom fabricated ዻ

HAND RESTORATION

Ⓐ **L6900** Hand restoration (casts, shading and measurements included), partial hand, with glove, thumb or one finger remaining ዻ

Ⓐ **L6905** Hand restoration (casts, shading and measurements included), partial hand, with glove, multiple fingers remaining ዻ

Ⓐ **L6910** Hand restoration (casts, shading and measurements included), partial hand, with glove, no fingers remaining ዻ

Ⓐ **L6915** Hand restoration (shading and measurements included), replacement glove for above ዻ

EXTERNAL POWER

BASE DEVICES

Ⓐ **L6920** Wrist disarticulation, external power, self-suspended inner socket, removable forearm shell, Otto Bock or equal switch, cables, two batteries and one charger, switch control of terminal device ⊘ ዻ

Ⓐ **L6925** Wrist disarticulation, external power, self-suspended inner socket, removable forearm shell, Otto Bock or equal electrodes, cables, two batteries and one charger, myoelectronic control of terminal device ⊘ ዻ

| Special Coverage Instructions | | Noncovered by Medicare | | Carrier Discretion | | ☑ Quality Alert | ● New Code | ○ Reinstated Code | ▲ Revised Code |

A — **L6930** Below elbow, external power, self-suspended inner socket, removable forearm shell, Otto Bock or equal switch, cables, two batteries and one charger, switch control of terminal device ⊘ &

A — **L6935** Below elbow, external power, self-suspended inner socket, removable forearm shell, Otto Bock or equal electrodes, cables, two batteries and one charger, myoelectronic control of terminal device ⊘ &

A — **L6940** Elbow disarticulation, external power, molded inner socket, removable humeral shell, outside locking hinges, forearm, Otto Bock or equal switch, cables, two batteries and one charger, switch control of terminal device ⊘ &

A — **L6945** Elbow disarticulation, external power, molded inner socket, removable humeral shell, outside locking hinges, forearm, Otto Bock or equal electrodes, cables, two batteries and one charger, myoelectronic control of terminal device ⊘ &

A — **L6950** Above elbow, external power, molded inner socket, removable humeral shell, internal locking elbow, forearm, Otto Bock or equal switch, cables, two batteries and one charger, switch control of terminal device ⊘ &

A — **L6955** Above elbow, external power, molded inner socket, removable humeral shell, internal locking elbow, forearm, Otto Bock or equal electrodes, cables, two batteries and one charger, myoelectronic control of terminal device ⊘ &

A — **L6960** Shoulder disarticulation, external power, molded inner socket, removable shoulder shell, shoulder bulkhead, humeral section, mechanical elbow, forearm, Otto Bock or equal switch, cables, two batteries and one charger, switch control of terminal device ⊘ &

A — **L6965** Shoulder disarticulation, external power, molded inner socket, removable shoulder shell, shoulder bulkhead, humeral section, mechanical elbow, forearm, Otto Bock or equal electrodes, cables, two batteries and one charger, myoelectronic control of terminal device ⊘ &

A — **L6970** Interscapular-thoracic, external power, molded inner socket, removable shoulder shell, shoulder bulkhead, humeral section, mechanical elbow, forearm, Otto Bock or equal switch, cables, two batteries and one charger, switch control of terminal device ⊘ &

A — **L6975** Interscapular-thoracic, external power, molded inner socket, removable shoulder shell, shoulder bulkhead, humeral section, mechanical elbow, forearm, Otto Bock or equal electrodes, cables, two batteries and one charger, myoelectronic control of terminal device ⊘ &

● A — **L7007** Electric hand, switch or myoelectric controlled, adult A

● A — **L7008** Electric hand, switch or myoelectric, controlled, pediatric A

● A — **L7009** Electric hook, switch or myoelectric controlled, adult A

~~L7010~~ ~~Electronic hand, Otto Bock, Steeper or equal, switch controlled~~
See code(s) L7007.

~~L7015~~ ~~Electronic hand, System Teknik, Variety Village or equal, switch controlled~~
See code(s) L7007.

~~L7020~~ ~~Electronic Greifer, Otto Bock or equal, switch controlled~~
See code L7009.

~~L7025~~ ~~Electronic hand, Otto Bock or equal, myoelectronically controlled~~
See code(s) L7007.

~~L7030~~ ~~Electronic hand, System Teknik, Variety Village or equal, myoelectronically controlled~~
See code(s) L7008.

~~L7035~~ ~~Electronic Greifer, Otto Bock or equal, myoelectronically controlled~~
See code(s) L7009.

▲ A — **L7040** Prehensile actuator, switch controlled ⊘ &

▲ A — **L7045** Electric hook, switch or myoelectric controlled, pediatric ⊘ &

ELBOW

A — **L7170** Electronic elbow, Hosmer or equal, switch controlled ⊘ &

A — **L7180** Electronic elbow, microprocessor sequential control of elbow and terminal device ⊘ &

A — **L7181** Electronic elbow, microprocessor simultaneous control of elbow and terminal device ⊘

A — **L7185** Electronic elbow, adolescent, Variety Village or equal, switch controlled ⊘ &

A — **L7186** Electronic elbow, child, Variety Village or equal, switch controlled ⊘ &

A — **L7190** Electronic elbow, adolescent, Variety Village or equal, myoelectronically controlled ⊘ &

A — **L7191** Electronic elbow, child, Variety Village or equal, myoelectronically controlled ⊘ &

A — **L7260** Electronic wrist rotator, Otto Bock or equal ⊘ &

A — **L7261** Electronic wrist rotator, for Utah arm ⊘ &

A — **L7266** Servo control, Steeper or equal ⊘ &

A — **L7272** Analogue control, UNB or equal ⊘ &

A — **L7274** Proportional control, 6–12 volt, Liberty, Utah or equal ⊘ &

BATTERY COMPONENTS

A — **L7360** Six volt battery, Otto Bock or equal, each &

A — **L7362** Battery charger, six volt, Otto Bock or equal ⊘ &

A — **L7364** Twelve volt battery, Utah or equal, each &

A — **L7366** Battery charger, twelve volt, Utah or equal ⊘ &

A — **L7367** Lithium ion battery, replacement ⊘ &

A — **L7368** Lithium ion battery charger ⊘ &

A — **L7400** Addition to upper extremity prosthesis, below elbow/wrist disarticulation, ultralight material (titanium, carbon fiber or equal) ⊘

A — **L7401** Addition to upper extremity prosthesis, above elbow disarticulation, ultralight material (titanium, carbon fiber or equal) ⊘

A — **L7402** Addition to upper extremity prosthesis, shoulder disarticulation/interscapular thoracic, ultralight material (titanium, carbon fiber or equal) ⊘

A — **L7403** Addition to upper extremity prosthesis, below elbow/wrist disarticulation, acrylic material ⊘

A — **L7404** Addition to upper extremity prosthesis, above elbow disarticulation, acrylic material ⊘

A — **L7405** Addition to upper extremity prosthesis, shoulder disarticulation/interscapular thoracic, acrylic material ⊘

Special Coverage Instructions   Noncovered by Medicare   Carrier Discretion   ☑ Quality Alert   ● New Code   ○ Reinstated Code   ▲ Revised Code

2007 HCPCS   **1**–**9** ASC Group   **MED:** Pub 100/NCD References   & DMEPOS Paid   ⊘ SNF Excluded   **L Codes — 119**

Prosthetic Procedures

L7499 — L8499

A   **L7499**   Upper extremity prosthesis, NOS

REPAIRS

A   **L7500**   Repair of prosthetic device, hourly rate
Medicare jurisdiction: local contractor if repair or implanted prosthetic device.
MED: 100-2,15,110.2; 100-2,15,120; 100-4,32,100

A   **L7510**   Repair of prosthetic device, repair or replace minor parts
Medicare jurisdiction: local contractor if repair of implanted prosthetic device.
MED: 100-2,15,110.2; 100-2,15,120; 100-4,32,100

A ☑   **L7520**   Repair prosthetic device, labor component, per 15 minutes
Medicare jurisdiction: local contractor if repair of implanted prosthetic device.

A   **L7600**   Prosthetic donning sleeve, any material, each

GENERAL

PROSTHESIS

A   **L8000**   Breast prosthesis, mastectomy bra   A ♀ &
MED: 100-2,15,120

A   **L8001**   Breast prosthesis, mastectomy bra, with integrated breast prosthesis form, unilateral   A ♀ &
MED: 100-2,15,120

A   **L8002**   Breast prosthesis, mastectomy bra, with integrated breast prosthesis form, bilateral   A ♀ &
MED: 100-2,15,120

A   **L8010**   Breast prosthesis, mastectomy sleeve   A ♀
MED: 100-2,15,120

A   **L8015**   External breast prosthesis garment, with mastectomy form, post-mastectomy   A ♀ &
MED: 100-2,15,120

A   **L8020**   Breast prosthesis, mastectomy form   A ♀ &
MED: 100-2,15,120

A   **L8030**   Breast prosthesis, silicone or equal   A ♀ &
MED: 100-2,15,120

A   **L8035**   Custom breast prosthesis, post mastectomy, molded to patient model   A ♀ &
MED: 100-2,15,120

A   **L8039**   Breast prosthesis, NOS   A ♀

Orbital and midfacial prosthesis (L8041-L8042)

Nasal prosthesis (L8040)

Frontal bone

Nasal bone

Maxilla

Zygoma

(L8043-L8044)

Facial prosthetics are typically custom manufactured from polymers and carefully matched to the original features. The maxilla, zygoma, frontal, and nasal bones are often involved, either singly or in combination (L8040-L8044)

A   **L8040**   Nasal prosthesis, provided by a nonphysician &

A   **L8041**   Midfacial prosthesis, provided by a nonphysician &

A   **L8042**   Orbital prosthesis, provided by a nonphysician &

A   **L8043**   Upper facial prosthesis, provided by a nonphysician &

A   **L8044**   Hemi-facial prosthesis, provided by a nonphysician &

A   **L8045**   Auricular prosthesis, provided by a nonphysician &

A   **L8046**   Partial facial prosthesis, provided by a nonphysician &

A   **L8047**   Nasal septal prosthesis, provided by a nonphysician &

A   **L8048**   Unspecified maxillofacial prosthesis, by report, provided by a nonphysician

A   **L8049**   Repair or modification of maxillofacial prosthesis, labor component, 15 minute increments, provided by a nonphysician

TRUSSES

A   **L8300**   Truss, single with standard pad &
MED: 100-2,15,120; 100-3,280.11; 100-3,280.12; 100-4,4,240

A   **L8310**   Truss, double with standard pads &
MED: 100-2,15,120; 100-3,280.11; 100-3,280.12; 100-4,4,240

A   **L8320**   Truss, addition to standard pad, water pad &
MED: 100-2,15,120; 100-3,280.11; 100-3,280.12; 100-4,4,240

A   **L8330**   Truss, addition to standard pad, scrotal pad   ♂ &
MED: 100-2,15,120; 100-3,280.11; 100-3,280.12; 100-4,4,240

PROSTHETIC SOCKS

A ☑   **L8400**   Prosthetic sheath, below knee, each &
MED: 100-2,15,120

A ☑   **L8410**   Prosthetic sheath, above knee, each &
MED: 100-2,15,120

A ☑   **L8415**   Prosthetic sheath, upper limb, each &
MED: 100-2,15,120

A ☑   **L8417**   Prosthetic sheath/sock, including a gel cushion layer, below knee or above knee, each &

A ☑   **L8420**   Prosthetic sock, multiple ply, below knee, each &
MED: 100-2,15,120

A ☑   **L8430**   Prosthetic sock, multiple ply, above knee, each &
MED: 100-2,15,120

A ☑   **L8435**   Prosthetic sock, multiple ply, upper limb, each &
MED: 100-2,15,120

A ☑   **L8440**   Prosthetic shrinker, below knee, each &
MED: 100-2,15,120

A ☑   **L8460**   Prosthetic shrinker, above knee, each &
MED: 100-2,15,120

A ☑   **L8465**   Prosthetic shrinker, upper limb, each &
MED: 100-2,15,120

A ☑   **L8470**   Prosthetic sock, single ply, fitting, below knee, each &
MED: 100-2,15,120

A ☑   **L8480**   Prosthetic sock, single ply, fitting, above knee, each &
MED: 100-2,15,120

A ☑   **L8485**   Prosthetic sock, single ply, fitting, upper limb, each &
MED: 100-2,15,120

A   **L8499**   Unlisted procedure for miscellaneous prosthetic services
Determine if an alternative HCPCS Level II or a CPT code better describes the service being reported. This code should be used only if a more specific code is unavailable.

Special Coverage Instructions   Noncovered by Medicare   Carrier Discretion   ☑ Quality Alert   ● New Code   ○ Reinstated Code   ▲ Revised Code

120 — L Codes   A Age Edit   M Maternity Edit   ♀ Female Only   ♂ Male Only   A - Y APC Status Indicators   *2007 HCPCS*

PROSTHETIC IMPLANTS

INTEGUMENTARY SYSTEM

Ⓐ **L8500** Artificial larynx, any type   ᵭ
MED: 100-2,15,120; 100-3,50.2; 100-4,4,240

Ⓐ **L8501** Tracheostomy speaking valve   ᵭ
MED: 100-3,50.4

Ⓐ **L8505** Artificial larynx replacement battery/accessory, any type

Ⓐ **L8507** Tracheo-esophageal voice prosthesis, patient inserted, any type, each   ᵭ

Ⓐ **L8509** Tracheo-esophageal voice prosthesis, inserted by a licensed health care provider, any type   ᵭ

Ⓐ **L8510** Voice amplifier   ᵭ
MED: 100-3,50.2

Ⓐ ☑ **L8511** Insert for indwelling tracheoesophageal prosthesis, with or without valve, replacement only, each   ᵭ

Ⓐ ☑ **L8512** Gelatin capsules or equivalent, for use with tracheoesophageal voice prosthesis, replacement only, per 10   ᵭ

Ⓐ ☑ **L8513** Cleaning device used with tracheoesophageal voice prosthesis, pipet, brush, or equal, replacement only, each   ᵭ

Ⓐ ☑ **L8514** Tracheoesophageal puncture dilator, replacement only, each   ᵭ

Ⓐ ☑ **L8515** Gelatin capsule, application device for use with tracheoesophageal voice prosthesis, each

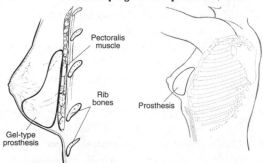

Pectoralis muscle

Rib bones

Prosthesis

Gel-type prosthesis

Ⓝ **L8600** Implantable breast prosthesis, silicone or equal   ᴬ♀ ᵭ
Medicare covers implants inserted in post-mastectomy reconstruction in a breast cancer patient. Always report concurrent to the implant procedure. Medicare jurisdiction: local contractor.
MED: 100-2,15,120; 100-3,140.2; 100-4,4,190; 100-4,4,240

Ⓝ ☑ **L8603** Injectable bulking agent, collagen implant, urinary tract, 2.5 ml syringe, includes shipping and necessary supplies   ᵭ
Medicare covers up to five separate collagen implant treatments in patients with intrinsic sphincter deficiency. Who have passed a collagen sensitivity test. Medicare jurisdiction: local contractor.
MED: 100-3,230.10; 100-4,4,190

Ⓝ ☑ **L8606** Injectable bulking agent, synthetic implant, urinary tract, 1 ml syringe, includes shipping and necessary supplies   ᵭ
MED: 100-3,230.10

Ⓝ **L8609** Artificial cornea

HEAD: SKULL, FACIAL BONES, AND TEMPOROMANDIBULAR JOINT

Ⓝ **L8610** Ocular implant   ᵭ
Medicare jurisdiction: local contractor.
MED: 100-2,15,120; 100-4,4,190; 100-4,4,240

Ⓝ **L8612** Aqueous shunt
Medicare jurisdiction: local contractor.
See code(s): Q0074
MED: 100-2,15,120; 100-4,4,190; 100-4,4,240

Ⓝ **L8613** Ossicular implant   ᵭ
Medicare jurisdiction: local contractor.
MED: 100-2,15,120; 100-4,4,190; 100-4,4,240

▲ Ⓝ **L8614** Cochlear device, includes all internal and external components   ᵭ
A cochlear implant is covered by Medicare when the patient has bilateral sensorineural deafness. Medicare jurisdiction: local contractor.
MED: 100-2,15,120; 100-3,50.3; 100-4,4,190; 100-4,4,240; 100-4,32,100
AHA: 4Q,'03,8; 3Q,'02,5

Ⓐ **L8615** Headset/headpiece for use with cochlear implant device, replacement

Ⓐ **L8616** Microphone for use with cochlear implant device, replacement

Ⓐ **L8617** Transmitting coil for use with cochlear implant device, replacement

Ⓐ **L8618** Transmitter cable for use with cochlear implant device, replacement

Ⓐ **L8619** Cochlear implant external speech processor, replacement   ᵭ
Medicare jurisdiction: local contractor.
MED: 100-3,50.3; 100-4,32,100

Ⓐ **L8621** Zinc air battery for use with cochlear implant device, replacement, each

Ⓐ ☑ **L8622** Alkaline battery for use with cochlear implant device, any size, replacement, each

Ⓐ **L8623** Lithium ion battery for use with cochlear implant device speech processor, other than ear level, replacement, each   ᵭ

Ⓐ **L8624** Lithium ion battery for use with cochlear implant device speech processor, ear level, replacement, each   ᵭ

UPPER EXTREMITY

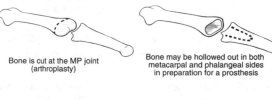

Bone is cut at the MP joint (arthroplasty)

Bone may be hollowed out in both metacarpal and phalangeal sides in preparation for a prosthesis

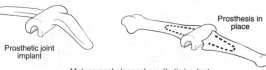

Prosthetic joint implant

Prosthesis in place

Metacarpophalangeal prosthetic implant

Ⓝ **L8630** Metacarpophalangeal joint implant   ᵭ
Medicare jurisdiction: local contractor.
MED: 100-2,15,120; 100-4,4,190; 100-4,4,240

Special Coverage Instructions   Noncovered by Medicare   Carrier Discretion   ☑ Quality Alert   ● New Code   ○ Reinstated Code   ▲ Revised Code

2007 HCPCS   1-9 ASC Group   **MED:** Pub 100/NCD References   ᵭ DMEPOS Paid   ⊘ SNF Excluded   **L Codes — 121**

L8500 — L8630

L8631 Metacarpal phalangeal joint replacement, two or more pieces, metal (e.g., stainless steel or cobalt chrome), ceramic-like material (e.g., pyrocarbon), for surgical implantation (all sizes, includes entire system)
MED: 100-2,15,120; 100-4,4,240

LOWER EXTREMITY - JOINT: KNEE, ANKLE, TOE

L8641 Metatarsal joint implant
Medicare jurisdiction: local contractor.
MED: 100-2,15,120; 100-4,4,190; 100-4,4,240

L8642 Hallux implant
Medicare jurisdiction: local contractor.
See code(s): Q0073
MED: 100-2,15,120; 100-4,4,190; 100-4,4,240

MISCELLANEOUS MUSCULAR-SKELETAL

L8658 Interphalangeal joint spacer, silicone or equal, each
Medicare jurisdiction: local contractor.
MED: 100-2,15,120; 100-4,4,190; 100-4,4,240

L8659 Interphalangeal finger joint replacement, two or more pieces, metal (e.g., stainless steel or cobalt chrome), ceramic-like material (e.g., pyrocarbon) for surgical implantation, any size
MED: 100-2,15,120; 100-4,4,240

CARDIOVASCULAR SYSTEM

L8670 Vascular graft material, synthetic, implant
Medicare jurisdiction: local contractor.
MED: 100-2,15,120; 100-4,4,190; 100-4,4,240

GENERAL

L8680 Implantable neurostimulator electrode, each
MED: 100-4,32,50

L8681 Patient programmer (external) for use with implantable programmable neurostimulator pulse generator

L8682 Implantable neurostimulator radiofrequency receiver

L8683 Radiofrequency transmitter (external) for use with implantable neurostimulator radiofrequency receiver

L8684 Radiofrequency transmitter (external) for use with implantable sacral root neurostimulator receiver for bowel and bladder management, replacement

L8685 Implantable neurostimulator pulse generator, single array, rechargeable, includes extension
MED: 100-4,32,50

L8686 Implantable neurostimulator pulse generator, single array, non-rechargeable, includes extension
MED: 100-4,32,50

L8687 Implantable neurostimulator pulse generator, dual array, rechargeable, includes extension
MED: 100-4,32,50

L8688 Implantable neurostimulator pulse generator, dual array, non-rechargeable, includes extension
MED: 100-4,32,50

▲ **L8689** External recharging system for battery (internal) for use with implantable neurostimulator

● **L8690** Auditory osseointegrated device, includes all internal and external components

● **L8691** Auditory osseointegrated device, external sound processor, replacement

● **L8695** External recharging system for battery (external) for use with implantable neurostimulator

L8699 Prosthetic implant, not otherwise specified
Determine if an alternative HCPCS Level II or a CPT code better describes the service being reported. This code should be used only if a more specific code is unavailable. Medicare jurisdiction: local contractor.
MED: 100-4,4,190

L9900 Orthotic and prosthetic supply, accessory, and/or service component of another HCPCS L code

---

Special Coverage Instructions   Noncovered by Medicare   Carrier Discretion   ☑ Quality Alert   ● New Code   ○ Reinstated Code   ▲ Revised Code

122 — L Codes   Age Edit   Maternity Edit   ♀ Female Only   ♂ Male Only   APC Status Indicators   **2007 HCPCS**

MEDICAL SERVICES M0000-M0301

OTHER MEDICAL SERVICES

M codes include office services, cellular therapy, prolotherapy, intragastric hypothermia, IV chelation therapy, and fabric wrapping of an abdominal aneurysm (MNP).

M codes fall under the jurisdiction of the local contractor

☒ **M0064** Brief office visit for the sole purpose of monitoring or changing drug prescriptions used in the treatment of mental psychoneurotic and personality disorders ⊘

MED: 100-4,12,210.1

Ⓔ **M0075** Cellular therapy
The therapeutic efficacy of injecting foreign proteins has not been established.

MED: 100-3,30.8

Ⓔ **M0076** Prolotherapy
The therapeutic efficacy of prolotherapy and joint sclerotherapy has not been established.

MED: 100-3,150.7

Ⓔ **M0100** Intragastric hypothermia using gastric freezing
Code with caution: This procedure is considered obsolete.

MED: 100-3,100.6

CARDIOVASCULAR SERVICES

Ⓔ **M0300** IV chelation therapy (chemical endarterectomy)
Chelation therapy is considered experimental in the United States.

MED: 100-3,20.21

Ⓔ **M0301** Fabric wrapping of abdominal aneurysm
Code with caution: This procedure has largely been replaced with more effective treatment modalities. Submit documentation.

MED: 100-3,20.23

Special Coverage Instructions   Noncovered by Medicare   Carrier Discretion   ☑ Quality Alert   ● New Code   ○ Reinstated Code   ▲ Revised Code

2007 HCPCS   🏽-🎱 ASC Group   **MED:** Pub 100/NCD References   🖧 DMEPOS Paid   ⊘ SNF Excluded   **M Codes — 123**

PATHOLOGY AND LABORATORY SERVICES P0000-P9999

P codes include chemistry, toxicology, and microbiology tests, screening Papanicolaou procedures, and various blood products.

CHEMISTRY AND TOXICOLOGY TESTS

P codes fall under the jurisdiction of the local contractor.

Ⓐ **P2028** Cephalin floculation, blood
Code with caution: This test is considered obsolete. Submit documentation.
MED: 100-3,300.1

Ⓐ **P2029** Congo red, blood
Code with caution: This test is considered obsolete. Submit documentation.
MED: 100-3,300.1

Ⓔ **P2031** Hair analysis (excluding arsenic)
For hair analysis for arsenic, see CPT codes 83015, 82175.
MED: 100-3,190.6

Ⓐ **P2033** Thymol turbidity, blood
Code with caution: This test is considered obsolete. Submit documentation.
MED: 100-3,300.1

Ⓐ **P2038** Mucoprotein, blood (seromucoid) (medical necessity procedure)
Code with caution: This test is considered obsolete. Submit documentation.
MED: 100-3,300.1

PATHOLOGY SCREENING TESTS

Ⓐ **P3000** Screening Papanicolaou smear, cervical or vaginal, up to three smears, by technician under physician supervision   Ⓐ ♀ ⊘
One Pap test is covered by Medicare every two years, unless the physician suspects cervical abnormalities and shortens the interval. See also G0123-G0124.
MED: 100-2,6,10; 100-3,190.2; 100-4,4,240

Ⓑ **P3001** Screening Papanicolaou smear, cervical or vaginal, up to three smears, requiring interpretation by physician   Ⓐ ♀ ⊘
One Pap test is covered by Medicare every two years, unless the physician suspects cervical abnormalities and shortens the interval. See also G0123-G0124.
MED: 100-2,6,10; 100-3,190.2; 100-4,4,240

MICROBIOLOGY TESTS

Ⓔ **P7001** Culture, bacterial, urine; quantitative, sensitivity study

MISCELLANEOUS

Ⓚ ☑ **P9010** Blood (whole), for transfusion, per unit
MED: 100-1,3,20.5; 100-2,1,10; 100-4,3,40.2.2

▲ Ⓚ ☑ **P9011** Blood, split unit
MED: 100-1,3,20.5; 100-2,1,10; 100-4,3,40.2.2

Ⓚ ☑ **P9012** Cryoprecipitate, each unit
MED: 100-1,3,20.5; 100-2,1,10; 100-4,3,40.2.2

Ⓚ ☑ **P9016** Red blood cells, leukocytes reduced, each unit
MED: 100-1,3,20.5; 100-2,1,10; 100-4,3,40.2.2

Ⓚ ☑ **P9017** Fresh frozen plasma (single donor), frozen within 8 hours of collection, each unit
MED: 100-1,3,20.5; 100-2,1,10; 100-4,3,40.2.2

Ⓚ ☑ **P9019** Platelets, each unit
MED: 100-1,3,20.5; 100-2,1,10; 100-4,3,40.2.2

Ⓚ ☑ **P9020** Platelet rich plasma, each unit
MED: 100-1,3,20.5; 100-4,3,40.2.2

Ⓚ ☑ **P9021** Red blood cells, each unit
MED: 100-1,3,20.5; 100-2,1,10; 100-4,3,40.2.2

Ⓚ ☑ **P9022** Red blood cells, washed, each unit
MED: 100-1,3,20.5; 100-2,1,10; 100-4,3,40.2.2

Ⓚ ☑ **P9023** Plasma, pooled multiple donor, solvent/detergent treated, frozen, each unit
MED: 100-1,3,20.5; 100-2,1,10; 100-4,3,40.2.2

Ⓚ ☑ **P9031** Platelets, leukocytes reduced, each unit
MED: 100-1,3,20.5; 100-1,3,20.5.2; 100-1,3,20.5.3; 100-2,1,10; 100-4,3,40.2.2

Ⓚ ☑ **P9032** Platelets, irradiated, each unit
MED: 100-1,3,20.5; 100-1,3,20.5.2; 100-1,3,20.5.3; 100-2,1,10; 100-4,3,40.2.2

Ⓚ ☑ **P9033** Platelets, leukocytes reduced, irradiated, each unit
MED: 100-1,3,20.5; 100-1,3,20.5.2; 100-1,3,20.5.3; 100-2,1,10; 100-4,3,40.2.2

Ⓚ ☑ **P9034** Platelets, pheresis, each unit
MED: 100-1,3,20.5; 100-1,3,20.5.2; 100-1,3,20.5.3; 100-2,1,10; 100-4,3,40.2.2

Ⓚ ☑ **P9035** Platelets, pheresis, leukocytes reduced, each unit
MED: 100-1,3,20.5; 100-1,3,20.5.2; 100-1,3,20.5.3; 100-2,1,10; 100-4,3,40.2.2

Ⓚ ☑ **P9036** Platelets, pheresis, irradiated, each unit
MED: 100-1,3,20.5; 100-1,3,20.5.2; 100-1,3,20.5.3; 100-2,1,10; 100-4,3,40.2.2

Ⓚ ☑ **P9037** Platelets, pheresis, leukocytes reduced, irradiated, each unit
MED: 100-1,3,20.5; 100-1,3,20.5.2; 100-1,3,20.5.3; 100-2,1,10; 100-4,3,40.2.2

Ⓚ ☑ **P9038** Red blood cells, irradiated, each unit
MED: 100-1,3,20.5; 100-1,3,20.5.2; 100-1,3,20.5.3; 100-2,1,10; 100-4,3,40.2.2

Ⓚ ☑ **P9039** Red blood cells, deglycerolized, each unit
MED: 100-1,3,20.5; 100-1,3,20.5.2; 100-1,3,20.5.3; 100-2,1,10; 100-4,3,40.2.2

Ⓚ ☑ **P9040** Red blood cells, leukocytes reduced, irradiated, each unit
MED: 100-1,3,20.5; 100-1,3,20.5.2; 100-1,3,20.5.3; 100-2,1,10; 100-4,3,40.2.2

Ⓚ ☑ **P9041** Infusion, albumin (human), 5%, 50 ml
Not considered a blood product for OPPS effective July 1, 2005.
MED: 100-2,1,10; 100-4,3,40.2.2

Ⓚ ☑ **P9043** Infusion, plasma protein fraction (human), 5%, 50 ml
MED: 100-1,3,20.5; 100-2,1,10; 100-4,3,40.2.2

Ⓚ ☑ **P9044** Plasma, cryoprecipitate reduced, each unit
MED: 100-1,3,20.5; 100-2,1,10; 100-4,3,40.2.2

Ⓚ ☑ **P9045** Infusion, albumin (human), 5%, 250 ml
Not considered a blood product for OPPS effective July 1, 2005.
MED: 100-2,1,10; 100-4,3,40.2.2

Ⓚ ☑ **P9046** Infusion, albumin (human), 25%, 20 ml
Not considered a blood product for OPPS effective July 1, 2005.
MED: 100-2,1,10; 100-4,3,40.2.2

Special Coverage Instructions   Noncovered by Medicare   Carrier Discretion   ☑ Quality Alert   ● New Code   ○ Reinstated Code   ▲ Revised Code

124 — P Codes   Ⓐ Age Edit   Ⓜ Maternity Edit   ♀ Female Only   ♂ Male Only   Ⓐ - ☑ APC Status Indicators   *2007 HCPCS*

K ☑ **P9047** Infusion, albumin (human), 25%, 50 ml
Not considered a blood product for OPPS effective July 1, 2005.
MED: 100-2,1,10; 100-4,3,40.2.2

K ☑ **P9048** Infusion, plasma protein fraction (human), 5%, 250 ml
MED: 100-2,1,10; 100-4,3,40.2.2

K ☑ **P9050** Granulocytes, pheresis, each unit
MED: 100-2,1,10; 100-4,3,40.2.2

K ☑ **P9051** Whole blood or red blood cells, leukocytes reduced, CMV-negative, each unit
MED: 100-2,1,10; 100-4,3,40.2.2

K ☑ **P9052** Platelets, HLA-matched leukocytes reduced, apheresis/pheresis, each unit
MED: 100-2,1,10; 100-4,3,40.2.2

K ☑ **P9053** Platelets, pheresis, leukocytes reduced, CMV-negative, irradiated, each unit
MED: 100-2,1,10; 100-4,3,40.2.2

K ☑ **P9054** Whole blood or red blood cells, leukocytes reduced, frozen, deglycerol, washed, each unit
MED: 100-2,1,10; 100-4,3,40.2.2

K ☑ **P9055** Platelets, leukocytes reduced, CMV-negative, apheresis/pheresis, each unit
MED: 100-2,1,10; 100-4,3,40.2.2

K ☑ **P9056** Whole blood, leukocytes reduced, irradiated, each unit
MED: 100-2,1,10; 100-4,3,40.2.2

K ☑ **P9057** Red blood cells, frozen/deglycerolized/washed, leukocytes reduced, irradiated, each unit
MED: 100-2,1,10; 100-4,3,40.2.2

K ☑ **P9058** Red blood cells, leukocytes reduced, CMV-negative, irradiated, each unit
MED: 100-2,1,10; 100-4,3,40.2.2

K ☑ **P9059** Fresh frozen plasma between 8–24 hours of collection, each unit
MED: 100-2,1,10; 100-4,3,40.2.2

K ☑ **P9060** Fresh frozen plasma, donor retested, each unit
MED: 100-2,1,10; 100-4,3,40.2.2

A ☑ **P9603** Travel allowance one way in connection with medically necessary laboratory specimen collection drawn from homebound or nursing home bound patient; prorated miles actually travelled
MED: 100-4,16,60

A ☑ **P9604** Travel allowance one way in connection with medically necessary laboratory specimen collection drawn from homebound or nursing home bound patient; prorated trip charge
MED: 100-4,16,60

A **P9612** Catheterization for collection of specimen, single patient, all places of service
See also new CPT catheterization codes 51701-51703
MED: 100-4,16,60

N **P9615** Catheterization for collection of specimen(s) (multiple patients)
See also new CPT catheterization codes 51701-51703
MED: 100-4,16,60

Special Coverage Instructions Noncovered by Medicare Carrier Discretion ☑ Quality Alert ● New Code ○ Reinstated Code ▲ Revised Code

2007 HCPCS **1**-**9** ASC Group **MED:** Pub 100/NCD References ᘒ DMEPOS Paid ⊘ SNF Excluded **P Codes — 125**

Q CODES (TEMPORARY) Q0000-Q9999

New temporary Q codes to pay health care providers for the supplies used in creating casts were established to replace the removal of the practice expense for all HCPCS codes, including the CPT codes for fracture management and for casts and splints. Coders should continue to use the appropriate CPT code to report the work and practice expenses involved with creating the cast or splint; the temporary Q codes replace less specific coding for the casting and splinting supplies.

Q codes fall under the jurisdiction of the local contractor unless they represent an incidental service or are otherwise specified.

⊠ **Q0035 Cardiokymography**
Covered only in conjunction with electrocardiographic stress testing in male patients with atypical angina or nonischemic chest pain, or female patients with angina.
MED: 100-3,20.24

B **Q0081 Infusion therapy, using other than chemotherapeutic drugs, per visit**
MED: 100-3,280.14
AHA: 1Q,'02,7; 4Q,'02,7

B **Q0083 Chemotherapy administration by other than infusion technique only (e.g., subcutaneous, intramuscular, push), per visit** ⊘

B ☑ **Q0084 Chemotherapy administration by infusion technique only, per visit** ⊘
MED: 100-3,280.14

B ☑ **Q0085 Chemotherapy administration by both infusion technique and other technique(s) (e.g., subcutaneous, intramuscular, push), per visit** ⊘

T **Q0091 Screening Papanicolaou smear; obtaining, preparing and conveyance of cervical or vaginal smear to laboratory** Ⓐ♀⊘
One pap test is covered by Medicare every two years for low risk patients and every one year for high risk patients. Q0091 can be reported with an E/M code when a separately identifiable E/M service is provided.
MED: 100-3, 190.2
MED: 100-3,190.2
AHA: 4Q,'02,8

N **Q0092 Set-up portable x-ray equipment**
MED: 100-4,13,90; 100-4,13,90.4

Ⓐ **Q0111 Wet mounts, including preparations of vaginal, cervical or skin specimens**

Ⓐ **Q0112 All potassium hydroxide (KOH) preparations**

Ⓐ **Q0113 Pinworm examination**

Ⓐ **Q0114 Fern test** ♀

Ⓐ **Q0115 Post-coital direct, qualitative examinations of vaginal or cervical mucous** Ⓐ♀

E **Q0144 Azithromycin dihydrate, oral, capsules/powder, 1 gm**
Use this code for Zithromax, Zithromax Z-PAK.

N **Q0163 Diphenhydramine HCl, 50 mg, oral, FDA approved prescription anti-emetic, for use as a complete therapeutic substitute for an IV anti-emetic at time of chemotherapy treatment not to exceed a 48-hour dosage regimen**
See also J1200. Medicare covers at the time of chemotherapy if regimen doesn't exceed 48 hours. Submit on the same claim as the chemotherapy. Use this code for Truxadryl.
MED: 100-2,6,10; 100-4,4,240; 100-4,17,80.2
AHA: 1Q,'02,2

N **Q0164 Prochlorperazine maleate, 5 mg, oral, FDA approved prescription anti-emetic, for use as a complete therapeutic substitute for an IV anti-emetic at the time of chemotherapy treatment, not to exceed a 48-hour dosage regimen**
Medicare covers at the time of chemotherapy if regimen doesn't exceed 48 hours. Submit on the same claim as the chemotherapy. Medicare jurisdiction: DME Medicare Administrative Contractor (DME MAC). Use this code for Compazine.
MED: 100-2,6,10; 100-4,4,240; 100-4,17,80.2

B **Q0165 Prochlorperazine maleate, 10 mg, oral, FDA approved prescription anti-emetic, for use as a complete therapeutic substitute for an IV anti-emetic at the time of chemotherapy treatment, not to exceed a 48-hour dosage regimen**
Medicare covers at the time of chemotherapy if regimen doesn't exceed 48 hours. Submit on the same claim as the chemotherapy. Medicare jurisdiction: DME Medicare Administrative Contractor (DME MAC). Use this code for Compazine.
MED: 100-2,6,10; 100-4,4,240; 100-4,17,80.2

K **Q0166 Granisetron HCl, 1 mg, oral, FDA approved prescription anti-emetic, for use as a complete therapeutic substitute for an IV anti-emetic at the time of chemotherapy treatment, not to exceed a 24-hour dosage regimen**
Medicare covers at the time of chemotherapy if regimen doesn't exceed 48 hours. Submit on the same claim as the chemotherapy. Medicare jurisdiction: DME Medicare Administrative Contractor (DME MAC). Use this code for Kytril.
MED: 100-2,6,10; 100-4,4,240; 100-4,17,80.2

N **Q0167 Dronabinol, 2.5 mg, oral, FDA approved prescription anti-emetic, for use as a complete therapeutic substitute for an IV anti-emetic at the time of chemotherapy treatment, not to exceed a 48-hour dosage regimen**
Medicare covers at the time of chemotherapy if regimen doesn't exceed 48 hours. Submit on the same claim as the chemotherapy. Medicare jurisdiction: DME Medicare Administrative Contractor (DME MAC). Use this code for Marinol.
MED: 100-2,6,10; 100-4,4,240; 100-4,17,80.2

B **Q0168 Dronabinol, 5 mg, oral, FDA approved prescription anti-emetic, for use as a complete therapeutic substitute for an IV anti-emetic at the time of chemotherapy treatment, not to exceed a 48-hour dosage regimen**
Medicare jurisdiction: DME Medicare Administrative Contractor (DME MAC). Use this code for Marinol.
MED: 100-2,6,10; 100-4,4,240; 100-4,17,80.2

N **Q0169 Promethazine HCl, 12.5 mg, oral, FDA approved prescription anti-emetic, for use as a complete therapeutic substitute for an IV anti-emetic at the time of chemotherapy treatment, not to exceed a 48-hour dosage regimen**
Medicare covers at the time of chemotherapy if regimen doesn't exceed 48 hours. Submit on the same claim as the chemotherapy. Medicare jurisdiction: DME Medicare Administrative Contractor (DME MAC). Use this code for Phenergan, Amergan.
MED: 100-2,6,10; 100-4,4,240; 100-4,17,80.2

Special Coverage Instructions   Noncovered by Medicare   Carrier Discretion   ☑ Quality Alert   ● New Code   ○ Reinstated Code   ▲ Revised Code

B **Q0170** Promethazine HCl, 25 mg, oral, FDA approved prescription anti-emetic, for use as a complete therapeutic substitute for an IV anti-emetic at the time of chemotherapy treatment, not to exceed a 48-hour dosage regimen
Medicare covers at the time of chemotherapy if regimen doesn't exceed 48 hours. Submit on the same claim as the chemotherapy. Medicare jurisdiction: DME Medicare Administrative Contractor (DME MAC). Use this code for Phenergan, Amergan.
MED: 100-2,6,10; 100-4,4,240; 100-4,17,80.2

N **Q0171** Chlorpromazine HCl, 10 mg, oral, FDA approved prescription anti-emetic, for use as a complete therapeutic substitute for an IV anti-emetic at the time of chemotherapy treatment, not to exceed a 48-hour dosage regimen
Medicare covers at the time of chemotherapy if regimen doesn't exceed 48 hours. Submit on the same claim as the chemotherapy. Medicare jurisdiction: DME Medicare Administrative Contractor (DME MAC). Use this code for Thorazine.
MED: 100-2,6,10; 100-4,4,240; 100-4,17,80.2

B **Q0172** Chlorpromazine HCl, 25 mg, oral, FDA approved prescription anti-emetic, for use as a complete therapeutic substitute for an IV anti-emetic at the time of chemotherapy treatment, not to exceed a 48-hour dosage regimen
Medicare covers at the time of chemotherapy if regimen doesn't exceed 48 hours. Submit on the same claim as the chemotherapy. Medicare jurisdiction: DME Medicare Administrative Contractor (DME MAC). Use this code for Thorazine.
MED: 100-2,6,10; 100-4,4,240; 100-4,17,80.2

N **Q0173** Trimethobenzamide HCl, 250 mg, oral, FDA approved prescription anti-emetic, for use as a complete therapeutic substitute for an IV anti-emetic at the time of chemotherapy treatment, not to exceed a 48-hour dosage regimen
Medicare covers at the time of chemotherapy if regimen doesn't exceed 48 hours. Submit on the same claim as the chemotherapy. Medicare jurisdiction: DME Medicare Administrative Contractor (DME MAC). Use this code for Tebamide, T-Gen, Ticon, Tigan, Triban, Thimazide.
MED: 100-2,6,10; 100-4,4,240; 100-4,17,80.2

N **Q0174** Thiethylperazine maleate, 10 mg, oral, FDA approved prescription anti-emetic, for use as a complete therapeutic substitute for an IV anti-emetic at the time of chemotherapy treatment, not to exceed a 48-hour dosage regimen
Medicare covers at the time of chemotherapy if regimen doesn't exceed 48 hours. Submit on the same claim as the chemotherapy. Medicare jurisdiction: DME Medicare Administrative Contractor (DME MAC). Use this code for Torecan.
MED: 100-2,6,10; 100-4,4,240; 100-4,17,80.2

N **Q0175** Perphenzaine, 4 mg, oral, FDA approved prescription anti-emetic, for use as a complete therapeutic substitute for an IV anti-emetic at the time of chemotherapy treatment, not to exceed a 48-hour dosage regimen
Medicare covers at the time of chemotherapy if regimen doesn't exceed 48 hours. Submit on the same claim as the chemotherapy. Medicare jurisdiction: DME Medicare Administrative Contractor (DME MAC). Use this code for Trilifon.
MED: 100-2,6,10; 100-4,4,240; 100-4,17,80.2

B **Q0176** Perphenzaine, 8 mg, oral, FDA approved prescription anti-emetic, for use as a complete therapeutic substitute for an IV anti-emetic at the time of chemotherapy treatment, not to exceed a 48-hour dosage regimen
Medicare covers at the time of chemotherapy if regimen doesn't exceed 48 hours. Submit on the same claim as the chemotherapy. Medicare jurisdiction: DME Medicare Administrative Contractor (DME MAC). Use this code for Trilifon.
MED: 100-2,6,10; 100-4,4,240; 100-4,17,80.2

N **Q0177** Hydroxyzine pamoate, 25 mg, oral, FDA approved prescription anti-emetic, for use as a complete therapeutic substitute for an IV anti-emetic at the time of chemotherapy treatment, not to exceed a 48-hour dosage regimen
Medicare covers at the time of chemotherapy if regimen doesn't exceed 48 hours. Submit on the same claim as the chemotherapy. Medicare jurisdiction: DME Medicare Administrative Contractor (DME MAC). Use this code for Vistaril.
MED: 100-2,6,10; 100-4,4,240; 100-4,17,80.2

B **Q0178** Hydroxyzine pamoate, 50 mg, oral, FDA approved prescription anti-emetic, for use as a complete therapeutic substitute for an IV anti-emetic at the time of chemotherapy treatment, not to exceed a 48-hour dosage regimen
Medicare covers at the time of chemotherapy if regimen doesn't exceed 48 hours. Submit on the same claim as the chemotherapy.
MED: 100-2,6,10; 100-4,4,240; 100-4,17,80.2

K **Q0179** Ondansetron HCl 8 mg, oral, FDA approved prescription anti-emetic, for use as a complete therapeutic substitute for an IV anti-emetic at the time of chemotherapy treatment, not to exceed a 48-hour dosage regimen
Medicare covers at the time of chemotherapy if regimen doesn't exceed 48 hours. Submit on the same claim as the chemotherapy. Medicare jurisdiction: DME Medicare Administrative Contractor (DME MAC). Use this code for Zofran.
MED: 100-2,6,10; 100-4,4,240; 100-4,17,80.2

K **Q0180** Dolasetron mesylate, 100 mg, oral, FDA approved prescription anti-emetic, for use as a complete therapeutic substitute for an IV anti-emetic at the time of chemotherapy treatment, not to exceed a 24-hour dosage regimen
Medicare covers at the time of chemotherapy if regimen doesn't exceed 24 hours. Submit on the same claim as the chemotherapy. Medicare jurisdiction: DME Medicare Administrative Contractor (DME MAC). Use this code for Anzemet.
MED: 100-2,6,10; 100-4,4,240; 100-4,17,80.2

E **Q0181** Unspecified oral dosage form, FDA approved prescription anti-emetic, for use as a complete therapeutic substitute for an IV anti-emetic at the time of chemotherapy treatment, not to exceed a 48-hour dosage regimen
Medicare covers at the time of chemotherapy if regimen doesn't exceed 48-hours. Submit on the same claim as the chemotherapy. Medicare jurisdiction: DME Medicare Administrative Contractor (DME MAC).
MED: 100-2,6,10; 100-4,4,240; 100-4,17,80.2

A **Q0480** Driver for use with pneumatic ventricular assist device, replacement only
AHA: 3Q,'05,2

Special Coverage Instructions   Noncovered by Medicare   Carrier Discretion   ☑ Quality Alert   ● New Code   ○ Reinstated Code   ▲ Revised Code

Q Codes (Temporary)

Q0481 — Q3020

[A] **Q0481** Microprocessor control unit for use with electric ventricular assist device, replacement only &
AHA: 3Q,'05,2

[A] **Q0482** Microprocessor control unit for use with electric/pneumatic combination ventricular assist device, replacement only &
AHA: 3Q,'05,2

[A] **Q0483** Monitor/display module for use with electric ventricular assist device, replacement only &
AHA: 3Q,'05,2

[A] **Q0484** Monitor/display module for use with electric or electric/pneumatic ventricular assist device, replacement only &
AHA: 3Q,'05,2

[A] **Q0485** Monitor control cable for use with electric ventricular assist device, replacement only &
AHA: 3Q,'05,2

[A] **Q0486** Monitor control cable for use with electric/pneumatic ventricular assist device, replacement only &
AHA: 3Q,'05,2

[A] **Q0487** Leads (pneumatic/electrical) for use with any type electric/pneumatic ventricular assist device, replacement only &
AHA: 3Q,'05,2

[A] **Q0488** Power pack base for use with electric ventricular assist device, replacement only &
AHA: 3Q,'05,2

[A] **Q0489** Power pack base for use with electric/pneumatic ventricular assist device, replacement only &
AHA: 3Q,'05,2

[A] **Q0490** Emergency power source for use with electric ventricular assist device, replacement only &
AHA: 3Q,'05,2

[A] **Q0491** Emergency power source for use with electric/pneumatic ventricular assist device, replacement only &
AHA: 3Q,'05,2

[A] **Q0492** Emergency power supply cable for use with electric ventricular assist device, replacement only &
AHA: 3Q,'05,2

[A] **Q0493** Emergency power supply cable for use with electric/pneumatic ventricular assist device, replacement only &
AHA: 3Q,'05,2

[A] **Q0494** Emergency hand pump for use with electric/pneumatic ventricular assist device, replacement only &
AHA: 3Q,'05,2

[A] **Q0495** Battery/power pack charger for use with electric or electric/pneumatic ventricular assist device, replacement only &
AHA: 3Q,'05,2

[A] **Q0496** Battery for use with electric or electric/pneumatic ventricular assist device, replacement only &
AHA: 3Q,'05,2

[A] **Q0497** Battery clips for use with electric or electric/pneumatic ventricular assist device, replacement only &
AHA: 3Q,'05,2

[A] **Q0498** Holster for use with electric or electric/pneumatic ventricular assist device, replacement only &
AHA: 3Q,'05,2

[A] **Q0499** Belt/vest for use with electric or electric/pneumatic ventricular assist device, replacement only &
AHA: 3Q,'05,2

[A] ☑ **Q0500** Filters for use with electric or electric/pneumatic ventricular assist device, replacement only &
The base unit for this code is for each filter.
AHA: 3Q,'05,2

[A] **Q0501** Shower cover for use with electric or electric/pneumatic ventricular assist device, replacement only &
AHA: 3Q,'05,2

[A] **Q0502** Mobility cart for pneumatic ventricular assist device, replacement only &
AHA: 3Q,'05,2

[A] **Q0503** Battery for pneumatic ventricular assist device, replacement only, each &
AHA: 3Q,'05,2

[A] **Q0504** Power adapter for pneumatic ventricular assist device, replacement only, vehicle type &
AHA: 3Q,'05,2

[A] **Q0505** Miscellaneous supply or accessory for use with ventricular assist device
AHA: 3Q,'05,2

[B] **Q0510** Pharmacy supply fee for initial immunosuppressive drug(s), first month following transplant
MED: 100-4,4,240

[B] **Q0511** Pharmacy supply fee for oral anti-cancer, oral anti-emetic or immunosuppressive drug(s); for the first prescription In a 30-day period
MED: 100-4,4,240

[B] **Q0512** Pharmacy supply fee for oral anti-cancer, oral anti-emetic or immunosuppressive drug(s); for a subsequent prescription in a 30-day period
MED: 100-4,4,240

[B] **Q0513** Pharmacy dispensing fee for inhalation drug(s); per 30 days

[B] **Q0514** Pharmacy dispensing fee for inhalation drug(s); per 90 days

[K] **Q0515** Injection, sermorelin acetate, 1 mcg
MED: 100-2,15,50; 100-4,4,230.1

▲ [N] **Q1003** New technology intraocular lens category 3 (reduced spherical aberration)

[N] **Q1004** New technology intraocular lens category 4 as defined in Federal Register notice

[N] **Q1005** New technology intraocular lens category 5 as defined in Federal Register notice

[N] ☑ **Q2004** Irrigation solution for treatment of bladder calculi, for example renacidin, per 500 ml
MED: 100-2,15,50

[K] ☑ **Q2009** Injection, fosphenytoin, 50 mg
Use this code for Cerebryx.

[K] ☑ **Q2017** Injection, teniposide, 50 mg
Use this code for Vumon.
MED: 100-2,15,50

[B] ☑ **Q3001** Radioelements for brachytherapy, any type, each ⊘
MED: 100-4,12,70; 100-4,13,20; 100-4,13,90

[A] **Q3014** Telehealth originating site facility fee
MED: 100-4,12,190

~~**Q3019** ALS vehicle used, emergency transport, no ALS level services furnished~~

~~**Q3020** ALS vehicle used, nonemergency transport, no ALS level service furnished~~

Special Coverage Instructions | Noncovered by Medicare | Carrier Discretion | ☑ Quality Alert | ● New Code | ○ Reinstated Code | ▲ Revised Code

128 — Q Codes | [A] Age Edit | [M] Maternity Edit | ♀ Female Only | ♂ Male Only | [A] - [Y] APC Status Indicators | 2007 HCPCS

K **Q3025** Injection, interferon beta-1A, 11 mcg for intramuscular use
Use this code for Avonex, Rebif. See also J1825.
MED: 100-2,15,50

E **Q3026** Injection, interferon beta-1A, 11 mcg for subcutaneous use
Use this code for Avonex Rebif. See also J1825.

N **Q3031** Collagen skin test
MED: 100-3,230.10

B **Q4001** Casting supplies, body cast adult, with or without head, plaster
MED: 100-4,4,240; 100-4,20,170

B **Q4002** Cast supplies, body cast adult, with or without head, fiberglass
MED: 100-4,4,240; 100-4,20,170

B **Q4003** Cast supplies, shoulder cast, adult (11 years +), plaster
MED: 100-4,4,240; 100-4,20,170

B **Q4004** Cast supplies, shoulder cast, adult (11 years +), fiberglass
MED: 100-4,4,240; 100-4,20,170

B **Q4005** Cast supplies, long arm cast, adult (11 years +), plaster
MED: 100-4,4,240; 100-4,20,170

B **Q4006** Cast supplies, long arm cast, adult (11 years +), fiberglass
MED: 100-4,4,240; 100-4,20,170

B **Q4007** Cast supplies, long arm cast, pediatric (0–10 years), plaster
MED: 100-4,4,240; 100-4,20,170

B **Q4008** Cast supplies, long arm cast, pediatric (0–10 years), fiberglass
MED: 100-4,4,240; 100-4,20,170

B **Q4009** Cast supplies, short arm cast, adult (11 years +), plaster
MED: 100-4,4,240; 100-4,20,170

B **Q4010** Cast supplies, short arm cast, adult (11 years +), fiberglass
MED: 100-4,4,240; 100-4,20,170

B **Q4011** Cast supplies, short arm cast, pediatric (0–10 years), plaster
MED: 100-4,4,240; 100-4,20,170

B **Q4012** Cast supplies, short arm cast, pediatric (0–10 years), fiberglass
MED: 100-4,4,240; 100-4,20,170

B **Q4013** Cast supplies, gauntlet cast (includes lower forearm and hand), adult (11 years +), plaster
MED: 100-4,4,240; 100-4,20,170

B **Q4014** Cast supplies, gauntlet cast (includes lower forearm and hand), adult (11 years +), fiberglass
MED: 100-4,4,240; 100-4,20,170

B **Q4015** Cast supplies, gauntlet cast (includes lower forearm and hand), pediatric (0–10 years), plaster
MED: 100-4,4,240; 100-4,20,170

B **Q4016** Cast supplies, gauntlet cast (includes lower forearm and hand), pediatric (0–10 years), fiberglass
MED: 100-4,4,240; 100-4,20,170

B **Q4017** Cast supplies, long arm splint, adult (11 years +), plaster
MED: 100-4,4,240; 100-4,20,170

B **Q4018** Cast supplies, long arm splint, adult (11 years +), fiberglass
MED: 100-4,4,240; 100-4,20,170

B **Q4019** Cast supplies, long arm splint, pediatric (0–10 years), plaster
MED: 100-4,4,240; 100-4,20,170

B **Q4020** Cast supplies, long arm splint, pediatric (0–10 years), fiberglass
MED: 100-4,4,240; 100-4,20,170

B **Q4021** Cast supplies, short arm splint, adult (11 years +), plaster
MED: 100-4,4,240; 100-4,20,170

B **Q4022** Cast supplies, short arm splint, adult (11 years +), fiberglass
MED: 100-4,4,240; 100-4,20,170

B **Q4023** Cast supplies, short arm splint, pediatric (0–10 years), plaster
MED: 100-4,4,240; 100-4,20,170

B **Q4024** Cast supplies, short arm splint, pediatric (0–10 years), fiberglass
MED: 100-4,4,240; 100-4,20,170

B **Q4025** Cast supplies, hip spica (one or both legs), adult (11 years +), plaster
MED: 100-4,4,240; 100-4,20,170

B **Q4026** Cast supplies, hip spica (one or both legs), adult (11 years +), fiberglass
MED: 100-4,4,240; 100-4,20,170

B **Q4027** Cast supplies, hip spica (one or both legs), pediatric (0–10 years), plaster
MED: 100-4,4,240; 100-4,20,170

B **Q4028** Cast supplies, hip spica (one or both legs), pediatric (0–10 years), fiberglass
MED: 100-4,4,240; 100-4,20,170

B **Q4029** Cast supplies, long leg cast, adult (11 years +), plaster
MED: 100-4,4,240; 100-4,20,170

B **Q4030** Cast supplies, long leg cast, adult (11 years +), fiberglass
MED: 100-4,4,240; 100-4,20,170

B **Q4031** Cast supplies, long leg cast, pediatric (0–10 years), plaster
MED: 100-4,4,240; 100-4,20,170

B **Q4032** Cast supplies, long leg cast, pediatric (0–10 years), fiberglass
MED: 100-4,4,240; 100-4,20,170

B **Q4033** Cast supplies, long leg cylinder cast, adult (11 years +), plaster
MED: 100-4,4,240; 100-4,20,170

B **Q4034** Cast supplies, long leg cylinder cast, adult (11 years +), fiberglass
MED: 100-4,4,240; 100-4,20,170

B **Q4035** Cast supplies, long leg cylinder cast, pediatric (0–10 years), plaster
MED: 100-4,4,240; 100-4,20,170

B **Q4036** Cast supplies, long leg cylinder cast, pediatric (0–10 years), fiberglass
MED: 100-4,4,240; 100-4,20,170

B **Q4037** Cast supplies, short leg cast, adult (11 years +), plaster
MED: 100-4,4,240; 100-4,20,170

Q Codes (Temporary)

Q4038 — Q9963

B   **Q4038** Cast supplies, short leg cast, adult (11 years +), fiberglass   A
MED: 100-4,4,240; 100-4,20,170

B   **Q4039** Cast supplies, short leg cast, pediatric (0–10 years), plaster   A
MED: 100-4,4,240; 100-4,20,170

B   **Q4040** Cast supplies, short leg cast, pediatric (0–10 years), fiberglass   A
MED: 100-4,4,240; 100-4,20,170

B   **Q4041** Cast supplies, long leg splint, adult (11 years +), plaster   A
MED: 100-4,4,240; 100-4,20,170

B   **Q4042** Cast supplies, long leg splint, adult (11 years +), fiberglass   A
MED: 100-4,4,240; 100-4,20,170

B   **Q4043** Cast supplies, long leg splint, pediatric (0–10 years), plaster   A
MED: 100-4,4,240; 100-4,20,170

B   **Q4044** Cast supplies, long leg splint, pediatric (0–10 years), fiberglass   A
MED: 100-4,4,240; 100-4,20,170

B   **Q4045** Cast supplies, short leg splint, adult (11 years +), plaster   A
MED: 100-4,4,240; 100-4,20,170

B   **Q4046** Cast supplies, short leg splint, adult (11 years +), fiberglass   A
MED: 100-4,4,240; 100-4,20,170

B   **Q4047** Cast supplies, short leg splint, pediatric (0–10 years), plaster   A
MED: 100-4,4,240; 100-4,20,170

B   **Q4048** Cast supplies, short leg splint, pediatric (0–10 years), fiberglass   A
MED: 100-4,4,240; 100-4,20,170

B   **Q4049** Finger splint, static
MED: 100-4,4,240; 100-4,20,170

B   **Q4050** Cast supplies, for unlisted types and materials of casts
MED: 100-4,4,240; 100-4,20,170

B   **Q4051** Splint supplies, miscellaneous (includes thermoplastics, strapping, fasteners, padding and other supplies)
MED: 100-4,4,240; 100-4,20,170

G   **Q4079** Injection, natalizumab, per 1 mg
AHA: 2Q,'05,11

▲ Y   **Q4080** Iloprost, inhalation solution, administered through DME, up to 20 mcg
AHA: 3Q,'05,7

● A   **Q4081** Injection, epoetin alfa, 100 units (for ESRD on dialysis)

● B   **Q4082** Drug or biological, not otherwise classified, Part B drug competitive acquisition program (CAP)

● B   **Q5001** Hospice care provided in patient's home/residence

● B   **Q5002** Hospice care provided in assisted living facility

● B   **Q5003** Hospice care provided in nursing long-term care facility (LTC) or nonskilled nursing facility (NF)

● B   **Q5004** Hospice care provided in skilled nursing facility (SNF)

● B   **Q5005** Hospice care provided in inpatient hospital

● B   **Q5006** Hospice care provided in inpatient hospice facility

● B   **Q5007** Hospice care provided in long-term care facility

● B   **Q5008** Hospice care provided in inpatient psychiatric facility

● B   **Q5009** Hospice care provided in place not otherwise specified (NOS)

K   **Q9945** Low osmolar contrast material, up to 149 mg/ml iodine concentration, per ml
MED: 100-4,13,20; 100-4,13,90

K   **Q9946** Low osmolar contrast material, 150–199 mg/ml iodine concentration, per ml
MED: 100-4,12,70; 100-4,13,20; 100-4,13,90

K   **Q9947** Low osmolar contrast material, 200–249 mg/ml iodine concentration, per ml
MED: 100-4,12,70; 100-4,13,20; 100-4,13,90

K   **Q9948** Low osmolar contrast material, 250–299 mg/ml iodine concentration, per ml
MED: 100-4,12,70; 100-4,13,20; 100-4,13,90

K   **Q9949** Low osmolar contrast material, 300-349 mg/ml iodine concentration, per ml
MED: 100-4,12,70; 100-4,13,20; 100-4,13,90

K   **Q9950** Low osmolar contrast material, 350–399 mg/ml iodine concentration, per ml
MED: 100-4,12,70; 100-4,13,20; 100-4,13,90

K   **Q9951** Low osmolar contrast material, 400 or greater mg/ml iodine concentration, per ml
MED: 100-4,12,70; 100-4,13,20; 100-4,13,90

K   **Q9952** Injection, gadolinium-based magnetic resonance contrast agent, per ml
MED: 100-4,12,70; 100-4,13,20; 100-4,13,90

K   **Q9953** Injection, iron-based magnetic resonance contrast agent, per ml
MED: 100-4,12,70; 100-4,13,20; 100-4,13,90

K   **Q9954** Oral magnetic resonance contrast agent, per 100 ml
MED: 100-4,12,70; 100-4,13,20; 100-4,13,90

K   **Q9955** Injection, perflexane lipid microspheres, per ml
MED: 100-4,4,230.1

K   **Q9956** Injection, octafluoropropane microspheres, per ml
MED: 100-4,4,230.1

K   **Q9957** Injection, perflutren lipid microspheres, per ml
MED: 100-4,4,230.1

N   **Q9958** High osmolar contrast material, up to 149 mg/ml iodine concentration, per ml
MED: 100-4,12,70; 100-4,13,20; 100-4,13,90
AHA: 3Q,'05,7

N   **Q9959** High osmolar contrast material, 150–199 mg/ml iodine concentration, per ml
MED: 100-4,12,70; 100-4,13,20; 100-4,13,90
AHA: 3Q,'05,7

N   **Q9960** High osmolar contrast material, 200–249 mg/ml iodine concentration, per ml
MED: 100-4,12,70; 100-4,13,20; 100-4,13,90
AHA: 3Q,'05,7

N   **Q9961** High osmolar contrast material, 250–299 mg/ml iodine concentration, per ml
MED: 100-4,12,70; 100-4,13,20; 100-4,13,90
AHA: 3Q,'05,7

N   **Q9962** High osmolar contrast material, 300–349 mg/ml iodine concentration, per ml
MED: 100-4,12,70; 100-4,13,20; 100-4,13,90
AHA: 3Q,'05,7

N   **Q9963** High osmolar contrast material, 350–399 mg/ml iodine concentration, per ml
MED: 100-4,12,70; 100-4,13,20; 100-4,13,90
AHA: 3Q,'05,7

Special Coverage Instructions   Noncovered by Medicare   Carrier Discretion   ☑ Quality Alert   ● New Code   ○ Reinstated Code   ▲ Revised Code

N ☐ **Q9964** High osmolar contrast material, 400 or greater mg/ml
iodine concentration, per ml
MED: 100-4,12,70; 100-4,13,20; 100-4,13,90
AHA: 3Q,'05,7

Special Coverage Instructions   Noncovered by Medicare   Carrier Discretion   ☑ Quality Alert   ● New Code   ○ Reinstated Code   ▲ Revised Code

2007 HCPCS   **1**-**9** ASC Group   **MED:** Pub 100/NCD References   ♿ DMEPOS Paid   ⊘ SNF Excluded   **Q Codes — 131**

DIAGNOSTIC RADIOLOGY SERVICES R0000-R5999

R codes are used for the transportation of portable x-ray and/or EKG equipment.

R codes fall under the jurisdiction of the local contractor.

B ☑ **R0070** Transportation of portable x-ray equipment and personnel to home or nursing home, per trip to facility or location, one patient seen

Only a single, reasonable transportation charge is allowed for each trip the portable x-ray supplier makes to a location. When more than one patient is x-rayed at the same location, prorate the single allowable transport charge among all patients.

MED: 100-4,13,90; 100-4,13,90.3

B ☑ **R0075** Transportation of portable x-ray equipment and personnel to home or nursing home, per trip to facility or location, more than one patient seen

Only a single, reasonable transportation charge is allowed for each trip the portable x-ray supplier makes to a location. When more than one patient is x-rayed at the same location, prorate the single allowable transport charge among all patients.

MED: 100-4,13,90; 100-4,13,90.3

B ☑ **R0076** Transportation of portable EKG to facility or location, per patient

Only a single, reasonable transportation charge is allowed for each trip the portable EKG supplier makes to a location. When more than one patient is tested at the same location, prorate the single allowable transport charge among all patients.

MED: 100-1,5,90.2; 100-2,15,80.1; 100-3,20.15; 100-4,13,90; 100-4,13,90.3; 100-4,16,10; 100-4,16,10.1; 100-4,16,110.4

| Special Coverage Instructions | Noncovered by Medicare | Carrier Discretion | ☑ Quality Alert | ● New Code | ○ Reinstated Code | ▲ Revised Code |

132 — R Codes   A Age Edit   M Maternity Edit   ♀ Female Only   ♂ Male Only   A - Y APC Status Indicators   *2007 HCPCS*

TEMPORARY NATIONAL CODES (NON-MEDICARE)
S0000-S9999

The S codes are used by the Blue Cross/Blue Shield Association (BCBSA) and the Health Insurance Association of America (HIAA) to report drugs, services, and supplies for which there are no national codes but for which codes are needed by the private sector to implement policies, programs, or claims processing. They are for the purpose of meeting the particular needs of the private sector. These codes are also used by the Medicaid program, but they are not payable by Medicare.

☑ **S0012** Butorphanol tartrate, nasal spray, 25 mg
Use this code for Stadol NS.

☑ **S0014** Tacrine HCl, 10 mg
Use this code for Cognex.

☑ **S0017** Injection, aminocaproic acid, 5 grams
Use this code for Amicar.

☑ **S0020** Injection, bupivicaine HCl, 30 ml
Use this code for Marcaine, Sensorcaine.

☑ **S0021** Injection, ceftoperazone sodium, 1 gram
Use this code for Cefobid.

☑ **S0023** Injection, cimetidine HCl, 300 mg
Use this code for Tagamet HCl.

☑ **S0028** Injection, famotidine, 20 mg
Use this code for Pepcid.

☑ **S0030** Injection, metronidazole, 500 mg
Use this code for Flagyl IV RTU.

☑ **S0032** Injection, nafcillin sodium, 2 grams
Use this code for Nallpen, Unipen.

☑ **S0034** Injection, ofloxacin, 400 mg
Use this code for Floxin IV.

☑ **S0039** Injection, sulfamethoxazole and trimethoprim, 10 ml
Use this code for Bactrim IV, Septra IV, SMZ-TMP, Sulfutrim.

☑ **S0040** Injection, ticarcillin disodium and clavulanate potassium, 3.1 grams
Use this code for Timentin.

☑ **S0073** Injection, aztreonam, 500 mg
Use this code for Azactam.

☑ **S0074** Injection, cefotetan disodium, 500 mg
Use this code for Cefotan.

☑ **S0077** Injection, clindamycin phosphate, 300 mg
Use this code for Cleocin Phosphate.

☑ **S0078** Injection, fosphenytoin sodium, 750 mg
Use this code for Cerebryx.

☑ **S0080** Injection, pentamidine isethionate, 300 mg
Use this code for NebuPent, Pentam 300, Pentacarinat. See also code J2545.

☑ **S0081** Injection, piperacillin sodium, 500 mg
Use this code for Pipracil.

☑ **S0088** Imatinib injection, 100 mg
Use this code for Gleevec.

☑ **S0090** Sildenafil citrate, 25 mg ▲
Use this code for Viagra.

☑ **S0091** Granisetron HCl, 1 mg (for circumstances falling under the Medicare statute, use Q0166)
Use this code for Kytril.

☑ **S0092** Injection, hydromorphone HCl, 250 mg (loading dose for infusion pump)
Use this code for Dilaudid, Hydromophone. See also J1170.

☑ **S0093** Injection, morphine sulfate, 500 mg (loading dose for infusion pump)
Use this code for Duramorph, MS Contin, Morphine Sulfate. See also J2270, J2271, J2275.

S0104 Zidovudine, oral 100 mg
See also J3485 for Retrovir.

☑ **S0106** Bupropion HCl sustained release tablet, 150 mg, per bottle of 60 tablets
Use this code for Wellbutrin SR tablets.

S0108 Mercaptopurine, oral, 50 mg
Use this code for Purinethol oral.

☑ **S0109** Methadone, oral, 5 mg
Use this code for Dolophine.

~~S0116 Bevacizumab, 100 mg~~

☑ **S0117** Tretinoin, topical 5 grams

S0122 Injection, menotropins, 75 IU
Use this code for Humegon, Pergonal, Repronex.

S0126 Injection, follitropin alfa, 75 IU
Use this code for Gonal-F.

S0128 Injection, follitropin beta, 75 IU ♀
Use this code for Follistim.

S0132 Injection, ganirelix acetate, 250 mcg ♀
Use this code for Antagon.

~~S0133 Histerelin, implant, 50 mg~~

☑ **S0136** Clozapine, 25 mg
Use this code for Clozaril.

☑ **S0137** Didanosine (ddI), 25 mg
Use this code for Videx.

☑ **S0138** Finasteride, 5 mg ♂
Use this code for Propecia (oral), Proscar (oral).

☑ **S0139** Minoxidil, 10 mg
Use this code for Loniten (oral).

☑ **S0140** Saquinavir, 200 mg
Use this code for Fortovase (oral), Invirase (oral).

☑ **S0141** Zalcitabine (ddC), 0.375 mg
Use this code for Hivid (oral).

S0142 Colistimethate sodium, inhalation solution administrated through DME, concentrated form, per mg

S0143 Aztreonam, inhalation solution administered through DME, concentrated form, per gram

S0145 Injection, pegylated interferon alfa-2a, 180 mcg per ml
Use this code for Pegasys.

S0146 Injection, pegylated interferon alfa-2b, 10 mcg per 0.5 ml

● **S0147** Injection, alglucosidase alfa, 20 mg
Use this code for Myozyme.

See also code: C9234.

☑ **S0155** Sterile dilutant for epoprostenol, 50 ml
Use this code for Flolan.

☑ **S0156** Exemestane, 25 mg
Use this code for Aromasin.

Special Coverage Instructions Noncovered by Medicare Carrier Discretion ☑ Quality Alert ● New Code ○ Reinstated Code ▲ Revised Code

2007 HCPCS 1-9 ASC Group **MED:** Pub 100/NCD References ᕐ DMEPOS Paid ⊘ SNF Excluded S Codes — 133

☑ **S0157** Becaplermin gel 0.01%, 0.5 gm
Use this code for Regraex Gel.

☑ **S0160** Dextroamphetamine sulfate, 5 mg

☑ **S0161** Calcitrol, 0.25 mcg

☑ **S0162** Injection, efalizumab, 125 mg
Use this code for Raptiva.

☑ **S0164** Injection, pantoprazole sodium, 40 mg
Use this code for Protonix IV.

☑ **S0166** Injection, olanzapine, 2.5 mg
Use this code for Zyprexa.

☑ **S0167** Injection, apomorphine HCl, 1 mg
See also code: J0364.

☑ **S0170** Anastrozole, oral, 1mg
Use this code for Arimidex.

☑ **S0171** Injection, bumetanide, 0.5 mg
Use this code for Bumex.

☑ **S0172** Chlorambucil, oral, 2 mg
Use this code for Leukeran.

☑ **S0174** Dolasetron mesylate, oral 50 mg (for circumstances falling under the Medicare statute, use Q0180)
Use this code for Anzemet.

☑ **S0175** Flutamide, oral, 125 mg
Use this code for Eulexin.

☑ **S0176** Hydroxyurea, oral, 500 mg
Use this code for Droxia, Hydrea, Mylocel.

☑ **S0177** Levamisole HCl, oral, 50 mg
Use this code for Ergamisol.

☑ **S0178** Lomustine, oral, 10 mg
Use this code for Ceenu.
MED: 100-4,17,80.2

☑ **S0179** Megestrol acetate, oral, 20 mg
Use this code for Megace.

● **S0180** Etonogestrel (contraceptive) implant system, including implants and supplies

☑ **S0181** Ondansetron HCl, oral, 4 mg (for circumstances falling under the Medicare statute, use Q0179)
Use this code for Zofran.

☑ **S0182** Procarbazine HCl, oral, 50 mg
Use this code for Matulane.

☑ **S0183** Prochlorperazine maleate, oral, 5 mg (for circumstances falling under the Medicare statute, use Q0164-Q0165)
Use this code for Compazine.

☑ **S0187** Tamoxifen citrate, oral, 10 mg
Use this code for Nolvadex.

☑ **S0189** Testosterone pellet, 75 mg

☑ **S0190** Mitepristone, oral, 200 mg   ♀
Use this code for Mifoprex 200 mg oral.

☑ **S0191** Misoprostol, oral, 200 mcg

☑ **S0194** Dialysis/stress vitamin supplement, oral, 100 capsules

S0195 Pneumococcal conjugate vaccine, polyvalent, intramuscular, for children from five years to nine years of age who have not previously received the vaccine   Ⓐ
Use this code for Pneumovax II.

☑ **S0196** Injectable poly-l-lactic acid, restorative implant, 1 ml, face (deep dermis, subcutaneous layers)

☑ **S0197** Prenatal vitamins, 30-day supply   Ⓜ ♀

~~S0198 Injection, pegaptanib sodium, 0.3 mg~~

S0199 Medically induced abortion by oral ingestion of medication including all associated services and supplies (e.g., patient counseling, office visits, confirmation of pregnancy by HCG, ultrasound to confirm duration of pregnancy, ultrasound to confirm completion of abortion) except drugs   ♀

S0201 Partial hospitalization services, less than 24 hours, per diem

S0207 Paramedic intercept, nonhospital based ALS service (nonvoluntary), nontransport

S0208 Paramedic intercept, hospital-based ALS service (nonvoluntary), nontransport

S0209 Wheelchair van, mileage, per mile

S0215 Nonemergency transportation; mileage, per mile
See also codes A0021-A0999 for transportation.

S0220 Medical conference by a physician with interdisciplinary team of health professionals or representatives of community agencies to coordinate activities of patient care (patient is present); approximately 30 minutes

S0221 Medical conference by a physician with interdisciplinary team of health professionals or representatives of community agencies to coordinate activities of patient care (patient is present); approximately 60 minutes

S0250 Comprehensive geriatric assessment and treatment planning performed by assessment team   Ⓐ

S0255 Hospice referral visit (advising patient and family of care options) performed by nurse, social worker, or other designated staff

S0257 Counseling and discussion regarding advance directives or end of life care planning and decisions, with patient and/or surrogate (list separately in addition to code for appropriate evaluation and management service)

S0260 History and physical (outpatient or office) related to surgical procedure (list separately in addition to code for appropriate evaluation and management service)

☑ **S0265** Genetic counseling, under physician supervision, each 15 minutes

S0302 Completed early periodic screening diagnosis and treatment (EPSDT) service (list in addition to code for appropriate evaluation and management service)

S0310 Hospitalist services (list separately in addition to code for appropriate evaluation and management service)

S0315 Disease management program; initial assessment and initiation of the program

▲ **S0316** Disease management program; follow-up/assessment

☑ **S0317** Disease management program; per diem

S0320 Telephone calls by a registered nurse to a disease management program member for monitoring purposes; per month

S0340 Lifestyle modification program for management of coronary artery disease, including all supportive services; first quarter/stage

S0341 Lifestyle modification program for management of coronary artery disease, including all supportive services; second or third quarter/stage

---

| Special Coverage Instructions | Noncovered by Medicare | Carrier Discretion | ☑ Quality Alert | ● New Code | ○ Reinstated Code | ▲ Revised Code |

S0342 Lifestyle modification program for management of coronary artery disease, including all supportive services; fourth quarter/stage

● **S0345** Electrocardiographic monitoring utilizing a home computerized telemetry station with automatic activation and real time notification of monitoring station, 24-hour attended monitoring, including recording, monitoring, receipt of transmissions, analysis, and physician review and interpretation; per 24-hour period

● **S0346** Electrocardiographic monitoring utilizing a home computerized telemetry station with automatic activation and real time notification of monitoring station, 24-hour attended monitoring, including recording, monitoring, receipt of transmissions, and analysis; per 24-hour period

● **S0347** Electrocardiographic monitoring utilizing a home computerized telemetry station with automatic activation and real time notification of monitoring station, 24-hour attended monitoring, including physician review and interpretation; per 24-hour period

S0390 Routine foot care; removal and/or trimming of corns, calluses and/or nails and preventive maintenance in specific medical conditions (e.g., diabetes), per visit
See also CPT code 11719-11721.

S0395 Impression casting of a foot performed by a practitioner other than the manufacturer of the orthotic

S0400 Global fee for extracorporeal shock wave lithotripsy treatment of kidney stone(s)
See CPT code 50590.

☑ **S0500** Disposable contact lens, per lens

☑ **S0504** Single vision prescription lens (safety, athletic, or sunglass), per lens

☑ **S0506** Bifocal vision prescription lens (safety, athletic, or sunglass), per lens

☑ **S0508** Trifocal vision prescription lens (safety, athletic, or sunglass), per lens

☑ **S0510** Nonprescription lens (safety, athletic, or sunglass), per lens

☑ **S0512** Daily wear specialty contact lens, per lens

☑ **S0514** Color contact lens, per lens

S0515 Scleral lens, liquid bandage device, per lens

S0516 Safety eyeglass frames

S0518 Sunglasses frames

S0580 Polycarbonate lens (list this code in addition to the basic code for the lens)

S0581 Nonstandard lens (list this code in addition to the basic code for the lens)

S0590 Integral lens service, miscellaneous services reported separately

S0592 Comprehensive contact lens evaluation

S0595 Dispensing new spectacle lenses for patient supplied frame

S0601 Screening proctoscopy ♂
MED: 100-4,4,240

S0605 Digital rectal examination, annual

S0610 Annual gynecological examination; new patient ♀
MED: 100-4,4,240

S0612 Annual gynecological examination; established patient ♀
MED: 100-4,4,240

S0613 Annual gynecological examination, clinical breast examination without pelvic examination ♀

S0618 Audiometry for hearing aid evaluation to determine the level and degree of hearing loss

S0620 Routine ophthalmological examination including refraction; new patient

S0621 Routine ophthalmological examination including refraction; established patient

S0622 Physical exam for college, new or established patient (list separately in addition to appropriate evaluation and management code) Ⓐ

S0625 Retinal telescreening by digital imaging of multiple different fundus areas to screen for vision threatening conditions, including imaging, interpretation and report

S0630 Removal of sutures by a physician other than the physician who originally closed the wound

S0800 Laser in situ keratomileusis (LASIK)

S0810 Photorefractive keratectomy (PRK)

S0812 Phototherapeutic keratectomy (PTK)

S0820 Computerized corneal topography, unilateral

S1001 Deluxe item, patient aware (list in addition to code for basic item)
MED: 100-2,1,10.1.4

S1002 Customized item (list in addition to code for basic item)

S1015 IV tubing extension set

S1016 Non-PVC (polyvinyl chloride) intravenous administration set, for use with drugs that are not stable in PVC e.g., Paclitaxel

S1025 Inhaled nitric oxide for the treatment of hypoxic respiratory failure in the neonate; per diem

S1030 Continuous noninvasive glucose monitoring device, purchase (for physician interpretation of data, use CPT code)

S1031 Continuous noninvasive glucose monitoring device, rental, including sensor, sensor replacement, and download to monitor (for physician interpretation of data, use CPT code)

▲ **S1040** Cranial remolding orthosis, pediatric, rigid, with soft interface material, custom fabricated, includes fitting and adjustment(s)

S2053 Transplantation of small intestine, and liver allografts

S2054 Transplantation of multivisceral organs

S2055 Harvesting of donor multivisceral organs, with preparation and maintenance of allografts; from cadaver donor

S2060 Lobar lung transplantation

S2061 Donor lobectomy (lung) for transplantation, living donor

S2065 Simultaneous pancreas kidney transplantation

S2068 Breast reconstruction with deep inferior epigastric perforator (deep) flap, including microvascular anastomosis and closure of donor site, unilateral ♀

Special Coverage Instructions   Noncovered by Medicare   Carrier Discretion   ☑ Quality Alert   ● New Code   ○ Reinstated Code   ▲ Revised Code

2007 HCPCS   1-9 ASC Group   MED: Pub 100/NCD References   ⅙ DMEPOS Paid   ⊘ SNF Excluded   S Codes — 135

Temporary National Codes (Non-Medicare)

S2070 — S2362

S2070 Cystourethroscopy, with ureteroscopy and/or pyeloscopy; with endoscopic laser treatment of ureteral calculi (includes ureteral catheterization)

S2075 Laparoscopy, surgical; repair incisional or ventral hernia

S2076 Laparoscopy, surgical; repair umbilical hernia

S2077 Laparoscopy, surgical; implantation of mesh or other prosthesis for incisional or ventral hernia repair (List separately in addition to code for the incisional or ventral hernia repair) ♀

S2078 Laparoscopic supracervical hysterectomy (subtotal hysterectomy), with or without removal of tube(s), with or without removal of ovary(s)

S2079 Laparoscopic esophagomyotomy (Heller type)

S2080 Laser-assisted uvulopalatoplasty (LAUP)

S2083 Adjustment of gastric band diameter via subcutanous port by injection or aspiration of saline

S2095 Transcatheter occlusion or embolization for tumor destruction, percutaneous, any method, using yttrium 90 microspheres

S2102 Islet cell tissue transplant from pancreas; allogeneic

S2103 Adrenal tissue transplant to brain

▲ **S2107** Adoptive immunotherapy, i.e., development of specific antitumor reactivity (e.g., tumor-infiltrating lymphocyte therapy) per course of treatment

S2112 Arthroscopy, knee, surgical for harvesting of cartilage (chondrocyte cells)

▲ **S2114** Arthroscopy, shoulder, surgical; tenodesis of biceps

▲ **S2115** Osteotomy, periacetabular, with internal fixation

S2117 Arthroereisis, subtalar

S2120 Low density lipoprotein (LDL) apheresis using heparin-induced extracorporeal LDL precipitation

S2135 Neurolysis, by injection, of metatarsal neuroma/interdigital neuritis, any interspace of the foot

S2140 Cord blood harvesting for transplantation, allogeneic

S2142 Cord blood-derived stem-cell transplantation, allogeneic

S2150 Bone marrow or blood-derived stem cells (peripheral or umbilical), allogeneic or autologous, harvesting, transplantation, and related complications; including: pheresis and cell preparation/storage; marrow ablative therapy; drugs, supplies, hospitalization with outpatient follow-up; medical/surgical, diagnostic, emergency, and rehabilitative services; and the number of days of pre- and post-transplant care in the global definition

S2152 Solid organ(s), complete or segmental, single organ or combination of organs; deceased or living donor(s), procurement, transplantation, and related complications including: drugs; supplies; hospitalization with outpatient follow-up; medical/surgical, diagnostic, emergency, and rehabilitative services; and the number of days of pre- and post-transplant care in the global definition

S2202 Echosclerotherapy

S2205 Minimally invasive direct coronary artery bypass surgery involving mini-thoracotomy or mini-sternotomy surgery, performed under direct vision; using arterial graft(s), single coronary arterial graft

S2206 Minimally invasive direct coronary artery bypass surgery involving mini-thoracotomy or mini-sternotomy surgery, performed under direct vision; using arterial graft(s), two coronary arterial grafts

S2207 Minimally invasive direct coronary artery bypass surgery involving mini-thoracotomy or mini-sternotomy surgery, performed under direct vision; using venous graft only, single coronary venous graft

S2208 Minimally invasive direct coronary artery bypass surgery involving mini-thoracotomy or mini-sternotomy surgery, performed under direct vision; using single arterial and venous graft(s), single venous graft

S2209 Minimally invasive direct coronary artery bypass surgery involving mini-thoracotomy or mini-sternotomy surgery, performed under direct vision; using two arterial grafts and single venous graft

S2213 Implantation of gastric electrical stimulation device

S2225 Myringotomy, laser-assisted

S2230 Implantation of magnetic component of semi-implantable hearing device on ossicles in middle ear

S2235 Implantation of auditory brain stem implant

S2250 Uterine artery embolization for uterine fibroids Ⓐ ♀

S2260 Induced abortion, 17 to 24 weeks Ⓜ ♀

~~**S2262** Abortion for maternal indication, 25 weeks or greater~~
See CPT code(s) 22523, 22524.

▲ **S2265** Induced abortion, 25 to 28 weeks Ⓜ ♀

▲ **S2266** Induced abortion, 29 to 31 weeks Ⓜ ♀

▲ **S2267** Induced abortion, 32 weeks or greater Ⓜ ♀

S2300 Arthroscopy, shoulder, surgical; with thermally-induced capsulorrhaphy

● **S2325** Hip core decompression

S2340 Chemodenervation of abductor muscle(s) of vocal cord

S2341 Chemodenervation of adductor muscle(s) of vocal cord

S2342 Nasal endoscopy for postoperative debridement following functional endoscopic sinus surgery, nasal and/or sinus cavity(s), unilateral or bilateral

● **S2344** Nasal/sinus endoscopy, surgical; with enlargement of sinus ostium opening using inflatable device (i.e., balloon sinuplasty)

S2348 Decompression procedure, percutaneous, of nucleus pulposus of intervertebral disc, using radiofrequency energy, single or multiple levels, lumbar

S2350 Diskectomy, anterior, with decompression of spinal cord and/or nerve root(s), including osteophytectomy; lumbar, single interspace

S2351 Diskectomy, anterior, with decompression of spinal cord and/or nerve root(s), including osteophytectomy; lumbar, each additional interspace (list separately in addition to code for primary procedure)

S2360 Percutaneous vertebroplasty, one vertebral body, unilateral or bilateral injection; cervical

S2361 Each additional cervical vertebral body (list separately in addition to code for primary procedure)

~~**S2362** Kyphoplasty, one vertebral body, unilateral or bilateral injection~~

Special Coverage Instructions   Noncovered by Medicare   Carrier Discretion   ☑ Quality Alert   ● New Code   ○ Reinstated Code   ▲ Revised Code

136 — S Codes   Ⓐ Age Edit   Ⓜ Maternity Edit   ♀ Female Only   ♂ Male Only   Ⓐ - Ⓨ APC Status Indicators   *2007 HCPCS*

~~S2363~~ ~~Kyphoplasty, one vertebral body, unilateral or bilateral injection; each additional vertebral body (list separately in addition to code for primary procedure)~~

S2400 Repair, congenital diaphragmatic hernia in the fetus using temporary tracheal occlusion, procedure performed in utero 　Ⓜ♀
Repair, congenital diaphragmatic hernia in the fetus using temporary tracheal occlusion, procedure performed in utero.

S2401 Repair, urinary tract obstruction in the fetus, procedure performed in utero 　Ⓜ♀

S2402 Repair, congenital cystic adenomatoid malformation in the fetus, procedure performed in utero 　Ⓜ♀

S2403 Repair, extralobar pulmonary sequestration in the fetus, procedure performed in utero 　Ⓜ♀

S2404 Repair, myelomeningocele in the fetus, procedure performed in utero 　Ⓜ♀

S2405 Repair of sacrococcygeal teratoma in the fetus, procedure performed in utero 　Ⓜ♀

S2409 Repair, congenital malformation of fetus, procedure performed in utero, not otherwise classified 　Ⓜ♀

S2411 Fetoscopic laser therapy for treatment of twin-to-twin transfusion syndrome 　Ⓜ♀

S2900 Surgical techniques requiring use of robotic surgical system (list separately in addition to code for primary procedure)

S3000 Diabetic indicator; retinal eye exam, dilated, bilateral

S3005 Performance measurement, evaluation of patient self assessment, depression

S3600 STAT laboratory request (situations other than S3601)

S3601 Emergency STAT laboratory charge for patient who is homebound or residing in a nursing facility

☑ S3620 Newborn metabolic screening panel, includes test kit, postage and the laboratory tests specified by the state for inclusion in this panel (e.g., galactose; hemoglobin, electrophoresis; hydroxyprogesterone, 17-d; phenylanine (PKU); and thyroxine, total) 　Ⓐ

S3625 Maternal serum triple marker screen including alpha-fetoprotein (APF), estriol, and human chorionic gonadotropin (hCG) 　Ⓜ♀

S3626 Maternal serum quadruple marker screen including alpha-fetoprotein (AFP), estriol, human chorionic gonadotropin (hcG), and inhibin A

S3630 Eosinophil count, blood, direct

S3645 HIV-1 antibody testing of oral mucosal transudate

S3650 Saliva test, hormone level; during menopause 　Ⓐ♀

S3652 Saliva test, hormone level; to assess preterm labor risk 　Ⓜ♀

S3655 Antisperm antibodies test (immunobead) 　Ⓐ♀

~~S3701~~ ~~Immunoassay for nuclear matrix protein 22 (NMP-22), quantitative~~

S3708 Gastrointestinal fat absorption study

S3818 Complete gene sequence analysis; BRCA 1 gene

S3819 Complete gene sequence analysis; BRCA 2 gene

S3820 Complete BRCA1 and BRCA2 gene sequence analysis for susceptibility to breast and ovarian cancer 　♀

S3822 Single mutation analysis (in individual with a known BRCA1 or BRCA2 mutation in the family) for susceptibility to breast and ovarian cancer 　♀

S3823 Three-mutation BRCA1 and BRCA2 analysis for susceptibility to breast and ovarian cancer in Ashkenazi individuals 　♀

S3828 Complete gene sequence analysis; MLH1 gene

S3829 Complete gene sequence analysis; MLH2 gene

S3830 Complete MLH1 and MLH2 gene sequence analysis for hereditary nonpolyposis colorectal cancer (HNPCC) genetic testing

S3831 Single-mutation analysis (in individual with a known MLH1 and MLH2 mutation in the family) for hereditary nonpolyposis colorectal cancer (HNPCC) genetic testing

S3833 Complete APC gene sequence analysis for susceptibility to familial adenomatous polyposis (FAP) and attenuated fap

S3834 Single-mutation analysis (in individual with a known APC mutation in the family) for susceptibility to familial adenomatous polyposis (FAP) and attenuated FAP

S3835 Complete gene sequence analysis for cystic fibrosis genetic testing

S3837 Complete gene sequence analysis for hemochromatosis genetic testing

S3840 DNA analysis for germline mutations of the RET proto-oncogene for susceptibility to multiple endocrine neoplasia type 2

S3841 Genetic testing for retinoblastoma

S3842 Genetic testing for Von Hippel-Lindau disease

S3843 DNA analysis of the F5 gene for susceptibility to factor V Leiden thrombophilia

S3844 DNA analysis of the connexin 26 gene (GJB2) for susceptibility to congenital, profound deafness

S3845 Genetic testing for alpha-thalassemia

S3846 Genetic testing for hemoglobin E beta-thalassemia

S3847 Genetic testing for Tay-Sachs disease

S3848 Genetic testing for Gaucher disease

S3849 Genetic testing for Niemann-Pick disease

S3850 Genetic testing for sickle cell anemia

S3851 Genetic testing for Canavan disease

S3852 DNA analysis for APOE epilson 4 allele for susceptibility to Alzheimer's disease

S3853 Genetic testing for myotonic muscular dystrophy

S3854 Gene expression profiling panel for use in the management of breast cancer treatment

S3855 Genetic testing for detection of mutations in the presenilin, 1 gene

S3890 DNA analysis, fecal, for colorectal cancer screening

S3900 Surface electromyography (EMG)

S3902 Ballistocardiogram

S3904 Masters two step

S4005 Interim labor facility global (labor occurring but not resulting in delivery) 　Ⓜ♀

● S4011 In vitro fertilization; including but not limited to identification and incubation of mature oocytes, fertilization with sperm, incubation of embryo(s), and subsequent visualization for determination of development 　Ⓜ♀

Special Coverage Instructions　　　Noncovered by Medicare　　　Carrier Discretion　　☑ Quality Alert　　● New Code　　○ Reinstated Code　　▲ Revised Code

2007 HCPCS　　　🔢-🔢 ASC Group　　MED: Pub 100/NCD References　　🔖 DMEPOS Paid　　⊘ SNF Excluded　　S Codes — 137

Temporary National Codes (Non-Medicare)

S4013 — S5501

S4013	Complete cycle, gamete intrafallopian transfer (GIFT), case rate	M ♀
S4014	Complete cycle, zygote intrafallopian transfer (ZIFT), case rate	M ♀
S4015	Complete in vitro fertilization cycle, not otherwise specified, case rate	M ♀
S4016	Frozen in vitro fertilization cycle, case rate	♀
S4017	Incomplete cycle, treatment cancelled prior to stimulation, case rate	♀
S4018	Frozen embryo transfer procedure cancelled before transfer, case rate	♀
S4020	In vitro fertilization procedure cancelled before aspiration, case rate	♀
S4021	In vitro fertilization procedure cancelled after aspiration, case rate	♀
S4022	Assisted oocyte fertilization, case rate	♀
S4023	Donor egg cycle, incomplete, case rate	♀
S4025	Donor services for in vitro fertilization (sperm or embryo), case rate	A
S4026	Procurement of donor sperm from sperm bank	A
S4027	Storage of previously frozen embryos	
S4028	Microsurgical epididymal sperm aspiration (MESA)	A ♂
S4030	Sperm procurement and cryopreservation services; initial visit	A ♂
S4031	Sperm procurement and cryopreservation services; subsequent visit	A ♂
S4035	Stimulated intrauterine insemination (IUI), case rate	♀
~~**S4036**~~	~~Intravaginal culture (IVC), case rate~~	
S4037	Cryopreserved embryo transfer, case rate	
S4040	Monitoring and storage of cryopreserved embryos, per 30 days	
S4042	Management of ovulation induction (interpretation of diagnostic tests and studies, non-face-to-face medical management of the patient), per cycle	
S4981	Insertion of levonorgestrel-releasing intrauterine system	♀
S4989	Contraceptive intrauterine device (e.g., Progestacert IUD), including implants and supplies	♀
☑ **S4990**	Nicotine patches, legend	
☑ **S4991**	Nicotine patches, nonlegend	
S4993	Contraceptive pills for birth control	♀
S4995	Smoking cessation gum	
☑ **S5000**	Prescription drug, generic	
☑ **S5001**	Prescription drug, brand name	
☑ **S5010**	5% dextrose and 45% normal saline, 1000 ml	
☑ **S5011**	5% dextrose in lactated ringer's, 1000 ml	
☑ **S5012**	5% dextrose with potassium chloride, 1000 ml	
☑ **S5013**	5% dextrose/45% normal saline with potassium chloride and magnesium sulfate, 1000 ml	
☑ **S5014**	5% dextrose/45% normal saline with potassium chloride and magnesium sulfate, 1500 ml	
S5035	Home infusion therapy, routine service of infusion device (e.g., pump maintenance)	
S5036	Home infusion therapy, repair of infusion device (e.g., pump repair)	

S5100	Day care services, adult; per 15 minutes	A
S5101	Day care services, adult; per half day	A
S5102	Day care services, adult; per diem	A
S5105	Day care services, center-based; services not included in program fee, per diem	
☑ **S5108**	Home care training to home care client, per 15 minutes	
☑ **S5109**	Home care training to home care client, per session	
S5110	Home care training, family; per 15 minutes	
S5111	Home care training, family; per session	
S5115	Home care training, nonfamily; per 15 minutes	
S5116	Home care training, nonfamily; per session	
S5120	Chore services; per 15 minutes	
S5121	Chore services; per diem	
S5125	Attendant care services; per 15 minutes	
S5126	Attendant care services; per diem	
S5130	Homemaker service, NOS; per 15 minutes	
S5131	Homemaker service, NOS; per diem	
S5135	Companion care, adult (e.g., IADL/ADL); per 15 minutes	A
S5136	Companion care, adult (e.g. IADL/ADL); per diem	A
S5140	Foster care, adult; per diem	A
S5141	Foster care, adult; per month	A
S5145	Foster care, therapeutic, child; per diem	A
S5146	Foster care, therapeutic, child; per month	A
S5150	Unskilled respite care, not hospice; per 15 minutes	
S5151	Unskilled respite care, not hospice; per diem	
S5160	Emergency response system; installation and testing	
S5161	Emergency response system; service fee, per month (excludes installation and testing)	
S5162	Emergency response system; purchase only	
S5165	Home modifications; per service	
S5170	Home delivered meals, including preparation; per meal	
S5175	Laundry service, external, professional; per order	
S5180	Home health respiratory therapy, initial evaluation	
S5181	Home health respiratory therapy, NOS, per diem	
S5185	Medication reminder services, non-face-to-face; per month	
S5190	Wellness assessment, performed by nonphysician	
S5199	Personal care item, NOS, each	
S5497	Home infusion therapy, catheter care/maintenance, not otherwise classified; includes administrative services, professional pharmacy services, care coordination, and all necessary supplies and equipment (drugs and nursing visits coded separately), per diem	
S5498	Home infusion therapy, catheter care/maintenance, simple (single lumen), includes administrative services, professional pharmacy services, care coordination and all necessary supplies and equipment, (drugs and nursing visits coded separately), per diem	
S5501	Home infusion therapy, catheter care/maintenance, complex (more than one lumen), includes administrative services, professional pharmacy services, care coordination, and all necessary supplies and equipment (drugs and nursing visits coded separately), per diem	

Special Coverage Instructions   Noncovered by Medicare   Carrier Discretion   ☑ Quality Alert   ● New Code   ○ Reinstated Code   ▲ Revised Code

138 — S Codes   A Age Edit   M Maternity Edit   ♀ Female Only   ♂ Male Only   A - ☑ APC Status Indicators   **2007 HCPCS**

S5502 Home infusion therapy, catheter care/maintenance, implanted access device, includes administrative services, professional pharmacy services, care coordination and all necessary supplies and equipment, (drugs and nursing visits coded separately), per diem (use this code for interim maintenance of vascular access not currently in use)

S5517 Home infusion therapy, all supplies necessary for restoration of catheter patency or declotting

S5518 Home infusion therapy, all supplies necessary for catheter repair

S5520 Home infusion therapy, all supplies (including catheter) necessary for a peripherally inserted central venous catheter (PICC) line insertion

S5521 Home infusion therapy, all supplies (including catheter) necessary for a midline catheter insertion

S5522 Home infusion therapy, insertion of peripherally inserted central venous catheter (PICC), nursing services only (no supplies or catheter included)

▲ S5523 Home infusion therapy, insertion of midline venous catheter, nursing services only (no supplies or catheter included)

☑ S5550 Insulin, rapid onset, 5 units

☑ S5551 Insulin, most rapid onset (Lispro or Aspart); 5 units

☑ S5552 Insulin, intermediate acting (NPH or LENTE); 5 units

☑ S5553 Insulin, long acting; 5 units

☑ S5560 Insulin delivery device, reusable pen; 1.5 ml size

☑ S5561 Insulin delivery device, reusable pen; 3 ml size

☑ S5565 Insulin cartridge for use in insulin delivery device other than pump; 150 units

☑ S5566 Insulin cartridge for use in insulin delivery device other than pump; 300 units

☑ S5570 Insulin delivery device, disposable pen (including insulin); 1.5 ml size

☑ S5571 Insulin delivery device, disposable pen (including insulin); 3 ml size

S8030 Scleral application of tantalum ring(s) for localization of lesions for proton beam therapy

S8035 Magnetic source imaging

S8037 Magnetic resonance cholangiopancreatography (MRCP)

S8040 Topographic brain mapping

S8042 Magnetic resonance imaging (MRI), low-field

S8049 Intraoperative radiation therapy (single administration)

S8055 Ultrasound guidance for multifetal pregnancy reduction(s), technical component (only to be used when the physician doing the reduction procedure does not perform the ultrasound. Guidance is included in the CPT code for multifetal pregnancy reduction — 59866) Ⓜ ♀

S8075 Computer analysis of full-field digital mammogram and further physician review for interpretation, mammography (list separately in addition to code for primary procedure)

S8080 Scintimammography (radioimmunoscintigraphy of the breast), unilateral, including supply of radiopharmaceutical

S8085 Fluorine-18 fluorodeoxyglucose (F-18 FDG) imaging using dual-head coincidence detection system (nondedicated PET scan)

S8092 Electron beam computed tomography (also known as Ultrafast CT, Cine CT)

S8093 Computed tomographic angiography, coronary arteries, with contrast material(s)

S8096 Portable peak flow meter

☑ S8097 Asthma kit (including but not limited to portable peak expiratory flow meter, instructional video, brochure, and/or spacer)

S8100 Holding chamber or spacer for use with an inhaler or nebulizer; without mask

S8101 Holding chamber or spacer for use with an inhaler or nebulizer; with mask

S8110 Peak expiratory flow rate (physician services)

☑ S8120 Oxygen contents, gaseous, 1 unit equals 1 cubic foot

☑ S8121 Oxygen contents, liquid, 1 unit equals 1 pound

S8185 Flutter device

S8186 Swivel adaptor

☑ S8189 Tracheostomy supply, not otherwise classified

S8190 Electronic spirometer (or microspirometer)

S8210 Mucus trap

S8260 Oral orthotic for treatment of sleep apnea, includes fitting, fabrication, and materials

S8262 Mandibular orthopedic repositioning device, each

S8265 Haberman feeder for cleft lip/palate

☑ S8270 Enuresis alarm, using auditory buzzer and/or vibration device

S8301 Infection control supplies, not otherwise specified

☑ S8415 Supplies for home delivery of infant Ⓜ ♀

S8420 Gradient pressure aid (sleeve and glove combination), custom made

☑ S8421 Gradient pressure aid (sleeve and glove combination), ready made

☑ S8422 Gradient pressure aid (sleeve), custom made, medium weight

☑ S8423 Gradient pressure aid (sleeve), custom made, heavy weight

☑ S8424 Gradient pressure aid (sleeve), ready made

☑ S8425 Gradient pressure aid (glove), custom made, medium weight

☑ S8426 Gradient pressure aid (glove), custom made, heavy weight

☑ S8427 Gradient pressure aid (glove), ready made

☑ S8428 Gradient pressure aid (gauntlet), ready made

☑ S8429 Gradient pressure exterior wrap

☑ S8430 Padding for compression bandage, roll

☑ S8431 Compression bandage, roll

Special Coverage Instructions   Noncovered by Medicare   Carrier Discretion   ☑ Quality Alert   ● New Code   ○ Reinstated Code   ▲ Revised Code

2007 HCPCS   ❶-❾ ASC Group   **MED:** Pub 100/NCD References   ℞ DMEPOS Paid   ⊘ SNF Excluded   **S Codes — 139**

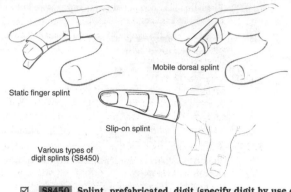

Static finger splint

Mobile dorsal splint

Slip-on splint

Various types of digit splints (S8450)

☑ **S8450** Splint, prefabricated, digit (specify digit by use of modifier)

☑ **S8451** Splint, prefabricated, wrist or ankle

☑ **S8452** Splint, prefabricated, elbow

S8460 Camisole, postmastectomy

☑ **S8490** Insulin syringes (100 syringes, any size)

S8940 Equestrian/hippotherapy, per session

☑ **S8948** Application of a modality (requiring constant provider attendance) to one or more areas; low-level laser; each 15 minutes

S8950 Complex lymphedema therapy, each 15 minutes

S8990 Physical or manipulative therapy performed for maintenance rather than restoration

S8999 Resuscitation bag (for use by patient on artificial respiration during power failure or other catastrophic event)

S9001 Home uterine monitor with or without associated nursing services   Ⓜ ♀

S9007 Ultrafiltration monitor

S9015 Automated EEG monitoring

~~S9022 Digital subtraction angiography (use in addition to CPT code for the procedure for further identification)~~

S9024 Paranasal sinus ultrasound

S9025 Omnicardiogram/cardiointegram

S9034 Extracorporeal shockwave lithotripsy for gall stones If performed with ERCP, use CPT code 43265.

S9055 Procuren or other growth factor preparation to promote wound healing

S9056 Coma stimulation per diem

S9061 Home administration of aerosolized drug therapy (e.g., Pentamidine); administrative services, professional pharmacy services, care coordination, all necessary supplies and equipment (drugs and nursing visits coded separately), per diem

S9075 Smoking cessation treatment

S9083 Global fee urgent care centers

S9088 Services provided in an urgent care center (list in addition to code for service)

S9090 Vertebral axial decompression, per session

S9092 Canolith repositioning, per visit

S9097 Home visit for wound care

S9098 Home visit, phototherapy services (e.g., Bili-lite), including equipment rental, nursing services, blood draw, supplies, and other services, per diem

S9109 Congestive heart failure telemonitoring, equipment rental, including telescale, computer system and software, telephone connections, and maintenance, per month

S9117 Back school, per visit

☑ **S9122** Home health aide or certified nurse assistant, providing care in the home; per hour

☑ **S9123** Nursing care, in the home; by registered nurse, per hour (use for general nursing care only, not to be used when CPT codes 99500–99602 can be used)

☑ **S9124** Nursing care, in the home; by licensed practical nurse, per hour

☑ **S9125** Respite care, in the home, per diem

☑ **S9126** Hospice care, in the home, per diem

☑ **S9127** Social work visit, in the home, per diem

☑ **S9128** Speech therapy, in the home, per diem

☑ **S9129** Occupational therapy, in the home, per diem

S9131 Physical therapy; in the home, per diem

☑ **S9140** Diabetic management program, follow-up visit to non-MD provider

☑ **S9141** Diabetic management program, follow-up visit to MD provider

S9145 Insulin pump initiation, instruction in initial use of pump (pump not included)

S9150 Evaluation by ocularist

S9208 Home management of preterm labor, including administrative services, professional pharmacy services, care coordination, and all necessary supplies or equipment (drugs and nursing visits coded separately), per diem (do not use this code with any home infusion per diem code)   Ⓜ ♀

S9209 Home management of preterm premature rupture of membranes (PPROM), including administrative services, professional pharmacy services, care coordination, and all necessary supplies or equipment (drugs and nursing visits coded separately), per diem (do not use this code with any home infusion per diem code)   Ⓜ ♀

S9211 Home management of gestational hypertension, includes administrative services, professional pharmacy services, care coordination and all necessary supplies and equipment (drugs and nursing visits coded separately); per diem (do not use this code with any home infusion per diem code)   Ⓜ ♀

S9212 Home management of postpartum hypertension, includes administrative services, professional pharmacy services, care coordination, and all necessary supplies and equipment (drugs and nursing visits coded separately), per diem (do not use this code with any home infusion per diem code)   ♀

S9213 Home management of preeclampsia, includes administrative services, professional pharmacy services, care coordination, and all necessary supplies and equipment (drugs and nursing services coded separately); per diem (do not use this code with any home infusion per diem code)   Ⓜ ♀

S9214 Home management of gestational diabetes, includes administrative services, professional pharmacy services, care coordination, and all necessary supplies and equipment (drugs and nursing visits coded separately); per diem (do not use this code with any home infusion per diem code)   Ⓜ ♀

Special Coverage Instructions   Noncovered by Medicare   Carrier Discretion   ☑ Quality Alert   ● New Code   ○ Reinstated Code   ▲ Revised Code

140 — S Codes   Ⓐ Age Edit   Ⓜ Maternity Edit   ♀ Female Only   ♂ Male Only   Ⓐ - Ⓨ APC Status Indicators   *2007 HCPCS*

S9325 Home infusion therapy, pain management infusion; administrative services, professional pharmacy services, care coordination, and all necessary supplies and equipment, (drugs and nursing visits coded separately), per diem (do not use this code with S9326, S9327 or S9328)

S9326 Home infusion therapy, continuous (24 hours or more) pain management infusion; administrative services, professional pharmacy services, care coordination and all necessary supplies and equipment (drugs and nursing visits coded separately), per diem

S9327 Home infusion therapy, intermittent (less than 24 hours) pain management infusion; administrative services, professional pharmacy services, care coordination, and all necessary supplies and equipment (drugs and nursing visits coded separately), per diem

S9328 Home infusion therapy, implanted pump pain management infusion; administrative services, professional pharmacy services, care coordination, and all necessary supplies and equipment (drugs and nursing visits coded separately), per diem

S9329 Home infusion therapy, chemotherapy infusion; administrative services, professional pharmacy services, care coordination, and all necessary supplies and equipment (drugs and nursing visits coded separately), per diem (do not use this code with S9330 or S9331)

S9330 Home infusion therapy, continuous (24 hours or more) chemotherapy infusion; administrative services, professional pharmacy services, care coordination, and all necessary supplies and equipment (drugs and nursing visits coded separately), per diem

S9331 Home infusion therapy, intermittent (less than 24 hours) chemotherapy infusion; administrative services, professional pharmacy services, care coordination, and all necessary supplies and equipment (drugs and nursing visits coded separately), per diem

☑ **S9335** Home therapy, hemodialysis; administrative services, professional pharmacy services, care coordination, and all necessary supplies and equipment (drugs and nursing services coded separately), per diem

S9336 Home infusion therapy, continuous anticoagulant infusion therapy (e.g., Heparin), administrative services, professional pharmacy services, care coordination and all necessary supplies and equipment (drugs and nursing visits coded separately), per diem

S9338 Home infusion therapy, immunotherapy, administrative services, professional pharmacy services, care coordination, and all necessary supplies and equipment (drugs and nursing visits coded separately), per diem

S9339 Home therapy; peritoneal dialysis, administrative services, professional pharmacy services, care coordination and all necessary supplies and equipment (drugs and nursing visits coded separately), per diem

S9340 Home therapy; enteral nutrition; administrative services, professional pharmacy services, care coordination, and all necessary supplies and equipment (enteral formula and nursing visits coded separately), per diem

S9341 Home therapy; enteral nutrition via gravity; administrative services, professional pharmacy services, care coordination, and all necessary supplies and equipment (enteral formula and nursing visits coded separately), per diem

S9342 Home therapy; enteral nutrition via pump; administrative services, professional pharmacy services, care coordination, and all necessary supplies and equipment (enteral formula and nursing visits coded separately), per diem

S9343 Home therapy; enteral nutrition via bolus; administrative services, professional pharmacy services, care coordination, and all necessary supplies and equipment (enteral formula and nursing visits coded separately), per diem

S9345 Home infusion therapy, anti-hemophilic agent infusion therapy (e.g., factor VIII); administrative services, professional pharmacy services, care coordination, and all necessary supplies and equipment (drugs and nursing visits coded separately), per diem

S9346 Home infusion therapy, alpha-1-proteinase inhibitor (e.g., Prolastin); administrative services, professional pharmacy services, care coordination, and all necessary supplies and equipment (drugs and nursing visits coded separately), per diem

S9347 Home infusion therapy, uninterrupted, long-term, controlled rate intravenous or subcutaneous infusion therapy (e.g., Epoprostenol); administrative services, professional pharmacy services, care coordination, and all necessary supplies and equipment (drugs and nursing visits coded separately), per diem

S9348 Home infusion therapy, sympathomimetic/inotropic agent infusion therapy (e.g., Dobutamine); administrative services, professional pharmacy services, care coordination, all necessary supplies and equipment (drugs and nursing visits coded separately), per diem

S9349 Home infusion therapy, tocolytic infusion therapy; administrative services, professional pharmacy services, care coordination, and all necessary supplies and equipment (drugs and nursing visits coded separately), per diem ⓜ ♀

S9351 Home infusion therapy, continuous antiemetic infusion therapy; administrative services, professional pharmacy services, care coordination, all necessary supplies and equipment (drugs and nursing visits coded separately), per diem

S9353 Home infusion therapy, continuous insulin infusion therapy; administrative services, professional pharmacy services, care coordination, and all necessary supplies and equipment (drugs and nursing visits coded separately), per diem

S9355 Home infusion therapy, chelation therapy; administrative services, professional pharmacy services, care coordination, and all necessary supplies and equipment (drugs and nursing visits coded separately), per diem

S9357 Home infusion therapy, enzyme replacement intravenous therapy; (e.g., Imiglucerase); administrative services, professional pharmacy services, care coordination, and all necessary supplies and equipment (drugs and nursing visits coded separately), per diem

S9359 Home infusion therapy, antitumor necrosis factor intravenous therapy; (e.g., Infliximab); administrative services, professional pharmacy services, care coordination, and all necessary supplies and equipment (drugs and nursing visits coded separately), per diem

S9361 Home infusion therapy, diuretic intravenous therapy; administrative services, professional pharmacy services, care coordination, and all necessary supplies and equipment (drugs and nursing visits coded separately), per diem

Special Coverage Instructions   Noncovered by Medicare   Carrier Discretion   ☑ Quality Alert   ● New Code   ○ Reinstated Code   ▲ Revised Code

2007 HCPCS   **1-9** ASC Group   **MED:** Pub 100/NCD References   ♿ DMEPOS Paid   ⊘ SNF Excluded   **S Codes — 141**

S9363 Home infusion therapy, antispasmotic therapy; administrative services, professional pharmacy services, care coordination, and all necessary supplies and equipment (drugs and nursing visits coded separately), per diem

S9364 Home infusion therapy, total parenteral nutrition (TPN); administrative services, professional pharmacy services, care coordination, and all necessary supplies and equipment including standard TPN formula (lipids, specialty amino acid formulas, drugs other than in standard formula and nursing visits coded separately), per diem (do not use with home infusion codes S9365–S9368 using daily volume scales)

S9365 Home infusion therapy, total parenteral nutrition (TPN); 1 liter per day, administrative services, professional pharmacy services, care coordination, and all necessary supplies and equipment including standard TPN formula (lipids, specialty amino acid formulas, drugs other than in standard formula and nursing visits coded separately), per diem

S9366 Home infusion therapy, total parenteral nutrition (TPN); more than 1 liter but no more than 2 liters per day, administrative services, professional pharmacy services, care coordination, and all necessary supplies and equipment including standard TPN formula (lipids, specialty amino acid formulas, drugs other than in standard formula and nursing visits coded separately), per diem

S9367 Home infusion therapy, total parenteral nutrition (TPN); more than 2 liters but no more than 3 liters per day, administrative services, professional pharmacy services, care coordination, and all necessary supplies and equipment including standard TPN formula (lipids, specialty amino acid formulas, drugs other than in standard formula and nursing visits coded separately), per diem

S9368 Home infusion therapy, total parenteral nutrition (TPN); more than 3 liters per day, administrative services, professional pharmacy services, care coordination, and all necessary supplies and equipment including standard TPN formula (lipids, specialty amino acid formulas, drugs other than in standard formula and nursing visits coded separately), per diem

S9370 Home therapy, intermittent antiemetic injection therapy; administrative services, professional pharmacy services, care coordination, and all necessary supplies and equipment (drugs and nursing visits coded separately), per diem

S9372 Home therapy; intermittent anticoagulant injection therapy (e.g., Heparin); administrative services, professional pharmacy services, care coordination, and all necessary supplies and equipment (drugs and nursing visits coded separately), per diem (do not use this code for flushing of infusion devices with Heparin to maintain patency)

S9373 Home infusion therapy, hydration therapy; administrative services, professional pharmacy services, care coordination, and all necessary supplies and equipment (drugs and nursing visits coded separately), per diem (do not use with hydration therapy codes S9374–S9377 using daily volume scales)

S9374 Home infusion therapy, hydration therapy; one liter per day, administrative services, professional pharmacy services, care coordination, and all necessary supplies and equipment (drugs and nursing visits coded separately), per diem

S9375 Home infusion therapy, hydration therapy; more than one liter but no more than two liters per day, administrative services, professional pharmacy services, care coordination, and all necessary supplies and equipment (drugs and nursing visits coded separately), per diem

S9376 Home infusion therapy, hydration therapy; more than two liters but no more than three liters per day, administrative services, professional pharmacy services, care coordination, and all necessary supplies and equipment (drugs and nursing visits coded separately), per diem

S9377 Home infusion therapy, hydration therapy; more than three liters per day, administrative services, professional pharmacy services, care coordination, and all necessary supplies (drugs and nursing visits coded separately), per diem

S9379 Home infusion therapy, infusion therapy, not otherwise classified; administrative services, professional pharmacy services, care coordination, and all necessary supplies and equipment (drugs and nursing visits coded separately), per diem

S9381 Delivery or service to high risk areas requiring escort or extra protection, per visit

S9401 Anticoagulation clinic, inclusive of all services except laboratory tests, per session

S9430 Pharmacy compounding and dispensing services

S9434 Modified solid food supplements for inborn errors of metabolism

S9435 Medical foods for inborn errors of metabolism

S9436 Childbirth preparation/Lamaze classes, nonphysician provider, per session Ⓐ ♀

S9437 Childbirth refresher classes, nonphysician provider, per session Ⓐ ♀

S9438 Cesarean birth classes, nonphysician provider, per session Ⓐ ♀

S9439 VBAC (vaginal birth after cesarean) classes, nonphysician provider, per session Ⓐ ♀

S9441 Asthma education, nonphysician provider, per session

S9442 Birthing classes, nonphysician provider, per session Ⓐ ♀

S9443 Lactation classes, nonphysician provider, per session Ⓐ ♀

S9444 Parenting classes, nonphysician provider, per session Ⓐ

S9445 Patient education, not otherwise classified, nonphysician provider, individual, per session

S9446 Patient education, not otherwise classified, nonphysician provider, group, per session

S9447 Infant safety (including CPR) classes, nonphysician provider, per session

S9449 Weight management classes, nonphysician provider, per session

S9451 Exercise classes, nonphysician provider, per session

S9452 Nutrition classes, nonphysician provider, per session

S9453 Smoking cessation classes, nonphysician provider, per session

S9454 Stress management classes, nonphysician provider, per session

S9455 Diabetic management program, group session

Special Coverage Instructions   Noncovered by Medicare   Carrier Discretion   ☑ Quality Alert   ● New Code   ○ Reinstated Code   ▲ Revised Code

142 — S Codes   Ⓐ Age Edit   Ⓜ Maternity Edit   ♀ Female Only   ♂ Male Only   Ⓐ - ☑ APC Status Indicators   *2007 HCPCS*

S9460 Diabetic management program, nurse visit

S9465 Diabetic management program, dietitian visit

S9470 Nutritional counseling, dietitian visit

S9472 Cardiac rehabilitation program, nonphysician provider, per diem

S9473 Pulmonary rehabilitation program, nonphysician provider, per diem

S9474 Enterostomal therapy by a registered nurse certified in enterostomal therapy, per diem

S9475 Ambulatory setting substance abuse treatment or detoxification services, per diem

☑ S9476 Vestibular rehabilitation program, nonphysician provider, per diem

S9480 Intensive outpatient psychiatric services, per diem

☑ S9482 Family stabilization services, per 15 minutes

S9484 Crisis intervention mental health services, per hour

S9485 Crisis intervention mental health services, per diem

S9490 Home infusion therapy, corticosteroid infusion; administrative services, professional pharmacy services, care coordination, and all necessary supplies and equipment (drugs and nursing visits coded separately), per diem

S9494 Home infusion therapy, antibiotic, antiviral, or antifungal therapy; administrative services, professional pharmacy services, care coordination, and all necessary supplies and equipment (drugs and nursing visits coded separately, per diem) (do not use this code with home infusion codes for hourly dosing schedules S9497–S9504)

S9497 Home infusion therapy, antibiotic, antiviral, or antifungal therapy; once every three hours; administrative services, professional pharmacy services, care coordination, and all necessary supplies and equipment (drugs and nursing visits coded separately), per diem

S9500 Home infusion therapy, antibiotic, antiviral, or antifungal therapy; once every 24 hours; administrative services, professional pharmacy services, care coordination, and all necessary supplies and equipment (drugs and nursing visits coded separately), per diem

S9501 Home infusion therapy, antibiotic, antiviral, or antifungal therapy; once every 12 hours; administrative services, professional pharmacy services, care coordination, and all necessary supplies and equipment (drugs and nursing visits coded separately), per diem

S9502 Home infusion therapy, antibiotic, antiviral, or antifungal therapy; once every eight hours, administrative services, professional pharmacy services, care coordination, and all necessary supplies and equipment (drugs and nursing visits coded separately), per diem

S9503 Home infusion therapy, antibiotic, antiviral, or antifungal; once every six hours; administrative services, professional pharmacy services, care coordination, and all necessary supplies and equipment (drugs and nursing visits coded separately), per diem

S9504 Home infusion therapy, antibiotic, antiviral, or antifungal; once every four hours; administrative services, professional pharmacy services, care coordination, and all necessary supplies and equipment (drugs and nursing visits coded separately), per diem

S9529 Routine venipuncture for collection of specimen(s), single home bound, nursing home, or skilled nursing facility patient

S9537 Home therapy; hematopoietic hormone injection therapy (e.g., erythropoietin, G-CSF, GM-CSF); administrative services, professional pharmacy services, care coordination, and all necessary supplies and equipment (drugs and nursing visits coded separately), per diem

S9538 Home transfusion of blood product(s); administrative services, professional pharmacy services, care coordination and all necessary supplies and equipment (blood products, drugs, and nursing visits coded separately), per diem

S9542 Home injectable therapy, not otherwise classified, including administrative services, professional pharmacy services, care coordination, and all necessary supplies and equipment (drugs and nursing visits coded separately), per diem

S9558 Home injectable therapy; growth hormone, including administrative services, professional pharmacy services, care coordination, and all necessary supplies and equipment (drugs and nursing visits coded separately), per diem

S9559 Home injectable therapy, interferon, including administrative services, professional pharmacy services, care coordination, and all necessary supplies and equipment (drugs and nursing visits coded separately), per diem

S9560 Home injectable therapy; hormonal therapy (e.g.; leuprolide, goserelin), including administrative services, professional pharmacy services, care coordination, and all necessary supplies and equipment (drugs and nursing visits coded separately), per diem

S9562 Home injectable therapy, palivizumab, including administrative services, professional pharmacy services, care coordination, and all necessary supplies and equipment (drugs and nursing visits coded separately), per diem

S9590 Home therapy, irrigation therapy (e.g., sterile irrigation of an organ or anatomical cavity); including administrative services, professional pharmacy services, care coordination, and all necessary supplies and equipment (drugs and nursing visits coded separately), per diem

S9810 Home therapy; professional pharmacy services for provision of infusion, specialty drug administration, and/or disease state management, not otherwise classified, per hour (do not use this code with any per diem code)

S9900 Services by authorized Christian Science practitioner for the process of healing, per diem; not to be used for rest or study; excludes in-patient services

S9970 Health club membership, annual

S9975 Transplant related lodging, meals and transportation, per diem

S9976 Lodging, per diem, not otherwise specified

S9977 Meals, per diem not otherwise specified

S9981 Medical records copying fee, administrative

S9982 Medical records copying fee, per page

S9986 Not medically necessary service (patient is aware that service not medically necessary)

S9988 Services provided as part of a Phase 1 clinical trial

S9989 Services provided outside of the United States of America (list in addition to code(s) for services(s))

S9990 Services provided as part of a Phase II clinical trial

S9991 Services provided as part of a Phase III clinical trial

Special Coverage Instructions | Noncovered by Medicare | Carrier Discretion | ☑ Quality Alert | ● New Code | ○ Reinstated Code | ▲ Revised Code

2007 HCPCS | 1-9 ASC Group | MED: Pub 100/NCD References | DMEPOS Paid | ○ SNF Excluded | S Codes — 143

Temporary National Codes (Non-Medicare)

S9992 — S9999

S9992 Transportation costs to and from trial location and local transportation costs (e.g., fares for taxicab or bus) for clinical trial participant and one caregiver/companion

S9994 Lodging costs (e.g., hotel charges) for clinical trial participant and one caregiver/companion

S9996 Meals for clinical trial participant and one caregiver/companion

S9999 Sales tax

Special Coverage Instructions   Noncovered by Medicare   Carrier Discretion   ☑ Quality Alert   ● New Code   ○ Reinstated Code   ▲ Revised Code

144 — S Codes   Ⓐ Age Edit   Ⓜ Maternity Edit   ♀ Female Only   ♂ Male Only   Ⓐ - Ⓨ APC Status Indicators   *2007 HCPCS*

NATIONAL T CODES ESTABLISHED FOR STATE MEDICAID AGENCIES T1000-T9999

The T codes are designed for use by Medicaid state agencies to establish codes for items for which there are no permanent national codes but for which codes are necessary to administer the Medicaid program (T codes are not accepted by Medicare but can be used by private insurers). This range of codes describes nursing and home health-related services, substance abuse treatment, and certain training-related procedures.

These codes are not valid for Medicare.

T1000 Private duty/independent nursing service(s) — licensed, up to 15 minutes

T1001 Nursing assessment/evaluation

T1002 RN services, up to 15 minutes

T1003 LPN/LVN services, up to 15 minutes

T1004 Services of a qualified nursing aide, up to 15 minutes

T1005 Respite care services, up to 15 minutes

T1006 Alcohol and/or substance abuse services, family/couple counseling

T1007 Alcohol and/or substance abuse services, treatment plan development and/or modification

T1009 Child sitting services for children of the individual receiving alcohol and/or substance abuse services

T1010 Meals for individuals receiving alcohol and/or substance abuse services (when meals not included in the program)

T1012 Alcohol and/or substance abuse services, skills development

T1013 Sign language or oral interpretive services, per 15 minutes

T1014 Telehealth transmission, per minute, professional services bill separately

T1015 Clinic visit/encounter, all-inclusive

T1016 Case management, each 15 minutes

T1017 Targeted case management, each 15 minutes

T1018 School-based individualized education program (IEP) services, bundled

T1019 Personal care services, per 15 minutes, not for an inpatient or resident of a hospital, nursing facility, ICF/MR or IMD, part of the individualized plan of treatment (code may not be used to identify services provided by home health aide or certified nurse assistant)

T1020 Personal care services, per diem, not for an inpatient or resident of a hospital, nursing facility, ICF/MR or IMD, part of the individualized plan of treatment (code may not be used to identify services provided by home health aide or certified nurse assistant)

T1021 Home health aide or certified nurse assistant, per visit

T1022 Contracted home health agency services, all services provided under contract, per day

T1023 Screening to determine the appropriateness of consideration of an individual for participation in a specified program, project or treatment protocol, per encounter

T1024 Evaluation and treatment by an integrated, specialty team contracted to provide coordinated care to multiple or severely handicapped children, per encounter

T1025 Intensive, extended multidisciplinary services provided in a clinic setting to children with complex medical, physical, mental and psychosocial impairments, per diem

T1026 Intensive, extended multidisciplinary services provided in a clinic setting to children with complex medical, physical, medical and psychosocial impairments, per hour

T1027 Family training and counseling for child development, per 15 minutes

T1028 Assessment of home, physical and family environment, to determine suitability to meet patient's medical needs

T1029 Comprehensive environmental lead investigation, not including laboratory analysis, per dwelling

T1030 Nursing care, in the home, by registered nurse, per diem

T1031 Nursing care, in the home, by licensed practical nurse, per diem

T1502 Administration of oral, intramuscular and/or subcutaneous medication by health care agency/professional, per visit

T1999 Miscellaneous therapeutic items and supplies, retail purchases, not otherwise classified; identify product in remarks

T2001 Nonemergency transportation; patient attendant/escort

T2002 Nonemergency transportation; per diem

T2003 Nonemergency transportation; encounter/trip

T2004 Nonemergency transport; commercial carrier, multipass

T2005 Nonemergency transportation; stretcher van

T2007 Transportation waiting time, air ambulance and nonemergency vehicle, one-half (1/2) hour increments

☑ **T2010** Preadmission screening and resident review (PASRR) level I identification screening, per screen

T2011 Preadmission screening and resident review (PASRR) level II evaluation, per evaluation

☑ **T2012** Habilitation, educational; waiver, per diem

☑ **T2013** Habilitation, educational, waiver; per hour

☑ **T2014** Habilitation, prevocational, waiver; per diem

☑ **T2015** Habilitation, prevocational, waiver; per hour

☑ **T2016** Habilitation, residential, waiver; per diem

☑ **T2017** Habilitation, residential, waiver; 15 minutes

☑ **T2018** Habilitation, supported employment, waiver; per diem

☑ **T2019** Habilitation, supported employment, waiver; per 15 minutes

☑ **T2020** Day habilitation, waiver; per diem

☑ **T2021** Day habilitation, waiver; per 15 minutes

☑ **T2022** Case management, per month

☑ **T2023** Targeted case management; per month

T2024 Service assessment/plan of care development, waiver

T2025 Waiver services; not otherwise specified (NOS)

Special Coverage Instructions   Noncovered by Medicare   Carrier Discretion   ☑ Quality Alert   ● New Code   ○ Reinstated Code   ▲ Revised Code

2007 HCPCS   **1-9** ASC Group   MED: Pub 100/NCD References   ℞ DMEPOS Paid   ⊘ SNF Excluded   **T Codes — 145**

National T Codes

T2026 — T5999

☑ **T2026** Specialized childcare, waiver; per diem

☑ **T2027** Specialized childcare, waiver; per 15 minutes

T2028 Specialized supply, not otherwise specified, waiver

T2029 Specialized medical equipment, not otherwise specified, waiver

☑ **T2030** Assisted living, waiver; per month

☑ **T2031** Assisted living; waiver, per diem

☑ **T2032** Residential care, not otherwise specified (NOS), waiver; per month

☑ **T2033** Residential care, not otherwise specified (NOS), waiver; per diem

☑ **T2034** Crisis intervention, waiver; per diem

T2035 Utility services to support medical equipment and assistive technology/devices, waiver

☑ **T2036** Therapeutic camping, overnight, waiver; each session

☑ **T2037** Therapeutic camping, day, waiver; each session

☑ **T2038** Community transition, waiver; per service

☑ **T2039** Vehicle modifications, waiver; per service

☑ **T2040** Financial management, self-directed, waiver; per 15 minutes

☑ **T2041** Supports brokerage, self-directed, waiver; per 15 minutes

☑ **T2042** Hospice routine home care; per diem

☑ **T2043** Hospice continuous home care; per hour

☑ **T2044** Hospice inpatient respite care; per diem

☑ **T2045** Hospice general inpatient care; per diem

☑ **T2046** Hospice long term care, room and board only; per diem

☑ **T2048** Behavioral health; long-term care residential (nonacute care in a residential treatment program where stay is typically longer than 30 days), with room and board, per diem

☑ **T2049** Nonemergency transportation; stretcher van, mileage; per mile

T2101 Human breast milk processing, storage and distribution only ♀

☑ **T4521** Adult sized disposable incontinence product, brief/diaper, small, each
MED: 100-3,230.10

☑ **T4522** Adult sized disposable incontinence product, brief/diaper, medium, each
MED: 100-3,230.10

☑ **T4523** Adult sized disposable incontinence product, brief/diaper, large, each
MED: 100-3,230.10

☑ **T4524** Adult sized disposable incontinence product, brief/diaper, extra large, each
MED: 100-3,230.10

☑ **T4525** Adult sized disposable incontinence product, protective underwear/pull-on, small size, each
MED: 100-3,230.10

☑ **T4526** Adult sized disposable incontinence product, protective underwear/pull-on, medium size, each
MED: 100-3,230.10

☑ **T4527** Adult sized disposable incontinence product, protective underwear/pull-on, large size, each
MED: 100-3,230.10

☑ **T4528** Adult sized disposable incontinence product, protective underwear/pull-on, extra large size, each
MED: 100-3,230.10

☑ **T4529** Pediatric sized disposable incontinence product, brief/diaper, small/medium size, each
MED: 100-3,230.10

☑ **T4530** Pediatric sized disposable incontinence product, brief/diaper, large size, each
MED: 100-3,230.10

☑ **T4531** Pediatric sized disposable incontinence product, protective underwear/pull-on, small/medium size, each
MED: 100-3,230.10

☑ **T4532** Pediatric sized disposable incontinence product, protective underwear/pull-on, large size, each
MED: 100-3,230.10

☑ **T4533** Youth sized disposable incontinence product, brief/diaper, each
MED: 100-3,230.10

☑ **T4534** Youth sized disposable incontinence product, protective underwear/pull-on, each
MED: 100-3,230.10

☑ **T4535** Disposable liner/shield/guard/pad/undergarment, for incontinence, each
MED: 100-3,230.10

☑ **T4536** Incontinence product, protective underwear/pull-on, reusable, any size, each
MED: 100-3,230.10

☑ **T4537** Incontinence product, protective underpad, reusable, bed size, each
MED: 100-3,230.10

☑ **T4538** Diaper service, reusable diaper, each diaper
MED: 100-3,230.10

☑ **T4539** Incontinence product, diaper/brief, reusable, any size, each
MED: 100-3,230.10

☑ **T4540** Incontinence product, protective underpad, reusable, chair size, each
MED: 100-3,230.10

☑ **T4541** Incontinence product, disposable underpad, large, each

☑ **T4542** Incontinence product, disposable underpad, small size, each

● **T4543** Disposable incontinence product, brief/diaper, bariatric, each

▲ **T5001** Positioning seat for persons with special orthopedic needs

T5999 Supply, not otherwise specified

Special Coverage Instructions   Noncovered by Medicare   Carrier Discretion   ☑ Quality Alert   ● New Code   ○ Reinstated Code ▲ Revised Code

146 — T Codes   Ⓐ Age Edit   Ⓜ Maternity Edit ♀ Female Only   ♂ Male Only   Ⓐ - ☑ APC Status Indicators   *2007 HCPCS*

VISION SERVICES V0000-V2999

These V codes include vision-related supplies, including spectacles, lenses, contact lenses, prostheses, intraocular lenses, and miscellaneous lenses.

FRAMES

V codes fall under the jurisdiction of the DME Medicare Administrative Contractor (DME MAC), unless incident to other services or otherwise noted.

Ⓐ   **V2020**   Frames, purchases   と
          MED: 100-2,15,120; 100-4,3,10.4

Ⓔ   **V2025**   Deluxe frame
          MED: 100-4,1,30.3.5

SPECTACLE LENSES

See S0500-S0592 for temporary vision codes.

SINGLE VISION, GLASS, OR PLASTIC

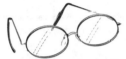
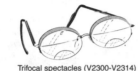

Monofocal spectacles (V2100-V2114)   Trifocal spectacles (V2300-V2314)

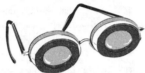

Low vision aids mounted to spectacles (V2610)   Telescopic or other compound lens fitted on spectacles as a low vision aid (V2615)

Ⓐ ☑ **V2100** Sphere, single vision, plano to plus or minus 4.00, per lens   と

Ⓐ ☑ **V2101** Sphere, single vision, plus or minus 4.12 to plus or minus 7.00d, per lens   と

Ⓐ ☑ **V2102** Sphere, single vision, plus or minus 7.12 to plus or minus 20.00d, per lens   と

Ⓐ ☑ **V2103** Spherocylinder, single vision, plano to plus or minus 4.00d sphere, 0.12 to 2.00d cylinder, per lens   と

Ⓐ ☑ **V2104** Spherocylinder, single vision, plano to plus or minus 4.00d sphere, 2.12 to 4.00d cylinder, per lens   と

Ⓐ ☑ **V2105** Spherocylinder, single vision, plano to plus or minus 4.00d sphere, 4.25 to 6.00d cylinder, per lens   と

Ⓐ ☑ **V2106** Spherocylinder, single vision, plano to plus or minus 4.00d sphere, over 6.00d cylinder, per lens   と

Ⓐ ☑ **V2107** Spherocylinder, single vision, plus or minus 4.25 to plus or minus 7.00 sphere, 0.12 to 2.00d cylinder, per lens   と

Ⓐ ☑ **V2108** Spherocylinder, single vision, plus or minus 4.25d to plus or minus 7.00d sphere, 2.12 to 4.00d cylinder, per lens   と

Ⓐ ☑ **V2109** Spherocylinder, single vision, plus or minus 4.25 to plus or minus 7.00d sphere, 4.25 to 6.00d cylinder, per lens   と

Ⓐ ☑ **V2110** Spherocylinder, single vision, plus or minus 4.25 to 7.00d sphere, over 6.00d cylinder, per lens   と

Ⓐ ☑ **V2111** Spherocylinder, single vision, plus or minus 7.25 to plus or minus 12.00d sphere, 0.25 to 2.25d cylinder, per lens   と

Ⓐ ☑ **V2112** Spherocylinder, single vision, plus or minus 7.25 to plus or minus 12.00d sphere, 2.25d to 4.00d cylinder, per lens   と

Ⓐ ☑ **V2113** Spherocylinder, single vision, plus or minus 7.25 to plus or minus 12.00d sphere, 4.25 to 6.00d cylinder, per lens   と

Ⓐ ☑ **V2114** Spherocylinder, single vision sphere over plus or minus 12.00d, per lens   と

Ⓐ ☑ **V2115** Lenticular (myodisc), per lens, single vision   と

Ⓐ   **V2118** Aniseikonic lens, single vision   と

Ⓐ   **V2121** Lenticular lens, per lens, single   と
         MED: 100-2,15,120; 100-4,3,10.4

Ⓐ   **V2199** Not otherwise classified, single vision lens

BIFOCAL, GLASS, OR PLASTIC

Ⓐ ☑ **V2200** Sphere, bifocal, plano to plus or minus 4.00d, per lens   と

Ⓐ ☑ **V2201** Sphere, bifocal, plus or minus 4.12 to plus or minus 7.00d, per lens   と

Ⓐ ☑ **V2202** Sphere, bifocal, plus or minus 7.12 to plus or minus 20.00d, per lens   と

Ⓐ ☑ **V2203** Spherocylinder, bifocal, plano to plus or minus 4.00d sphere, 0.12 to 2.00d cylinder, per lens   と

Ⓐ ☑ **V2204** Spherocylinder, bifocal, plano to plus or minus 4.00d sphere, 2.12 to 4.00d cylinder, per lens   と

Ⓐ ☑ **V2205** Spherocylinder, bifocal, plano to plus or minus 4.00d sphere, 4.25 to 6.00d cylinder, per lens   と

Ⓐ ☑ **V2206** Spherocylinder, bifocal, plano to plus or minus 4.00d sphere, over 6.00d cylinder, per lens

Ⓐ ☑ **V2207** Spherocylinder, bifocal, plus or minus 4.25 to plus or minus 7.00d sphere, 0.12 to 2.00d cylinder, per lens   と

Ⓐ ☑ **V2208** Spherocylinder, bifocal, plus or minus 4.25 to plus or minus 7.00d sphere, 2.12 to 4.00d cylinder, per lens   と

Ⓐ ☑ **V2209** Spherocylinder, bifocal, plus or minus 4.25 to plus or minus 7.00d sphere, 4.25 to 6.00d cylinder, per lens   と

Ⓐ ☑ **V2210** Spherocylinder, bifocal, plus or minus 4.25 to plus or minus 7.00d sphere, over 6.00d cylinder, per lens   と

Ⓐ ☑ **V2211** Spherocylinder, bifocal, plus or minus 7.25 to plus or minus 12.00d sphere, 0.25 to 2.25d cylinder, per lens   と

Ⓐ ☑ **V2212** Spherocylinder, bifocal, plus or minus 7.25 to plus or minus 12.00d sphere, 2.25 to 4.00d cylinder, per lens   と

Ⓐ ☑ **V2213** Spherocylinder, bifocal, plus or minus 7.25 to plus or minus 12.00d sphere, 4.25 to 6.00d cylinder, per lens   と

Ⓐ ☑ **V2214** Spherocylinder, bifocal, sphere over plus or minus 12.00d, per lens   と

Ⓐ ☑ **V2215** Lenticular (myodisc), per lens, bifocal   と

Ⓐ ☑ **V2218** Aniseikonic, per lens, bifocal   と

Ⓐ ☑ **V2219** Bifocal seg width over 28mm   と

Ⓐ ☑ **V2220** Bifocal add over 3.25d   と

Ⓐ   **V2221** Lenticular lens, per lens, bifocal   と
         MED: 100-2,15,120; 100-4,3,10.4

Ⓐ   **V2299** Specialty bifocal (by report)
         Pertinent documentation to evaluate medical appropriateness should be included when this code is reported.

Special Coverage Instructions   Noncovered by Medicare   Carrier Discretion   ☑ Quality Alert   ● New Code   ○ Reinstated Code   ▲ Revised Code

2007 HCPCS   1-9 ASC Group   MED: Pub 100/NCD References   と DMEPOS Paid   Ⓢ SNF Excluded   **V Codes — 147**

TRIFOCAL, GLASS, OR PLASTIC

Ⓐ ☑ **V2300** Sphere, trifocal, plano to plus or minus 4.00d, per lens

Ⓐ ☑ **V2301** Sphere, trifocal, plus or minus 4.12 to plus or minus 7.00d per lens

Ⓐ ☑ **V2302** Sphere, trifocal, plus or minus 7.12 to plus or minus 20.00, per lens

Ⓐ ☑ **V2303** Spherocylinder, trifocal, plano to plus or minus 4.00d sphere, 0.12 to 2.00d cylinder, per lens

Ⓐ ☑ **V2304** Spherocylinder, trifocal, plano to plus or minus 4.00d sphere, 2.25 to 4.00d cylinder, per lens

Ⓐ ☑ **V2305** Spherocylinder, trifocal, plano to plus or minus 4.00d sphere, 4.25 to 6.00 cylinder, per lens

Ⓐ ☑ **V2306** Spherocylinder, trifocal, plano to plus or minus 4.00d sphere, over 6.00d cylinder, per lens

Ⓐ ☑ **V2307** Spherocylinder, trifocal, plus or minus 4.25 to plus or minus 7.00d sphere, 0.12 to 2.00d cylinder, per lens

Ⓐ ☑ **V2308** Spherocylinder, trifocal, plus or minus 4.25 to plus or minus 7.00d sphere, 2.12 to 4.00d cylinder, per lens

Ⓐ ☑ **V2309** Spherocylinder, trifocal, plus or minus 4.25 to plus or minus 7.00d sphere, 4.25 to 6.00d cylinder, per lens

Ⓐ ☑ **V2310** Spherocylinder, trifocal, plus or minus 4.25 to plus or minus 7.00d sphere, over 6.00d cylinder, per lens

Ⓐ ☑ **V2311** Spherocylinder, trifocal, plus or minus 7.25 to plus or minus 12.00d sphere, 0.25 to 2.25d cylinder, per lens

Ⓐ ☑ **V2312** Spherocylinder, trifocal, plus or minus 7.25 to plus or minus 12.00d sphere, 2.25 to 4.00d cylinder, per lens

Ⓐ ☑ **V2313** Spherocylinder, trifocal, plus or minus 7.25 to plus or minus 12.00d sphere, 4.25 to 6.00d cylinder, per lens

Ⓐ ☑ **V2314** Spherocylinder, trifocal, sphere over plus or minus 12.00d, per lens

Ⓐ ☑ **V2315** Lenticular (myodisc), per lens, trifocal

Ⓐ **V2318** Aniseikonic lens, trifocal

Ⓐ ☑ **V2319** Trifocal seg width over 28 mm

Ⓐ ☑ **V2320** Trifocal add over 3.25d

Ⓐ **V2321** Lenticular lens, per lens, trifocal
MED: 100-2,15,120; 100-4,3,10.4

Ⓐ **V2399** Specialty trifocal (by report)
Pertinent documentation to evaluate medical appropriateness should be included when this code is reported.

VARIABLE ASPHERICITY LENS, GLASS, OR PLASTIC

Ⓐ ☑ **V2410** Variable asphericity lens, single vision, full field, glass or plastic, per lens

Ⓐ ☑ **V2430** Variable asphericity lens, bifocal, full field, glass or plastic, per lens

Ⓐ **V2499** Variable sphericity lens, other type

CONTACT LENS

If procedure code 92391 or 92396 is reported, recode with specific lens type listed below (per lens).

Ⓐ ☑ **V2500** Contact lens, PMMA, spherical, per lens

Ⓐ ☑ **V2501** Contact lens, PMMA, toric or prism ballast, per lens

Ⓐ ☑ **V2502** Contact lens, PMMA, bifocal, per lens

Ⓐ ☑ **V2503** Contact lens, PMMA, color vision deficiency, per lens

Ⓐ ☑ **V2510** Contact lens, gas permeable, spherical, per lens

Ⓐ ☑ **V2511** Contact lens, gas permeable, toric, prism ballast, per lens

Ⓐ ☑ **V2512** Contact lens, gas permeable, bifocal, per lens

Ⓐ ☑ **V2513** Contact lens, gas permeable, extended wear, per lens

Ⓐ ☑ **V2520** Contact lens, hydrophilic, spherical, per lens
Hydrophilic contact lenses are covered by Medicare only for aphakic patients. Local contractor if incident to physician services.
MED: 100-3,80.1; 100-3,80.4

Ⓐ ☑ **V2521** Contact lens, hydrophilic, toric, or prism ballast, per lens
Hydrophilic contact lenses are covered by Medicare only for aphakic patients. Local contractor if incident to physician services.
MED: 100-3,80.1; 100-3,80.4

Ⓐ ☑ **V2522** Contact lens, hydrophilic, bifocal, per lens
Hydrophilic contact lenses are covered by Medicare only for aphakic patients. Local contractor if incident to physician services.
MED: 100-3,80.1; 100-3,80.4

Ⓐ ☑ **V2523** Contact lens, hydrophilic, extended wear, per lens
Hydrophilic contact lenses are covered by Medicare only for aphakic patients.
MED: 100-3,80.1; 100-3,80.4

Ⓐ ☑ **V2530** Contact lens, scleral, gas impermeable, per lens (for contact lens modification, see CPT Level I code 92325)

Ⓐ ☑ **V2531** Contact lens, scleral, gas permeable, per lens (for contact lens modification, see CPT Level I code 92325)
MED: 100-3,80.5

Ⓐ **V2599** Contact lens, other type
Local contractor if incident to physician services.

VISION AIDS

If procedure code 92392 is reported, recode with specific systems below.

Ⓐ **V2600** Hand held low vision aids and other nonspectacle mounted aids

Ⓐ **V2610** Single lens spectacle mounted low vision aids

Ⓐ **V2615** Telescopic and other compound lens system, including distance vision telescopic, near vision telescopes and compound microscopic lens system

---

Special Coverage Instructions   Noncovered by Medicare   Carrier Discretion   ☑ Quality Alert   ● New Code   ○ Reinstated Code   ▲ Revised Code

PROSTHETIC EYE

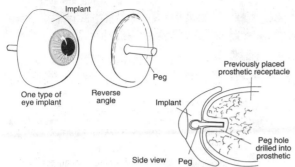

One type of eye implant | Reverse angle | Implant | Peg | Previously placed prosthetic receptacle | Peg hole drilled into prosthetic | Side view | Peg

A **V2623** Prosthetic eye, plastic, custom   ♿
MED: 100-2,15,120; 100-4,3,10.4

A **V2624** Polishing/resurfacing of ocular prosthesis   ♿

A **V2625** Enlargement of ocular prosthesis   ♿

A **V2626** Reduction of ocular prosthesis   ♿

A **V2627** Scleral cover shell   ♿
A scleral shell covers the cornea and the anterior sclera. Medicare covers a scleral shell when it is prescribed as an artificial support to a shrunken and sightless eye or as a barrier in the treatment of severe dry eye.
MED: 100-3,80.5

A **V2628** Fabrication and fitting of ocular conformer   ♿

A **V2629** Prosthetic eye, other type

INTRAOCULAR LENSES

N **V2630** Anterior chamber intraocular lens
The IOL must be FDA-approved for reimbursement. Medicare payment for an IOL is included in the payment for ASC facility services. Medicare jurisdiction: local contractor.
MED: 100-2,15,120; 100-4,3,10.4

N **V2631** Iris supported intraocular lens
The IOL must be FDA-approved for reimbursement. Medicare payment for an IOL is included in the payment for ASC facility services. Medicare jurisdiction: local contractor.
MED: 100-2,15,120; 100-4,3,10.4

N **V2632** Posterior chamber intraocular lens
The IOL must be FDA-approved for reimbursement. Medicare payment for an IOL is included in the payment for ASC facility services. Medicare jurisdiction: local contractor.
MED: 100-2,15,120; 100-4,3,10.4

MISCELLANEOUS

A ☑ **V2700** Balance lens, per lens   ♿

E **V2702** Deluxe lens feature
MED: 100-2,15,120; 100-4,3,10.4

A ☑ **V2710** Slab off prism, glass or plastic, per lens   ♿

A ☑ **V2715** Prism, per lens   ♿

A ☑ **V2718** Press-on lens, fresnell prism, per lens   ♿

A ☑ **V2730** Special base curve, glass or plastic, per lens   ♿

A ☑ **V2744** Tint, photochromatic, per lens   ♿
MED: 100-2,15,120; 100-4,3,10.4

A ☑ **V2745** Addition to lens; tint, any color, solid, gradient or equal, excludes photochromatic, any lens material, per lens   ♿
MED: 100-2,15,120; 100-4,3,10.4

A ☑ **V2750** Antireflective coating, per lens   ♿
MED: 100-2,15,120; 100-4,3,10.4

A ☑ **V2755** U-V lens, per lens   ♿
MED: 100-2,15,120; 100-4,3,10.4

E **V2756** Eye glass case

A ☑ **V2760** Scratch resistant coating, per lens   ♿

B ☑ **V2761** Mirror coating, any type, solid, gradient or equal, any lens material, per lens
MED: 100-2,15,120; 100-4,3,10.4

A ☑ **V2762** Polarization, any lens material, per lens   ♿
MED: 100-2,15,120; 100-4,3,10.4

A ☑ **V2770** Occluder lens, per lens   ♿

A ☑ **V2780** Oversize lens, per lens   ♿

B ☑ **V2781** Progressive lens, per lens

A ☑ **V2782** Lens, index 1.54 to 1.65 plastic or 1.60 to 1.79 glass, excludes polycarbonate, per lens   ♿
MED: 100-2,15,120; 100-4,3,10.4

A ☑ **V2783** Lens, index greater than or equal to 1.66 plastic or greater than or equal to 1.80 glass, excludes polycarbonate, per lens   ♿
MED: 100-2,15,120; 100-4,3,10.4

A ☑ **V2784** Lens, polycarbonate or equal, any index, per lens   ♿
MED: 100-2,15,120; 100-4,3,10.4

F **V2785** Processing, preserving and transporting corneal tissue
Medicare jurisdiction: local contractor.

A ☑ **V2786** Specialty occupational multifocal lens, per lens   ♿
MED: 100-2,15,120; 100-4,3,10.4

E **V2788** Presbyopia correcting function of intraocular lens

N **V2790** Amniotic membrane for surgical reconstruction, per procedure
Medicare jurisdiction: local contractor.

A **V2797** Vision supply, accessory and/or service component of another HCPCS vision code

A **V2799** Vision service, miscellaneous
Determine if an alternative HCPCS Level II or a CPT code better describes the service being reported. This code should be used only if a more specific code is unavailable.

HEARING SERVICES V5000-V5999

This range of codes describes hearing tests and related supplies and equipment, speech-language pathology screenings, and repair of augmentative communicative system.

Hearing services fall under the jurisdiction of the local contractor unless incidental or otherwise noted.

E **V5008** Hearing screening
MED: 100-2,16,90

E **V5010** Assessment for hearing aid

E **V5011** Fitting/orientation/checking of hearing aid

E **V5014** Repair/modification of a hearing aid

E **V5020** Conformity evaluation

E **V5030** Hearing aid, monaural, body worn, air conduction

Special Coverage Instructions   Noncovered by Medicare   Carrier Discretion   ☑ Quality Alert   ● New Code   ○ Reinstated Code   ▲ Revised Code

Hearing Services

V5040 — V5364

E	V5040	Hearing aid, monaural, body worn, bone conduction
E	V5050	Hearing aid, monaural, in the ear
E	V5060	Hearing aid, monaural, behind the ear
E	V5070	Glasses, air conduction
E	V5080	Glasses, bone conduction
E	V5090	Dispensing fee, unspecified hearing aid
E	V5095	Semi-implantable middle ear hearing prosthesis Use this code for Vibrant Soundbridge Implantable Middle Ear Prosthesis.
E	V5100	Hearing aid, bilateral, body worn
E	V5110	Dispensing fee, bilateral
E	V5120	Binaural, body
E	V5130	Binaural, in the ear
E	V5140	Binaural, behind the ear
E	V5150	Binaural, glasses
E	V5160	Dispensing fee, binaural
E	V5170	Hearing aid, CROS, in the ear
E	V5180	Hearing aid, CROS, behind the ear
E	V5190	Hearing aid, CROS, glasses
E	V5200	Dispensing fee, CROS
E	V5210	Hearing aid, BICROS, in the ear
E	V5220	Hearing aid, BICROS, behind the ear
E	V5230	Hearing aid, BICROS, glasses
E	V5240	Dispensing fee, BICROS
E	V5241	Dispensing fee, monaural hearing aid, any type
E	V5242	Hearing aid, analog, monaural, CIC (completely in the ear canal)
E	V5243	Hearing aid, analog, monaural, ITC (in the canal)
E	V5244	Hearing aid, digitally programmable analog, monaural, CIC
E	V5245	Hearing aid, digitally programmable, analog, monaural, ITC
E	V5246	Hearing aid, digitally programmable analog, monaural, ITE (in the ear)
E	V5247	Hearing aid, digitally programmable analog, monaural, BTE (behind the ear)
E	V5248	Hearing aid, analog, binaural, CIC
E	V5249	Hearing aid, analog, binaural, ITC
E	V5250	Hearing aid, digitally programmable analog, binaural, CIC
E	V5251	Hearing aid, digitally programmable analog, binaural, ITC
E	V5252	Hearing aid, digitally programmable, binaural, ITE
E	V5253	Hearing aid, digitally programmable, binaural, BTE
E	V5254	Hearing aid, digital, monaural, CIC
E	V5255	Hearing aid, digital, monaural, ITC
E	V5256	Hearing aid, digital, monaural, ITE
E	V5257	Hearing aid, digital, monaural, BTE
E	V5258	Hearing aid, digital, binaural, CIC
E	V5259	Hearing aid, digital, binaural, ITC
E	V5260	Hearing aid, digital, binaural, ITE
E	V5261	Hearing aid, digital, binaural, BTE
E	V5262	Hearing aid, disposable, any type, monaural
E ☑	V5263	Hearing aid, disposable, any type, binaural
E ☑	V5264	Ear mold/insert, not disposable, any type
E ☑	V5265	Ear mold/insert, disposable, any type
E ☑	V5266	Battery for use in hearing device
E ☑	V5267	Hearing aid supplies/accessories
E ☑	V5268	Assistive listening device, telephone amplifier, any type
E	V5269	Assistive listening device, alerting, any type
E	V5270	Assistive listening device, television amplifier, any type
E	V5271	Assistive listening device, television caption decoder
E	V5272	Assistive listening device, TDD
E	V5273	Assistive listening device, for use with cochlear implant
E	V5274	Assistive listening device, not otherwise specified
E	V5275	Ear impression, each
E	V5298	Hearing aid, not otherwise classified
B	V5299	Hearing service, miscellaneous ⊘ Determine if an alternative HCPCS Level II or a CPT code better describes the service being reported. This code should be used only if a more specific code is unavailable. MED: 100-2,16,90

SPEECH-LANGUAGE PATHOLOGY SERVICES

E	V5336	Repair/modification of augmentative communicative system or device (excludes adaptive hearing aid) Medicare jurisdiction: DME regional contractor.
E	V5362	Speech screening
E	V5363	Language screening
E	V5364	Dysphagia screening

Special Coverage Instructions   Noncovered by Medicare   Carrier Discretion   ☑ Quality Alert   ● New Code   ○ Reinstated Code   ▲ Revised Code

150 — V Codes   A Age Edit   M Maternity Edit   ♀ Female Only   ♂ Male Only   A - Y APC Status Indicators   *2007 HCPCS*

APPENDIX 1 — TABLE OF DRUGS

Introduction and Directions

The HCPCS 2007 Table of Drugs is designed to quickly and easily direct the user to drug names and their corresponding codes. Both generic and brand or trade names are alphabetically listed in the "Drug Name" column of the table. The associated A, C, J, K, Q, or S code is given only for the generic name of the drug.

The "Unit Per" column lists the stated amount for the referenced generic drug as provided by CMS. "Up to" listings are inclusive of all quantities up to and including the listed amount. All other listings are for the amount of the drug as listed. The editors recognize that the availability of some drugs in the quantities listed is dependent on many variables beyond the control of the clinical ordering clerk. The availability in your area of regularly used drugs in the most cost-effective quantities should be relayed to your third-party payers.

The "Route of Administration" column addresses the most common methods of delivering the referenced generic drug as described in current pharmaceutical literature. The official definitions for Level II drug codes generally describe administration other than by oral method. Therefore, with a handful of exceptions, oral-delivered options for most drugs are omitted from the Route of Administration column.

Intravenous administration includes all methods, such as gravity infusion, injections, and timed pushes. When several routes of administration are listed, the first listing is simply the first, or most common, method as described in current reference literature. The "VAR" posting denotes various routes of administration and is used for drugs that are commonly administered into joints, cavities, tissues, or topical applications, in addition to other parenteral administrations. Listings posted with "OTH" alert the user to other administration methods, such as suppositories or catheter injections.

Please be reminded that the Table of Drugs, as well as all HCPCS Level II national definitions and listings, constitutes a post-treatment medical reference for billing purposes only. Although the editors have exercised all normal precautions to ensure the accuracy of the table and related material, the use of any of this information to select medical treatment is entirely inappropriate.

See Appendix 3 for abbreviations.

Drug Name	Unit Per:	Route	Code
10% LMD	500 ML	IV	J7100
5% DEXTROSE/NORMAL SALINE	5%	VAR	J7042
5% DEXTROSE/WATER	500 ML	IV	J7060
A-HYDROCORT	100 MG	IV, IM, SC	J1720
A-METHAPRED	125 MG	IM, IV	J2930
A-METHAPRED	40 MG	IM, IV	J2920
ABARELIX	10 MG	IM	J0128
ABATACEPT	10 MG	IV	J0129 ▲
ABBOKINASE	250,000 IU	IV	J3365
ABBOKINASE	5,000 IU	IV	J3364
ABCIXIMAB	10 MG	IV	J0130
ABELCET	50 MG	IV	J0285
ABRAXANE	1 MG	IV	J9264
ACCUNEB ▶NONCOMPOUNDED,◀ CONCENTRATED	1 MG	INH	J7611
ACCUNEB ▶NONCOMPOUNDED, UNIT DOSE◀	1 MG	INH	J7613
~~ACELLULAR SKIN SUBSTITUTE~~	~~PER 16 SQ CM~~	~~OTH~~	~~C9221~~
ACETADOTE	1 G	INH	J7608
ACETADOTE	100 MG	IV	J0132
ACETAZOLAMIDE SODIUM	500 MG	IM, IV	J1120
ACETYLCYSTEINE	1 G	INH	J7608
ACTHREL	1 MCG	IV	J0795
ACTIMMUNE	0.25 MG	SC	J1830
ACTIMMUNE	3 MU	SC	J9216
ACTIVASE	1 MG	IV	J2997
ACUTECT	DOSE	IV	A9504
ACYCLOVIR	5 MG	IV	J0133
ADAGEN	25 IU	IM	J2504

Drug Name	Unit Per:	Route	Code
ADALIMUMAB	20 MG	SC	J0135
ADBEON	4 MG	IM, IV	J0704
ADENOCARD	6 MG	IV	J0150
ADENOSCAN	30 MG	IV	J0152
ADENOSINE	30 MG	IV	J0152
ADENOSINE	6 MG	IV	J0150
ADRENALIN	1 MG	IM, IV, SC	J0170
ADRENALIN CHLORIDE	1 MG	IM, IV, SC	J0170
ADRIAMYCIN	10 MG	IV	J9000
ADRUCIL	500 MG	IV	J9190
AEROBID	1 MG	INH	J7641
AGALSIDASE BETA	1 MG	IV	J0180
AGGRASTAT	12.5 MG	IM, IV	J3246
ALATROFLOXACIN MESYLATE	100 MG	IV	J0200
ALBUTEROL AND IPRATROPIUM BROMIDE NONCOMPOUNDED	2.5MG/0.5 MG	INH	J7620 ●
ALBUTEROL COMPOUNDED, CONCENTRATED	1 MG	INH	J7610 ●
ALBUTEROL COMPOUNDED, UNIT DOSE	1 MG	INH	J7609 ●
ALBUTEROL ▶NONCOMPOUNDED,◀ CONCENETRATED FORM	1 MG	INH	J7611
ALBUTEROL ▶NONCOMPOUNDED,◀ UNIT DOSE FORM	1 MG	INH	J7613
ALDESLEUKIN	1 VIAL	IV	J9015
ALDURAZYME	0.1 MG	IV	J1931
ALEFACEPT	0.5 MG	IV, IM	J0215
ALEMTUZUMAB	10 MG	IV	J9010
ALFERON N	250,000 IU	IM	J9215
ALGLUCERASE	10 U	IV	J0205
ALGLUCOSIDASE ALFA	10 MG	IV	C9234 ●
ALGLUCOSIDASE ALFA	20 MG	IV	S0147 ●
ALIMTA	10 MG	IV	J9305
ALKERAN	2 MG	ORAL	J8600
ALKERAN	50 MG	IV	J9245
ALOXI	25 MCG	IV	J2469
ALPHA 1 - PROTEINASE INHIBITOR — HUMAN	10 MG	IV	J0256
ALPHANATE	1 IU	IV	J7190
ALPHANINE SD	1 IU	IV	J7194
ALPROSTADIL	1.25 MCG	VAR	J0270
ALPROSTADIL	EA	OTH	J0275
ALTEPLASE RECOMBINANT	1 MG	IV	J2997
ALUPENT, ▶NONCOMPOUNDED,◀ CONCENTRATED	10 MG	INH	J7668
ALUPENT, ▶NONCOMPOUNDED, UNIT DOSE◀	10 MG	INH	J7669
AMANTADINE HYDROCHLORIDE (BRAND NAME)	100 MG	ORAL	G9033
AMANTADINE HYDROCHLORIDE (GENERIC)	100 MG	ORAL	G9017
AMBISOME	10 MG	IV	J0289
AMCORT	5 MG	IM	J3302
AMERGAN	12.5 MG	ORAL	Q0169
AMEVIVE	0.5 MG	IV, IM	J0215
AMICAR	5 G	IV	S0017
AMIFOSTINE	500 MG	IV	J0207
AMIKACIN SULFATE	100 MG	IM, IV	J0278
AMIKIN	100 MG	IM, IV	S0072

Drug Name	Unit Per:	Route	Code
AMINOCAPRIOC ACID	5 G	IV	S0017
AMINOPHYLLINE	250 MG	IV	J0280
AMIODARONE HCL	30 MG	IV	J0282
AMITRIPTYLINE HCL	20 MG	IM	J1320
AMMONIA N-13	DOSE	IV	A9526
AMOBARBITAL	125 MG	IM, IV	J0300
AMPHOCIN	50 MG	IV	J0285
AMPHOTEC	10 MG	IV	J0287
AMPHOTERICIN B	50 MG	IV	J0285
AMPHOTERICIN B CHOLESTERYL SULFATE COMPLEX	10 MG	IV	J0288
AMPHOTERICIN B LIPID COMPLEX	10 MG	IV	J0287
AMPHOTERICIN B LIPOSOME	10 MG	IV	J0289
AMPICILLIN SODIUM	500 MG	IM, IV	J0290
AMPICILLIN SODIUM/SULBACTAM SODIUM	1.5 G	IM, IV	J0295
AMYTAL	125 MG	IM, IV	J0300
ANABOLIN LA 100	100 MG	IM	J2321
ANASTROZOLE	1 MG	ORAL	S0170
ANCEF	500 MG	IV, IM	J0690
ANDRO LA 200	200 MG	IM	J3130
ANDROLONE-D 100	100 MG	IM	J2321
ANDRONAQ 50	50 MG	IM	J3140
ANDROPOSITORY 100	100 MG	IM	J3120
ANECTINE	20 MG	IM, IV	J0330
ANERGAN 25	50 MG	IM, IV	J2550
ANERGAN 50	50 MG	IM, IV	J2550
ANGIOMAX	1 MG	IV	J0583
ANIDULAFUNGIN	1 MG	IV	J0348 ●
ANISTREPLASE	30 U	IV	J0350
ANTAGON	250 MCG	SC	S0132
ANTI-INHIBITOR	1 IU	IV	J7198
ANTI-THYMOCYTE GLOBULIN,EQUINE	250 MG	OTH	J7504
ANTIFLEX	60 MG	IV, IM	J2360
ANTIHEMOPHILIC FACTOR HUMAN METHOD M MONOCLONAL PURIFIED	1 IU	IV	J7192
ANTIHEMOPHILIC FACTOR PORCINE	1 IU	IV	J7191
ANTINAUS	50 MG	IM, IV	J2550
ANTITHROMBIN III	1 IU	IV	J7195
ANTIZOL	15 MG	IV	J1451
ANZEMET	10 MG	IV	J1260
ANZEMET	100 MG	ORAL	Q0180
ANZEMET	50 MG	ORAL	S0174
APLIGRAF	SQ CM	OTH	J7340
APOKYN	1 MG	SC	J0364 ●
APOKYN	1 MG	SC	S0167
APOMORPHINE HYDROCHLORIDE	1 MG	SC	J0364 ●
APOMORPHINE HYDROCHLORIDE	1 MG	SC	S0167
APREPITANT, ORAL, 5 MG	5 MG	ORAL	J8501
APROTININ	10,000 KIU	IV	J0365
AQUAMEPHYTON	1 MG	IM, SC, IV	J3430
ARA-C	100 MG	SC, IV	J9100
ARAMINE	10 MG	IV, IM, SC	J0380
ARANESP, ESRD USE	1 MCG	SC, IV	J0882
ARANESP, NON-ESRD USE	1 MCG	SC, IV	J0881
ARBUTAMINE HCL	1 MG	IV	J0395

Drug Name	Unit Per:	Route	Code
AREDIA	30 MG	IV	J2430
ARGATROBAN	5 MG	IV	C9121
ARIMIDEX	1 MG	ORAL	S0170
ARISTOCORT	5 MG	IM	J3302
ARISTOCORTE FORTE	5 MG	IM	J3302
ARISTOCORTE INTRALESIONAL	5 MG	OTH	J3302
ARISTOSPAN	5 MG	VAR	J3303
ARIXTRA	0.5 MG	SC	J1652
AROMASIN	25 MG	ORAL	S0156
ARRANON	50 MG	IV	J9261 ●
ARRESTIN	200 MG	IM	J3250
ARSENIC TRIOXIDE	1 MG	IV	J9017
ASPARAGINASE	10,000 U	VAR	J9020
ASTRAMORPH PF	10 MG	IM, IV, SC	J2275
ATGAM	250 MG	OTH	J7504
ATIVAN	2 MG	IM, IV	J2060
ATOPICLAIR	ANY SIZE	OTH	A6250 ●
ATROPEN	0.3 MG	IV, IM, SC	J0460
ATROPINE SULFATE	0.3 MG	IV, IM, SC	J0460
ATROPINE, COMPOUNDED, CONCENTRATED	I MG	INH	J7635 ●
ATROPINE, ▶COMPOUNDED, UNIT DOSE◀	▶1 MG◀	INH	J7636
ATROVENT, ▶NONCOMPOUNDED, UNIT DOSE◀	▶1 MG◀	INH	J7644
AUROTHIOGLUCOSE	50 MG	IM	J2910
AUTOPLEX T	1 IU	IV	J7198
AVASTIN	10 MG	IV	J9035
AVELOX	100 MG	IV	J2280
AVONEX	11 MCG	IM	Q3025
AVONEX	33 MCG	IM	J1825
AZACITIDINE	1 MG	SC	J9025
AZACTAM	500 MG	IV	S0073
AZASAN	50 MG	ORAL	J7500
AZATHIOPRINE	100 MG	OTH	J7501
AZATHIOPRINE	50 MG	ORAL	J7500
AZATHIOPRINE SODIUM	100 MG	OTH	J7501
AZITHROMYCIN	500 MG	IV	J0456
AZMACORT	PER MG	INH	J7684
AZMACORT CONCENTRATED	PER MG	INH	J7683
AZTREONAM	500 MG	IV	S0073
AZTREONAM	PER MG	INH	S0143
BACLOFEN	10 MG	IT	J0475
BACLOFEN	50 MCG	OTH	J0476
BACTERIOSTATIC WATER	5%	VAR	J7051
BACTOCILL	250 MG	IM, IV	J2700
BACTRIM IV	10 ML	IV	S0039
BAL	100 MG	IM	J0470
BANFLEX	60 MG	IV, IM	J2360
BASILIXIMAB	20 MG	IV	J0480
BAYGAM	1 CC	IM	J1460
BAYRHO D	50 MCG	IM	J2788
BAYRHO-D	100 IU	IM	J2792
BAYRHO-D	300 MCG	IM	J2790
BAYTET	250 U	IM	J1670
BCG VACCINE LIVE	VIAL	IV	J9031
BEBULIN VH	1 IU	IV	J7194
BECAPLERMIN GEL 0.01%	0.5 G	OTH	S0157

Drug Name	Unit Per:	Route	Code
BECLOMETHASONE ▶COMPOUNDED◀	1 MG	INH	J7622
BECLOVENT ▶COMPOUNDED◀	1 MG	INH	J7622
BECONASE ▶COMPOUNDED◀	1 MG	INH	J7622
BENA-D 10	50 MG	IV, IM	J1200
BENA-D 50	50 MG	IV, IM	J1200
BENADRYL	50 MG	IV, IM	J1200
BENAHIST 10	50 MG	IV, IM	J1200
BENAHIST 50	50 MG	IV, IM	J1200
BENEFIX	1 IU	IV	J7195
BENOJECT-10	50 MG	IV, IM	J1200
BENOJECT-50	50 MG	IV, IM	J1200
BENTYL	20 MG	IM	J0500
BENZTROPINE MESYLATE	1 MG	IM, IV	J0515
BERUBIGEN	1,000 MCG	SC, IM	J3420
BETA-2	1 MG	INH	J7648
BETALIN 12	1,000 MCG	SC, IM	J3420
BETAMETHASONE ACETATE AND BETAMETHASONE SODIUM PHOSPHATE	3 MG, OF EACH	IM	J0702
BETAMETHASONE SODIUM PHOSPHATE	4 MG	IM, IV	J0704
BETAMETHASONE ▶COMPOUNDED, UNIT DOSE◀	1 MG	INH	J7624
BETASERON	0.25 MG	SC	J1830
BETHANECHOL CHLORIDE, MYOTONACHOL OR URECHOLINE	5 MG	SC	J0520
BEVACIZUMAB	10 MG	IV	J9035
BEXXAR THERAPEUTIC	TX DOSE	IV	A9545
BICILLIN CR	1,200,000 U	IM	J0540
BICILLIN CR	600,000 U	IM	J0530
BICILLIN CR 900/300	1,200,000 U	IM, IV	J0540
BICILLIN CR 900/300	2,400,000 U	IM, IV	J0550
BICILLIN LA	1,200,000 U	IM	J0570
BICILLIN LA	2,400,000 U	INJ	J0580
BICILLIN LA	600,000 U	IM	J0560
BICNU	100 MG	IV	J9050
BIOCLATE	1 IU	IV	J7192
BIOTROPIN	1 MG	SC	J2941
BITOLTEROL MESYLATE, ▶COMPOUNDED◀ CONCENTRATED	PER MG	INH	J7628
BITOLTEROL MESYLATE, ▶COMPOUNDED UNIT DOSE◀	PER MG	INH	J7629
BIVALIRUDIN	1 MG	IV	J0583
BLENOXANE	15 U	IM, IV, SC	J9040
BLEOMYCIN LYOPHILLIZED	15 U	IM, IV, SC	J9040
BLEOMYCIN SULFATE	15 U	IM, IV, SC	J9040
BONIVA	1 MG	IV	J1740 ▲
BORTEZOMIB	0.1 MG	IV	J9041
BOTOX	1 U	IM	J0585
BOTULINUM TOXIN TYPE A	1 U	OTH	J0585
BOTULINUM TOXIN TYPE B	100 U	OTH	J0587
BRAVELLE	75 IU	SC, IM	J3355
BRETHINE	1 MG	SC, IV	J3105
BRETHINE	PER MG	INH	J7681
BRETHINE CONCENTRATED	PER MG	INH	J7680
BRICANYL	PER MG	INH	J7681
BRICANYL CONCENTRATED	PER MG	INH	J7680
BRICANYL SUBCUTANEOUS	1 MG	SC	J3105

Drug Name	Unit Per:	Route	Code
BROM-A-COT	10 MG	IM, SC, IV	J0945
BROMPHENIRAMINE MALEATE	10 MG	IM, SC, IV	J0945
BRONCHO SALINE	5 CC	VAR	J7051
BUDESONIDE COMPOUNDED, CONCETRATED	0.25 MG	INH	J7634 ●
BUDESONIDE, COMPOUNDED, ▶UNIT DOSE◀	0.5 MG	INH	J7627
BUDESONIDE, NONCOMPOUNDED, ▶UNIT DOSE◀	0.5 MG	INH	J7626
BUDESONIDE, ▶NONCOMPOUNDED, CONCENTRATED◀	0.25 MG	INH	J7633
BUMETANIDE	0.5 MG	IM, IV	S0171
BUPIVACAINE HCL	30 ML	OTH	S0020
BUPRENEX	0.1 MG	IM, IV	J0592
BUPRENORPHINE HCL	0.1 MG	IM, IV	J0592
BUPROPION HCL	150 MG	ORAL	S0106
BUSULFAN	▶1 MG◀	IV	J0594 ▲
BUSULFAN	2 MG	OTH	J8510
BUSULFEX	▶1 MG◀	IV	J0594 ▲
BUSULFEX	2 MG	ORAL	J8510
BUTORPHANOL TARTRATE	2 MG	IM, IV	J0595
BUTORPHANOL TARTRATE	25 MG	OTH	S0012
CABERGOLINE	0.25 MG	ORAL	J8515
CAFCIT	5 MG	IV	J0706
CAFFEINE CITRATE	5 MG	IV	J0706
CALCIJEX	0.1 MCG	IM	J0636
CALCIMAR	UP TO 400 U	SC, IM	J0630
CALCITONIN SALMON	400 U	SC, IM	J0630
CALCITRIOL	0.1 MCG	IM	J0636
CALCITROL	0.25 MCG	ORAL	S0161
CALCIUM DISODIUM VERSENATE	1,000 MG	IV, SC, IM	J0600
CALCIUM GLUCONATE	10 ML	IV	J0610
CALCIUM GLYCEROPHOSPHATE AND CALCIUM LACTATE	10 ML	IM, SC	J0620
CAMPATH	10 MG	IV	J9010
CAMPTOSAR	20 MG	IV	J9206
CANCIDAS	5 MG	IV	J0637
CAPECITABINE	150 MG	ORAL	J8520
CAPROMAB PENDETIDE	DOSE	IV	A9507
CARBACOT	10 ML	IV, IM	J2800
CARBOCAINE	10 ML	VAR	J0670
CARBOPLATIN	50 MG	IV	J9045
CARDIOGEN 82	60 MCI	IV	A9555
CARDIOLITE	DOSE	IV	A9500
CARIMUNE	1 GM	IV	J1563
CARMUSTINE	100 MG	IV	J9050
CARNITOR	1 G	IV	J1955
CARTICEL		OTH	J7330
CASPOFUNGIN ACETATE	5 MG	IV	J0637
CATAPRES	1 MG	OTH	J0735
CATHFLO	1 MG	IV	J2997
CAVERJECT	1.25 MCG	VAR	J0270
CEENU	10 MG	ORAL	S0178
CEFAZOLIN SODIUM	500 MG	IV, IM	J0690
CEFEPIME HCL	500 MG	IV	J0692
CEFIZOX	500 MG	IV, IM	J0715
CEFOBID	1 G	IV	S0021
CEFOPERAZONE SODIUM	1 G	IV	S0021

Appendix 1 — Table of Drugs

Drug Name	Unit Per:	Route	Code
CEFOTAN	500 MG	IM, IV	S0074
CEFOTAXIME SODIUM	1 GM	IV, IM	J0698
CEFOTETAN DISODIUM	500 MG	IM. IV	S0074
CEFOXITIN	1 GM	IV, IM	J0694
CEFOXITIN SODIUM	1 GM	IV, IM	J0694
CEFTAZIDIME	500 MG	IM, IV	J0713
CEFTIZOXIME SODIUM	500 MG	IV, IM	J0715
CEFTRIAXONE	250 MG	IV, IM	J0696
CEFTRIAXONE SODIUM	250 MG	IV, IM	J0696
CEFUROXIME	750 MG	IM, IV	J0697
CEFUROXIME SODIUM STERILE	750 MG	IM, IV	J0697
CELESTONE SOLUSPAN	3 MG	IM	J0702
CELLCEPT	250 MG	ORAL	J7517
CENACORT A-40	10 MG	IM	J3301
CENACORT FORTE	5 MG	IM	J3302
CEPHALOTHIN SODIUM	1 G	IM, IV	J1890
CEPTAZ	500 MG	IM, IV	J0713
CEREBRYX	50 MG	IM, IV	Q2009
CEREBRYX	750 MG	IM, IV	S0078
CEREDASE	10 U	IV	J0205
CERETEC	DOSE	IV	A9521
CEREZYME	1 U	IV	J1785
CERUBIDINE	10 MG	IV	J9150
CESAMET	1 MG	ORAL	J8650 ●
CETUXIMAB	10 MG	IV	J9055
CHLORAMBUCIL	2 MG	ORAL	S0172
CHLORAMPHENICOL SODIUM SUCCINATE	1 G	IV	J0720
CHLORDIAZEPOXIDE HCL	100 MG	IM, IV	J1990
CHLOROMYCETIN	1 G	IV	J0720
CHLOROPROCAINE HCL	30 ML	VAR	J2400
CHLOROTHIAZIDE SODIUM	500 MG	IV	J1205
CHLORPROMAZINE HCL	10 MG	ORAL	Q0171
CHLORPROMAZINE HCL	25 MG	ORAL	Q0172
CHLORPROMAZINE HCL	50 MG	IM, IV	J3230
CHORIONIC GONADOTROPIN	1,000 USP U	IM	J0725
CHROMIC PHOSPHATE P32	1 MCI	IV	A9564
CHROMITOPE	250 UCI	IV	A9553
CHROMIUM CR-51 SODIUM IOTHALAMATE, DIAGNOSTIC	10 UCI	IV	A9553
CIDOFOVIR	375 MG	IV	J0740
CILASTATIN SODIUM	250 MG	IV, IM	J0743
CIMETIDINE HCL	300 MG	IM, IV	S0023
CIPRO	200 MG	IV	J0744
CIPROFLOXACIN FOR INTRAVENOUS INFUSION	200 MG	IV	J0744
CISPLATIN	10 MG	IV	J9060
CLADRIBINE	1 MG	IV	J9065
CLAFORAN	1 GM	IV, IM	J0698
CLEOCIN PHOSPHATE	300 MG	IV	S0077
CLINAGEN LA	UP TO 40 MG	IM	J0970
CLINDAMYCIN PHOSPHATE	300 MG	IV	S0077
CLOFARABINE	1 MG	IV	J9027
CLOLAR	1 MG	IV	J9027
CLONIDINE HCL	1 MG	OTH	J0735
CLOSTRIDIUM BOTULINUM TOXIN	1 U	OTH	J0585
CLOZAPINE	25 MG	ORAL	S0136
CLOZARIL	25 MG	ORAL	S0136

Drug Name	Unit Per:	Route	Code
COBAL	1,000 MCG	IM, SC	J3420
COBALT CO-57 CYNOCOBALAMIN, DIAGNOSTIC	1 UCI	ORAL	A9559
COBATOPE 57	1 UCI	ORAL	A9559
COBEX	1,000 MCG	SC, IM	J3420
CODEINE PHOSPHATE	30 MG	IM, IV, SC	J0745
COGENTIN	1 MG	IM, IV	J0515
COGNEX	10 MG	ORAL	30014
COLCHICINE	1 MG	IV	J0760
COLHIST	10 MG	IM, SC, IV	J0945
COLISTIMETHATE SODIUM	150 MG	IM, IV	J0770
COLISTIMETHATE SODIUM	PER MG	INH	S0142
COLLAGEN, MICROPOROUS NONHUMAN	SQ CM	OTH	C9351 ●
COLLAGEN-GLYCOSAMINOGLYCAN SKIN SUBSTITUTE	SQ CM	OTH	J7343
COLY-MYCIN M	150 MG	IM, IV	J0770
COMPAZINE	10 MG	IM, IV	J0780
COMPAZINE	10 MG	ORAL	Q0165
COMPAZINE	5 MG	ORAL	Q0164
COMPAZINE	5 MG	ORAL	S0183
CONTRACEPTIVE SUPPLY, HORMONE CONTAINING PATCH	EACH	OTH	J7304
COPAXONE	20 MG	SC	J1595
COPPER T MODEL TCU380A IUD COPPER WIRE/COPPER COLLAR	EA	OTH	J7300
CORDARONE	30 MG	IV	J0282
CORTASTAT	1 MG	IM, IV, OTH	J1100
CORTASTAT LA	1 MG	IM	J1094
CORTICORELIN OVINE TRIFLUTATE	1 MCG	IV	J0795
CORTICOTROPIN	40 U	IV, IM, SC	J0800
CORTIMED	80 MG	IM	J1040
CORTROSYN	0.25 MG	IM, IV	J0835
CORVERT	1 MG	IV	J1742
COSMEGEN	0.5 MG	IV	J9120
COSYNTROPIN	0.25 MG	IM, IV	J0835
COTOLONE	1 ML	IM	J2650
COTOLONE	5 MG	ORAL	J7510
CROMOLYN SODIUM	10 MG	INH	J7631
CRYSTAL B12	1,000 MCG	IM, SC	J3420
CRYSTICILLIN 300 A.S.	600,000 UNITS	IM, IV	J2510
CRYSTICILLIN 600 A.S.	600,000 UNITS	IM, IV	J2510
CUBICIN	1 MG	IV	J0878
CYANO	1,000 MCG	IM, SC	J3420
CYANOCOBALAMIN	1,000 MCG	IM, SC	J3420
CYANOCOBALAMIN COBALT 58/57	1 UCI	IV	A9546
CYANOCOBALAMIN COBALT CO-57	1 UCI	ORAL	A9559
CYCLOPHOSPHAMIDE	1 G	IV	J9091
CYCLOPHOSPHAMIDE	100 MG	IV	J9070
CYCLOPHOSPHAMIDE	2 G	IV	J9092
CYCLOPHOSPHAMIDE	200 MG	IV	J9080
CYCLOPHOSPHAMIDE	25 MG	ORAL	J8530
CYCLOPHOSPHAMIDE	500 MG	IV	J9090
CYCLOPHOSPHAMIDE LYOPHILIZED	1 G	IV	J9096
CYCLOPHOSPHAMIDE LYOPHILIZED	100 MG	IV	J9093
CYCLOPHOSPHAMIDE LYOPHILIZED	2 G	IV	J9097
CYCLOPHOSPHAMIDE LYOPHILIZED	200 MG	IV	J9094
CYCLOPHOSPHAMIDE LYOPHILIZED	500 MG	IV	J9095

APPENDIX 1 — TABLE OF DRUGS

Drug Name	Unit Per:	Route	Code	Drug Name	Unit Per:	Route	Code
CYCLOSPORINE	100 MG	ORAL	J7502	DELTA-CORTEF	5 MG	ORAL	J7510
CYCLOSPORINE	25 MG	ORAL	J7515	DELTASONE	5 MG	ORAL	J7506
CYCLOSPORINE	250 MG	OTH	J7516	DELTASONE	5 MG	OTH	J7506
CYTARABINE	100 MG	SC, IV	J9100	DEMADEX	10 MG	IV	J3265
CYTARABINE	500 MG	SC, IV	J9110	DEMEROL	100 MG	IM, IV, SC	J2175
CYTARABINE LIPOSOME	10 MG	IT	J9098	DENILEUKIN DIFTITOX	300 MCG	IV	J9160
CYTOGAM	VIAL	IV	J0850	DEPANDRATE	1 CC, 200 MG	IM	J1080
CYTOMEGALOVIRUS IMMUNE GLOB	VIAL	IV	J0850	DEPANDROGYN	1 ML	IM	J1060
CYTOSAR-U	100 MG	SC, IV	J9100	DEPGYNOGEN	UP TO 5 MG	IM	J1000
CYTOSAR-U	500 MG	SC, IV	J9110	DEPHENACEN-50	50 MG	IM, IV	J1200
CYTOTEC	200 MCG	ORAL	S0191	DEPMEDALONE	40 MG	IM	J1030
CYTOVENE	500 MG	IV	J1570	DEPMEDALONE	80 MG	IM	J1040
CYTOXAN	1 G	IV	J9091	DEPO-ESTRADIOL CYPIONATE	UP TO 5 MG	IM	J1000
CYTOXAN	100 MG	IV	J9070	DEPO-MEDROL	20 MG	IM	J1020
CYTOXAN	2 G	IV	J9092	DEPO-MEDROL	40 MG	IM	J1030
CYTOXAN	200 MG	IV	J9080	DEPO-MEDROL	80 MG	IM	J1040
CYTOXAN	25 MG	ORAL	J8530	DEPO-PROVERA	150 MG	IM	J1055
CYTOXAN	500 MG	IV	J9090	DEPO-PROVERA	50 MG	IM	J1051
CYTOXAN LYOPHILIZED	1 G	IV	J9096	DEPO-TESTADIOL	1 ML	IM	J1060
CYTOXAN LYOPHILIZED	100 MG	IV	J9093	DEPO-TESTOSTERONE	1 CC, 200 MG	IM	J1080
CYTOXAN LYOPHILIZED	2 G	IV	J9097	DEPO-TESTOSTERONE	UP TO 100 MG	IM	J1070
CYTOXAN LYOPHILIZED	200 MG	IV	J9094	DEPO-TESTOSTERONE CYPIONATE	UP TO 100 MG	IM	J1070
CYTOXAN LYOPHILIZED	500 MG	IV	J9095	DEPOCYT	10 MG	IT	J9098
D.H.E. 45	1 MG	IM, IV	J1110	DEPOGEN	UP TO 5 MG	IM	J1000
DACARBAZINE	100 MG	IV	J9130	DEPTESTROGEN	UP TO 100 MG	IM	J1070
DACARBAZINE	200 MG	IV	J9140	DERMAGRAFT	SQ CM	OTH	J7342
DACLIZUMAB	25 MG	OTH	J7513	DERMAL AND EPIDERMAL, TISSUE OF NON-HUMAN ORIGIN, WITH OR WITHOUT OTHER BIOENGINEERED OR PROCESSED ELEMENTS, WITHOUT METABOLICALLY ACTIVE ELEMENTS	SQ CM	EA	J7343
DACOGEN	1 MG	IV	J0894 ▲				
DACTINOMYCIN	0.5 MG	IV	J9120				
DALALONE	1 MG	IM, IV, OTH	J1100				
DALALONE LA	1 MG	IM	J1094	DERMAL TISSUE, OF HUMAN ORIGIN, WITH OR WITHOUT OTHER BIOENGINEERED OR PROCESSED ELEMENTS, WITH METABOLICALLY ACTIVE ELEMENTS	SQ CM	EA	J7342
DALTEPARIN SODIUM	2,500 IU	SC	J1645				
DAPTOMYCIN	1 MG	IV	J0878				
DARBEPOETIN ALFA, ESRD USE	1 MCG	SC, IV	J0882				
DARBEPOETIN ALFA, NON-ESRD USE	1 MCG	SC, IV	J0881	DERMAL TISSUE, OF HUMAN ORIGIN, WITH OR WITHOUT OTHER BIOENGINEERED OR PROCESSED ELEMENTS, WITHOUT METABOLICALLY ACTIVE ELEMENTS	SQ CM	EA	J7344
DAUNORUBICIN CITRATE	10 MG	IV	J9151				
DAUNORUBICIN HCL	10 MG	IV	J9150				
DAUNOXOME	10 MG	IV	J9151	DESFERAL	500 MG	IM, SC, IV	J0895
DDAVP	1 MCG	IV, SC	J2597	DESMOPRESSIN ACETATE	1 MCG	IV, SC	J2597
DECA-DURABOLIN	100 MG	IM	J2321	DEXAMETHASONE	0.25 MG	ORAL	J8540
DECA-DURABOLIN	200 MG	IM	J2322	DEXAMETHASONE ACETATE	1 MG	IM	J1094
DECA-DURABOLIN	50 MG	IM	J2320	DEXAMETHASONE ACETATE ANHYDROUS	1 MG	IM	J1094
DECADRON	0.25 MG	ORAL	J8540	DEXAMETHASONE SODIUM PHOSPHATE	1 MG	IM, IV, OTH	J1100
DECADRON LA	1 MG	IM	J1094				
DECADRON PHOSPHATE	1 MG	IM, IV, OTH	J1100	DEXAMETHASONE, ▶COMPOUNDED, CONCENTRATED◀	PER MG	INH	J7637
~~DECELLURIZED SKIN SUBSTITUTE~~	~~1 CC~~	~~OTH~~	~~C9222~~				
DECITABINE	1 MG	IV	J0894 ▲	DEXAMETHASONE, ▶COMPOUNDED, UNIT DOSE◀	PER MG	INH	J7638
DECOLONE-100	100 MG	IM	J2321				
DECOLONE-50	50 MG	IM	J2320	DEXEDRINE	5 MG	ORAL	S0160
DEFEROXAMINE MESYLATE	500 MG	IM, SC, IV	J0895	DEXFERRUM	50 MG	IM, IV	J1752
DELATEST	100 MG	IM	J3120	DEXONE	0.25 MG	ORAL	J8540
DELATESTRYL	100 MG	IM	J3120	DEXONE LA	1 MG	IM	J1094
DELATESTRYL	200 MG	IM	J3130	DEXRAZOXANE	250 MG	IV	J1190
DELESTROGEN	10 MG	IM	J1380	DEXRAZOXANE HYDROCHLORIDE	250 MG	IV	J1190
DELESTROGEN	20 MG	IM	J1390	DEXTRAN 40	500 ML	IV	J7100
DELESTROGEN	UP TO 40 MG	IM	J0970	DEXTROAMPHETAMINE SULFATE	5 MG	ORAL	S0160

Appendix 1 — Table of Drugs

Drug Name	Unit Per:	Route	Code
DEXTROSE	500 ML	IV	J7060
DEXTROSE, STERILE WATER, AND/OR DEXTROSE DILUENT/FLUSH	10 ML	VAR	A46216 ●
DEXTROSE/SODIUM CHLORIDE	5%	VAR	J7042
DEXTROSE/THEOPHYLLINE	40 MG	IV	J2810
DEXTROSTAT	5 MG	ORAL	S0160
DIALYSIS/STRESS VITAMINS	100 CAPS	ORAL	S0194
DIAMOX	500 MG	IM, IV	J1120
DIASTAT	5 MG	IV, IM	J3360
DIAZEPAM	5 MG	IV, IM	J3360
DIAZOXIDE	300 MG	IV	J1730
DICYCLOMINE HCL	20 MG	IM	J0500
DIDANOSINE (DDI)	25 MG	ORAL	S0137
DIDRONEL	300 MG	IV	J1436
DIETHYLSTILBESTROL DIPHSPHATE	250 MG	INJ	J9165
DIFLUCAN	200 MG	IV	J1450
DIGIBIND	VIAL	IV	J1162
DIGIFAB	VIAL	IV	J1162
DIGOXIN	0.5 MG	IM, IV	J1160
DIGOXIN IMMUNE FAB	VIAL	IV	J1162
DIHYDROERGOTAMINE MESYLATE	1 MG	IM, IV	J1110
DILANTIN	50 MG	IM, IV	J1165
DILAUDID	250 MG	OTH	S0092
DILAUDID	4 MG	SC, IM, IV	J1170
DILOR	500 MG	IM	J1180
DIMENHYDRINATE	50 MG	IM, IV	J1240
DIMERCAPROL	100 MG	IM	J0470
DIMINE	50 MG	IV, IM	J1200
DINATE	50 MG	IM, IV	J1240
DIOVAL	10 MG	IM	J1380
DIOVAL	20 MG	IM	J1390
DIOVAL 40	10 MG	IM	J1380
DIOVAL 40	20 MG	IM	J1390
DIOVAL XX	10 MG	IM	J1380
DIOVAL XX	20 MG	IM	J1390
DIPHENHYDRAMINE HCL	50 MG	IV, IM	J1200
DIPHENHYDRAMINE HCL	50 MG	ORAL	Q0163
DIPYRIDAMOLE	10 MG	IV	J1245
DISOTATE	150 MG	IV	J3520
DIURIL	500 MG	IV	J1205
DIURIL SODIUM	500 MG	IV	J1205
DIZAC	5 MG	IV, IM	J3360
DMSA	VIAL	IV	C1201
DMSA KIT	VIAL	IV	C1201
DMSO, DIMETHYL SULFOXIDE	50%, 50 ML	OTH	J1212
DOBUTAMINE HCL	250 MG	IV	J1250
DOBUTREX	250 MG	IV	J1250
DOCETAXEL	20 MG	IV	J9170
DOLASETRON MESYLATE	10 MG	IV	J1260
DOLASETRON MESYLATE	100 MG	ORAL	Q0180
DOLASETRON MESYLATE	50 MG	ORAL	S0174
DOLOPHINE	5 MG	ORAL	S0109
DOLOPHINE HCL	10 MG	IM, SC	J1230
DOMMANATE	50 MG	IM, IV	J1240
DOPAMINE HCL	40 MG	IV	J1265
DORNASE ALPHA	PER MG	INH	J7639
DOSTINEX	0.25 MG	ORAL	J8515

Drug Name	Unit Per:	Route	Code
DOXERCALCIFEROL	1 MG	IV	J1270
DOXIL	10 MG	IV	J9001
DOXORUBICIN HCL	10 MG	IV	J9000
DRAMAMINE	50 MG	IM, IV	J1240
DRAMILIN	50 MG	IM, IV	J1240
DRAMOCEN	50 MG	IM, IV	J1240
DRAMOJECT	50 MG	IM, IV	J1240
DRONABINAL	2.5 MG	ORAL	Q0167
DRONABINAL	5 MG	ORAL	Q0168
DROPERIDOL	5 MG	IM, IV	J1790
DROPERIDOL AND FENTANYL CITRATE	2 ML	IM, IV	J1810
DROXIA	500 MG	ORAL	S0176
DTIC-DOME	100 MG	IV	J9130
DTIC-DOME	200 MG	IV	J9140
DUO-SPAN	1 ML	IM	J1060
DUO-SPAN II	1 ML	IM	J1060
DURACILLIN A.S.	600,000 UNITS	IM, IV	J2510
DURACLON	1 MG	OTH	J0735
DURAGEN-10	10 MG	IM	J1380
DURAGEN-10	20 MG	IM	J1390
DURAGEN-20	10 MG	IM	J1380
DURAGEN-20	20 MG	IM	J1390
DURAGEN-40	10 MG	IM	J1380
DURAGEN-40	20 MG	IM	J1390
DURAMORPH	10 MG	IM, IV, SC	J2275
DURAMORPH	500 MG	OTH	S0093
DURATHATE-200	100 MG	IM	J3130
DURO CORT	80 MG	IM	J1040
DYMENATE	50 MG	IM, IV	J1240
DYPHYLLINE	500 MG	IM	J1180
ECHOCARDIOGRAM IMAGE ENHANCER	1 ML	IV	Q9955
ECHOCARDIOGRAM IMAGE ENHANCER	1 ML	INJ	Q9956
EDETATE CALCIUM DISODIUM	1,000 MG	IV, SC, IM	J0600
EDETATE DISODIUM	150 MG	IV	J3520
EDEX	1.25 MCG	VAR	J0270
EFALIZUMAB	125 MG	SC	S0162
ELAPRASE	1 MG	IV	C9232 ●
ELAVIL	20 MG	IM	J1320
ELIGARD	1 MG	IM	J9218
ELIGARD	7.5 MG	IM	J9217
ELITEK	50 MCG	IM	J2783
ELLENCE	2 MG	IV	J9178
ELLIOTTS B SOLUTION	1 ML	IV, IT	J9175
ELOXATIN	0.5 MG	IV	J9263
ELSPAR	10,000 U	VAR	J9020
EMEND	5 MG	ORAL	J8501
EMINASE	30 U	IV	J0350
ENBREL	25 MG	IM, IV	J1438
ENDOXAN-ASTA	1 G	IV	J9091
ENDOXAN-ASTA	100 MG	IV	J9070
ENDOXAN-ASTA	200 MG	IV	J9080
ENDOXAN-ASTA	500 MG	IV	J9090
ENDRATE	150 MG	IV	J3520
ENFUVIRTIDE	1 MG	SC	J1324 ●
ENOVIL	20 MG	IM	J1320

Drug Name	Unit Per:	Route	Code	Drug Name	Unit Per:	Route	Code
ENOXAPARIN SODIUM	10 MG	SC	J1650	FACTOR VIII RECOMBINANT	1 IU	IV	J7192
EPINEPHRINE	1 MG	IM, IV, SC, VAR	J0170	FACTOR VIII, HUMAN	1 IU	IV	J7190
EPIPEN	0.3 MG	IM	J0170	FACTREL	100 MCG	SC, IV	J1620
EPIRUBICIN HCL	2 MG	IV	J9178	FAMOTIDINE	20 MG	IV	S0028
EPOETIN ALFA, ESRD USE	1,000 U	SC, IV	J0886	FASLODEX	25 MG	IM	J9395
EPOETIN ALFA, NON-ESRD USE	1,000 U	SC, IV	J0885	FDG	STUDY DOSE		A9552
EPOGEN, ESRD USE	1,000 U	SC, IV	J0886	FEIBA-VH AICC	1 IU	IV	J7198
EPOGEN, NON-ESRD USE	1,000 U	SC, IV	J0885	FENTANYL CITRATE	0.1 MG	IM, IV	J3010
EPOPROSTENOL	0.5 MG	IV	J1325	FERIDEX IV	1 ML	IV	Q9953
EPOPROSTENOL STERILE DILUTANT	50 ML	IV	S0155	FERRLECIT	12.5 MG	IV	J2916
EPTIFIBATIDE	5 MG	IM, IV	J1327	FERTINEX	75 IU	SC	J3355
ERAXIS	1 MG	IV	J0348 ●	FILGRASTIM	300 MCG	SC, IV	J1440
ERBITUX	10 MG	IV	J9055	FILGRASTIM	480 MCG	SC, IV	J1441
ERGAMISOL	50 MG	ORAL	S0177	FINASTERIDE	5 MG	ORAL	S0138
ERGONOVINE MALEATE	0.2 MG	IM, IV	J1330	FLAGYL	500 MG	IV	S0030
ERTAPENEM SODIUM	500 MG	IM, IV	J1335	~~FLEBOGAMMA~~	~~1 CC~~	~~IM~~	~~J1460~~
ERYTHROCIN LACTOBIONATE	500 MG	IV	J1364	~~FLEBOGAMMA~~	~~1 G~~	~~IV~~	~~J1563~~
ESTONE AQUEOUS	1 MG	IM, IV	J1435	FLEXOJECT	60 MG	IV, IM	J2360
ESTRA-L 20	10 MG	IM	J1380	FLEXON	60 MG	IV, IM	J2360
ESTRA-L 20	20 MG	IM	J1390	FLOLAN	0.5 MG	IV	J1325
ESTRA-L 40	10 MG	IM	J1380	FLOXIN IV	400 MG	IV	S0034
ESTRA-L 40	20 MG	IM	J1390	FLOXURIDINE	500 MG	IV	J9200
ESTRADIOL CYPIONATE	UP TO 5 MG	IM	J1000	FLUCONAZOLE	200 MG	IV	J1450
ESTRADIOL L.A.	10 MG	IM	J1380	FLUDARA	50 MG	IV	J9185
ESTRADIOL L.A.	20 MG	IM	J1390	FLUDARABINE PHOSPHATE	50 MG	IV	J9185
ESTRADIOL L.A. 20	10 MG	IM	J1380	FLUDEOXYGLUCOSE F18	STUDY DOSE	IV	A9552
ESTRADIOL L.A. 20	20 MG	IM	J1390	FLUNISOLIDE, ▶COMPOUNDED, UNIT DOSE◀	1 MG	INH	J7641
ESTRADIOL L.A. 40	10 MG	IM	J1380	FLUOCINOLONE ACETONIDE ▶INTRAVITREAL◀	▶IMPLANT◀	OTH	J7311 ▲
ESTRADIOL L.A. 40	20 MG	IM	J1390	FLUORODEOXYGLUCOSE F-18 FDG, DIAGNOSTIC	45 MCI	IV	A9552
ESTRADIOL VALERATE	10 MG	IM	J1380				
ESTRADIOL VALERATE	20 MG	IM	J1390	FLUOROURACIL	500 MG	IV	J9190
ESTRADIOL VALERATE	UP TO 40 MG	IM	J0970	FLUPHENAZINE DECANOATE	25 MG	SC, IM	J2680
ESTRAGYN	1 MG	IV, IM	J1435	FLUTAMIDE	125 MG	ORAL	S0175
ESTRO-A	1 MG	IV, IM	J1435	FOLEX	5 MG	IV, IM, IT, IA	J9250
ESTROGEN CONJUGATED	25 MG	IV, IM	J1410	FOLEX	50 MG	IV, IM, IT, IA	J9260
ESTRONE	1 MG	IV, IM	J1435	FOLEX PFS	5 MG	IV, IM, IT, IA	J9250
ESTRONOL	1 MG	IM, IV	J1435	FOLEX PFS	50 MG	IV, IM, IT, IA	J9260
ETANERCEPT	25 MG	IM, IV	J1438	FOLLISTIM	75 IU	SC, IM	S0128
ETHAMOLIN	100 MG	IV	J1430	FOLLITROPIN ALFA	75 IU	SC	S0126
ETHANOLAMINE OLEATE	100 MG	IV	J1430	FOLLITROPIN BETA	75 IU	SC, IM	S0128
ETHYOL	500 MG	IV	J0207	FOMEPIZOLE	15 MG	IV	J1451
ETIDRONATE DISODIUM	300 MG	IV	J1436	FOMIVIRSEN SODIUM	1.65 MG	OTH	J1452
ETOPOSIDE	10 MG	IV	J9181	FONDAPARINUX SODIUM	0.5 MG	SC	J1652
ETOPOSIDE	100 MG	IV	J9182	FORMOTEROL, ▶COMPOUNDED, UNIT DOSE◀	12 MCG	INH	J7640
ETOPOSIDE	50 MG	ORAL	J8560				
EUFLEXXA	20-25 MG	OTH	J7319 ▲	FORTAZ	500 MG	IM, IV	J0713
~~EUFLEXXA~~	~~30 MG~~	~~OTH~~	~~G9220~~	FORTEO	10 MCG	SC	J3110
EULEXIN	125 MG	ORAL	S0175	FORTOVASE	200 MG	ORAL	S0140
EVERONE	100 MG	IM	J3120	FOSCARNET SODIUM	1,000 MG	IV	J1455
EVERONE	100 MG	IM	J3130	FOSCAVIR	1,000 MG	IV	J1455
EXMESTANE	25 MG	ORAL	S0156	FOSPHENYTOIN	50 MG	IM, IV	Q2009
FABRAZYME	1 MG	IV	J0180	FOSPHENYTOIN SODIUM	750 MG	IM, IV	S0078
FACTOR IX NON-RECOMBINANT	1 IU	IV	J7193	FRAGMIN	2,500 IU	SC	J1645
FACTOR IX RECOMBINANT	1 IU	IV	J7195	FUDR	500 MG	IV	J9200
FACTOR IX+ COMPLEX	1 IU	IV	J7194	FULVESTRANT	25 MG	IM	J9395
FACTOR VIIA RECOMBINANT	1 MCG	IV	J7189	FUNGIZONE	50 MG	IV	J0285
FACTOR VIII PORCINE	1 IU	IV	J7191				

Appendix 1 — Table of Drugs

Drug Name	Unit Per:	Route	Code	Drug Name	Unit Per:	Route	Code
FUROCOT	20 MG	IM, IV	J1940	GEMTUZUMAB	5 MG	IV	J9300
FUROMIDE M.D.	20 MG	IM, IV	J1940	GEMZAR	200 MG	IV	J9201
FUROSEMIDE	20 MG	IM, IV	J1940	GENARC	1 IU	IV	J7192
FUZEON	1 MG	SC	J1324 ●	GENGRAF	100 MG	ORAL	J7502
GADOLINIUM-BASED MAGNETIC RESONANCE CONTRAST AGENT	1 ML	IV	Q9952	GENGRAF	25 MG	ORAL	J7515
				GENOTROPIN	1 MG	SC	J2941
GALLIUM GA-67	1 MCI	IV	A9556	GENOTROPIN MINIQUICK	1 MG	SC	J2941
GALLIUM NITRATE	1 MG	IV	J1457	GENOTROPIN NUTROPIN	1 MG	SC	J2941
GALSULFASE	▶1 MG◀	IV	J1458 ▲	GENTAMICIN	80 MG	IM, IV	J1580
GAMASTAN	1 CC	IM	J1460	GENTAMICIN SULFATE	80 MG	IM, IV	J1580
GAMASTAN	2 CC	IM	J1470	GENTRAN	500 ML	IV	J7100
GAMASTAN	3 CC	IM	J1480	GENTRAN 75	500 ML	IV	J7110
GAMASTAN	4 CC	IM	J1490	GEODON	10 MG	IM	J3486
GAMASTAN	5 CC	IM	J1500	GEREF	1MCG	SC	Q0515
GAMASTAN	6 CC	IM	J1510	GESTERONE	50 MG	IM	J2675
GAMASTAN	7 CC	IM	J1520	GESTRIN	50 MG	IM	J2675
GAMASTAN	8 CC	IM	J1530	GLATIRAMER ACETATE	20 MG	SC	J1595
GAMASTAN	9 CC	IM	J1540	GLEEVEC	100 MG	ORAL	S0088
GAMASTAN	10 CC	IM	J1550	GLOFIL-125	10 UCI	IV	A9554
GAMASTAN	OVER 10 CC	IM	J1560	GLUCAGEN	1 MG	SC, IM, IV	J1610
GAMIMMUNE N	500 MG	IV	J1567	GLUCAGON	1 MG	SC, IM, IV	J1610
GAMMA GLOBULIN	1 CC	IM	J1460	GLUCOTOPE	STUDY DOSE	IV	A9552
GAMMA GLOBULIN	2 CC	IM	J1470	GLYCOPYRROLATE, ▶COMPOUNDED◀ CONCENTRATED	PER MG	INH	J7642
GAMMA GLOBULIN	3 CC	IM	J1480				
GAMMA GLOBULIN	4 CC	IM	J1490	GLYCOPYRROLATE, ▶COMPOUNDED, UNIT DOSE◀	1 MG	INH	J7643
GAMMA GLOBULIN	5 CC	IM	J1500				
GAMMA GLOBULIN	6 CC	IM	J1510	GOLD SODIUM THIOMALATE	50 MG	IM	J1600
GAMMA GLOBULIN	7 CC	IM	J1520	GONADORELIN HCL	100 MCG	SC, IV	J1620
GAMMA GLOBULIN	8 CC	IM	J1530	GONAL-F	75 IU	SC	S0126
GAMMA GLOBULIN	9 CC	IM	J1540	GOSERELIN ACETATE	3.6 MG	SC	J9202
GAMMA GLOBULIN	10 CC	IM	J1550	GRAFTJACKET REGULAR MATRIX	PER 16 SQ CM	OTH	C9221
GAMMA GLOBULIN	OVER 10 CC	IM	J1560	GRAFTJACKET SOFT TISSUE MATRIX	1 CC	OTH	C9222
GAMMAGARD S/D	500 MG	IV	J1566				
GAMMAR	1 CC	IM	J1460	GRANISETRON HCL	1 MG	ORAL	Q0166
GAMMAR	2 CC	IM	J1470	GRANISETRON HCL	1 MG	IV	S0091
GAMMAR	3 CC	IM	J1480	GRANISETRON HCL	100 MCG	IV	J1626
GAMMAR	4 CC	IM	J1490	GYNOGEN L.A. 10	10 MG	IM	J1380
GAMMAR	5 CC	IM	J1500	GYNOGEN L.A. 10	20 MG	IM	J1390
GAMMAR	6 CC	IM	J1510	GYNOGEN L.A. 20	10 MG	IM	J1380
GAMMAR	7 CC	IM	J1520	GYNOGEN L.A. 20	20 MG	IM	J1390
GAMMAR	8 CC	IM	J1530	GYNOGEN L.A. 40	10 MG	IM	J1380
GAMMAR	9 CC	IM	J1540	GYNOGEN L.A. 40	20 MG	IM	J1390
GAMMAR	10 CC	IM	J1550	GYNOGEN LA	20 MG	IM	J1390
GAMMAR	OVER 10 CC	IM	J1560	H.P. ACTHAR	40 U	VAR	J0800
GAMMAR P	500 MG	IV	J1566	HALDOL	5 MG	IM, IV	J1630
GAMULIN RH	300 MCG	IM	J2790	HALDOL DECANOATE	50 MG	IM	J1631
GAMUNEX	500 MG	IV	J1567	HALOPERIDOL	5 MG	IM, IV	J1630
GANCICLOVIR	4.5 MG	OTH	J7310	HAVID	0.375 MG	ORAL	S0141
GANCICLOVIR SODIUM	500 MG	IV	J1570	HECTOROL	1 MG	IV	J1270
GANIRELIX ACETATE	250 MCG	SC	S0132	HELIXATE	1 IU	IV	J7192
GANITE	1 MG	IV	J1457	HEMIN	1 MG	IV	J1640
GARAMYCIN	80 MG	IM, IV	J1580	HEMOFIL-M	1 IU	IV	J7190
GASTROCROM	10 MG	INH	J7631	HEP LOCK	10 U	IV	J1642
GASTROMARK	1 ML	ORAL	Q9954	HEPARIN SODIUM	1,000 U	IV, SC	J1644
GATIFLOXACIN	10 MG	IV	J1590	HEPARIN SODIUM	10 U	IV	J1642
GEFITINIB	250 MG	ORAL	J8565	HERCEPTIN	10 MG	IV	J9355
GEMCITABINE HCL	200 MG	IV	J9201	HEXABRIX 320	1 ML	IV	Q9949

APPENDIX 1 — TABLE OF DRUGS

Drug Name	Unit Per:	Route	Code	Drug Name	Unit Per:	Route	Code
HEXADROL	0.25 MG	ORAL	J8540	HYDROXYZINE HCL	25 MG	IM	J3410
HIGH OSMOLAR CONTRAST MATERIAL, UP TO 149 MG/ML IODINE CONCENTRATION	1 ML	IV	Q9958	HYDROXYZINE PAMOATE	25 MG	ORAL	Q0177
				HYDROXYZINE PAMOATE	50 MG	ORAL	Q0178
HIGH OSMOLAR CONTRAST MATERIAL, UP TO 150-199 MG/ML IODINE CONCENTRATION	1 ML	IV	Q9959	HYLAN G-F 20	16 MG	OTH	J7319 ▲
				HYLENEX	1 USP UNIT	SC	J3473 ●
				HYOSCYAMINE SULFATE	0.25 MG	SC, IM, IV	J1980
HIGH OSMOLAR CONTRAST MATERIAL, UP TO 200-249 MG/ML IODINE CONCENTRATION	1 ML	IV	Q9960	HYPERSTAT	300 MG	IV	J1730
				HYPRHO-D	300 MCG	IM	J2790
HIGH OSMOLAR CONTRAST MATERIAL, UP TO 250-299 MG/ML IODINE CONCENTRATION	1 ML	IV	Q9961	HYPRHO-D	50 MCG	IM	J2788
				HYREXIN	50 MG	IV, IM	J1200
HIGH OSMOLAR CONTRAST MATERIAL, UP TO 300-349 MG/ML IODINE CONCENTRATION	1 ML	IV	Q9962	HYZINE	25 MG	IM	J3410
				HYZINE-50	25 MG	IM	J3410
				I-131 TOSITUMOMAB DIAGNOSTIC	DOSE	IV	A9544
HIGH OSMOLAR CONTRAST MATERIAL, UP TO 350-399 MG/ML IODINE CONCENTRATION	1 ML	IV	Q9963	I-131 TOSITUMOMAB THERAPEUTIC	DOSE	IV	A9545
				IBANDRONATE SODIUM	1 MG	IV	J1740 ▲
HIGH OSMOLAR CONTRAST MATERIAL, UP TO 400 OR GREATER MG/ML IODINE CONCENTRATION	1 ML	IV	Q9964	IBRITUMOMAB TUXETAN	5 MCI	IV	A9542
				IBUTILIDE FUMARATE	1 MG	IV	J1742
HISTERONE 100	50 MG	IM	J3140	IDAMYCIN	5 MG	IV	J9211
HISTERONE 50	50 MG	IM	J3140	IDAMYCIN PFS	5 MG	IV	J9211
HISTRELIN ACETATE	10 MG	INJ	J1675	IDARUBICIN HCL	5 MG	IV	J9211
HISTRELIN IMPLANT	50 MG	OTH	J9225	IDURSULFASE	1 MG	IV	J1740 ●
HUMALOG	5 U	SC	J1815	IFEX	1 G	IV	J9208
HUMALOG	5 U	SC	S5551	IFOSFAMIDE	1 G	IV	J9208
HUMALOG	50 U	SC	J1817	IL-2	1 VIAL	IV	J9015
HUMATE-P	1 IU	IV	J7187 ▲	ILETIN	5 UNITS	SC	J1815
HUMATROPE	1 MG	SC	J2941	ILETIN II NPH PORK	50 U	SC	J1817
HUMIRA	20 MG	SC	J0135	ILETIN II REGULAR PORK	5 U	SC	J1815
HUMULIN	5 U	SC	J1815	ILOPROST INHALATION SOLUTION	▶20 UCI◀	INH	Q4080
HUMULIN	50 U	SC	J1817	IMAGENT	1 ML	IV	Q9955
HUMULIN R	5 U	SC	J1815	IMATINIB	100 MG	ORAL	S0088
HUMULIN R U-500	5 U	SC	J1815	IMIGLUCERASE	1 U	IV	J1785
HYALGAN	20-25 MG	OTH	J7317	IMITREX	6 MG	SC	J3030
HYALGAN	30 MG	OTH	C9220	IMMUNE GLOBULIN LYOPHILIZED	500 MG	IV	J1566
HYALURONIDASE	150 UNITS	VAR	J3470	IMMUNE GLOBULIN NONLYOPHILIZED	500 MG	IV	J1567
HYALURONIDASE RECOMBINANT	1 USP UNIT	SC	J3473 ●				
HYALURONIDASE, OVINE, PRESERVATIVE FREE	1 USP	OTH	J3471	IMMUNE GLOBULIN SUBCUTANEOUS	100 MG	SC	J1562 ●
HYALURONIDASE, OVINE, PRESERVATIVE FREE	1000 USP	OTH	J3472	IMURAN	100 MG	OTH	J7501
				IMURAN	50 MG	ORAL	J7500
HYATE C	1 IU	IV	J7191	IN-111 SATUMOMAB PENDETIDE	DOSE	IV	A4642
HYBOLIN DECANOATE	100 MG	IM	J2321	INAPSINE	5 MG	IM, IV	J1790
HYBOLIN DECANOATE	50 MG	IM	J2320	INDERAL	1 MG	IV	J1800
HYCAMTIN	4 MG	IV	J9350	INDIUM IN-111 IBRITUMOMAB TIUXETAN, DIAGNOSTIC	5 MCI	IV	A9542
HYDRALAZINE HCL	20 MG	IV, IM	J0360				
HYDRATE	50 MG	IM, IV	J1240	INDIUM IN-111 OXYQUINOLINE	0.5 MCI	IV	A9547
HYDREA	500 MG	ORAL	S0176	INDIUM IN-111 PENTETREOTIDE	1 MCI	IV	A9565
HYDROCORTISONE ACETATE	25 MG	IV, IM, SC	J1700	INFED	50 MG	IM, IV	J1751
HYDROCORTISONE SODIUM PHOSPHATE	50 MG	IV, IM, SC	J1710	INFERGEN	1 MCG	SC	J9212
				INFLIXIMAB	100 MG	IV	J1745
HYDROCORTISONE SODIUM SUCCINATE	100 MG	IV, IM, SC	J1720	INFUMORPH	10 MG	IM, IV, SC	J2270
				INFUMORPH	10 MG	OTH	J2275
HYDROCORTONE PHOSPHATE	50 MG	SC, IM, IV	J1710	INFUMORPH PRESERVATIVE FREE	100 MG	IM, IV, SC	J2271
HYDROMORPHONE HCL	4 MG	SC, IM, IV	J1170	INNOHEP	1,000 IU	SC	J1655
HYDROMORPHONE HYDROCHLORIDE	250 MG	OTH	S0092	INNOVAR	2 ML	IM, IV	J1810
				INSULIN	5 U	SC	J1815
HYDROXOCOBALAMIN	1,000 MCG	IM, SC	J3420	INSULIN	50 U	SC	J1817
HYDROXYCOBAL	1,000 MCG	IM, SC	J3420	INSULIN LISPRO	5 U	SC	J1815
HYDROXYUREA	500 MG	ORAL	S0176	INSULIN LISPRO	5 U	SC	S5551

Appendix 1 — Table of Drugs

Drug Name	Unit Per:	Route	Code
INSULIN PURIFIED REGULAR PORK	5 U	SC	J1815
INTAL	10 MG	INH	J7631
INTEGRA BILAYER MATRIX	SQ CM	OTH	J3743
INTEGRILIN	5 MG	IM, IV	J1327
INTERFERON ALFA-2A	3,000,000 U	SC, IM	J9213
INTERFERON ALFA-2B	1,000,000 U	SC, IM	J9214
INTERFERON ALFA-N3	250,000 IU	IM	J9215
INTERFERON ALFACON-1	1 MCG	SC	J9212
INTERFERON BETA-1A	11 MCG	IM	Q3025
INTERFERON BETA-1A	11 MCG	SC	Q3026
INTERFERON BETA-1A	33 MCG	IM	J1825
INTERFERON BETA-1B	0.25 MG	SC	J1830
INTERFERON, ALFA-2A, RECOMBINANT	3,000,000 U	SC, IM	J9213
INTERFERON, ALFA-2B, RECOMBINANT	1,000,000 U	SC, IM	J9214
INTERFERON, ALFA-N3, (HUMAN LEUKOCYTE DERIVED)	250,000 IU	IM	J9215
INTERFERON, GAMMA 1-B	3 MU	SC	J9216
INTERLUEKIN	1 VIAL	IV	J9015
INTRON A	1,000,000 U	SC, IM	J9214
INTROPIN	40 MG	IV	J1265
INVANZ	500 MG	IM, IV	J1335
INVIRASE	200 MG	ORAL	S0140
IOBENGUANE SULFATE I-131	0.5 MCI	IV	A9508
IODINE I-123 SODIUM IODIDE CAPSULE(S), DIAGNOSTIC	100 UCI	ORAL	A9516
IODINE I-125 SERUM ALBUMIN, DIAGNOSTIC	10 UCI	IV	A9554
IODINE I-125 SODIUM IOTHALAMATE, DIAGNOSTIC	10 UCI	IV	A9554
IODINE I-125, SODIUM IODIDE SOLUTION, THERAPEUTIC	1 UCI	ORAL	A9527 ●
IODINE I-131 IODINATED SERIUM ALBUMIN, DIAGNOSTIC	PER 5 UCI	ORAL	A9524
IODINE I-131 SERUM ALBUMIN, DIAGNOSTIC	5 UCI	IV	A9532
IODINE I-131 SODIUM IODIDE CAPSULE(S), DIAGNOSTIC	1 MCI	ORAL	A9528
IODINE I-131 SODIUM IODIDE CAPSULE(S), THERAPEUTIC	1 MCI	ORAL	A9517
IODINE I-131 SODIUM IODIDE SOLUTION, DIAGNOSTIC	1 MCI	ORAL	A9529
IODINE I-131 SODIUM IODIDE SOLUTION, THERAPEUTIC	1 MCI	ORAL	A9530
IODINE I-131 SODIUM IODIDE, DIAGNOSTIC	100 UCI	IV	A9531
IODINE I-131 TOSITUMOMAB, DIAGNOSTIC	STUDY DOSE	IV	A9544
IODINE I-131 TOSITUMOMAB, THERAPEUTIC	STUDY DOSE	IV	A9545
IODOTOPE THERAPEUTIC CAPSULE(S)	1 MCI	ORAL	A9517
IODOTOPE THERAPEUTIC SOLUTION	1 MCI	ORAL	A9530
ION-BASED MAGNETIC RESONANCE CONTRAST AGENT	1 ML	IV	Q9953
IOTHALAMATE SODIUM I-125	STUDY DOSE	IV	A9554
IPLEX	1 MG	SC	J2170 ●
IPRATROPIUM BROMIDE, ▶NONCOMPOUNDED, UNIT DOSE◀	1 MG	INH	J7644
IPTRATROPIUM BROMIDE COMPOUNDED, UNIT DOSE	1 MG	INH	J7645 ●
IRESSA	250 MG	ORAL	J8565

Drug Name	Unit Per:	Route	Code
IRINOTECAN	20 MG	IV	J9206
IRON DEXTRAN 165	50 MG	IM, IV	J1751
IRON DEXTRAN 237	50 MG	IM, IV	J1752
IRON SUCROSE	1 MG	IV	J1756
ISOCAINE	10 ML	VAR	J0670
ISOETHARINE HCL COMPOUNDED, CONCENTRATED	1 MG	INH	J7647 ●
ISOETHARINE HCL NONCOMPOUNDED, CONCENTRATED	1 MG	INH	J7650 ●
ISOETHARINE HCL, ▶NONCOMPOUNDED◀ CONCENTRATED	PER MG	INH	J7648
ISOETHARINE HCL, ▶NONCOMPOUNDED, UNIT DOSE◀	1 MG	INH	J7649
ISOJEX	▶5 MCI◀	IV	A9532
ISOPROTERENOL HCL COMPOUNDED, CONCENTRATED	1 MG	INH	J7657 ●
ISOPROTERENOL HCL COMPOUNDED, UNIT DOSE	1 MG	INH	J7660 ●
ISOPROTERENOL HCL, ▶NONCOMPOUNDED◀ CONCENTRATED	1 MG	INH	J7658
ISOPROTERNOL HCL, ▶NONCOMPOUNDED, UNIT DOSE◀	PER MG	INH	J7659
ISOVUE 200	1 ML	IV	Q9947
ISOVUE 250	1 ML	IV	Q9948
ISOVUE 300	1 ML	IV	Q9949
ISOVUE 370	1 ML	IV	Q9950
ISOVUE-M 200	1 ML	IV	Q9947
ISOVUE-M 300	1 ML	IV	Q9949
ITRACONAZOLE	50 MG	IV	J1835
IVEEGAM	500 MG	IV	J1566
JENAMICIN	80 MG	IM, IV	J1580
K-FLEX	60 MG	IV, IM	J2360
KABIKINASE	250,000 IU	IV	J2995
KANAMYCIN	500 MG	IM, IV	J1840
KANTREX	500 MG	IM, IV	J1840
KANTREX	75 MG	IM, IV	J1850
KEFZOL	500 MG	IV, IM	J0690
KENAJECT-40	10 MG	IM	J3301
KENALOG-10	10 MG	IM	J3301
KENALOG-40	10 MG	IM	J3301
KEPIVANCE	50 MCG	IV	J2425
KESTRONE	1 MG	IV, IM	J1435
KETOROLAC TROMETHAMINE	15 MG	IM, IV	J1885
KEY-PRED 25	1 ML	IM	J2650
KEY-PRED 50	1 ML	IM	J2650
KINEVAC	5 MCG	IV	J2805
KOATE-DVI	1 IU	IV	J7190
KOGENATE	1 IU	IV	J7190
KOGENATE	1 IU	IV	J7192
KONAKION	1 MG	SC, IM, IV	J3430
KONYNE 80	1 IU	IV	J7194
KYTRIL	1 MG	ORAL	Q0166
KYTRIL	1 MG	IV	S0091
KYTRIL	100 MCG	IV	J1626
L-CARNITINE	1 G	IV	J1955
L-PHENYLALANINE MUSTARD	50 MG	IV	J9245
L.A.E. 20	10 MG	IM	J1380

Drug Name	Unit Per:	Route	Code
L.A.E. 20	20 MG	IM	J1390
LANOXIN	0.5 MG	IM, IV	J1160
LANTUS	50 U	SC	J1817
LARONIDASE	0.1 MG	IV	J1931
LASIX	20 MG	IM, IV	J1940
LENTE ILETIN I	5 U	SC	J1815
LEPIRUDIN	50 MG	IV	J1945
LEUCOVORIN CALCIUM	50 MG	IM, IV	J0640
LEUKERAN	2 MG	ORAL	S0172
LEUKINE	50 MCG	IV	J2820
LEUPROLIDE ACETATE	1 MG	IM	J9218
LEUPROLIDE ACETATE	7.5 MG	IM	J9217
LEUPROLIDE ACETATE (FOR DEPOT SUSPENSION)	3.75 MG	IM	J1950
LEUPROLIDE ACETATE DEPOT	7.5 MG	IM	J9217
LEUPROLIDE ACETATE IMPLANT	65 MG	OTH	J9219
LEUSTATIN	1 MG	IV	J9065
LEVABUTEROL COMPOUNDED, UNIT DOSE	1 MG	INH	J7615 ●
LEVABUTEROL, COMPOUNDED, CONCENTRATED	0.5 MG	INH	J7607 ●
LEVALBUTEROL ►NONCOMPOUNDED,◄ CONCENTRATED FORM	0.5 MG	INH	J7612
LEVALBUTEROL, ►NONCOMPOUNED UNIT DOSE◄	0.5 MG	INH	J7614
LEVAMISOLE HCL	50 MG	ORAL	S0177
LEVAQUIN	1 G	IV	J1956
LEVOCARNITINE	1 G	IV	J1955
LEVOFLOXACIN	1 G	IV	J1956
LEVONORGESTREL	52 MG	OTH	J7302
LEVORPHANOL TARTRATE	2 MG	SC, IV, IM	J1960
LEVOXYL	5 MG	ORAL	J7506
LEVSIN	0.25 MG	SC, IM, IV	J1980
LEVULAN KERASTICK	SINGLE UNIT DOSE (354 MG)	OTH	J7308
LIBRIUM	100 MG	IM, IV	J1990
LIDOCAINE HCL	10 MG	IV	J2001
LINCOCIN HCL	300 MG	IV	J2010
LINCOMYCIN HCL	300 MG	IM, IV	J2010
LINEZOLID	200 MG	IV	J2020
LIORESAL	10 MG	IT	J0475
LIORESAL INTRATHECAL REFILL	50 MCG	IT	J0476
LIQUAEMIN SODIUM	1,000 UNITS	SC, IV	J1644
LIQUID PRED SYRUP	5 MG	OTH	J7506
LISPRO-PFC	50 U	SC	J1817
LOMUSTINE	10 MG	ORAL	S0178
LONITEN	10 MG	ORAL	S0139
LORAZEPAM	2 MG	IM, IV	J2060
LOVENOX	10 MG	SC	J1650
LOW OSMOLAR CONTRAST MATERIAL, 400 OR GREATER MG/ML IODINE CONCENTRATION	1 ML	IV	Q9951
LOW OSMOLAR CONTRAST MATERIAL, UP TO 150-199 MG/ML IODINE CONCENTRATION	1 ML	IV	Q9946
LOW OSMOLAR CONTRAST MATERIAL, UP TO 200-249 MG/ML IODINE CONCENTRATION	1 ML	IV	Q9947
LOW OSMOLAR CONTRAST MATERIAL, UP TO 250-299 MG/ML IODINE CONCENTRATION	1 ML	IV	Q9948

Drug Name	Unit Per:	Route	Code
LOW OSMOLAR CONTRAST MATERIAL, UP TO 300-349 MG/ML IODINE CONCENTRATION	1 ML	IV	Q9949
LOW OSMOLAR CONTRAST MATERIAL, UP TO 350-399 MG/ML IODINE CONCENTRATION	1 ML	IV	Q9950
LUCENTIS	0.5 MG	OTH	C9233 ●
LUFYLLIN	500 MG	IM	J1180
LUMINAL SODIUM	120 MG	IM, IV	J2560
LUNELLE	5 MG/25 MG	IM	J1056
LUPRON	1 MG	IM	J9218
LUPRON	7.5 MG	IM	J9217
LUPRON DEPOT	3.75 MG	IM	J1950
LUPRON DEPOT	7.5 MG	IM	J9217
LUPRON IMPLANT	65 MG	OTH	J9219
LUTREPULSE	100 MCG	SC, IV	J1620
LYMPHOCYTE IMMUNE GLOBULIN, ANTITHYMOCYTE GLOBULIN, EQUINE	250 MG	OTH	J7504
LYMPHOCYTE IMMUNE GLOBULIN, ANTITHYMOCYTE GLOBULIN, RABBIT	25 MG	OTH	J7511
MACUGEN	0.3 MG	OTH	J2503
MAGNESIUM SULFATE	10 MG	IV	J3475
MAGNETIC RESONANCE CONTRAST AGENT	1 ML	ORAL	Q9954
MAGNEVIST 46.9%	1 ML	IV	Q9952
MAGROTEC	10 MCI	IV	A9540
MANNITOL	25% IN 50 ML	IV	J2150
MARCAINE HCL	30 ML	VAR	S0200
MARINOL	2.5 MG	ORAL	Q0167
MARINOL	5 MG	ORAL	Q0168
MARMINE	50 MG	IM, IV	J1240
MATULANE	50 MG	ORAL	S0182
MAXIPIME	500 MG	IV	J0692
MECASERMIN	1 MG	SC	J2170 ●
MECHLORETHAMINE HYDROCHLORIDE	10 MG	IV	J9230
MEDROL	4 MG	ORAL	J7509
MEDROXYPROGESTERONE ACETATE	150 MG	IM	J1055
MEDROXYPROGESTERONE ACETATE	50 MG	IM	J1051
MEDROXYPROGESTERONE ACETATE/ESTRADIOL CYPIONATE	5 MG/25 MG	IM	J1056
MEFOXIN	1 G	IV	J0694
MEGACE	20 MG	ORAL	S0179
MEGESTROL ACETATE	20 MG	ORAL	S0179
MELPHALAN HCL	2 MG	ORAL	J8600
MELPHALAN HCL	50 MG	IV	J9245
MENADIONE	1 MG	IM, SC, IV	J3430
MENOTROPINS	75 IU	SC, IM, IV	S0122
MEPERGAN	50 MG	IM, IV	J2180
MEPERIDINE AND PROMETHAZINE HCL	50 MG	IM, IV	J2180
MEPERIDINE HCL	100 MG	IM, IV, SC	J2175
MEPIVACAINE HCL	10 ML	VAR	J0670
MERCAPTOPURINE	50 MG	ORAL	S0108
MERITATE	150 MG	IV	J3520
MEROPENEM	100 MG	IV	J2185
MERREM	100 MG	IV	J2185
MESNA	200 MG	IV	J9209
MESNEX	200 MG	IV	J9209

Appendix 1 — Table of Drugs

Drug Name	Unit Per:	Route	Code
METAPROTERENOL SULFATE COMPOUNDED, UNIT DOSE	10 MG	INH	J7670 ●
METAPROTERENOL SULFATE, ▶NONCOMPOUNDED, UNIT DOSE◀	10 MG	INH	J7669
METAPROTERENOL SULFATE, ▶NONCOMPOUNDED,◀ CONCENTRATED	10 MG	INH	J7668
METARAMINOL BITARTRATE	10 MG	IV, IM, SC	J0380
METASTRON STRONTIUM 89 CHLORIDE	1 MCI	IV	A9600
METATRACE	STUDY DOSE	IV	A9552
METHACHOLINE CHLORIDE	1 MG	INH	J7674
METHADONE	5 MG	ORAL	S0109
METHADONE HCL	10 MG	IM, SC	J1230
METHAPREL, ▶COMPOUNDED,◀ UNIT DOSE	10 MG	INH	J7670 ●
METHAPREL, ▶NONCOMPOUNDED,◀ CONCENTRATED	10 MG	INH	J7668
METHAPREL, ▶NONCOMPOUNDED, UNIT DOSE◀	10 MG	INH	J7669
METHERGINE	0.2 MG	IM, IV	J2210
METHOCARBAMOL	10 ML	IV, IM	J2800
METHOTREXATE	5 MG	IV, IM, IT, IA	J9250
METHOTREXATE	50 MG	IV, IM, IT, IA	J9260
METHOTREXATE LPF	5 MG	IV, IM, IT, IA	J9250
METHOTREXATE LPF	50 MG	IV, IM, IT, IA	J9260
METHOTREXATE SODIUM	2.5 MG	ORAL	J8610
METHOTREXATE SODIUM	5 MG	IV, IM, IT, IA	J9250
METHOTREXATE SODIUM	50 MG	IV, IM, IT, IA	J9260
METHYLCOTOLONE	80 MG	IM	J1040
METHYLDOPA HCL	250 MG	IV	J0210
METHYLDOPATE HCL	5 MG	IV	J0210
METHYLENE BLUE	1 ML	IV	A9535
METHYLERGONOVINE MALEATE	0.2 MG	IM, IV	J2210
METHYLPRED	4 MG	ORAL	J7509
METHYLPREDNISOLONE	125 MG	IM, IV	J2930
METHYLPREDNISOLONE	4 MG	ORAL	J7509
METHYLPREDNISOLONE	UP TO 40 MG	IM, IV	J2920
METHYLPREDNISOLONE ACETATE	20 MG	IM	J1020
METHYLPREDNISOLONE ACETATE	40 MG	IM	J1030
METHYLPREDNISOLONE ACETATE	80 MG	IM	J1040
METOCLOPRAMIDE	10 MG	IV	J2765
METRONIDAZOLE	500 MG	IV	S0030
MIACALCIN	400 U	SC, IM	J0630
MIBG	0.5 MCI	IV	A9508
MICAFUNGIN SODIUM	1 MG	IV	J2248 ▲
MIDAZOLAM HCl	1 MG	IM, IV	J2250
MILRINONE LACTATE	5 MG	IV	J2260
MINOXIDIL	10 MG	ORAL	S0139
MIO REL	60 MG	IV, IM	J2360
MIRENA	52 MG	OTH	J7302
MISOPROSTOL	200 MG	ORAL	S0191
MITHRACIN	2,500 MCG	IV	J9270
MITOMYCIN	20 MG	IV	J9290
MITOMYCIN	40 MG	IV	J9291
MITOMYCIN	5 MG	IV	J9280
MITOXANA	1 G	IV	J9208
MITOXANTRONE HYDROCHLORIDE	5 MG	IV	J9293
MONARC-M	1 IU	IV	J7190

Drug Name	Unit Per:	Route	Code
MONOCLATE-P	1 IU	IV	J7190
MONONINE	1 IU	IV	J7193
MONOPUR	75 IU	SC, IM	S0122
MORPHINE SULFATE	10 MG	IM, IV, SC	J2270
MORPHINE SULFATE	100 MG	IM, IV, SC	J2271
MORPHINE SULFATE	500 MG	OTH	S0093
MORPHINE SULFATE, PRESERVATIVE FREE, STERILE SOLUTION	10 MG	IM, IV, SC	J2275
MOXIFLOXACIN	100 MG	IV	J2280
MPI INDIUM DTPA	0.5 MCI	IV	A9548
MS CONTIN	500 MG	OTH	S0093
MUCOMYST	1 G	INH	J7608
MUCOSIL	1 G	INH	J7608
MULTIHANCE	1 ML	IV	Q9952
MUROMONAB-CD3	5 MG	OTH	J7505
MUSE	EA	OTH	J0275
MUSTARGEN	10 MG	IV	J9230
MUTAMYCIN	20 MG	IV	J9290
MUTAMYCIN	40 MG	IV	J9291
MUTAMYCIN	5 MG	IV	J9280
MYCAMINE	1 MG	IV	J2248 ▲
MYCOPHENOLATE MOFETIL	250 MG	ORAL	J7517
MYCOPHENOLIC ACID	180 MG	ORAL	J7518
MYFORTIC DELAYED RELEASE	180 MG	ORAL	J7518
MYLERAN	2 MG	ORAL	J8510
MYLOCEL	500 MG	ORAL	S0176
MYLOTARG	5 MG	IV	J9300
MYOBLOC	100 U	IM	J0587
MYOCHRYSINE	50 MG	IM	J1600
MYOLIN	60 MG	IV, IM	J2360
MYOPHEN	60 MG	IV, IM	J2360
MYOVIEW	DOSE	IV	A9502
MYOZYME	10 MG	IV	C9234 ●
MYOZYME	20 MG	IV	S0147 ●
NABILONE	1 MG	ORAL	J8650 ●
NAFCILLIN SODIUM	2 GM	IM, IV	S0032
NAGLAZYME	▶1 MG◀	IV	J1458 ▲
NALBUPHINE HCL	10 MG	IM, IV, SC	J2300
NALLPEN	2 GM	IM, IV	S0032
NALOXONE HCL	1 MG	IM, IV, SC	J2310
NALTREXONE, DEPOT FORM	1 MG	IM	J2315 ●
NANDROBOLIC L.A.	100 MG	IM	J2321
NANDROLONE DECANOATE	100 MG	IM	J2321
NANDROLONE DECANOATE	200 MG	IM	J2322
NANDROLONE DECANOATE	50 MG	IM	J2320
NARCAN	1 MG	IM, IV, SC	J2310
NAROPIN	1 MG	VAR	J2795
NASAHIST B	10 MG	IM	J0945
NASALCROM	10 MG	INH	J7631
NATALIZUMAB	1 MG	IV	Q4079
NATRECOR	0.1 MG	IV	J2325
NATURAL ESTROGENIC SUBSTANCE	1 MG	IM, IV	J1410
NAVELBINE	10 MG	IV	J9390
ND-STAT	10 MG	IM, SC, IV	J0945
NEBCIN	80 MG	IM, IV	J3260
NEBUPENT	300 MG	INH	J2545

Drug Name	Unit Per:	Route	Code	Drug Name	Unit Per:	Route	Code
NEBUPENT	300 MG	IM, IV	S0080	NUTROPIN	1 MG	SC	J2941
NELARABINE	50 MG	IV	J9261 ●	NUTROPIN A.Q.	1 MG	SC	J2941
NEMBUTAL SODIUM	120 MG	IM, IV	J2560	NUVARING VAGINAL RING	EA	OTH	J7303
NEMBUTAL SODIUM	50 MG	IM, IV, OTH	J2515	O-FLEX	60 MG	IV, IM	J2360
NEO SYNEPHRINE HCL	1 ML	SC, IM, IV	J2370	OCATMIDE PFS	10 MG	IV	J2765
NEO-DURABOLIC	100 MG	IM	J2321	OCTAFLUOROPROPANE UCISPHERES	1 ML	IV	Q9956
NEO-DURABOLIC	200 MG	IM	J2322	OCTAGAM IMMUNE GLOBULIN	1 GM	IV	J1563
NEO-DURABOLIC	50 MG	IM	J2320	OCTREOSCAN	1 MCI	IV	A9565
NEOCYTEN	60 MG	IV, IM	J2360	OCTREOTIDE ACETATE DEPOT	1 MG	IM	J2353
NEORAL	25 MG	ORAL	J7515	OCTREOTIDE, NON-DEPOT FORM	25 MCG	SC, IV	J2354
NEORAL	250 MG	ORAL	J7516	OFLOXACIN	400 MG	IV	S0034
NEOSAR	1 G	IV	J9091	OLANZAPINE	2.5 MG	IM	S0166
NEOSAR	100 MG	IV	J9070	OMALIZUMAB	5 MG	SC	J2357
NEOSAR	2 G	IV	J9092	OMNIPAQUE 140	1 ML	IV	Q9945
NEOSAR	200 MG	IV	J9080	OMNIPAQUE 180	1 ML	IV	Q9946
NEOSAR	500 MG	IV	J9090	OMNIPAQUE 240	1 ML	IV	Q9947
NEOSCAN	1 MCI	IV	A9556	OMNIPAQUE 300	1 ML	IV	Q9949
NEOSTIGMINE METHYLSULFATE	250 MG	IM, IV	J2710	OMNIPAQUE 350	1 ML	IV	Q9950
NEOTECT	STUDY DOSE	IV	A9536	OMNISCAN	1 ML	IV	Q9952
NESACAINE	30 ML	VAR	J2400	ONCASPAR	VIAL	IM, IV	J9266
NESACAINE-MPF	30 ML	VAR	J2400	ONCOSCINT	DOSE	IV	A4642
NESIRITIDE	0.1 MG	IV	J2325	ONDANSETRON HCL	4 MG	ORAL	S0181
NEULASTA	6 MG	SC, SQ	J2505	ONDANSETRON HCL	8 MG	ORAL	Q0179
NEUMEGA	5 MG	SC	J2355	ONDANSETRON HYDROCHLORIDE	1 MG	IV	J2405
NEUPOGEN	300 MCG	SC, IV	J1440	ONTAK	300 MCG	IV	J9160
NEUPOGEN	480 MCG	SC, IV	J1441	ONXOL	30 MG	IV	J9265
NEUROLITE	25 MCI	IV	A9557	OPRELVEKIN	5 MG	SC	J2355
NEUTREXIN	25 MG	IV	J3305	OPTIMARK	1 ML	IV	Q9952
NEUTROSPEC	25 MCI	IV	A9566	OPTIRAY	1 ML	IV	Q9950
NIPENT	10 MG	IV	J9268	OPTIRAY 160	1 ML	IV	Q9946
NITROGEN N-13 AMMONIA, DIAGNOSTIC	STUDY DOSE, UP TO 40 MCI	INJ	A9526	OPTIRAY 240	1 ML	IV	Q9947
NOC DRUGS, INHALATION SOLUTION ADMINISTERED THROUGH DME	1 EA		J7699	OPTIRAY 300	1 ML	IV	Q9949
				OPTIRAY 320	1 ML	IV	Q9949
NOLVADEX	10 MG	ORAL	S0187	OPTISON	1 ML	IV	Q9957
NOLVADEX	10 MG	ORAL	S0187	ORAL MAGNETIC RESONANCE CONTRAST AGENT, PER 100 ML	100 ML	ORAL	Q9954
NORDITROPIN	1 MG	SC	J2941	ORCEL	SQ CM	OTH	J7340
NORDYL	50 MG	IV, IM	J1200	ORENCIA	10 MG	IV	J0129 ▲
NORFLEX	60 MG	IV, IM	J2360	ORPHENADRINE CITRATE	60 MG	IV, IM	J2360
~~NORMAL SALINE~~	~~2 ML~~	~~IV~~	~~J2912~~	ORPHENATE	60 MG	IV, IM	J2360
NORPLANT	EA	OTH	J7306	ORTHOCLONE OKT3	5 MG	OTH	J7505
NORZINE	10 MG	IM	J3280	ORTHOVISC	30 MG	OTH	J7318
NOT OTHERWISE CLASSIFIED, ANTINEOPLASTIC DRUGS			J9999	OSELTAMIVIR PHOSPHATE (BRAND NAME)	75 MG	ORAL	G9035
NOV-ONXOL	30 MG	IV	J9265	OSELTAMIVIR PHOSPHATE (GENERIC)	75 MG	ORAL	G9019
NOVANTRONE	5 MG	IV	J9293	OSMITROL	25% IN 50 ML	IV	J2150
NOVAREL	1,000 USP U	IM	J0725	OXACILLIN SODIUM	250 MG	IM, IV	J2700
NOVO NORDISK	5 UNITS	SC	J1815	OXALIPLATIN	0.5 MG	IV	J9263
NOVOLIN	50 U	SC	J1817	OXILAN 300	1 ML	IV	Q9949
NOVOLIN R	5 U	SC	J1815	OXILAN 350	1 ML	IV	Q9950
NOVOLOG	50 U	SC	J1817	OXYMORPHONE HCL	1 MG	IV, SC, IM	J2410
NOVOSEVEN	1 MCG	IV	J7189	OXYTETRACYCLINE HCL	50 MG	IM	J2460
NPH	5 UNITS	SC	J1815	OXYTOCIN	10 U	IV, IM	J2590
NUBAIN	10 MG	IM, IV, SC	J2300	PACIS BCG	VIAL	OTH	J9031
NUMORPHAN	1 MG	IV, SC, IM	J2410	PACLITAXEL	30 MG	IV	J9265
NUMORPHAN H.P.	1 MG	IV, SC, IM	J2410				
NUTRI-TWELVE	1,000 MCG	IM, SC	J3420				

Appendix 1 — Table of Drugs

Drug Name	Unit Per:	Route	Code
PACLITAXEL PROTEIN-BOUND PARTICLES	1 MG	IV	J9264
PALIFERMIN	50 MCG	IV	J2425
PALIVIZUMAB-RSV-IGM	50 MG	IM	C9003
PALONOSETRON HCL	25 MCG	IV	J2469
PAMIDRONATE DISODIUM	30 MG	IV	J2430
PANGLOBULIN	1 G	IV	J1563
PANHEMATIN	1 MG	IV	J1640
PANITUMUMAB	10 MG	IV	C9235 ●
PANTOPRAZOLE SODIUM	40 MG	IV	S0164
PANTOPRAZOLE SODIUM	VIAL	IV	C9113
PAPAVERINE HCL	60 MG	IV, IM	J2440
PARAGARD T380A	EA	OTH	J7300
PARAPLANTIN	50 MG	IV	J9045
PARICALCITOL	1 MCG	IV, IM	J2501
PEDIAPRED	5 MG	ORAL	J7510
PEG-INTRON	10 MCG	SC	S0146
PEG-INTRON	180 MCG	SC	S0145
PEGADEMASE BOVINE	25 IU	IM	J2504
PEGAPTANIB SODIUM	0.3 MG	OTH	J2503
PEGASPARGASE	VIAL	IM, IV	J9266
PEGASYS	10 MCG	SC	S0146
PEGFILGRASTIM	6 MG	SC	J2505
PEGINTERFERON ALFA-2A	180 MCG	SC	S0145
PEGYLATED INTERFERON ALFA-2A	180 MCG	SC	S0145
PEGYLATED INTERFERON ALFA-2B	10 MCG	SC	S0146
PEMETREXED	10 MG	IV	J9305
PEN G BENZ/PEN G PROCAINE	600,000 U	IM	J0530
PENICILLIN G BENZATHINE	1,200,000 U	IM	J0570
PENICILLIN G BENZATHINE	2,400,000 U	IM	J0580
PENICILLIN G BENZATHINE	600,000 U	IM	J0560
PENICILLIN G BENZATHINE AND PENICILLIN G PROCAINE	1,200,000 U	IM	J0540
PENICILLIN G POTASSIUM	600,000 U	IM, IV	J2540
PENICILLIN G PROCAINE	600,000 U	IM, IV	J2510
PENTACARINAT	300 MG	INH	J2545
PENTACARINAT	300 MG	IM, IV	S0080
PENTAM	300 MG	IM, IV	J2545
PENTAM 300	300 MG	IM, IV	S0080
PENTAMIDINE ISETHIONATE	300 MG	INH	J2545
PENTAMIDINE ISETHIONATE	300 MG	IM, IV	S0080
PENTASPAN	100 ML	IV	J2513
PENTASTARCH 10% SOLUTION	100 ML	IV	J2513
PENTAZOCINE	30 MG	IM, SC, IV	J3070
PENTOBARBITAL SODIUM	50 MG	IM, IV, OTH	J2515
PENTOSTATIN	10 MG	IV	J9268
PEPCID	20 MG	IV	S0028
PERFLEXANE LIPID UCISPHERE	1 ML	IV	Q9955
PERFLUTREN LIPID UCISPHERE	1 ML	IV	Q9957
PERMAPEN	600,000	IM	J0560
PERMAPEN	> 2,400,000 U	IM	J0580
PERMAPEN	>1,200,000 U	IM	J0570
PERPHENAZINE	4 MG	ORAL	Q0175
PERPHENAZINE	5 MG	IM, IV	J3310
PERSANTINE	10 MG	IV	J1245
PFIZERPEN A.S.	600,000 UNITS	IM, IV	J2510
PHENAZINE 25	50 MG	IM, IV	J2550

Drug Name	Unit Per:	Route	Code
PHENAZINE 50	50 MG	IM, IV	J2550
PHENERGAN	12.5 MG	ORAL	Q0169
PHENERGAN	50 MG	IM, IV	J2550
PHENOBARBITAL SODIUM	120 MG	IM, IV	J2560
PHENTOLAMINE MESYLATE	5 MG	IM, IV	J2760
PHENYLEPHRINE HCL	1 ML	SC, IM, IV	J2370
PHENYTOIN SODIUM	50 MG	IM, IV	J1165
PHOSPHOCOL	1 MCI	IV	A9563
PHOSPHOTEC	25 MCI	IV	A9538
PHOTOFRIN	75 MG	IV	J9600
PHYTONADIONE	1 MG	IM, SC, IV	J3430
PIPERACILLIN SODIUM	500 MG	IM, IV	S0081
PIPERACILLIN SODIUM/TAZOBACTAM SODIUM	1 G/1.125 GM	IV	J2543
PITOCIN	10 U	IV, IM	J2590
PLATINOL AQ	10 MG	IV	J9060
PLATINOL AQ	50 MG	IV	J9062
PLENAXIS	10 MG	IM	J0128
PLICAMYCIN	2,500 MCG	IV	J9270
PNEUMOCOCCAL CONJUGATE	EA	IM	S0195
PNEUMOVAX II	EA	IM	S0195
POLOCAINE	10 ML	VAR	J0670
POLY-L-LACTIC ACID	1 ML	SC	S0196
POLYGAM	500 MG	IV	J1566
POLYGAM S/D	500 MG	IV	J1566
PORFIMER SODIUM	75 MG	IV	J9600
PORK INSULIN	5 UNITS	SC	J1815
POTASSIUM CHLORIDE	2 MEQ	IV	J3480
PRALIDOXIME CHLORIDE	1 MG	IV, IM, SC	J2730
PREDACORT	1 ML	IM	J2650
PREDALONE-50	1 ML	IM	J2650
PREDCOR-25	1 ML	IM	J2650
PREDCOR-50	1 ML	IM	J2650
PREDICORT-50	1 ML	IM	J2650
PREDNICOT	5 ML	ORAL	J7506
PREDNISOLONE	5 MG	ORAL	J7510
PREDNISOLONE ACETATE	1 ML	IM	J2650
PREDNISONE	5 MG	ORAL	J7506
PREDNORAL	5 MG	ORAL	J7510
PREDOJECT-50	1 ML	IM	J2650
PREDONE	5 MG	ORAL	J7506
PREGNYL	1,000 USP U	IM	J0725
PRELONE	5 MG	ORAL	J7510
PREMARIN	25 MG	IV, IM	J1410
PRENATAL VITAMINS	30 TABS	ORAL	S0197
PRI-ANDRIOL LA	50 MG	IM	J2320
PRI-METHYLATE	80 MG	IM	J1040
PRIALT	1 MCG	IV	J2278
PRIMACOR	5 MG	IV	J2260
PRIMAXIN	250 MG	IV, IM	J0743
PRIMESTRIN AQUEOUS	1 MG	IM, IV	J1410
PRISCOLINE HCL	25 MG	IV	J2670
PROCAINAMIDE HCL	1 G	IM, IV	J2690
PROCARBAZINE HCL	50 MG	ORAL	S0182
PROCHLOPERAZINE MALEATE	5 MG	ORAL	S0183
PROCHLORPERAZINE	10 MG	IM, IV	J0780
PROCHLORPERAZINE MALEATE	10 MG	ORAL	Q0165

Drug Name	Unit Per:	Route	Code
PROCHLORPERAZINE MALEATE	5 MG	ORAL	Q0164
PROCRIT, ESRD USE	1,000 U	SC, IV	J0886
PROCRIT, NON-ESRD USE	1,000 U	SC, IV	J0885
PROFILNINE HEAT-TREATED	1 IU	IV	J7194
PROFILNINE SD	1 IU	IV	J7194
PROFONIX	VIAL	INJ	C9113
PROGESTERONE	50 MG	IM	J2675
PROGRAF	1 MG	ORAL	J7507
PROGRAF	5 MG	OTH	J7525
PROHANCE	1 ML	IV	Q9952
PROKINE	50 MCG	IV	J2820
PROLASTIN	10 MG	IV	J0256
PROLEUKIN	1 VIAL	VAR	J9015
PROLIXIN DECANOATE	25 MG	SC, IM	J2680
PROMAZINE HCL	25 MG	IM	J2950
PROMETHAZINE HCL	12.5 MG	ORAL	Q0169
PROMETHAZINE HCL	50 MG	IM, IV	J2550
PRONESTYL	1 G	IM, IV	J2690
PROPECIA	5 MG	ORAL	S0138
PROPLEX SX-T	1 IU	IV	J7194
PROPLEX T	1 IU	IV	J7194
PROPRANOLOL HCL	1 MG	IV	J1800
PROREX	50 MG	IM, IV	J2550
PROSCAR	5 MG	ORAL	S0138
PROSTAPHLIN	250 MG	IM, IV	J2700
PROSTASCINT	DOSE	IV	A9507
PROSTIGMIN	0.5 MG	IM, IV	J2710
PROSTIN VR	1.25 MCG	INJ	J0270
PROTAMINE SULFATE	10 MG	IV	J2720
PROTEINASE INHIBITOR (HUMAN)	10 MG	IV	J0256
PROTHAZINE	50 MG	IM, IV	J2550
PROTIRELIN	250 MCG	IV	J2725
PROTONIX IV	40 MG	IV	S0164
PROTONIX IV	VIAL	IV	C9113
PROTOPAM CHLORIDE	1 G	SC, IM, IV	J2730
PROTROPIN	1 MG	SC, IM	J2940
PROVENTIL ▶NONCOMPOUNDED,◀ CONCENTRATED	1 MG	INH	J7611
PROVENTIL ▶NONCOMPOUNDED, UNIT DOSE◀	1 MG	INH	J7613
PROVOCHOLINE POWDER	1 MG	INH	J7674
PROZINE-50	25 MG	IM	J2950
PULMICORT	0.25 MG	INH	J7633
PULMICORT RESPULES	0.5 MG	INH	J7627
PULMICORT RESPULES NONCOMPOUNDED, CONCETRATED	0.25 MG	INH	J7626 ●
PULMOZYME	1 MG	INH	J7639
PURINETHOL	50 MG	ORAL	S0108
PYRIDOXINE HCL	100 MG	INJ	J3415
QUADRAMET	50 MCI	IV	A9605
QUELICIN	20 MG	IM, IV	J0330
QUINUPRISTIN/DALFOPRISTIN	500 MG	IV	J2770
RANIBIZUMAB	0.5 MG	OTH	C9233 ●
RANITIDINE HCL	25 MG	INJ	J2780
RAPAMUNE	1 MG	ORAL	J7520
RAPTIVA	125 MG	SC	S0162
RASBURICASE	50 MCG	IM	J2783

Drug Name	Unit Per:	Route	Code
REBETRON KIT	1,000,000 UNITS	SC, IM	J9214
REBIF	11 MCG	SC	Q3026
REBIF	33 MCG	SC	J1825
RECOMBINATE	1 IU	IV	J7192
REDISOL	1,000 MCG	SC. IM	J3420
REFACTO	1 IU	IV	J7192
REFLUDAN	50 MG	IM, IV	J1945
REGITINE	5 MG	IM, IV	J2760
REGLAN	10 MG	IV	J2765
REGRANEX GEL	0.5 G	OTH	J0157
REGRANEX GEL	0.5 G	OTH	S0157
REGULAR INSULIN	5 UNITS	SC	J1815
RELAXIN	10 ML	IV, IM	J2800
RELION	5 U	SC	J1815
RELION NOVOLIN	50 U	SC	J1817
REMICADE	10 MG	IV	J1745
REMODULIN	1 MG	SC	J3285
REODULIN	1 MG	SC	J3285
REOPRO	10 MG	IV	J0130
REPRONEX	75 IU	SC, IM, IV	S0122
RESP SYNCYTIAL VIR IMMUNE GLOB	50 MG	IV	J1565
RESPIGAM	50 MG	IV	J1565
RESPIROL ▶NONCOMPOUNDED,◀ CONCENTRATED	1 MG	INH	J7611
RESPIROL ▶NONCOMPOUNDED, UNIT DOSE◀	1 MG	INH	J7613
RETAVASE	18.1 MG	IV	J2993
RETEPLASE	18.1 MG	IV	J2993
RETISERT	IMPLANT	OTH	J7311 ●
RETROVIR	10 MG	IV	J3485
RETROVIR	100 MG	ORAL	S0104
RHEOMACRODEX	500 ML	IV	J7100
RHEUMATREX DOSE PACK	2.5 MG	ORAL	J8610
RHO D IMMUNE GLOBULIN	100 IU	IV	J2792
RHO D IMMUNE GLOBULIN	50 MCG	IM	J2788
RHOGAM	300 MCG	IM	J2790
RHOGAM	50 MCG	IM	J2788
RHOPHYLAC	100 IU	IV	J2792
RHOPHYLAC	300 MCG	IM	J2790
RIMANTADINE HYDROCHLORIDE	100 MG	ORAL	G9036
RIMANTADINE HYDROCHLORIDE (GENERIC)	100 MG	ORAL	G9020
RIMSO	50 ML	OTH	J1212
RINGERS LACTATE INFUSION	1,000 ML	VAR	J7120
RISPERDAL COSTA LONG ACTING	0.5 MG	IM	J2794
RISPERIDONE, LONG ACTING	0.5 MG	IM	J2794
RITUXAN	100 MG	IV	J9310
RITUXIMAB	100 MG	IV	J9310
ROBAXIN	10 ML	IV, IM	J2800
ROBINUL	1 MG	INH	J7643
ROCEPHIN	250 MG	IV, IM	J0696
ROFERON-A	3,000,000 U	SC, IM	J9213
ROPIVACAINE HYDROCHLORIDE	1 MG	VAR	J2795
RUBEX	10 MG	IV	J9000
RUBIDIUM RB-82	60 MCI	IV	A9555
RUBRAMIN PC	1,000 MCG	SC, IM	J3420

Appendix 1 — Table of Drugs

Drug Name	Unit Per:	Route	Code
RUBRATOPE 57	1 MCI	ORAL	A9559
SAIZEN	1 MG	SC	J2941
SAIZEN SOMATROPIN RDNA ORIGIN	1 MG	SC	J2941
SALINE OR STERILE WATER, METERED DOSE DISPENSER	10 ML	INH	A4218 ●
SALINE, STERILE WATER, AND/OR DEXTROSE DILUENT/FLUSH	10 ML	VAR	A4216 ●
SALINE/STERILE WATER	500 ML	VAR	A4217 ●
SAMARIUM LEXIDRONAMM	50 MCI	IV	A9605
SANDIMMUNE	100 MG	ORAL	J7502
SANDIMMUNE	25 MG	ORAL	J7515
SANDIMMUNE	250 MG	OTH	J7516
SANDOGLOBULIN	1 G	IV	J1563
SANDOSTATIN	25 MCG	SC, IV	J2354
SANDOSTATIN LAR	1 MG	IM	J2353
SANGCYA	100 MG	ORAL	J7502
SANO-DROL	40 MG	IM	J1030
SANO-DROL	80 MG	IM	J1040
SAQUINAVIR	200 MG	ORAL	S0140
SARGRAMOSTIM (GM-CSF)	50 MCG	IV	J2820
SECREFLO	1 MCG	IV	J2850
SECRETIN, SYNTHETIC, HUMAN	1 MCG	IV	J2850
SENSORCAINE	30 ML	VAR	S0200
SEPTRA IV	10 ML	IV	S0039
SERMORELIN ACETATE	1 MCG	IV	Q0515
SEROSTIM	1 MG	SC	J2941
SEROSTIM RDNA ORIGIN	1 MG	SC	J2941
SILDENAFIL CITRATE	25 MG	ORAL	S0090
SIMULECT	20 MG	IV	J0480
SINCALIDE	5 MCG	IV	J2805
SIROLIMUS	1 MG	ORAL	J7520
SMZ-TMP	10 ML	IV	S0039
~~SODIUM CHLORIDE~~	~~2 ML~~	~~IV~~	~~J2912~~
SODIUM CHLORIDE	5 CC	VAR	J7051
SODIUM FERRIC GLUCONATE COMPLEX IN SUCROSE	12.5 MG	IV	J2916
SODIUM HYALURONATE	1 MG	OTH	J7318
SODIUM HYALURONATE	INJ	▶OTH◀	J7319 ▲
~~SODIUM HYALURONATE~~	~~30 MG~~	~~OTH~~	~~C9220~~
SODIUM IODIDE I-131 CAPSULE DIAGNOSTIC	1 MCI	ORAL	A9528
SODIUM IODIDE I-131 CAPSULE THERAPEUTIC	1 MCI	ORAL	A9517
SODIUM IODIDE I-131 SOLUTION THERAPEUTIC	1 MCI	ORAL	A9530
SODIUM PHOSPHATE P32	1 MCI	IV	A9563
SOLGANAL	50 MG	IM	J2910
SOLTAMOX	10 MG	ORAL	S0187
SOLU-CORTEF	100 MG	IV, IM, SC	J1720
SOLU-MEDROL	125 MG	IM, IV	J2930
SOLU-MEDROL	40 MG	IM, IV	J2920
SOMATREM	1 MG	SC, IM	J2940
SOMATROPIN	1 MG	SC	J2941
SPARINE	25 MG	IM	J2950
SPECTINOMYCIN DIHYDROCHLORIDE	2 G	IM	J3320
SPORANOX	50 MG	IV	J1835
STADOL	1 MG	IM, IV	J0595
STADOL NS	25 MG	OTH	S0012

Drug Name	Unit Per:	Route	Code
STERAPRED	5 MG	ORAL	J7506
~~STERILE SALINE OR WATER~~	~~5 CC~~	~~VAR~~	~~J7051~~
STERILE WATER OR SALINE, METERED DOSE DISPENSER	10 ML	INH	A4218 ●
STERILE WATER, SALINE, AND/OR DEXTROSE DILUENT/FLUSH	10 ML	VAR	A4216 ●
STERILE WATER/SALINE	500 ML	VAR	A4217 ●
STREPTASE	250,000 IU	IV	J2995
STREPTOKINASE	250,000 IU	IV	J2995
STREPTOMYCIN	1 G	IM	J3000
STREPTOZOCIN	1 GM	IV	J9320
STRONTIUM 89 CHLORIDE	1 MCI	IV	A9600
SUBLIMAZE	0.1 MG	IM, IV	J3010
SUCCINYLCHOLINE CHLORIDE	20 MG	IM, IV	J0330
SULFAMETHOXAZOLE AND TRIMETHOPRIM	10 ML	IV	S0039
SULFUTRIM	10 ML	IV	S0039
SUMATRIPTAN SUCCINATE	6 MG	SC	J3030
~~SUPARTZ~~	~~30 MG~~	~~OTH~~	~~C9220~~
SUPARTZ	▶INJ◀	OTH	J7319 ▲
SUS-PHRINE	UP TO 1 ML	VAR	J0170
SYNAGIS	50 MG	IM	C9003
SYNERCID	500 MG	IV	J2770
SYNTOCINON	10 UNITS	IV	J2590
SYNVISC	16 MG	OTH	J7320
~~SYREX~~	~~2 ML~~	~~IV~~	~~J2912~~
SYTOBEX	1,000 MCG	SC, IM	J3420
T-GEN	250 MG	ORAL	Q0173
TACRINE HCL	10 MG	ORAL	S0014
TACROLIMUS	1 MG	ORAL	J7507
TACROLIMUS	5 MG	OTH	J7525
TAGAMET HCL	300 MG	IM, IV	S0023
TALWIN	30 MG	IM, SC, IV	J3070
TAMOXIFEN CITRATE	10 MG	ORAL	S0187
TAXOL	30 MG	IV	J9265
TAXOTERE	20 MG	IV	J9170
TAZICEF	500 MG	IM, IV	J0713
TEBAMIDE	250 MG	ORAL	Q0173
TECHNEPLEX	25 MCI	IV	A9539
TECHNESCAN	1 MCI	IV	A9512
TECHNESCAN FANOLESOMAB	STUDY DOSE	IV	A9566
TECHNESCAN MAA	10 MCI	IV	A9540
TECHNESCAN MAG3	STUDY DOSE	IV	A9562
TECHNESCAN PYP	25 MCI	IV	A9538
TECHNETIUM SESTAMBI	40 MCI	IV	A9500
TECHNETIUM TC 99M ACRCITUMOMAB	25 MCI	IV	A9549
TECHNETIUM TC 99M APCITIDE	20 MCI	IV	A9504
TECHNETIUM TC 99M ARCITUMOMAB, DIAGNOSTIC	45 MCI	IV	A9568 ●
TECHNETIUM TC 99M BICISATE	25 MCI	IV	A9557
TECHNETIUM TC 99M DEPREOTIDE	35 MCI	IV	A9536
TECHNETIUM TC 99M EXAMETAZIME	25 MCI	IV	A9521
TECHNETIUM TC 99M FANOLESOMAB	25 MCI	IV	A9566
TECHNETIUM TC 99M LABELED RED BLOOD CELLS	30 MCI	IV	A9560
TECHNETIUM TC 99M MACROAGGREGATED ALBUMIN	10 MCI	IV	A9540

APPENDIX 1 — TABLE OF DRUGS

Drug Name	Unit Per:	Route	Code	Drug Name	Unit Per:	Route	Code
TECHNETIUM TC 99M MEBROFENIN	15 MCI	IV	A9537	THORAZINE	10 MG	ORAL	Q0171
TECHNETIUM TC 99M MERTIATIDE	15 MCI	IV	A9562	THORAZINE	25 MG	ORAL	Q0172
TECHNETIUM TC 99M OXIDRONATE	30 MCI	IV	A9561	THORAZINE	50 MG	IM, IV	J3230
TECHNETIUM TC 99M PENTETATE	25 MCI	IV	A9539	THROMBATE III	1 IU	IV	J7197
TECHNETIUM TC 99M PENTETATE	75 MCI	INH	A9539	THYMOGLOBULIN	25 MG	OTH	J7511
TECHNETIUM TC 99M PYROPHOSPHATE	25 MCI	IV	A9538	THYROGEN	0.9 MG	IM, SC	J3240
TECHNETIUM TC 99M SODIUM GLUCEPATATE	25 MCI	IV	A9550	THYROTROPIN ALPHA	0.9 MG	IM, SC	J3240
TECHNETIUM TC 99M SUCCIMER	10 MCI	IV	A9551	THYTROPAR	0.9 MG	SC, IM	J3240
TECHNETIUM TC 99M SULFUR COLLOID	20 MCI	IV	A9541	TICARCILLIN DISODIUM AND CLAVULANATE	3.1 G	IV	S0040
TECHNETIUM TC 99M TETROFOSMIN	40 MCI	IV	A9502	TICE BCG	VIAL	OTH	J9031
TEMODAR	100 MG	ORAL	J8700	TICON	200 MG	IM	J3250
TEMOZOLOMIDE	100 MG	ORAL	J8700	TICON	250 MG	ORAL	Q0173
TENECTEPLASE	50 MG	IV	J3100	TIGAN	200 MG	IM	J3250
TENIPOSIDE	50 MG	IV	Q2017	TIGECYCLINE	1 MG	IV	J3243 ▲
TEQUIN	10 MG	IV	J1590	TIJECT-20	200 MG	IM	J3250
TERBUTALINE SULFATE	1 MG	SC, IV	J3105	TIMENTIN	3.1 G	IV	S0040
TERBUTALINE SULFATE, ▶COMPOUNDED, CONCENTRATED◀	▶1 MG◀	▶INH◀	J7680 ▲	TINZAPARIN	1,000 IU	SC	J1655
				TIROFIBAN HCL	0.25 MG	IM, IV	J3246
TERBUTALINE SULFATE, ▶COMPOUNDED, UNIT DOSE◀	1 MG	INH	J7681	TIROFIBAN HYDROCHLORIDE	12.5 MG	IM, IV	J3246
				TNKASE	50 MG	IV	J3100
TERIPARATIDE	10 MCG	SC	J3110	TOBI	300 MG	INH	J7682
TERRAMYCIN	50 MG	IM	J2460	TOBRAMYCIN COMPOUNDED, UNIT DOSE	300 MG	INH	J7685 ●
TESTAQUA	50 MG	IM	J3140				
TESTERONE	50 MG	IM	J3140	TOBRAMYCIN SULFATE	80 MG	IM, IV	J3260
TESTEX	50 MG	IM	J3150	TOBRAMYCIN, ▶NONCOMPOUNDED, UNIT DOSE◀	300 MG	INH	J7682
TESTOJECT-50	50 MG	IM	J3140				
TESTONE LA 100	100 MG	IM	J3120	TOLAZOLINE HCL	25 MG	IV	J2670
TESTONE LA 200	100 MG	IM	J3130	TOPOSAR	10 MG	IV	J9181
TESTOSTERONE AQUEOUS	50 MG	IM	J3140	TOPOSAR	100 MG	IV	J9182
TESTOSTERONE CYPIONATE	1 CC, 200 MG	IM	J1080	TOPOTECAN	4 MG	IV	J9350
TESTOSTERONE CYPIONATE	UP TO 100 MG	IM	J1070	TORADOL IV/IM	15 MG	IM, IV	J1885
TESTOSTERONE CYPIONATE & ESTRADIOL CYPIONATE	1 ML	IM	J1060	TORECAN	10 MG	IM	J3280
				TORECAN	10 MG	ORAL	Q0174
TESTOSTERONE ENANTHATE	100 MG	IM	J3120	TORNALATE	PER MG	INH	J7629
TESTOSTERONE ENANTHATE	200 MG	IM	J3130	TORNALATE CONCENTRATE	PER MG	INH	J7628
TESTOSTERONE ENANTHATE & ESTRADIOL VALERATE	UP TO 1 CC	IM	J0900	TORSEMIDE	10 MG	IV	J3265
				TOSITUMOMAB DIAGNOSTIC	DOSE	IV	A9544
TESTOSTERONE PELLET	75 MG	OTH	S0189	TOSITUMOMAB THERAPEUTIC	DOSE	IV	A9545
TESTOSTERONE PROPIONATE	100 MG	IM	J3150	TRANSCYTE	PER 247 SQ CM	OTH	J7340
TESTOSTERONE SUSPENSION	50 MG	IM	J3140	TRASTUZUMAB	10 MG	IV	J9355
TESTRIIN PA	100 MG	IM	J3130	TRASYLOL	10,000 KIU	IV	J0365
TESTRO AQ	50 MG	IM	J3140	TRELSTAR DEPOT	3.75 MG	IM	J3315
TETANUS IMMUNE GLOBULIN	250 U	IM	J1670	TRELSTAR DEPOT PLUS DEBIOCLIP KIT	3.75 MG	IM	J3315
TETRACYCLINE HCL	250 MG	IV	J0120				
THALLOUS CHLORIDE	1 MCI	IV	A9505	TRELSTAR LA	3.75 MG	IM	J3315
THALLOUS CHLORIDE TL-201	1 MCI	IV	A9505	TREPROSTINIL	1 MG	SC	J3285
THALLOUS CHLORIDE USP	1 MCI	IV	A9505	TRETINOIN	5 G	OTH	S0117
THEELIN AQUEOUS	1 MG	IM, IV	J1435	TRI-KORT	10 MG	IM	J3301
THEOPHYLLINE	40 MG	IV	J2810	TRIAM-A	10 MG	IM	J3301
THERACYS	VIAL	IV	J9031	TRIAMCINOLONE ACETONIDE	10 MG	IM	J3301
THIAMINE HCL	100 MG	INJ	J3411	TRIAMCINOLONE DIACETATE	5 MG	IM	J3302
THIETHYLPERAZINE MALEATE	10 MG	IM	J3280	TRIAMCINOLONE HEXACETONIDE	5 MG	VAR	J3303
THIETHYLPERAZINE MALEATE	10 MG	ORAL	Q0174	TRIAMCINOLONE, COMPOUNDED, CONCENTRATED	1 MG	INH	J7683 ●
THIMAZIDE	250 MG	ORAL	Q0173	TRIAMCINOLONE, ▶COMPOUNDED, UNIT DOSE◀	1 MG	INH	J7684
THIOTEPA	15 MG	IV	J9340	TRIBAN	250 MG	ORAL	Q0173

Appendix 1 — Table of Drugs

Drug Name	Unit Per:	Route	Code
TRILIFON	4 MG	ORAL	Q0175
TRILOG	10 MG	IM	J3301
TRILONE	5 MG	IM	J3302
TRIMETHOBENZAMIDE HCL	200 MG	IM	J3250
TRIMETHOBENZAMIDE HCL	250 MG	ORAL	Q0173
TRIMETREXATE GLUCURONATE	25 MG	IV	J3305
TRIPTORELIN PAMOATE	3.75 MG	IM	J3315
TRISENOX	1 MG	IV	J9017
TROBICIN	2 G	IM	J3320
TRUXADRYL	50 MG	IV, IM	J1200
TRYPTANOL	20 MG	IM	J1320
~~TYGACIL~~	~~1 MG~~	~~IV~~	~~C9228~~
TYGACIL	1 MG	IV	J3243
TYPE A BOTOX	1 U	OTH	J0585
ULTRALENTE	5 UNITS	SC	J1815
ULTRATAG	30 MCI	IV	A9560
ULTRAVIST	1 ML	IV	Q9949
ULTRAVIST 150	1 ML	IV	Q9946
ULTRAVIST 240	1 ML	IV	Q9947
ULTRAVIST 370	1 ML	IV	Q9950
UNASYN	1.5 G	IM, IV	J0295
UNCLASSIFIED BIOLOGICS			J3590
UREA	40 G	IV	J3350
UREAPHIL	40 G	IV	J3350
UROFOLLITROPIN	75 IU	SC, IM	J3355
UROKINASE	250,000 IU	IV	J3365
UROKINASE	5,000 IU	IV	J3364
V-GAN 25	50 MG	IM, IV	J2550
V-GAN 50	50 MG	IM, IV	J2550
VALERGEN	10 MG	IM	J1380
VALERGEN	20 MG	IM	J1390
VALIUM	5 MG	IV, IM	J3360
VALRUBICIN	200 MG	OTH	J9357
VALSTAR	200 MG	OTH	J9357
VANCOLET	500 MG	IM, IV	J3370
VANCOMYCIN HCL	500 MG	IV, IM	J3370
VANTAS	50 MG	OTH	J9225
VAROCIN	500 MG	IM, IV	J3370
VECTIBIX	10 MG	IV	C9235 ●
VELCADE	0.1 MG	IV	J9041
VELOSULIN	5 UNITS	SC	J1815
VELOSULIN BR	5 U	SC	J1815
VENOFER	1 MG	IV	J1756
VENOGLOBULIN-S	1 G	IV	J1563
VENTOLIN ▶NONCOMPOUNDED,◀ CONCENTRATED	1 MG	INH	J7611
VENTOLIN ▶NONCOMPOUNDED, UNIT DOSE◀	1 MG	INH	J7613
VEPESID	10 MG	IV	J9181
VEPESID	100 MG	IV	J9182
VEPESID	50 MG	ORAL	J8560
VERSED	1 MG	IM, IV	J2250
VERTEPORFIN	0.1 MG	IV	J3396
VFEND	200 MG	IV	J3465
VIAGRA	25 MG	ORAL	S0090
VIDAZA	1 MG	SC	J9025
VIDEX	25 MG	ORAL	S0137

Drug Name	Unit Per:	Route	Code
VINBLASTINE SULFATE	1 MG	IV	J9360
VINCRISTINE SULFATE	1 MG	IV	J9370
VINCRISTINE SULFATE	2 MG	IV	J9375
VINORELBINE TARTRATE	10 MG	IV	J9390
VIRILON	1 CC, 200 MG	IM	J1080
VISIPAQUE 270	1 ML	IV	Q9948
VISIPAQUE 320	1 ML	IV	Q9949
VISTAJECT-25	25 MG	IM	J3410
VISTARIL	25 MG	IM	J3410
VISTARIL	25 MG	ORAL	Q0177
VISTIDE	375 MG	IV	J0740
VISUDYNE	0.1 MG	IV	J3396
VITAMIN B-12 CYANOCOBALAMIN	1,000 MCG	IM, SC	J3420
VITRASE	1 USP	OTH	J3471
VITRASE	1,000 USP	OTH	J3472
VITRASERT	4.5 MG	OTH	J7310
VITRAVENE	1.65 MG	OTH	J1452
VIVITROL	1 MG	IM	J2315 ●
~~VON WILLEBRAND FACTOR COMPLEX, HUMAN~~	~~IU~~	~~IV~~	~~J7188~~
VON WILLEBRAND FACTOR COMPLEX, RISTOCETIN COFACTOR	IU	IV	J7187 ●
VORICONAZOLE	200 MG	IV	J3465
VUMON	50 MG	IV	Q2017
WEHAMINE	50 MG	IM, IV	J1240
WEHDRYL	50 MG	IM, IV	J1200
WELBUTRIN SR	150 MG	ORAL	S0106
WINRHO SDF	100 IU	IV	J2792
WYCILLIN	600,000 U	IM, IV	J2510
WYDASE	150 UNITS	VAR	J3470
XELODA	150 MG	ORAL	J8520
XELODA	500 MG	ORAL	J8521
XENON XE-133	10 MCI	OTH	A9558
XOLAIR	5 MG	SC	J2357
XOPENENEX ▶HFA NONCOMPOUNDED,◀ CONCENTRATED	0.5 MG	INH	J7612
XOPENEX ▶NONCOMPOUNDED, UNIT DOSE◀	0.5 MG	INH	J7614
XYLOCAINE	10 MG	IV	J2001
YTTRIUM 90 IBRITUMOMAB TIUXETAN	TX DOSE	IV	A9543
ZALCITABINE (DDC)	0.375 MG	ORAL	S0141
ZANAMIVIR (BRAND NAME)	10 MG	INH	G9034
ZANAMIVIR (GENERIC)	10 MG	INH	G9018
ZANOSAR	1 GM	IV	J9320
ZANTAC	25 MG	INJ	J2780
ZEMAIRA	10 MG	IV	J0256
ZEMPLAR	1 MCG	IV, IM	J2501
ZENAPAX	25 MG	OTH	J7513
ZETRAN	5 MG	IM, IV	J3360
ZEVALIN DIAGNOSTIC	TX DOSE	IV	A9542
ZEVALIN THERAPEUTIC	TX DOSE	IV	A9543
ZICONOTIDE	1 MCG	IT	J2278
ZIDOVUDINE	10 MG	IV	J3485
ZIDOVUDINE	100 MG	ORAL	S0104
ZINECARD	250 MG	IV	J1190
ZIPRASIDONE MESYLATE	10 MG	IM	J3486
ZITHROMAX	1 G	ORAL	Q0144

APPENDIX 1 — TABLE OF DRUGS

Drug Name	Unit Per:	Route	Code
ZITHROMAX	500 MG	IV	J0456
ZOFRAN	1 MG	IV	J2405
ZOFRAN	4 MG	ORAL	S0181
ZOFRAN	8 MG	ORAL	Q0179
ZOLADEX	3.6 MG	SC	J9202
ZOLEDRONIC ACID	1 MG	IV	J3487
ZOMETA	1 MG	IV	J3487
ZORBTIVE	1 MG	SC	J2941
ZOSYN	1 G/1.125 GM	IV	J2543
ZOVIRAX	5 MG	IV	J0133
ZOVIRAX	50 MG	IV	S0071
ZYPREXA	2.5 MG	IM	S0166
ZYVOX	200 MG	IV	J2020

UNCLASSIFIED DRUGS

Drug Name	Unit Per:	Route	Code
~~ABATACEPT~~	~~250 MG~~	~~IV~~	~~J3490~~
ALLOPURINOL SODIUM	500 MG	IV	J3490
ALOPRIM	500 MG	IV	J3490
AMICAR	250 MG	IV	J3490
AMIDATE	2 MG	IV	J3490
AMINOCAPROIC ACID	250 MG	IV	J3490
~~APOKYN~~	~~10 MG~~	~~SC~~	~~J3490~~
~~APOMORPHINE HYDROCHLORIDE~~	~~10 MG~~	~~SC~~	~~J3490~~
ARGININE HYDROCHLORIDE	300 ML	IV	J3490
~~ARIMIDEX~~	~~1 EA~~		~~J8999~~
ASCORBIC ACID	250 MG	IV	J3490
ATROPINE SULFATE/EDROPHONIUM CHLORIDE	10 MG	IV	J3490
AZTREONAM	500 MG	IV	J3490
BUMETANIDE	0.25 MG	IM, IV	J3490
BUPIVACAINE, 0.25%	1 ML	OTH	J3490
BUPIVACAINE, 0.50%	1 ML	OTH	J3490
BUPIVACAINE, 0.75%	1 ML	OTH	J3490
CALCIUM CHLORIDE	100 MG	IV	J3490
CEENU	1 EA		J8999
~~CHLORAMBUCIL~~		~~ORAL~~	~~J8999~~
CIMETIDINE HCL	150 MG	IM, IV	J3490
CLAVULANTE POTASSIUM/TICARCILLIN DISODIUM	0.1-3 GM	IV	J3490
CLINDAMYCIN PHOSPHATE	150 MG	IV	J3490
COPPER SULFATE	0.4 MG	INJ	J3490
DEXTROSE 50%	50 ML	IV	J3490
DILTIAZEM HCL	5 MG	IV	J3490

Drug Name	Unit Per:	Route	Code
DIPRIVAN	10 MG		J3490
DOXYCYCLINE HYCLATE	100 MG	INJ	J3490
EDROPHONIUM CHLORIDE	10 MG	IM, IV	J3490
ENALAPRILAT	1.25 MG	IV	J3490
ENLON PLUS	10 MG	IV	J3490
ESMOLOL HCL	10 MG	IV	J3490
ETOMIDATE	2 MG	IV	J3490
FAMOTIDINE	10 MG	IV	J3490
FLUMAZENIL	0.1 MG	IV	J3490
FOLIC ACID	5 MG	SC, IM, IV	J3490
GLYCOPYRROLATE	0.2 MG	IM, IV	J3490
KETAMINE HCL	10 MG	IM, IV	J3490
LABETALOL HCL	5 MG	INJ	J3490
~~LEUKERAN~~	~~1 EA~~		~~J8999~~
LIDOCAINE	1 ML	VAR	J3490
~~LYSODREN~~	~~1 EA~~	~~ORAL~~	~~J8999~~
METOPROLOL TARTRATE	1 MG	IV	J3490
METRONIDAZOLE IN NACL	500 MG	IV	J3490
~~MITOTANE~~	~~1 EA~~	~~ORAL~~	~~J8999~~
MORRHUATE SODIUM	50 MG	OTH	J3490
NAFCILLIN SODIUM	1 GM	IM, IV	J3490
NITROGLYCERIN	5 MG	IV	J3490
PEGASYS	180 MCG	SC	J3490
PEGINTERFERON ALFA-2A	180 MCG	SC	J3490
POTASSIUM ACETATE	2 MEQ	IV	J3490
POTASSIUM POSPHATE	3 MMOL	IV	J3490
~~PRESCRIPTION DRUG, ORAL, CHEMOTHERAPEUTIC, NOS~~	~~1 EA~~		~~J8999~~
~~PRESCRIPTION DRUG, ORAL, NON CHEMOTHERAPEUTIC, NOS~~	~~1 EA~~		~~J8499~~
PROPOFOL	10 MG	IV	J3490
PROTONIX	40 MG	IV	J3490
RIFAMPIN	600 MG	IV	J3490
SARRACENIA PURPURA	1 ML	INJ	J3490
SODIUM ACETATE	2 MEQ		J3490
SODIUM BICARBONATE, 8.4%	50 ML	IV	J3490
SODIUM CHLORIDE, HYPERTONIC	250 CC	IV	J3490
SODIUM THIOSULFATE	100 MG	IV	J3490
VALPROATE SODIUM	100 MG	IV	J3490
VASOPRESSIN	20 UNITS	SC, IM	J3490
VASOTEC	1.25 MG	IV	J3490
VECURONIUM BROMIDE	1 MG	IV	J3490
VERAPAMIL HCL	2.5 MG	IV	J3490

APPENDIX 2 — MODIFIERS

A1	Dressing for one wound
A2	Dressing for two wounds
A3	Dressing for three wounds
A4	Dressing for four wounds
A5	Dressing for five wounds
A6	Dressing for six wounds
A7	Dressing for seven wounds
A8	Dressing for eight wounds
A9	Dressing for nine or more wounds
AA	Anesthesia services performed personally by anesthesiologist
AD	Medical supervision by a physician: more than four concurrent anesthesia procedures
AE	Registered dietician
AF	Specialty physician
AG	Primary physician
AH	Clinical psychologist
AJ	Clinical social worker
AK	Nonparticipating physician
AM	Physician, team member service
AP	Determination of refractive state was not performed in the course of diagnostic ophthalmological examination
AQ	Physician providing a service in an unlisted health professional shortage area (HPSA)
AR	Physician scarcity area
AS	PA, nurse practitioner, or clinical nurse specialist services for assistant at surgery
AT	Acute treatment (this modifier should be used when reporting service 98940, 98941, 98942)
AU	Item furnished in conjunction with a urological, ostomy, or tracheostomy supply
AV	Item furnished in conjunction with a prosthetic device, prosthetic or orthotic
AW	Item furnished in conjunction with a surgical dressing
AX	Item furnished in conjunction with dialysis services
BA	Item furnished in conjunction with parenteral enteral nutrition (PEN) services
BL	Special acquisition of blood and blood products
BO	Orally administered nutrition, not by feeding tube
BP	The beneficiary has been informed of the purchase and rental options and has elected to purchase the item
BR	The beneficiary has been informed of the purchase and rental options and has elected to rent the item
BU	The beneficiary has been informed of the purchase and rental options and after 30 days has not informed the supplier of his/her decision
CA	Procedure payable only in the inpatient setting when performed emergently on an outpatient who expires prior to admission
CB	Service ordered by a renal dialysis facility (RDF) physician as part of the beneficiary's benefit, is not part of the composite rate, and is separately reimbursable
CC	Procedure code change (use CC when the procedure code submitted was changed either for administrative reasons or because an incorrect code was filed)
CD	AMCC test has been ordered by an ESRD facility or MCP physician that is a part of the composite rate and is not separately billable
CE	AMCC test has been ordered by an ESRD facility or MCP physician that is a composite rate test but is beyond the normal frequency covered under the rate and is separately reimbursable based on medically necessary
CF	AMCC test has been ordered by an ESRD facility or MCP physician that is not part of the composite rate and is separately billable

CR	Catastrophe/Disaster related
E1	Upper left, eyelid
E2	Lower left, eyelid
E3	Upper right, eyelid
E4	Lower right, eyelid
EJ	Subsequent claims for a defined course of therapy, e.g., EPO, sodium hyaluronate, infliximab
EM	Emergency reserve supply (for ESRD benefit only)
EP	Service provided as part of Medicaid early periodic screening diagnosis and treatment (EPSDT) program
ET	Emergency services
EY	No physician or other licensed health care provider order for this item or service
F1	Left hand, second digit
F2	Left hand, third digit
F3	Left hand, fourth digit
F4	Left hand, fifth digit
F5	Right hand, thumb
F6	Right hand, second digit
F7	Right hand, third digit
F8	Right hand, fourth digit
F9	Right hand, fifth digit
FA	Left hand, thumb
FB	Item provided without cost to provider, supplier or practitioner, or credit received for replaced device (examples, but not limited to, covered under warranty, replaced due to defect, free samples)
FP	Service provided as part of family planning program
G1	Most recent URR reading of less than 60
G2	Most recent URR reading of 60 to 64.9
G3	Most recent URR reading of 65 to 69.9
G4	Most recent URR reading of 70 to 74.9
G5	Most recent URR reading of 75 or greater
G6	ESRD patient for whom less than six dialysis sessions have been provided in a month
G7	Pregnancy resulted from rape or incest or pregnancy certified by physician as life threatening
G8	Monitored anesthesia care (MAC) for deep complex, complicated, or markedly invasive surgical procedure
G9	Monitored anesthesia care (MAC) for patient who has history of severe cardiopulmonary condition
GA	Waiver of liability statement on file
GB	Claim being resubmitted for payment because it is no longer covered under a global payment demonstration
GC	This service has been performed in part by a resident under the direction of a teaching physician
GE	This service has been performed by a resident without the presence of a teaching physician under the primary care exception
GF	Nonphysician (e.g., nurse practitioner (NP), certified registered nurse anesthetist (CRNA), certified registered nurse (CRN), clinical nurse specialist (CNS), physician assistant (PA)) services in a critical access hospital
GG	Performance and payment of a screening mammogram and diagnostic mammogram on the same patient, same day
GH	Diagnostic mammogram converted from screening mammogram on same day
GJ	Opt out physician or practitioner emergency or urgent service
GK	Actual item/service ordered by physician, item associated with GA or GZ modifier
GL	Medically unnecessary upgrade provided instead of standard item, no charge, no advance beneficiary notice (ABN)
GM	Multiple patients on one ambulance trip

GN	Service delivered under an outpatient speech-language pathology plan of care
GO	Service delivered under an outpatient occupational therapy plan of care
GP	Service delivered under an outpatient physical therapy plan of care
GQ	Via asynchronous telecommunications system
GR	This service was performed in whole or in part by a resident in a department of veterans affairs medical center or clinic, supervised in accordance with VA policy
GS	Dosage of EPO or darbepoetin alfa has been reduced and maintained in response to hematocrit or hemoglobulin level
GT	Via interactive audio and video telecommunication systems
GV	Attending physician not employed or paid under arrangement by the patient's hospice provider
GW	Service not related to the hospice patient's terminal condition
GY	Item or service statutorily excluded or does not meet the definition of any Medicare benefit
GZ	Item or service expected to be denied as not reasonable and necessary
H9	Court-ordered
HA	Child/adolescent program
HB	Adult program, nongeriatric
HC	Adult program, geriatric
HD	Pregnant/parenting womens' program
HE	Mental health program
HF	Substance abuse program
HG	Opioid addiction treatment program
HH	Integrated mental health substance abuse program
HI	Integrated mental health and mental retardation/developmental disabilities program
HJ	Employee assistance program
HK	Specialized mental health programs for high-risk populations
HL	Intern
HM	Less than bachelor degree level
HN	Bachelors degree level
HO	Masters degree level
HP	Doctoral level
HQ	Group setting
HR	Family/couple with client present
HS	Family/couple without client present
HT	Multi-disciplinary team
HU	Funded by child welfare agency
HV	Funded state addictions agency
HW	Funded by state mental health agency
HX	Funded by county/local agency
HY	Funded by juvenile justice agency
HZ	Funded by criminal justice agency
J1	Competitive acquisition program (CAP) no-pay submission for a prescription number
J2	Competitive acquisition program (CAP), restocking of emergency drugs after emergency administration
J3	Competitive acquisition program (CAP), drug not available through CAP as written, reimbursed under average sales price methodology
JA	Administered intravenously
JB	Administered subcutaneously
JW	Drug amount discarded/not administered to any patient

K0	Lower extremity prosthesis functional level 0-does not have the ability or potential to ambulate or transfer safely with or without assistance and a prosthesis does not enhance their quality of life or mobility
K1	Lower extremity prosthesis functional level 1-does have the ability or potential to use a prosthesis for transfer or ambulation on level surfaces at fixed cadence, typical of the limited and unlimited household ambulator.
K2	Lower extremity prosthesis functional level 2-has the ability or potential for ambulation with the ability to traverse low level environmental barriers such as curbs, stairs, or uneven surfaces, typical of limited community ambulator
K3	Lower extremity prosthesis functional level 3-has the ability or potential for ambulation with variable cadence, typical of the community ambulator who has the ability to traverse most environmental barriers and may have vocational, therapeutic, or exercise activity that demands prosthetic utilization beyond simple locomotion
K4	Lower extremity prosthesis functional level 4-has the ability or potential for prosthetic ambulation that exceeds basic ambulation skills, exhibiting high impact, stress, or energy levels, typical of the prosthetic demands of the child, active adult, or athlete
KA	Add-on option/accessory for wheelchair
KB	Beneficiary requested upgrade for ABN, more than four modifiers identified on claim
KC	Replacement of special power wheelchair interface
KD	Drug or biological infused through DME
KF	Item designated by FDA as class III device
KH	DMEPOS item, initial claim, purchase or first month rental
KI	DMEPOS item, second or third month rental
KJ	DMEPOS item, parenteral enteral nutrition (PEN) pump or capped rental, months four to 15
KM	Replacement of facial prosthesis including new impression/moulage
KN	Replacement of facial prosthesis using previous master model
KO	Single drug unit dose formulation
KP	First drug of a multiple drug unit dose formulation
KQ	Second or subsequent drug of a multiple drug unit dose formulation
KR	Rental item, billing for partial month
KS	Glucose monitor supply for diabetic beneficiary not treated with insulin
KX	Specific required documentation on file
KZ	New coverage not implemented by managed care
LC	Left circumflex coronary artery
LD	Left anterior descending coronary artery
LL	Lease/rental (use the LL modifier when DME equipment rental is to be applied against the purchase price)
LR	Laboratory round trip
LS	FDA-monitored intraocular lens implant
LT	Left side (used to identify procedures performed on the left side of the body)
M2	Medicare secondary payer (MSP)
MS	Six month maintenance and servicing fee for reasonable and necessary parts and labor which are not covered under any manufacturer or supplier warranty
NR	New when rented (use the NR modifier when DME which was new at the time of rental is subsequently purchased)
NU	New equipment
P1	Anesthesia physical status-Normal, healthy patient
P2	Anesthesia physical status-Patient with mild, systemic disease
P3	Anesthesia physical status-Patient with severe, systemic disease
P4	Anesthesia physical status-Patient with severe, systemic disease that is a constant threat to life

Appendix 2 — Modifiers

P5 Anesthesia physical status-Moribund patient who is not expected to survive without the operation

P6 Anesthesia physical status-Declared brain-dead patient whose organs are being removed for donor purposes

PL Progressive addition lenses

Q2 HCFA/ORD demonstration project procedure/service

Q3 Live kidney donor surgery and related services

Q4 Service for ordering/referring physician qualifies as a service exemption

Q5 Service furnished by a substitute physician under a reciprocal billing arrangement

Q6 Service furnished by a locum tenens physician

Q7 One Class A finding

Q8 Two Class B findings

Q9 One Class B and two Class C findings

QA FDA investigational device exemption

QC Single channel monitoring

QD Recording and storage in solid state memory by a digital recorder

QE Prescribed amount of oxygen is less than one liter per minute (LPM)

QF Prescribed amount of oxygen exceeds four LPM and portable oxygen is prescribed

QG Prescribed amount of oxygen is greater than four liters per minute (LPM)

QH Oxygen conserving device is being used with an oxygen delivery system

QJ Services/items provided to a prisoner or patient in state or local custody, however the state or local government, as applicable, meets the requirements in 42 CFR 411.4(B)

QK Medical direction of two, three or four concurrent anesthesia procedures involving qualified individuals

QL Patient pronounced dead after ambulance called

QM Ambulance service provided under arrangement by a provider of services

QN Ambulance service furnished directly by a provider of services

QP Documentation is on file showing that the laboratory test(s) was ordered individually or ordered as a CPT-recognized panel other than automated profile codes 80002-80019, G0058, G0059, and G0060

QR Item or service provided in a Medicare specified study

QS Monitored anesthesia care service

QT Recording and storage on tape by an analog tape recorder

QV Item or service provided as routine care in a Medicare qualifying clinical trial

QW CLIA waived test

QX CRNA service: with medical direction by a physician

QY Medical direction of one certified registered nurse anesthetist (CRNA) by an anesthesiologist

QZ CRNA service: without medical direction by a physician

RC Right coronary artery

RD Drug provided to beneficiary, but not administered incident to

RP Replacement and repair -RP may be used to indicate replacement of DME, orthotic and prosthetic devices which have been in use for sometime. The claim shows the code for the part, followed by the 'RP' modifier and the charge for the part.

RR Rental (use the RR modifier when DME is to be rented)

RT Right side (used to identify procedures performed on the right side of the body)

SA Nurse practitioner rendering service in collaboration with a physician

SB Nurse midwife

SC Medically necessary service or supply

SD Services provided by registered nurse with specialized, highly technical home infusion training

SE State and/or federally-funded programs/services

SF Second opinion ordered by a professional review organization (PRO) per section 9401, p.l. 99-272 (100% reimbursement - no Medicare deductible or coinsurance)

SG Ambulatory surgical center (ASC) facility service

SH Second concurrently administered infusion therapy

SJ Third or more concurrently administered infusion therapy

SK Member of high risk population (use only with codes for immunization)

SL State supplied vaccine

SM Second surgical opinion

SN Third surgical opinion

SQ Item ordered by home health

SS Home infusion services provided in the infusion suite of the IV therapy provider

ST Related to trauma or injury

SU Procedure performed in physician's office (to denote use of facility and equipment)

SV Pharmaceuticals delivered to patient's home but not utilized

SW Services provided by a certified diabetic educator

SY Persons who are in close contact with member of high-risk population (use only with codes for immunization)

T1 Left foot, second digit

T2 Left foot, third digit

T3 Left foot, fourth digit

T4 Left foot, fifth digit

T5 Right foot, great toe

T6 Right foot, second digit

T7 Right foot, third digit

T8 Right foot, fourth digit

T9 Right foot, fifth digit

TA Left foot, great toe

TC Technical component. Under certain circumstances, a charge may be made for the technical component alone. Under those circumstances the technical component charge is identified by adding modifier 'TC' to the usual procedure number. Technical component charges are institutional charges and not billed separately by physicians. However, portable x-ray suppliers only bill for technical component and should utilize modifier TC. The charge data from portable x-ray suppliers will then be used to build customary and prevailing profiles.

TD RN

TE LPN/LVN

TF Intermediate level of care

TG Complex/high tech level of care

TH Obstetrical treatment/services, prenatal or postpartum

TJ Program group, child and/or adolescent

TK Extra patient or passenger, nonambulance

TL Early intervention/individualized family service plan (IFSP)

TM Individualized education program (IEP)

TN Rural/outside providers' customary service area

TP Medical transport, unloaded vehicle

TQ Basic life support by volunteer ambulance provider

TR School-based individualized education program (IEP) services provided outside the public school district responsible for the student

TS Follow-up service

TT	Individualized service provided to more than one patient in same setting
TU	Special payment rate, overtime
TV	Special payment rates, holidays/weekends
TW	Back-up equipment
U1	Medicaid level of care 1, as defined by each state
U2	Medicaid level of care 2, as defined by each state
U3	Medicaid level of care 3, as defined by each state
U4	Medicaid level of care 4, as defined by each state
U5	Medicaid level of care 5, as defined by each state
U6	Medicaid level of care 6, as defined by each state
U7	Medicaid level of care 7, as defined by each state
U8	Medicaid level of care 8, as defined by each state
U9	Medicaid level of care 9, as defined by each state
UA	Medicaid level of care 10, as defined by each state
UB	Medicaid level of care 11, as defined by each state
UC	Medicaid level of care 12, as defined by each state
UD	Medicaid level of care 13, as defined by each state
UE	Used durable medical equipment
UF	Services provided in the morning
UG	Services provided in the afternoon
UH	Services provided in the evening
UJ	Services provided at night
UK	Services provided on behalf of the client to someone other than the client (collateral relationship)
UN	Two patients served
UP	Three patients served
UQ	Four patients served
UR	Five patients served
US	Six or more patients served
VP	Aphakic patient

APPENDIX 3 — ABBREVIATIONS AND ACRONYMS

HCPCS Abbreviations and Acronyms

The following abbreviations and acronyms are used in the HCPCS descriptions:

/	or
<	less than
<=	less than equal to
>	greater than
>=	greater than equal to
AC	alternating current
AFO	ankle-foot orthosis
AICC	anti-inhibitor coagulant complex
AK	above the knee
AKA	above knee amputation
ALS	advanced life support
AMP	ampule
ART	artery
ART	Arterial
ASC	ambulatory surgery center
ATT	attached
A-V	Arteriovenous
AVF	arteriovenous fistula
BICROS	bilateral routing of signals
BK	below the knee
BLS	basic life support
BP	blood pressure
BTE	behind the ear (hearing aid)
CAPD	continuous ambulatory peritoneal dialysis
Carb	carbohydrate
CBC	complete blood count
cc	cubic centimeter
CCPD	continuous cycling peritoneal analysis
CHF	congestive heart failure
CIC	completely in the canal (hearing aid)
CIM	Coverage Issue Manual
Clsd	closed
cm	centimeter
CMN	certificate of medical necessity
CMS	Centers for Medicare and Medicaid Services
CMV	Cytomegalovirus
Conc	concentrate
Conc	concentrated
Cont	continuous
CP	clinical psychologist
CPAP	continuous positive airway pressure
CPT	Current Procedural Terminology
CRF	chronic renal failure
CRNA	certified registered nurse anesthetist
CROS	contralateral routing of signals
CSW	clinical social worker
CT	computed tomography
CTLSO	cervical-thoracic-lumbar-sacral orthosis
cu	cubic
DC	direct current
DI	diurnal rhythm
Dx	diagnosis
DLI	donor leukocyte infusion
DME	durable medical equipment
DME MAC	durable medical equipment Medicare administrative contractor
DMEPOS	Durable Medical Equipment, Prosthestics, Orthotics and Other Supplies
DMERC	durable medical equipment regional carrier
DR	diagnostic radiology
DX	diagnostic
e.g.	for example
Ea	each
ECF	extended care facility
EEG	electroencephalogram
EKG	electrocardiogram
EMG	electromyography
EO	elbow orthosis
EP	electrophysiologic
EPO	epoetin alfa
EPSDT	early periodic screening, diagnosis and treatment
ESRD	end-stage renal disease
Ex	extended
Exper	experimental
Ext	external
F	french
FDA	Food and Drug Administration
FDG-PET	Positron emission with tomography with 18 fluorodeoxyglucose
Fem	female
FO	finger orthosis
FPD	fixed partial denture
Fr	french
ft	foot
G-CSF	filgrastim (granulocyte colony-stimulating factor)
gm	gram (g)
H2O	water
HCl	hydrochloric acid, hydrochloride
HCPCS	Healthcare Common Procedural Coding System
HCT	hematocrit
HFO	hand-finger orthosis
HHA	home health agency
HI	high
HI-LO	high-low
HIT	home infusion therapy
HKAFO	hip-knee-ankle foot orthosis
HLA	human leukocyte antigen
HMES	heat and moisture exchange system
HNPCC	hereditary non-polyposis colorectal cancer
HO	hip orthosis
HPSA	health professional shortage area
IA	intra-arterial administration
ip	interphalangeal
I-131	Iodine 131
ICF	intermediate care facility
ICU	intensive care facility
IM	intramuscular
in	inch
INF	infusion
INH	inhalation solution
INJ	injection
IOL	intraocular lens
IPD	intermittent peritoneal dialysis
IPPB	intermittent positive pressure breathing
IT	intrathecal administration
ITC	in the canal (hearing aid)
ITE	in the ear (hearing aid)
IU	international units

IV	intravenous		PHP	physician hospital plan
IVF	in vitro fertilization		PI	paramedic intercept
KAFO	knee-ankle-foot orthosis		PICC	peripherally inserted central venous catheter
KO	knee orthosis		PKR	photorefractive keratotomy
KOH	potassium hydroxide		Pow	powder
L	left		PRK	photoreactive keratectomy
LASIK	laser in situ keratomileusis		PRO	peer review organization
LAUP	laser assisted uvulopalatoplasty		PSA	prostate specific antigen
lbs	pounds		PTB	patellar tendon bearing
LDL	low density lipoprotein		PTK	phototherapeutic keratectomy
Lo	low		PVC	polyvinyl chloride
LPM	liters per minute		R	right
LPN/LVN	Licensed Practical Nurse/Licensed Vocational Nurse		Repl	replace
LSO	lumbar-sacral orthosis		RN	registered nurse
MAC	Medicare administrative contractor		RP	retrograde pyelogram
mp	metacarpophalangeal		Rx	prescription
mcg	microgram		SACH	solid ankle, cushion heel
mCi	millicurie		SC	subcutaneous
MCM	Medicare Carriers Manual		SCT	specialty care transport
MCP	metacarparpophalangeal joint		SEO	shoulder-elbow orthosis
MCP	monthly capitation payment		SEWHO	shoulder-elbow-wrist-hand orthosis
mEq	milliequivalent		SEXA	single energy x-ray absorptiometry
MESA	microsurgical epididymal sperm aspiration		SGD	speech generating device
mg	milligram		SGD	sinus rhythm
mgs	milligrams		SM	samarium
MHT	megahertz		SNCT	sensory nerve conduction test
ml	milliliter		SNF	skilled nursing facility
mm	millimeter		SO	sacroilliac othrosis
mmHg	millimeters of Mercury		SO	shoulder orthosis
MRA	magnetic resonance angiography		Sol	solution
MRI	magnetic resonance imaging		SQ	square
NA	sodium		SR	screen
NCI	National Cancer Institute		ST	standard
NEC	not elsewhere classified		ST	sustained release
NG	nasogastric		Syr	syrup
NH	nursing home		TABS	tablets
NMES	neuromuscular electrical stimulation		Tc	Technetium
NOC	not otherwise classified		Tc 99m	technetium isotope
NOS	not otherwise specified		TENS	transcutaneous electrical nerve stimulator
O2	oxygen		THKAO	thoracic-hip-knee-ankle orthosis
OBRA	Omnibus Budget Reconciliation Act		TLSO	thoracic-lumbar-sacral-orthosis
OMT	osteopathic manipulation therapy		TM	temporomandibular
OPPS	outpatient prospective payment system		TMJ	temporomandibular joint
ORAL	oral administration		TPN	total parenteral nutrition
OSA	obstructive sleep apnea		U	unit
Ost	ostomy		uCi	microcurie
OTH	other routes of administration		VAR	various routes of administration
oz	ounce		w	with
PA	physician's assistant		w/	with
PAR	parenteral		w/o	with or without
PCA	patient controlled analgesia		WAK	wearable artificial kidney
PCH	pouch		wc	wheelchair
PEN	parenteral and enteral nutrition		WHFO	wrist-hand-finger orthotic
PENS	percutaneous electrical nerve stimulation		Wk	week
PET	positron emission tomography		w/o	without
PHP	pre-paid health plan		Xe	xenon (isotope mass of xenon 133)

Appendix 3 — Abbreviations and Acronyms

APPENDIX 4 — PUB 100 REFERENCES
REVISIONS TO THE CMS MANUAL SYSTEM

The Centers for Medicare and Medicaid Services (CMS) initiated its long awaited transition from a paper-based manual system to a Web-based system on October 1, 2003, which updates and restructures all manual instructions. The new system, called the online CMS Manual system, combines all of the various program instructions into an electronic manual, which can be found at http://www.cms.hhs.gov/manuals.

Effective September 30, 2003, the former method of publishing program memoranda (PMs) to communicate program instructions was replaced by the following four templates:

- One-time notification:
- Manual revisions:
- Business requirement:
- Confidential requirements:

The Office of Strategic Operations and Regulatory Affairs (OSORA), Division of Issuances, will continue to communicate advanced program instructions to the regions and contractor community every Friday as it currently does. These instructions will also contain a transmittal sheet to identify changes pertaining to a specific manual, requirement, or notification.

The Web-based system has been organized by functional area (e.g., eligibility, entitlement, claims processing, benefit policy, program integrity) in an effort to eliminate redundancy within the manuals, simplify the updating process, and make CMS program instructions available in a more timely manner. The initial release will include Pub. 100, Pub. 100-02, Pub. 100-03, Pub. 100-04, Pub. 100-05, Pub. 100-09, Pub. 100-15, and Pub. 100-20.

The Web-based system contains the functional areas included in the table below:

Publication #	Title
Pub. 100	Introduction
Pub. 100-1	Medicare General Information, Eligibility, and Entitlement
Pub. 100-2	Medicare Benefit Policy (basic coverage rules)
Pub. 100-3	Medicare National Coverage Determinations (national coverage decisions)
Pub. 100-4	Medicare Claims Processing (includes appeals, contractor interface with CWF, and MSN)
Pub. 100-5	Medicare Secondary Payer
Pub. 100-6	Medicare Financial Management (includes Intermediary Desk Review and Audit)
Pub. 100-7	Medicare State Operations
Pub. 100-8	Medicare Program Integrity
Pub. 100-9	Medicare Contractor Beneficiary and Provider Communications
Pub. 100-10	Medicare Quality Improvement Organization
Pub. 100-11	Reserved
Pub. 100-12	State Medicaid
Pub. 100-13	Medicaid State Children's Health Insurance Program
Pub. 100-14	Medicare End Stage Renal Disease Network
Pub. 100-15	Medicare State Buy-In
Pub. 100-16	Medicare Managed Care
Pub. 100-17	Medicare Business Partners Systems Security
Pub. 100-18	Medicare Business Partners Security Oversight
Pub. 100-19	Demonstrations
Pub. 100-20	One-Time Notification

Table of Contents

The table below shows the paper-based manuals used to construct the Web-based system. Although this is just an overview, CMS is in the process of developing detailed crosswalks to guide you from a specific section of the old manuals to the appropriate area of the new manual, as well as to show how the information in each section was derived.

Paper-Based Manuals	Internet-Only Manuals
Pub. 06 — Medicare Coverage Issues	Pub. 100-01 — Medicare General Information, Eligibility, and Entitlement
Pub. 09 — Medicare Outpatient Physical Therapy	Pub. 100-02 — Medicare Benefit Policy
Pub. 10 — Medicare Hospital	Pub. 100-03 — Medicare National Coverage Determinations
Pub. 11 — Medicare Home Health Agency	Pub. 100-04 — Medicare Claims Processing
Pub. 12 — Medicare Skilled Nursing Facility	Pub. 100-05 — Medicare Secondary Payer
Pub. 13 — Medicare Intermediary Manual, Parts 1, 2, 3, and 4	Pub. 100-06 — Medicare Financial Management
Pub. 14 — Medicare Carriers Manual, Parts 1, 2, 3, and 4	Pub. 100-08 — Medicare Program Integrity
Pub. 21 — Medicare Hospice	Pub. 100-09 — Medicare Contractor Beneficiary and Provider Communications
Pub. 27 — Medicare Rural Health Clinic and Federally Qualified Health Center	
Pub. 29 — Medicare Renal Dialysis Facility	

Program Memoranda
Pub. 60A — Intermediaries
Pub. 60B — Carriers
Pub. 60AB — Intermediaries/Carriers
NOTE: Information derived from Pub. 06 to Pub. 60AB was used to develop Pub. 100-01 to Pub. 100-09 for the Internet-only manual.

Paper-Based Manuals	Internet-Only Manuals
Pub. 19 — Medicare Peer Review	Pub. 100-10 — Medicare Quality Organization Improvement Organization
Pub. 07 — Medicare State Operations	Pub. 100-07 — Medicare State Operations
Pub. 45 — State Medicaid	Pub. 100-12 — State Medicaid
Pub. 81 — Medicare End Stage Renal Disease	Pub. 100-13 — Medicaid State Children's Health Insurance Program
Pub. 24 — Medicare State Buy-In	Pub. 100-14 — Medicare End Stage Renal Disease Network Organizations Network Organizations
Pub. 75 — Health Maintenance Organization/Competitive Medical Plan Care	Pub. 100-15 — Medicare State Buy-In
Pub. 76 — Health Maintenance Organization/Competitive Medical Plan (PM)	Pub. 100-16 — Medicare Managed

Paper-Based Manuals	Internet-Only Manuals
Pub. 77 — Manual for Federally Qualified Health Maintenance Organizations	Pub. 100-17 — Business Partners Systems Security
Pub. 13 — Medicare Intermediaries Manual, Part 2	Pub. 100-18 — Business Partners Security Oversight
Pub. 14 — Medicare Carriers Manual, Part 2	Pub 100-19 — Demonstrations
Pub. 13 — Medicare Intermediaries Manual, Part 2	Pub 100-20 — One-Time
Pub. 14 — Medicare Carriers Manual, Part 2	
Demonstrations (PMs)	

Program instructions that impact multiple manuals or have no manual impact.

NATIONAL COVERAGE DETERMINATIONS MANUAL

The National Coverage Determinations Manual (NCD), which is the electronic replacement for the Coverage Issues Manual (CIM), is organized according to categories such as diagnostic services, supplies, and medical procedures. The table of contents lists each category and subject within that category. A revision transmittal sheet will identify any new material and recap the changes as well as provide an effective date for the change and any background information. At any time, one can refer to a transmittal indicated on the page of the manual to view this information.

By the time it is complete, the book will contain two chapters. Chapter 1 includes a description of national coverage determinations that have been made by CMS. When available, chapter 2 will contain a list of HCPCS codes related to each coverage determination. To make the manual easier to use, it is organized in accordance with CPT category sequences. Where there is no national coverage determination that affects a particular CPT category, the category is listed as reserved in the table of contents.

The following table is the crosswalk of the NCD to the CIM. However, at this time, many of the NCD policies are not yet available. The CMS Web site also contains a crosswalk of the CIM to the NCD.

MEDICARE BENEFIT POLICY MANUAL

The Medicare Benefit Policy Manual replaces current Medicare general coverage instructions that are not national coverage determinations. As a general rule, in the past these instructions have been found in chapter II of the Medicare Carriers Manual, the Medicare Intermediary Manual, other provider manuals, and program memoranda. New instructions will be published in this manual. As new transmittals are included they will be identified.

On the CMS Web site, a crosswalk from the new manual to the source manual is provided with each chapter and may be accessed from the chapter table of contents. In addition, the crosswalk for each section is shown immediately under the section heading.

The list below is the table of contents for the Medicare Benefit Policy Manual:

Chapter	Title
One	Inpatient Hospital Services
Two	Inpatient Psychiatric Hospital Services
Three	Duration of Covered Inpatient Services
Four	Inpatient Psychiatric Benefit Days Reduction and Lifetime Limitation
Five	Lifetime Reserve Days
Six	Hospital Services Covered Under Part B
Seven	Home Health Services
Eight	Coverage of Extended Care (SNF) Services Under Hospital Insurance

Chapter	Title
Nine	Coverage of Hospice Services Under Hospital Insurance
Ten	Ambulance Services
Eleven	End Stage Renal Disease (ESRD)
Twelve	Comprehensive Outpatient Rehabilitation Facility (CORF) Coverage
Thirteen	Rural Health Clinic (RHC) and Federally Qualified Health Center (FQHC) Services
Fourteen	Medical Devices
Fifteen	Covered Medical and Other Health Services
Sixteen	General Exclusions from Coverage

PUB100 REFERENCES

Pub. 100-1, Chapter 1, Section 10.1

A Brief Description

Hospital Insurance is designed to help patients defray the expenses incurred by hospitalization and related care. In addition to inpatient hospital benefits, hospital insurance covers posthospital extended care in SNFs and posthospital care furnished by a home health agency in the patient's home. Blood clotting factors, for hemophilia patients competent to use such factors to control bleeding without medical or other supervision, and items related to the administration of such factors, are also a Part A benefit for beneficiaries in a covered Part A stay. The purpose of these additional benefits is to provide continued treatment after hospitalization and to encourage the appropriate use of more economical alternatives to inpatient hospital care. Program payments for services rendered to beneficiaries by providers (i.e., hospitals, SNFs, and home health agencies) are generally made to the provider.

In each benefit period, payment may be made for up to 90 inpatient hospital days, and 100 days of posthospital extended care services. Under the latter benefit, the beneficiary must have been in a hospital receiving inpatient hospital services for at least 3 consecutive days (counting the day of admission but not the day of discharge) and be admitted to a SNF or to the SNF level of care in a swing bed hospital within 30 days after the date of hospital discharge. (Under certain circumstances, the 30 days may be extended.)

Where the person became entitled to HI at or after age 65, the hospital discharge must have occurred on or after the first day of the month in which he attained age 65. If his or her current entitlement began before age 65; i.e., he became entitled to HI under the disability or chronic renal disease provisions of the law, the hospital discharge must have occurred while he was so entitled. The 3 consecutive calendar days requirement can be met by stays totaling 3 consecutive days in one or more hospitals.

A SNF provides skilled nursing care and related services for patients who require medical or nursing care, or rehabilitation services. A SNF may be either a separate institution (e.g., a nursing home) or a part of an institution (e.g., a convalescent wing of a hospital). It must be licensed or approved under State or local law, meet the health and safety conditions prescribed by the Secretary of the Department of Health and Human Services (DHHS), and have a written transfer agreement with one or more participating hospitals providing for the transfer of patients between the hospital and the facility, and for the interchange of medical and other information. If an otherwise qualified SNF has attempted in good faith but without success to enter into a transfer agreement, this requirement may be waived by the State agency.

For Medicare purposes, the term SNF does not include any institution which is primarily for the care and treatment of mental diseases. Extended care services include room and board; skilled nursing care by or under the supervision of a registered nurse; physical therapy, occupational therapy, or speech-language pathology services; medical social services; drugs, biologicals, supplies, appliances, and equipment; and other services ordinarily furnished by or under arrangements made by the facility. No payment may be made for items or services which would not be covered in a hospital, or for custodial care when that is the only type of care that the beneficiary needs.

The services of residents and interns of a hospital with which the facility has a swing bed "transfer" agreement and other diagnostic and therapeutic services furnished by such a hospital are covered, but only if billed through the SNF.

Under §4005(b)(2) of the Omnibus Budget Reconciliation Act of 1987, effective for swing bed agreements entered into after March 31, 1988, hospitals with more than 49 beds (but less than 100 beds) are subject to the following conditions. However, these conditions were eliminated by section 408 of the Balanced Budget Refinement Act of 1999 (BBRA), effective with the start of the facility's fourth cost reporting period that begins on or after July 1, 1998. (For those facilities that received no Medicare payment prior to October 1, 1995, this change is effective as of the date of BBRA's enactment, November 29, 1999.)

If there is an available SNF bed in the geographic region, the hospital must transfer the extended care patient within 5 days of the availability date (excluding weekends and holidays) unless the patient's physician certifies within that 5-day period, that transfer of that patient to that facility is not medically appropriate on the availability date. In order to do this, the hospital must identify all SNFs in the geographic region and enter into agreements with them for the transfer of extended care patients. The agreement must call for the SNF to notify the hospital of the availability of beds and the dates these beds will be available for extended care patients.

For each cost reporting period, payment may not be made for patient days of extended care services that exceed 15 percent of the total number of available patient days (except that such payment shall continue to be made for those patients who are receiving extended care services at the time the hospital reaches the 15% limit). The limit is calculated by multiplying the average number of licensed beds by the total number of days in the cost reporting period.

Hospitals having fewer than 50 beds and rural hospitals which entered into transfer agreements before March 31, 1988 (i.e., those which were licensed for more than 49 beds but who were operating as a 50 or less bed facility), are not subject to the 5-weekday transfer requirement or the payment limitation for extended care days. (See section 2230.10 of the Provider Reimbursement Manual, Part 1, for the explanation of the payment limitation.)

"Geographic region" is an area which includes the SNFs with which a hospital has traditionally arranged transfers and all other SNFs within the same proximity to the hospital. In the case of a hospital without existing transfer practices upon which to base a determination, the geographic region is an area which includes all the SNFs within 50 miles of the hospital unless the hospital can demonstrate that the SNFs are inaccessible to its patients. In the event of a dispute as to whether a SNF is within this region or the SNF is inaccessible to hospital patients, the CMS regional office shall make a determination.

Hospices also provide Part A hospital insurance services such as short-term inpatient care. In order to be eligible to elect hospice care under Medicare, an individual must be entitled to Part A of Medicare and be certified as being terminally ill. An individual is considered to be terminally ill if the individual has a medical prognosis that his or her life expectancy is 6 months or less if the illness runs its normal course.

Pub. 100-1, Chapter 3, Section 20.5

Blood Deductibles (Part A and Part B)

Program payment may not be made for the first 3 pints of whole blood or equivalent units of packed red cells received under Part A and Part B combined in a calendar year. However, blood processing (e.g., administration, storage) is not subject to the deductible.

The blood deductibles are in addition to any other applicable deductible and coinsurance amounts for which the patient is responsible.

The deductible applies only to the first 3 pints of blood furnished in a calendar year, even if more than one provider furnished blood.

Pub. 100-1, Chapter 3, Section 20.5.2

Part B Blood Deductible

Blood is furnished on an outpatient basis or is subject to the Part B blood deductible and is counted toward the combined limit. It should be noted that payment for blood may be made to the hospital under Part B only for blood furnished in an outpatient setting. Blood is not covered for inpatient Part B services.

Pub. 100-1, Chapter 3, Section 20.5.3

Items Subject to Blood Deductibles

The blood deductibles apply only to whole blood and packed red cells. The term whole blood means human blood from which none of the liquid or cellular components have been removed. Where packed red cells are furnished, a unit of packed red cells is considered equivalent to a pint of whole blood. Other components of blood such as platelets, fibrinogen, plasma, gamma globulin, and serum albumin are not subject to the blood deductible. However, these components of blood are covered as biologicals.

Refer to Pub. 100-04, Medicare Claims Processing Manual, chapter 4, §231 regarding billing for blood and blood products under the Hospital Outpatient Prospective Payment System (OPPS).

Pub. 100-1, Chapter 5, Section 90.2

Laboratory means a facility for the biological, microbiological, serological, chemical, immuno-hematological, hematological, biophysical, cytological, pathological, or other examination of materials derived from the human body for the purpose of providing information for the diagnosis, prevention, or treatment of any disease or impairment of, or the assessment of the health of, human beings. These examinations also include procedures to determine, measure, or otherwise describe the presence or absence of various substances or organisms in the body. Facilities only collecting or preparing specimens (or both) or only serving as a mailing service and not performing testing are not considered laboratories.

Pub. 100-2, Chapter 1, Section 10

Covered Inpatient Hospital Services Covered Under Part A

A3-3101, HO-210

Patients covered under hospital insurance are entitled to have payment made on their behalf for inpatient hospital services. (Inpatient hospital services do not include extended care services provided by hospitals pursuant to swing bed approvals. See Pub. 100-1, Chapter 8, §10.1, "Hospital Providers of Extended Care Services."). However, both inpatient hospital and inpatient SNF benefits are provided under Part A - Hospital Insurance Benefits for the Aged and Disabled, of Title XVIII).

Additional information concerning the following topics can be found in the following manual chapters:

• Benefit periods is found in Chapter 3, "Duration of Covered Inpatient Services";

• Copayment days is found in Chapter 2, "Duration of Covered Inpatient Services";

• Lifetime reserve days is found in Chapter 5, "Lifetime Reserve Days";

• Related payment information is housed in the Provider Reimbursement Manual.

Blood must be furnished on a day which counts as a day of inpatient hospital services to be covered as a Part A service and to count toward the blood deductible. Thus, blood is not covered under Part A and does not count toward the Part A blood deductible when furnished to an inpatient after the inpatient has exhausted all benefit days in a benefit period, or where the individual has elected not to use lifetime reserve days. However, where the patient is discharged on their first day of entitlement or on the hospital's first day of participation, the hospital is permitted to submit a billing form with no accommodation charge, but with ancillary charges including blood.

The records for all Medicare hospital inpatient discharges are maintained in CMS for statistical analysis and use in determining future PPS DRG classifications and rates.

Non-PPS hospitals do not pay for noncovered services generally excluded from coverage in the Medicare Program. This may result in denial of a part of the billed charges or in denial of the entire admission, depending upon circumstance. In PPS hospitals, the following are also possible:

1. In appropriately admitted cases where a noncovered procedure was performed, denied services may result in payment of a different DRG (i.e., one which excludes payment for the noncovered procedure); or

2. In appropriately admitted cases that become cost outlier cases, denied services may lead to denial of some or all of an outlier payment.

The following examples illustrate this principle. If care is noncovered because a patient does not need to be hospitalized, the intermediary denies the admission and makes no Part A (i.e., PPS) payment unless paid under limitation on liability. Under limitation on liability, Medicare payment may be made when the provider and the beneficiary were not aware the services were not necessary and could not reasonably be expected to know that he services were not necessary. For detailed instructions, see the Medicare Claims Processing Manual, Chapter 30, "Limitation on Liability." If a patient is appropriately hospitalized but receives (beyond routine services) only noncovered care, the admission is denied.

NOTE: The intermediary does not deny an admission that includes covered care, even if noncovered care was also rendered. Under PPS, Medicare assumes that it is paying for only the covered care rendered whenever covered services needed to treat and/or diagnose the illness were in fact provided.

If a noncovered procedure is provided along with covered nonroutine care, a DRG change rather than an admission denial might occur. If noncovered procedures are elevating costs into the cost outlier category, outlier payment is denied in whole or in part.

When the hospital is included in PPS, most of the subsequent discussion regarding coverage of inpatient hospital services is relevant only in the context of determining the appropriateness of admissions, which DRG, if any, to pay, and the appropriateness of payment for any outlier cases.

If a patient receives items or services in excess of, or more expensive than, those for which payment can be made, payment is made only for the covered items or services or for only the appropriate prospective payment amount. This provision applies not only to inpatient services, but also to all hospital services under Parts A and B of the program. If the items or services were requested by the patient, the hospital may charge him the difference between the amount customarily charged for the services requested and the amount customarily charged for covered services.

An inpatient is a person who has been admitted to a hospital for bed occupancy for purposes of receiving inpatient hospital services. Generally, a patient is considered an inpatient if formally admitted as inpatient with the expectation that he or she will remain at least overnight and occupy a bed even though it later develops that the patient can be discharged or transferred to another hospital and not actually use a hospital bed overnight.

The physician or other practitioner responsible for a patient's care at the hospital is also responsible for deciding whether the patient should be admitted as an inpatient. Physicians should use a 24-hour period as a benchmark, i.e., they should order admission for patients who are expected to need hospital care for 24 hours or more, and treat other patients on an outpatient basis. However, the decision to admit a patient is a complex medical judgment which can be made only after the physician has considered a number of factors, including the patient's medical history and current medical needs, the types of facilities available to inpatients and to outpatients, the hospital's by-laws and admissions policies, and the relative appropriateness of treatment in each setting. Factors to be considered when making the decision to admit include such things as:

The severity of the signs and symptoms exhibited by the patient;

The medical predictability of something adverse happening to the patient;

The need for diagnostic studies that appropriately are outpatient services (i.e., their performance does not ordinarily require the patient to remain at the hospital for 24 hours or more) to assist in assessing whether the patient should be admitted; and

The availability of diagnostic procedures at the time when and at the location where the patient presents.

Admissions of particular patients are not covered or noncovered solely on the basis of the length of time the patient actually spends in the hospital. In certain specific situations coverage of services on an inpatient or outpatient basis is determined by the following rules:

Minor Surgery or Other Treatment - When patients with known diagnoses enter a hospital for a specific minor surgical procedure or other treatment that is expected to keep them in the hospital for only a few hours (less than 24), they are considered outpatients for coverage purposes regardless of: the hour they came to the hospital, whether they used a bed, and whether they remained in the hospital past midnight.

Renal Dialysis - Renal dialysis treatments are usually covered only as outpatient services but may under certain circumstances be covered as inpatient services depending on the patient's condition. Patients staying at home, who are ambulatory, whose conditions are stable and who come to the hospital for routine chronic dialysis treatments, and not for a diagnostic workup or a change in therapy, are considered outpatients. On the other hand, patients undergoing short-term dialysis until their kidneys recover from an acute illness (acute dialysis), or persons with borderline renal failure who develop acute renal failure every time they have an illness and require dialysis (episodic dialysis) are usually inpatients. A patient may begin dialysis as an inpatient and then progress to an outpatient status.

Under original Medicare, the Quality Improvement Organization (QIO), for each hospital is responsible for deciding, during review of inpatient admissions on a case-by-case basis, whether the admission was medically necessary. Medicare law authorizes the QIO to make these judgments, and the judgments are binding for purposes of Medicare coverage. In making these judgments, however, QIOs consider only the medical evidence which was available to the physician at the time an admission decision had to be made. They do not take into account other information (e.g., test results) which became available only

after admission, except in cases where considering the post-admission information would support a finding that an admission was medically necessary.

Refer to Parts 4 and 7 of the QIO Manual with regard to initial determinations for these services. The QIO will review the swing bed services in these PPS hospitals as well.

NOTE: When patients requiring extended care services are admitted to beds in a hospital, they are considered inpatients of the hospital. In such cases, the services furnished in the hospital will not be considered extended care services, and payment may not be made under the program for such services unless the services are extended care services furnished pursuant to a swing bed agreement granted to the hospital by the Secretary of Health and Human Services.

Pub. 100-2, Chapter 1, Section 10.1.4

Charges for Deluxe Private Room
A3-3101.1.D, HO-210.1.D

Beneficiaries found to need a private room (either because they need isolation for medical reasons or because they need immediate admission when no other accommodations are available) may be assigned to any of the provider's private rooms. They do not have the right to insist on the private room of their choice, but their preferences should be given the same consideration as if they were paying all provider charges themselves. The program does not, under any circumstances, pay for personal comfort items. Thus, the program does not pay for deluxe accommodations and/or services. These would include a suite, or a room substantially more spacious than is required for treatment, or specially equipped or decorated, or serviced for the comfort and convenience of persons willing to pay a differential for such amenities. If the beneficiary (or representative) requests such deluxe accommodations, the provider should advise that there will be a charge, not covered by Medicare, of a specified amount per day (not exceeding the differential defined in the next sentence); and may charge the beneficiary that amount for each day he/she occupies the deluxe accommodations. The maximum amount the provider may charge the beneficiary for such accommodations is the differential between the most prevalent private room rate at the time of admission and the customary charge for the room occupied. Beneficiaries may not be charged this differential if they (or their representative) do not request the deluxe accommodations.

The beneficiary may not be charged such a differential in private room rates if that differential is based on factors other than personal comfort items. Such factors might include differences between older and newer wings, proximity to lounge, elevators or nursing stations, desirable view, etc. Such rooms are standard 1-bed units and not deluxe rooms for purposes of these instructions, even though the provider may call them deluxe and have a higher customary charge for them. No additional charge may be imposed upon the beneficiary who is assigned to a room that may be somewhat more desirable because of these factors.

Pub. 100-2, Chapter 1, Section 40

Supplies, Appliances, and Equipment
A3-3101.4, HO-210.4

Supplies, appliances, and equipment, which are ordinarily furnished by the hospital for the care and treatment of the beneficiary solely during the inpatient hospital stay, are covered inpatient hospital services.

Under certain circumstances, supplies, appliances, and equipment used during the beneficiary's inpatient stay are covered under Part A even though the supplies, appliances and equipment leave the hospital with the patient upon discharge. These are circumstances in which it would be unreasonable or impossible from a medical standpoint to limit the patient's use of the item to the periods during which the individual is an inpatient. Examples of items covered under this rule are:

Items permanently installed in or attached to the patient's body while an inpatient, such as cardiac valves, cardiac pacemakers, and artificial limbs; and

Items which are temporarily installed in or attached to the patient's body while an inpatient, and which are also necessary to permit or facilitate the patient's release from the hospital, such as tracheotomy or drainage tubes.

Hospital "admission packs" containing primarily toilet articles, such as soap, toothbrushes, toothpaste, and combs, are covered under Part A if routinely furnished by the hospital to all its inpatients. If not routinely furnished to all patients, the packs are not covered. In that situation, the hospital may charge beneficiaries for the pack, but only if they request it with knowledge of what they are requesting and what the charge to them will be.

Supplies, appliances, and equipment furnished to an inpatient for use only outside the hospital are not, in general, covered as inpatient hospital services. However, a temporary or disposable item, which is medically necessary to permit or facilitate the patient's departure from the hospital and is required until the patient can obtain a continuing supply, is covered as an inpatient hospital service.

Oxygen furnished to hospital inpatients is covered under Part A as an inpatient supply.

Pub. 100-2, Chapter 6, Section 10

Medical and Other Health Services Furnished to Inpatients of Participating Hospitals

Payment may be made under Part B for physician services and for the nonphysician medical and other health services listed below when furnished by a participating hospital (either directly or under arrangements) to an inpatient of the hospital, but only if payment for these services cannot be made under Part A.

In PPS hospitals, this means that Part B payment could be made for these services if:

• No Part A prospective payment is made at all for the hospital stay because of patient exhaustion of benefit days before admission;

• The admission was disapproved as not reasonable and necessary (and waiver of liability payment was not made);

• The day or days of the otherwise covered stay during which the services were provided were not reasonable and necessary (and no payment was made under waiver of liability);

• The patient was not otherwise eligible for or entitled to coverage under Part A (See the Medicare Benefit Policy Manual, Chapter 1, §150, for services received as a result of noncovered services); or

• No Part A day outlier payment is made (for discharges before October 1997) for one or more outlier days due to patient exhaustion of benefit days after admission but before the case's arrival at outlier status, or because outlier days are otherwise not covered and waiver of liability payment is not made.

However, if only day outlier payment is denied under Part A (discharges before October 1997), Part B payment may be made for only the services covered under Part B and furnished on the denied outlier days.

In non-PPS hospitals, Part B payment may be made for services on any day for which Part A payment is denied (i.e., benefit days are exhausted; services are not at the hospital level of care; or patient is not otherwise eligible or entitled to payment under Part A).

Services payable are:

• Diagnostic x-ray tests, diagnostic laboratory tests, and other diagnostic tests;

• X-ray, radium, and radioactive isotope therapy, including materials and services of technicians;

• Surgical dressings, and splints, casts, and other devices used for reduction of fractures and dislocations;

• Prosthetic devices (other than dental) which replace all or part of an internal body organ (including contiguous tissue), or all or part of the function of a permanently inoperative or malfunctioning internal body organ, including replacement or repairs of such devices;

• Leg, arm, back, and neck braces, trusses, and artificial legs, arms, and eyes including adjustments, repairs, and replacements required because of breakage, wear, loss, or a change in the patient's physical condition;

• Outpatient physical therapy, outpatient speech-language pathology services, and outpatient occupational therapy (see the Medicare Benefit Policy Manual, Chapter 15, "Covered Medical and Other Health Services," §§220 and 230);

• Screening mammography services;

• Screening pap smears;

• Influenza, pneumococcal pneumonia, and hepatitis B vaccines;

• Colorectal screening;

• Bone mass measurements;

• Diabetes self-management;

• Prostate screening;

• Ambulance services;

• Hemophilia clotting factors for hemophilia patients competent to use these factors without supervision);

• Immunosuppressive drugs;

• Oral anti-cancer drugs;

• Oral drug prescribed for use as an acute anti-emetic used as part of an anti-cancer chemotherapeutic regimen; and

• Epoetin Alfa (EPO).

Coverage rules for these services are described in the Medicare Benefit Policy Manual, Chapters: 11, "End Stage Renal Disease (ESRD);" 14, "Medical Devices;" or 15, "Medical and Other Health Services."

For services to be covered under Part A or Part B, a hospital must furnish nonphysician services to its inpatients directly or under arrangements. A nonphysician service is one which does not meet the criteria defining physicians' services specifically provided for in regulation at 42 CFR 415.102. Services "incident to" physicians' services (except for the services of nurse anesthetists employed by anesthesiologists) are nonphysician services for purposes of this provision. This provision is applicable to all hospitals participating in Medicare, including those paid under alternative arrangements such as State cost control systems, and to emergency hospital services furnished by nonparticipating hospitals.

In all hospitals, every service provided to a hospital inpatient other than those listed in the next paragraph must be treated as an inpatient hospital service to be paid for under Part A, if Part A coverage is available and the beneficiary is entitled to Part A. This is because every hospital must provide directly or arrange for any nonphysician service rendered to its inpatients, and a hospital can be paid under Part B for a service provided in this manner only if Part A coverage does not exist.

These services, when provided to a hospital inpatient, may be covered under Part B, even though the patient has Part A coverage for the hospital stay. This is because these services are covered under Part B and not covered under Part A. They are:

Physicians' services (including the services of residents and interns in unapproved teaching programs);

Influenza vaccine;

Pneumococcal vaccine and its administration;

Hepatitis B vaccine and its administration;

Screening mammography services;

Screening pap smears and pelvic exams;

Colorectal screening;

Bone mass measurements;

Diabetes self management training services; and

Prostate screening.

However, note that in order to have any Medicare coverage at all (Part A or Part B), any nonphysician service rendered to a hospital inpatient must be provided directly or arranged for by the hospital.

Pub. 100-2, Chapter 6, Section 20.5

Outpatient Observation Services

A. Outpatient Observation Services Defined

Observation care is a well-defined set of specific, clinically appropriate services, which include ongoing short term treatment, assessment, and reassessment before a decision can be made regarding whether patients will require further treatment as hospital inpatients or if they are able to be discharged from the hospital. Observation status is commonly assigned to patients who present to the emergency department and who then require a significant period of treatment or monitoring before a decision is made concerning their admission or discharge.

Observation services are covered only when provided by the order of a physician or another individual authorized by State licensure law and hospital staff bylaws to admit patients to the hospital or to order outpatient tests. In the majority of cases, the decision whether to discharge a patient from the hospital following resolution of the reason for the observation care or to admit the patient as an inpatient can be made in less than 48 hours, usually in less than 24 hours. In only rare and exceptional cases do reasonable and necessary outpatient observation services span more than 48 hours.

Hospitals may bill for patients who are "direct admissions" to observation. A "direct admission" occurs when a physician in the community refers a patient to the hospital for observation, bypassing the clinic or emergency department (ED). Effective for services furnished on or after January 1, 2003, hospitals may bill for patients directly admitted for observation services.

See Pub. 100-04, Medicare Claims Processing Manual, Chapter 4, §290, at http://www.cms.hhs.gov/manuals/downloads/clm104c04.pdf for billing and payment instructions for outpatient observation services.

B. Coverage of Outpatient Observation Services

When a physician orders that a patient be placed under observation, the patient's status is that of an outpatient. The purpose of observation is to determine the need for further treatment or for inpatient admission. Thus, a patient in observation may improve and be released, or be admitted as an inpatient (see Pub. 100-02, Medicare Benefit Policy Manual, Chapter 1, §10 "Covered Inpatient Hospital Services Covered Under Part A" at http://www.cms.hhs.gov/manuals/Downloads/bp102c01.pdf).

C. Notification of Beneficiary

All hospital observation services, regardless of the duration of the observation care, that are medically reasonable and necessary are covered by Medicare, and hospitals receive OPPS payments for such observation services. A separate APC payment is made for outpatient observation services involving three specific conditions: chest pain, asthma, and congestive heart failure (see the Medicare Claims Processing Manual, §290.4.2) for additional criteria which must be met. Payments for all other reasonable and necessary observation services are packaged into the payments for other separately payable services provided to the patient on the same day. An ABN should not be issued in the context of reasonable and necessary observation services, whether packaged or paid separately.

If a hospital intends to place or retain a beneficiary in observation for a noncovered service, it must give the beneficiary proper written advance notice of noncoverage under limitation on liability procedures (see Pub. 100-04, Medicare Claims Processing Manual; Chapter 30, "Financial Liability Protections," §20, at http://www.cms.hhs.gov/manuals/downloads/clm104c30.pdf for information regarding Limitation On Liability (LOL) Under §1879 Where Medicare Claims Are Disallowed).

"Noncovered," in this context, refers to such services as those listed in paragraph D, below.

D. Services That Are Not Covered as Outpatient Observation

The following types of services are not covered as outpatient observation services:

• Services that are not reasonable or necessary for the diagnosis or treatment of the patient.

• Services that are provided for the convenience of the patient, the patient's family, or a physician, (e.g., following an uncomplicated treatment or a procedure, physician busy when patient is physically ready for discharge, patient awaiting placement in a long term care facility).

• Services that are covered under Part A, such as a medically appropriate inpatient admission, or services that are part of another Part B service, such as postoperative monitoring during a standard recovery period, (e.g., 4-6 hours), which should be billed as recovery room services. Similarly, in the case of patients who undergo diagnostic testing in a hospital outpatient department, routine preparation services furnished prior to the testing and recovery afterwards are included in the payment for those diagnostic services. Observation should not be billed concurrently with therapeutic services such as chemotherapy.

• Standing orders for observation following outpatient surgery.

Claims for the preceding services are to be denied as not reasonable and necessary, under §1862(a)(1)(A) of the Act.

Pub. 100-2, Chapter 10, Section 10.1

Vehicle and Crew Requirement
B3-2120.1, A3-3114, HO-236.1

Pub. 100-2, Chapter 10, Section 20

Coverage Guidelines for Ambulance Service Claims
B3-2125

Payment may be made for expenses incurred by a patient for ambulance service provided conditions l, 2, and 3 in the left-hand column have been met. The right-hand column indicates the documentation needed to establish that the condition has been met.

Conditions	*Review Action*
1. Patient was transported by an approved supplier of ambulance services.	1. Ambulance supplier is listed in the table of approved ambulance companies (§10.1.3)
2. The patient was suffering from an illness or injury, which contraindicated transportation by other means. (§10.2)	2. (a) The contractor presumes the requirement was met if the submitted documentation indicates that the patient:
	• Was transported in an emergency situation, e.g., as a result of an accident, injury or acute illness, or
	• Needed to be restrained to prevent injury to the beneficiary or others; or
	• Was unconscious or in shock; or
	• Required oxygen or other emergency treatment during transport to the nearest appropriate facility; or
	• Exhibits signs and symptoms of acute respiratory distress or cardiac distress such as shortness of breath or chest pain; or
	• Exhibits signs and symptoms that indicate the possibility of acute stroke; or
	• Had to remain immobile because of a fracture that had not been set or the possibility of a fracture; or
	• Was experiencing severe hemorrhage; or
	• Could be moved only by stretcher; or
	• Was bed-confined before and after the ambulance trip.

(b)

In the absence of any of the conditions listed in (a)above additional documentation should be obtained to establish medical need where the evidence indicates the existence of the circumstances listed below:

(i) Patient's condition would not ordinarily require movement by stretcher, or

(ii) The individual was not admitted as a hospital inpatient (except in accident cases), or

(iii) The ambulance was used solely because other means of transportation were unavailable, or

(iv) The individual merely needed assistance in getting from his room or home to a vehicle.

(c) Where the information indicates a situation not listed in 2(a) or 2(b) above, refer the case to your supervisor.

Conditions	*Review Action*
3. The patient was transported from and to points listed below.	3. Claims should show the ZIP code of the point of pickup.
(a) From patient's residence (or other place where need arose) to hospital or skilled nursing facility.	(a) i. Condition met if trip began within the institution's service area as shown in the carrier's locality guide. ii. Condition met where the trip began outside the institution's service area if the institution was the nearest one with appropriate facilities.

NOTE: A patient's residence is the place where he or she makes his/her home and dwells permanently, or for an extended period of time. A skilled nursing facility is one, which is listed in the Directory of Medical Facilities as a participating SNF or as an institution which meets §1861(j)(1) of the Act.

NOTE: A claim for ambulance service to a participating hospital or skilled nursing facility should not be denied on the grounds that there is a nearer nonparticipating institution having appropriate facilities.

(b) Skilled nursing facility to a hospital or hospital to a skilled nursing facility.	(b) (i) Condition met if the ZIP code of the pickup point is within the service area of the destination as shown in the carrier's locality guide. (ii) Condition met where the ZIP code of the pickup point is outside the service area of the destination if the destination institution was the nearest appropriate facility.
(c) Hospital to hospital or skilled nursing facility to skilled nursing facility.	(c) Condition met if the discharging institution was not an appropriate facility and the admitting institution was the nearest appropriate facility.
(d) From a hospital or skilled nursing facility to patient's residence.	(d) (i) Condition met if patient's residence is within the institution's service area as shown in the carrier's locality guide. (ii) Condition met where the patient's residence is outside the institution's service area if the institution was the nearest appropriate facility.
(e) Round trip for hospital or participating skilled nursing facility inpatients to the nearest hospital or nonhospital treatment facility.	(e) Condition met if the reasonable and necessary diagnostic or therapeutic service required by patient's condition is not available at the institution where the beneficiary is an inpatient.

NOTE: Ambulance service to a physician's office or a physician-directed clinic is not covered. See §10.3.7 above, where a stop is made at a physician's office en route to a hospital and §10.3.3 for additional exceptions.)

4. Ambulance services involving hospital admissions in Canada or Mexico are covered (Medicare Claims Processing Manual, Chapter 1, "General Billing Requirements, " §§10.1.3.) if the following conditions are met:	(a) The foreign hospitalization has been determined to be covered; and (b) The ambulance service meets the coverage requirements set forth in §§10-10.3. If the foreign hospitalization has been determined to be covered on the basis of emergency services (See the Medicare Claims Processing Manual, Chapter 1, "General Billing Requirements," §10.1.3), the necessity requirement (§10.2) and the destination requirement (§10.3) are considered met.
5. The carrier will make partial payment for otherwise covered ambulance service, which exceeded limits defined in item 6. The carrier will base the payment on the amount payable had the patient been transported:	(a) From the pickup point to the nearest appropriate facility, or (b) From the nearest appropriate facility to the beneficiary's residence where he or she is being returned home from a distant institution.

Pub. 100-2, Chapter 11, Section 130.1

Inpatient Dialysis in Nonparticipating Hospitals
A3-3173.3

Emergency inpatient dialysis services provided by a nonparticipating U.S. hospital are covered if the requirements in §130 above are met.

Pub. 100-2, Chapter 15, Section 50

Drugs and Biologicals
B3-2049, A3-3112.4.B, HO-230.4.B

The Medicare program provides limited benefits for outpatient drugs. The program covers drugs that are furnished "incident to" a physician's service provided that the drugs are not usually self-administered by the patients who take them.

Generally, drugs and biologicals are covered only if all of the following requirements are met:

- They meet the definition of drugs or biologicals (see §50.1);
- They are of the type that are not usually self-administered. (see §50.2);
- They meet all the general requirements for coverage of items as incident to a physician's services (see §§50.1 and 50.3);
- They are reasonable and necessary for the diagnosis or treatment of the illness or injury for which they are administered according to accepted standards of medical practice (see §50.4);
- They are not excluded as noncovered immunizations (see §50.4.4.2); and
- They have not been determined by the FDA to be less than effective. (See §§50.4.4.)

Medicare Part B does generally not cover drugs that can be self-administered, such as those in pill form, or are used for self-injection. However, the statute provides for the coverage of some self-administered drugs. Examples of self-administered drugs that are covered include blood-clotting factors, drugs used in immunosuppressive therapy, erythropoietin for dialysis patients, osteoporosis drugs for certain homebound patients, and certain oral cancer drugs. (See §110.3 for coverage of drugs, which are necessary to the effective use of Durable Medical Equipment (DME) or prosthetic devices.)

Pub. 100-2, Chapter 15, Section 50.2

Administration of Drug or Biological
AB-02-072, AB-02-139, B3-2049.2

The Medicare program provides limited benefits for outpatient prescription drugs. The program covers drugs that are furnished "incident to" a physician's service provided that the drugs are not usually self-administered by the patients who take them. Section 112 of the Benefits, Improvements & Protection Act of 2000 (BIPA) amended sections 1861(s)(2)(A) and 1861(s)(2)(B) of the Act to redefine this exclusion. The prior statutory language referred to those drugs "which cannot be self-administered." Implementation of the BIPA provision requires interpretation of the phrase "not usually self-administered by the patient".

A. Policy

Fiscal intermediaries and carriers are instructed to follow the instructions below when applying the exclusion for drugs that are usually self-administered by the patient. Each individual contractor must make its own individual determination on each drug. Contractors must continue to apply the policy that not only the drug is medically reasonable and necessary for any individual claim, but also that the route of administration is medically reasonable and necessary. That is, if a drug is available in both oral and injectable forms, the injectable form of the drug must be medically reasonable and necessary as compared to using the oral form.

For certain injectable drugs, it will be apparent due to the nature of the condition(s) for which they are administered or the usual course of treatment for those conditions, they are, or are not, usually self-administered. For example, an injectable drug used to treat migraine headaches is usually self-administered. On the other hand, an injectable drug, administered at the same time as chemotherapy, used to treat anemia secondary to chemotherapy is not usually self-administered.

B. Administered

The term "administered" refers only to the physical process by which the drug enters the patient's body. It does not refer to whether the process is supervised by a medical professional (for example, to observe proper technique or side-effects of the drug). Only injectable (including intravenous) drugs are eligible for inclusion under the "incident to" benefit. Other routes of administration including, but not limited to, oral drugs, suppositories, topical medications are all considered to be usually self-administered by the patient.

C. Usually

For the purposes of applying this exclusion, the term "usually" means more than 50 percent of the time for all Medicare beneficiaries who use the drug. Therefore, if a drug is self-administered by more than 50 percent of Medicare beneficiaries, the drug is excluded from coverage and the contractor may not make any Medicare payment for it. In arriving at a single determination as to whether a drug is usually self-administered, contractors should make a separate determination for each indication for a drug as to whether that drug is usually self-administered.

After determining whether a drug is usually self-administered for each indication, contractors should determine the relative contribution of each indication to total use of the drug (i.e., weighted average) in order to make an overall determination as to whether the drug is usually self-administered. For example, if a drug has three indications, is not self-administered for the first indication, but is self administered for the second and third indications, and the first indication makes up 40 percent of total usage, the second indication makes up 30 percent of total usage, and the third indication makes up 30 percent of total usage, then the drug would be considered usually self-administered.

Reliable statistical information on the extent of self-administration by the patient may not always be available. Consequently, CMS offers the following guidance for each contractor's consideration in making this determination in the absence of such data:

1. Absent evidence to the contrary, presume that drugs delivered intravenously are not usually self-administered by the patient.

2. Absent evidence to the contrary, presume that drugs delivered by intramuscular injection are not usually self-administered by the patient. (Avonex, for example, is delivered by intramuscular injection, not usually self-administered by the patient.) The contractor may consider the depth and nature of the particular intramuscular injection in applying this presumption. In applying this presumption, contractors should examine the use of the particular drug and consider the following factors:

3. Absent evidence to the contrary, presume that drugs delivered by subcutaneous injection are self-administered by the patient. However, contractors should examine the use of the particular drug and consider the following factors:

A. Acute Condition - Is the condition for which the drug is used an acute condition? If so, it is less likely that a patient would self-administer the drug. If the condition were longer term, it would be more likely that the patient would self-administer the drug.

B. Frequency of Administration - How often is the injection given? For example, if the drug is administered once per month, it is less likely to be self-administered by the patient. However, if it is administered once or more per week, it is likely that the drug is self-administered by the patient.

In some instances, carriers may have provided payment for one or perhaps several doses of a drug that would otherwise not be paid for because the drug is usually self-administered. Carriers may have exercised this discretion for limited coverage, for example, during a brief time when the patient is being trained under the supervision of a physician in the proper technique for self-administration. Medicare will no longer pay for such doses. In addition, contractors may no longer pay for any drug when it is administered on an outpatient emergency basis, if the drug is excluded because it is usually self-administered by the patient.

D. Definition of Acute Condition

For the purposes of determining whether a drug is usually self-administered, an acute condition means a condition that begins over a short time period, is likely to be of short duration and/or the expected course of treatment is for a short, finite interval. A course of treatment consisting of scheduled injections lasting less than two weeks, regardless of frequency or route of administration, is considered acute. Evidence to support this may include Food and Drug administration (FDA) approval language, package inserts, drug compendia, and other information.

E. By the Patient

The term "by the patient" means Medicare beneficiaries as a collective whole. The carrier includes only the patients themselves and not other individuals (that is, spouses, friends, or other care-givers are not considered the patient). The determination is based on whether the drug is self-administered by the patient a majority of the time that the drug is used on an outpatient basis by Medicare beneficiaries for medically necessary indications. The carrier ignores all instances when the drug is administered on an inpatient basis.

The carrier makes this determination on a drug-by-drug basis, not on a beneficiary-by-beneficiary basis. In evaluating whether beneficiaries as a collective whole self-administer, individual beneficiaries who do not have the capacity to self-administer any drug due to a condition other than the condition for which they are taking the drug in question are not considered. For example, an individual afflicted with paraplegia or advanced dementia would not have the capacity to self-administer any injectable drug, so such individuals would not be included in the population upon which the determination for self-administration by the patient was based. Note that some individuals afflicted with a less severe stage of an otherwise debilitating condition would be included in the population upon which the determination for "self-administered by the patient" was based; for example, an early onset of dementia.

F. Evidentiary Criteria

Contractors are only required to consider the following types of evidence: peer reviewed medical literature, standards of medical practice, evidence-based practice guidelines, FDA approved label, and package inserts. Contractors may also consider other evidence submitted by interested individuals or groups subject to their judgment.

Contractors should also use these evidentiary criteria when reviewing requests for making a determination as to whether a drug is usually self-administered, and requests for reconsideration of a pending or published determination.

Please note that prior to the August 1, 2002, one of the principal factors used to determine whether a drug was subject to the self-administered exclusion was whether the FDA label contained instructions for self-administration. However, CMS notes that under the new standard, the fact that the FDA label includes instructions for self-administration is not, by itself, a determining factor that a drug is subject to this exclusion.

G. Provider Notice of Noncovered Drugs

Contractors must describe on their Web site the process they will use to determine whether a drug is usually self-administered and thus does not meet the "incident to" benefit category. Contractors must publish a list of the injectable drugs that are subject to the self-administered exclusion on their Web site, including the data and rationale that led to the determination. Contractors will report the workload associated with developing new coverage statements in CAFM 21208.

Contractors must provide notice 45 days prior to the date that these drugs will not be covered. During the 45-day time period, contractors will maintain existing medical review and payment procedures. After the 45-day notice, contractors may deny payment for the drugs subject to the notice.

Contractors must not develop local medical review policies (LMRPs) for this purpose because further elaboration to describe drugs that do not meet the 'incident to' and the 'not usually self-administered' provisions of the statute are unnecessary. Current LMRPs based solely on these provisions must be withdrawn. LMRPs that address the self-administered exclusion and other information may be reissued absent the self-administered drug exclusion material. Contractors will report this workload in CAFM 21206. However, contractors may continue to use and write

LMRPs to describe reasonable and necessary uses of drugs that are not usually self-administered.

H. Conferences Between Contractors

Contractors' Medical Directors may meet and discuss whether a drug is usually self-administered without reaching a formal consensus. Each contractor uses its discretion as to whether or not it will participate in such discussions. Each contractor must make its own individual determinations, except that fiscal intermediaries may, at their discretion, follow the determinations of the local carrier with respect to the self-administered exclusion.

I. Beneficiary Appeals

If a beneficiary's claim for a particular drug is denied because the drug is subject to the "self-administered drug" exclusion, the beneficiary may appeal the denial. Because it is a "benefit category" denial and not a denial based on medical necessity, an Advance Beneficiary Notice (ABN) is not required. A "benefit category" denial (i.e., a denial based on the fact that there is no benefit category under which the drug may be covered) does not trigger the financial liability protection provisions of Limitation On Liability (under §1879 of the Act). Therefore, physicians or providers may charge the beneficiary for an excluded drug.

J. Provider and Physician Appeals

A physician accepting assignment may appeal a denial under the provisions found in Chapter 29 of the Medicare Claims Processing Manual.

K. Reasonable and Necessary

Carriers and fiscal intermediaries will make the determination of reasonable and necessary with respect to the medical appropriateness of a drug to treat the patient's condition. Contractors will continue to make the determination of whether the intravenous or injection form of a drug is appropriate as opposed to the oral form. Contractors will also continue to make the determination as to whether a physician's office visit was reasonable and necessary. However, contractors should not make a determination of whether it was reasonable and necessary for the patient to choose to have his or her drug administered in the physician's office or outpatient hospital setting. That is, while a physician's office visit may not be reasonable and necessary in a specific situation, in such a case an injection service would be payable.

L. Reporting Requirements

Each carrier and intermediary must report to CMS, every September 1 and March 1, its complete list of injectable drugs that the contractor has determined are excluded when furnished incident to a physician's service on the basis that the drug is usually self-administered. The CMS anticipates that contractors will review injectable drugs on a rolling basis and publish their list of excluded drugs as it is developed. For example, contractors should not wait to publish this list until every drug has been reviewed. Contractors must send their exclusion list to the following e-mail address: drugdata@cms.hhs.gov a template that CMS will provide separately, consisting of the following data elements in order:

1. Carrier Name

2. State

3. Carrier ID#

4. HCPCS

5. Descriptor

6. Effective Date of Exclusion

7. End Date of Exclusion

8. Comments

Any exclusion list not provided in the CMS mandated format will be returned for correction.

To view the presently mandated CMS format for this report, open the file located at: http://cms.hhs.gov/manuals/pm_trans/AB02_139a.zip

Pub. 100-2, Chapter 15, Section 50.4

Reasonableness and Necessity
B3-2049.4

Pub. 100-2, Chapter 15, Section 50.4.2

Unlabeled Use of Drug
B3-2049.3

An unlabeled use of a drug is a use that is not included as an indication on the drug's label as approved by the FDA. FDA approved drugs used for indications other than what is indicated on the official label may be covered under Medicare if the carrier determines the use to be medically accepted, taking into consideration the major drug compendia, authoritative medical literature and/or accepted standards of medical practice. In the case of drugs used in an anti-cancer chemotherapeutic regimen, unlabeled uses are covered for a medically accepted indication as defined in §50.5.

These decisions are made by the contractor on a case-by-case basis.

Pub. 100-2, Chapter 15, Section 50.5

Administered Drugs and Biologicals
B3-2049.5

Medicare Part B does not cover drugs that are usually self-administered by the patient unless the statute provides for such coverage. The statute explicitly provides coverage, for blood clotting factors, drugs used in immunosuppressive therapy, erythropoietin for dialysis patients, certain oral anti-cancer drugs and anti-emetics used in certain situations.

Pub. 100-2, Chapter 15, Section 80.1

Clinical Laboratory Services

B3-2070.1

Section 1833 and 1861 of the Act provides for payment of clinical laboratory services under Medicare Part B. Clinical laboratory services involve the biological, microbiological, serological, chemical, immunohematological, hematological, biophysical, cytological, pathological, or other examination of materials derived from the human body for the diagnosis, prevention, or treatment of a disease or assessment of a medical condition. Laboratory services must meet all applicable requirements of the Clinical Laboratory Improvement Amendments of 1988 (CLIA), as set forth at 42 CFR part 493. Section 1862(a)(1)(A) of the Act provides that Medicare payment may not be made for services that are not reasonable and necessary. Clinical laboratory services must be ordered and used promptly by the physician who is treating the beneficiary as described in 42 CFR 410.32(a), or by a qualified nonphysician practitioner, as described in 42 CFR 410.32(a)(3).

See the Medicare Claims Processing Manual Chapter 16 for related claims processing instructions.

Pub. 100-2, Chapter 15, Section 100

Surgical Dressings, Splints, Casts, and Other Devices Used for Reductions of Fractures and Dislocations

B3-2079, A3-3110.3, HO-228.3,

Surgical dressings are limited to primary and secondary dressings required for the treatment of a wound caused by, or treated by, a surgical procedure that has been performed by a physician or other health care professional to the extent permissible under State law. In addition, surgical dressings required after debridement of a wound are also covered, irrespective of the type of debridement, as long as the debridement was reasonable and necessary and was performed by a health care professional acting within the scope of his/her legal authority when performing this function. Surgical dressings are covered for as long as they are medically necessary.

Primary dressings are therapeutic or protective coverings applied directly to wounds or lesions either on the skin or caused by an opening to the skin. Secondary dressing materials that serve a therapeutic or protective function and that are needed to secure a primary dressing are also covered. Items such as adhesive tape, roll gauze, bandages, and disposable compression material are examples of secondary dressings. Elastic stockings, support hose, foot coverings, leotards, knee supports, surgical leggings, gauntlets, and pressure garments for the arms and hands are examples of items that are not ordinarily covered as surgical dressings. Some items, such as transparent film, may be used as a primary or secondary dressing.

If a physician, certified nurse midwife, physician assistant, nurse practitioner, or clinical nurse specialist applies surgical dressings as part of a professional service that is billed to Medicare, the surgical dressings are considered incident to the professional services of the health care practitioner. (See §§60.1, 180, 190, 200, and 210.) When surgical dressings are not covered incident to the services of a health care practitioner and are obtained by the patient from a supplier (e.g., a drugstore, physician, or other health care practitioner that qualifies as a supplier) on an order from a physician or other health care professional authorized under State law or regulation to make such an order, the surgical dressings are covered separately under Part B.

Splints and casts, and other devices used for reductions of fractures and dislocations are covered under Part B of Medicare. This includes dental splints.

Pub. 100-2, Chapter 15, Section 110

General

B3-2100, A3-3113, HO-235, HHA-220

Expenses incurred by a beneficiary for the rental or purchases of durable medical equipment (DME) are reimbursable if the following three requirements are met:

• The equipment meets the definition of DME (§110.1);

• The equipment is necessary and reasonable for the treatment of the patient's illness or injury or to improve the functioning of his or her malformed body member (§110.1); and

• The equipment is used in the patient's home.

The decision whether to rent or purchase an item of equipment generally resides with the beneficiary, but the decision on how to pay rests with CMS. For some DME, program payment policy calls for lump sum payments and in others for periodic payment. Where covered DME is furnished to a beneficiary by a supplier of services other than a provider of services, the DMERC makes the reimbursement. If a provider of services furnishes the equipment, the intermediary makes the reimbursement. The payment method is identified in the annual fee schedule update furnished by CMS.

The CMS issues quarterly updates to a fee schedule file that contains rates by HCPCS code and also identifies the classification of the HCPCS code within the following categories:

Category Code	Definition
IN	Inexpensive and Other Routinely Purchased Items
FS	Frequently Serviced Items
CR	Capped Rental Items
OX	Oxygen and Oxygen Equipment
OS	Ostomy, Tracheostomy & Urological Items
SD	Surgical Dressings

Category Code	Definition
PO	Prosthetics & Orthotics
SU	Supplies
TE	Transcutaneous Electrical Nerve Stimulators

The DMERCs, carriers, and intermediaries, where appropriate, use the CMS files to determine payment rules. See the Medicare Claims Processing Manual, Chapter 20, "Durable Medical Equipment, Surgical Dressings and Casts, Orthotics and Artificial Limbs, and Prosthetic Devices," for a detailed description of payment rules for each classification.

Payment may also be made for repairs, maintenance, and delivery of equipment and for expendable and nonreusable items essential to the effective use of the equipment subject to the conditions in §110.2.

See the Medicare Benefit Policy Manual, Chapter 11, "End Stage Renal Disease," for hemodialysis equipment and supplies.

Pub. 100-2, Chapter 15, Section 110.1

Definition of Durable Medical Equipment

B3-2100.1, A3-3113.1, HO-235.1, HHA-220.1, B3-2100.2, A3-3113.2, HO-235.2, HHA-220.2

Durable medical equipment is equipment which:

• Can withstand repeated use;

• Is primarily and customarily used to serve a medical purpose;

• Generally is not useful to a person in the absence of an illness or injury; and

• Is appropriate for use in the home.

All requirements of the definition must be met before an item can be considered to be durable medical equipment.

The following describes the underlying policies for determining whether an item meets the definition of DME and may be covered.

A. Durability

An item is considered durable if it can withstand repeated use, i.e., the type of item that could normally be rented. Medical supplies of an expendable nature, such as incontinent pads, lambs wool pads, catheters, ace bandages, elastic stockings, surgical facemasks, irrigating kits, sheets, and bags are not considered "durable" within the meaning of the definition. There are other items that, although durable in nature, may fall into other coverage categories such as supplies, braces, prosthetic devices, artificial arms, legs, and eyes.

B. Medical Equipment

Medical equipment is equipment primarily and customarily used for medical purposes and is not generally useful in the absence of illness or injury. In most instances, no development will be needed to determine whether a specific item of equipment is medical in nature. However, some cases will require development to determine whether the item constitutes medical equipment. This development would include the advice of local medical organizations (hospitals, medical schools, medical societies) and specialists in the field of physical medicine and rehabilitation. If the equipment is new on the market, it may be necessary, prior to seeking professional advice, to obtain information from the supplier or manufacturer explaining the design, purpose, effectiveness and method of using the equipment in the home as well as the results of any tests or clinical studies that have been conducted.

1. Equipment Presumptively Medical

Items such as hospital beds, wheelchairs, hemodialysis equipment, iron lungs, respirators, intermittent positive pressure breathing machines, medical regulators, oxygen tents, crutches, canes, trapeze bars, walkers, inhalators, nebulizers, commodes, suction machines, and traction equipment presumptively constitute medical equipment. (Although hemodialysis equipment is covered as a prosthetic device (§120), it also meets the definition of DME, and reimbursement for the rental or purchase of such equipment for use in the beneficiary's home will be made only under the provisions for payment applicable to DME. See the Medicare Benefit Policy Manual, Chapter 11, "End Stage Renal Disease," §30.1, for coverage of home use of hemodialysis.) NOTE: There is a wide variety in types of respirators and suction machines. The DMERC's medical staff should determine whether the apparatus specified in the claim is appropriate for home use.

2. Equipment Presumptively Nonmedical

Equipment which is primarily and customarily used for a nonmedical purpose may not be considered "medical" equipment for which payment can be made under the medical insurance program. This is true even though the item has some remote medically related use. For example, in the case of a cardiac patient, an air conditioner might possibly be used to lower room temperature to reduce fluid loss in the patient and to restore an environment conducive to maintenance of the proper fluid balance. Nevertheless, because the primary and customary use of an air conditioner is a nonmedical one, the air conditioner cannot be deemed to be medical equipment for which payment can be made.

Other devices and equipment used for environmental control or to enhance the environmental setting in which the beneficiary is placed are not considered covered DME. These include, for example, room heaters, humidifiers, dehumidifiers, and electric air cleaners. Equipment which basically serves comfort or convenience functions or is primarily for the convenience of a person caring for the patient, such as elevators, stairway elevators, and posture chairs, do not constitute medical equipment. Similarly, physical fitness equipment (such as an exercycle), first-aid or precautionary-type equipment (such as preset portable oxygen units), self-help devices (such as safety grab bars), and training equipment (such as Braille training texts) are considered nonmedical in nature.

HCPCS — APPENDIXES

Appendix 4 — Pub 100 References

3. Special Exception Items

Specified items of equipment may be covered under certain conditions even though they do not meet the definition of DME because they are not primarily and customarily used to serve a medical purpose and/or are generally useful in the absence of illness or injury. These items would be covered when it is clearly established that they serve a therapeutic purpose in an individual case and would include:

a. Gel pads and pressure and water mattresses (which generally serve a preventive purpose) when prescribed for a patient who had bed sores or there is medical evidence indicating that they are highly susceptible to such ulceration; and

b. Heat lamps for a medical rather than a soothing or cosmetic purpose, e.g., where the need for heat therapy has been established.

In establishing medical necessity for the above items, the evidence must show that the item is included in the physician's course of treatment and a physician is supervising its use.

NOTE: The above items represent special exceptions and no extension of coverage to other items should be inferred

C. Necessary and Reasonable

Although an item may be classified as DME, it may not be covered in every instance. Coverage in a particular case is subject to the requirement that the equipment be necessary and reasonable for treatment of an illness or injury, or to improve the functioning of a malformed body member. These considerations will bar payment for equipment which cannot reasonably be expected to perform a therapeutic function in an individual case or will permit only partial therapeutic function in an individual case or will permit only partial payment when the type of equipment furnished substantially exceeds that required for the treatment of the illness or injury involved.

See the Medicare Claims Processing Manual, Chapter 1, "General Billing Requirements;" §60, regarding the rules for providing advance beneficiary notices (ABNs) that advise beneficiaries, before items or services actually are furnished, when Medicare is likely to deny payment for them. ABNs allow beneficiaries to make an informed consumer decision about receiving items or services for which they may have to pay out-of-pocket and to be more active participants in their own health care treatment decisions.

1. Necessity for the Equipment

Equipment is necessary when it can be expected to make a meaningful contribution to the treatment of the patient's illness or injury or to the improvement of his or her malformed body member. In most cases the physician's prescription for the equipment and other medical information available to the DMERC will be sufficient to establish that the equipment serves this purpose.

2. Reasonableness of the Equipment

Even though an item of DME may serve a useful medical purpose, the DMERC or intermediary must also consider to what extent, if any, it would be reasonable for the Medicare program to pay for the item prescribed. The following considerations should enter into the determination of reasonableness:

1. Would the expense of the item to the program be clearly disproportionate to the therapeutic benefits which could ordinarily be derived from use of the equipment?

2. Is the item substantially more costly than a medically appropriate and realistically feasible alternative pattern of care?

3. Does the item serve essentially the same purpose as equipment already available to the beneficiary?

3. Payment Consistent With What is Necessary and Reasonable

Where a claim is filed for equipment containing features of an aesthetic nature or features of a medical nature which are not required by the patient's condition or where there exists a reasonably feasible and medically appropriate alternative pattern of care which is less costly than the equipment furnished, the amount payable is based on the rate for the equipment or alternative treatment which meets the patient's medical needs.

The acceptance of an assignment binds the supplier-assignee to accept the payment for the medically required equipment or service as the full charge and the supplier-assignee cannot charge the beneficiary the differential attributable to the equipment actually furnished.

4. Establishing the Period of Medical Necessity

Generally, the period of time an item of durable medical equipment will be considered to be medically necessary is based on the physician's estimate of the time that his or her patient will need the equipment. See the Medicare Program Integrity Manual, Chapters 5 and 6, for medical review guidelines.

D. Definition of a Beneficiary's Home

For purposes of rental and purchase of DME a beneficiary's home may be his/her own dwelling, an apartment, a relative's home, a home for the aged, or some other type of institution. However, an institution may not be considered a beneficiary's home if it:

- Meets at least the basic requirement in the definition of a hospital, i.e., it is primarily engaged in providing by or under the supervision of physicians, to inpatients, diagnostic and therapeutic services for medical diagnosis, treatment, and care of injured, disabled, and sick persons, or rehabilitation services for the rehabilitation of injured, disabled, or sick persons; or

- Meets at least the basic requirement in the definition of a skilled nursing facility, i.e., it is primarily engaged in providing to inpatients skilled nursing care and related services for patients who require medical or nursing care, or rehabilitation services for the rehabilitation of injured, disabled, or sick persons.

Thus, if an individual is a patient in an institution or distinct part of an institution which provides the services described in the bullets above, the individual is not entitled to have separate Part B payment made for rental or purchase of DME. This is because such an institution may not be considered the individual's home. The same concept applies even if the patient resides in a bed or portion of the institution not certified for Medicare.

If the patient is at home for part of a month and, for part of the same month is in an institution that cannot qualify as his or her home, or is outside the U.S., monthly payments may be made for the entire month. Similarly, if DME is returned to the provider before the end of a payment month because the beneficiary died in that month or because the equipment became unnecessary in that month, payment may be made for the entire month.

Pub. 100-2, Chapter 15, Section 110.2

Repairs, Maintenance, Replacement, and Delivery

Under the circumstances specified below, payment may be made for repair, maintenance, and replacement of medically required DME, including equipment which had been in use before the user enrolled in Part B of the program. However, do not pay for repair, maintenance, or replacement of equipment in the frequent and substantial servicing or oxygen equipment payment categories. In addition, payments for repair and maintenance may not include payment for parts and labor covered under a manufacturer's or supplier's warranty.

A. Repairs

To repair means to fix or mend and to put the equipment back in good condition after damage or wear. Repairs to equipment which a beneficiary owns are covered when necessary to make the equipment serviceable. However, do not pay for repair of previously denied equipment or equipment in the frequent and substantial servicing or oxygen equipment payment categories. If the expense for repairs exceeds the estimated expense of purchasing or renting another item of equipment for the remaining period of medical need, no payment can be made for the amount of the excess. (See subsection C where claims for repairs suggest malicious damage or culpable neglect.)

Since renters of equipment recover from the rental charge the expenses they incur in maintaining in working order the equipment they rent out, separately itemized charges for repair of rented equipment are not covered. This includes items in the frequent and substantial servicing, oxygen equipment, capped rental, and inexpensive or routinely purchased payment categories which are being rented.

A new Certificate of Medical Necessity (CMN) and/or physician's order is not needed for repairs.

For replacement items, see Subsection C below.

B. Maintenance

Routine periodic servicing, such as testing, cleaning, regulating, and checking of the beneficiary's equipment, is not covered. The owner is expected to perform such routine maintenance rather than a retailer or some other person who charges the beneficiary. Normally, purchasers of DME are given operating manuals which describe the type of servicing an owner may perform to properly maintain the equipment. It is reasonable to expect that beneficiaries will perform this maintenance. Thus, hiring a third party to do such work is for the convenience of the beneficiary and is not covered. However, more extensive maintenance which, based on the manufacturers' recommendations, is to be performed by authorized technicians, is covered as repairs for medically necessary equipment which a beneficiary owns. This might include, for example, breaking down sealed components and performing tests which require specialized testing equipment not available to the beneficiary. Do not pay for maintenance of purchased items that require frequent and substantial servicing or oxygen equipment.

Since renters of equipment recover from the rental charge the expenses they incur in maintaining in working order the equipment they rent out, separately itemized charges for maintenance of rented equipment are generally not covered. Payment may not be made for maintenance of rented equipment other than the maintenance and servicing fee established for capped rental items. For capped rental items which have reached the 15-month rental cap, contractors pay claims for maintenance and servicing fees after 6 months have passed from the end of the final paid rental month or from the end of the period the item is no longer covered under the supplier's or manufacturer's warranty, whichever is later. See the Medicare Claims Processing Manual, Chapter 20, "Durable Medical Equipment, Prosthetics and Orthotics, and Supplies (DMEPOS)," for additional instruction and an example.

A new CMN and/or physician's order is not needed for covered maintenance.

C. Replacement

Replacement refers to the provision of an identical or nearly identical item. Situations involving the provision of a different item because of a change in medical condition are not addressed in this section.

Equipment which the beneficiary owns or is a capped rental item may be replaced in cases of loss or irreparable damage. Irreparable damage refers to a specific accident or to a natural disaster (e.g., fire, flood). A physician's order and/or new Certificate of Medical Necessity (CMN), when required, is needed to reaffirm the medical necessity of the item.

Irreparable wear refers to deterioration sustained from day-to-day usage over time and a specific event cannot be identified. Replacement of equipment due to irreparable wear takes into consideration the reasonable useful lifetime of the equipment. If the item of equipment has been in continuous use by the patient on either a rental or purchase basis for the equipment's useful lifetime, the beneficiary may elect to obtain a new piece of equipment. Replacement may be reimbursed when a new physician order and/or new CMN, when required, is needed to reaffirm the medical necessity of the item.

The reasonable useful lifetime of durable medical equipment is determined through program instructions. In the absence of program instructions, carriers may determine the reasonable useful lifetime of equipment, but in no case can it be less than 5 years. Computation of the useful lifetime is based on when the equipment is delivered to the beneficiary, not the age of the equipment. Replacement due to wear is not covered during the reasonable useful lifetime of the equipment. During the reasonable useful lifetime, Medicare does cover repair up to the cost of replacement (but not actual replacement) for medically necessary equipment owned by the beneficiary. (See subsection A.)

Charges for the replacement of oxygen equipment, items that require frequent and substantial servicing or inexpensive or routinely purchased items which are being rented are not covered.

Cases suggesting malicious damage, culpable neglect, or wrongful disposition of equipment should be investigated and denied where the DMERC determines that it is unreasonable to make program payment under the circumstances. DMERCs refer such cases to the program integrity specialist in the RO.

D. Delivery

Payment for delivery of DME whether rented or purchased is generally included in the fee schedule allowance for the item. See Pub. 100-04, Medicare Claims Processing Manual, Chapter 20, "Durable Medical Equipment, Prosthetics and Orthotics, and Supplies (DMEPOS)," for the rules that apply to making reimbursement for exceptional cases.

Pub. 100-2, Chapter 15, Section 110.3

Coverage of Supplies and Accessories

B3-2100.5, A3-3113.4, HO-235.4, HHA-220.5

Payment may be made for supplies, e.g., oxygen, that are necessary for the effective use of durable medical equipment. Such supplies include those drugs and biologicals which must be put directly into the equipment in order to achieve the therapeutic benefit of the durable medical equipment or to assure the proper functioning of the equipment, e.g., tumor chemotherapy agents used with an infusion pump or heparin used with a home dialysis system. However, the coverage of such drugs or biologicals does not preclude the need for a determination that the drug or biological itself is reasonable and necessary for treatment of the illness or injury or to improve the functioning of a malformed body member.

In the case of prescription drugs, other than oxygen, used in conjunction with durable medical equipment, prosthetic, orthotics, and supplies (DMEPOS) or prosthetic devices, the entity that dispenses the drug must furnish it directly to the patient for whom a prescription is written. The entity that dispenses the drugs must have a Medicare supplier number, must possess a current license to dispense prescription drugs in the State in which the drug is dispensed, and must bill and receive payment in its own name. A supplier that is not the entity that dispenses the drugs cannot purchase the drugs used in conjunction with DME for resale to the beneficiary. Reimbursement may be made for replacement of essential accessories such as hoses, tubes, mouthpieces, etc., for necessary DME, only if the beneficiary owns or is purchasing the equipment.

Pub. 100-2, Chapter 15, Section 120

Prosthetic Devices

B3-2130, A3-3110.4, HO-228.4, A3-3111, HO-229

A. General

Prosthetic devices (other than dental) which replace all or part of an internal body organ (including contiguous tissue), or replace all or part of the function of a permanently inoperative or malfunctioning internal body organ are covered when furnished on a physician's order. This does not require a determination that there is no possibility that the patient's condition may improve sometime in the future. If the medical record, including the judgment of the attending physician, indicates the condition is of long and indefinite duration, the test of permanence is considered met. (Such a device may also be covered under §60.I as a supply when furnished incident to a physician's service.)

Examples of prosthetic devices include artificial limbs, parenteral and enteral (PEN) nutrition, cardiac pacemakers, prosthetic lenses (see subsection B), breast prostheses (including a surgical brassiere) for postmastectomy patients, maxillofacial devices, and devices which replace all or part of the ear or nose. A urinary collection and retention system with or without a tube is a prosthetic device replacing bladder function in case of permanent urinary incontinence. The foley catheter is also considered a prosthetic device when ordered for a patient with permanent urinary incontinence. However, chucks, diapers, rubber sheets, etc., are supplies that are not covered under this provision. Although hemodialysis equipment is a prosthetic device, payment for the rental or purchase of such equipment in the home is made only for use under the provisions for payment applicable to durable medical equipment.

An exception is that if payment cannot be made on an inpatient's behalf under Part A, hemodialysis equipment, supplies, and services required by such patient could be covered under Part B as a prosthetic device, which replaces the function of a kidney. See the Medicare Benefit Policy Manual, Chapter 11, "End Stage Renal Disease," for payment for hemodialysis equipment used in the home. See the Medicare Benefit Policy Manual, Chapter 1, "Inpatient Hospital Services," §10, for additional instructions on hospitalization for renal dialysis.

NOTE: Medicare does not cover a prosthetic device dispensed to a patient prior to the time at which the patient undergoes the procedure that makes necessary the use of the device. For example, the carrier does not make a separate Part B payment for an intraocular lens (IOL) or pacemaker that a physician, during an office visit prior to the actual surgery, dispenses to the patient for his or her use. Dispensing a prosthetic device in this manner raises health and safety issues. Moreover, the need for the device cannot be clearly established until the procedure that makes its use possible is successfully performed. Therefore, dispensing a prosthetic device in this manner is not considered reasonable and necessary for the treatment of the patient's condition.

Colostomy (and other ostomy) bags and necessary accouterments required for attachment are covered as prosthetic devices. This coverage also includes irrigation and flushing equipment and other items and supplies directly related to ostomy care, whether the attachment of a bag is required.

Accessories and/or supplies which are used directly with an enteral or parenteral device to achieve the therapeutic benefit of the prosthesis or to assure the proper functioning of the device

may also be covered under the prosthetic device benefit subject to the additional guidelines in the Medicare National Coverage Determinations Manual.

Covered items include catheters, filters, extension tubing, infusion bottles, pumps (either food or infusion), intravenous (I.V.) pole, needles, syringes, dressings, tape, Heparin Sodium (parenteral only), volumetric monitors (parenteral only), and parenteral and enteral nutrient solutions. Baby food and other regular grocery products that can be blenderized and used with the enteral system are not covered. Note that some of these items, e.g., a food pump and an I.V. pole, qualify as DME. Although coverage of the enteral and parenteral nutritional therapy systems is provided on the basis of the prosthetic device benefit, the payment rules relating to lump sum or monthly payment for DME apply to such items.

The coverage of prosthetic devices includes replacement of and repairs to such devices as explained in subsection D.

Finally, the Benefits Improvement and Protection Act of 2000 amended §1834(h)(1) of the Act by adding a provision (1834 (h)(1)(G)(i)) that requires Medicare payment to be made for the replacement of prosthetic devices which are artificial limbs, or for the replacement of any part of such devices, without regard to continuous use or useful lifetime restrictions if an ordering physician determines that the replacement device, or replacement part of such a device, is necessary.

Payment may be made for the replacement of a prosthetic device that is an artificial limb, or replacement part of a device if the ordering physician determines that the replacement device or part is necessary because of any of the following:

1. A change in the physiological condition of the patient;

2. An irreparable change in the condition of the device, or in a part of the device, or

3. The condition of the device, or the part of the device, requires repairs and the cost of such repairs would be more than 60 percent of the cost of a replacement device, or, as the case may be, of the part being replaced.

This provision is effective for items replaced on or after April 1, 2001. It supersedes any rule that that provided a 5-year or other replacement rule with regard to prosthetic devices.

B. Prosthetic Lenses

The term "internal body organ" includes the lens of an eye. Prostheses replacing the lens of an eye include post-surgical lenses customarily used during convalescence from eye surgery in which the lens of the eye was removed. In addition, permanent lenses are also covered when required by an individual lacking the organic lens of the eye because of surgical removal or congenital absence. Prosthetic lenses obtained on or after the beneficiary's date of entitlement to supplementary medical insurance benefits may be covered even though the surgical removal of the crystalline lens occurred before entitlement.

1. Prosthetic Cataract Lenses

One of the following prosthetic lenses or combinations of prosthetic lenses furnished by a physician (see §30.4 for coverage of prosthetic lenses prescribed by a doctor of optometry) may be covered when determined to be reasonable and necessary to restore essentially the vision provided by the crystalline lens of the eye:

• Prosthetic bifocal lenses in frames;

• Prosthetic lenses in frames for far vision, and prosthetic lenses in frames for near vision; or

• When a prosthetic contact lens(es) for far vision is prescribed (including cases of binocular and monocular aphakia), make payment for the contact lens(es) and prosthetic lenses in frames for near vision to be worn at the same time as the contact lens(es), and prosthetic lenses in frames to be worn when the contacts have been removed.

Lenses which have ultraviolet absorbing or reflecting properties may be covered, in lieu of payment for regular (untinted) lenses, if it has been determined that such lenses are medically reasonable and necessary for the individual patient.

Medicare does not cover cataract sunglasses obtained in addition to the regular (untinted) prosthetic lenses since the sunglasses duplicate the restoration of vision function performed by the regular prosthetic lenses.

2. Payment for Intraocular Lenses (IOLs) Furnished in Ambulatory Surgical Centers (ASCs)

Effective for services furnished on or after March 12, 1990, payment for intraocular lenses (IOLs) inserted during or subsequent to cataract surgery in a Medicare certified ASC is included with the payment for facility services that are furnished in connection with the covered surgery.

Refer to the Medicare Claims Processing Manual, Chapter 14, "Ambulatory Surgical Centers," for more information.

3. Limitation on Coverage of Conventional Lenses

One pair of conventional eyeglasses or conventional contact lenses furnished after each cataract surgery with insertion of an IOL is covered.

C. Dentures

Dentures are excluded from coverage. However, when a denture or a portion of the denture is an integral part (built-in) of a covered prosthesis (e.g., an obturator to fill an opening in the palate), it is covered as part of that prosthesis.

D. Supplies, Repairs, Adjustments, and Replacement

Supplies are covered that are necessary for the effective use of a prosthetic device (e.g., the batteries needed to operate an artificial larynx). Adjustment of prosthetic devices required by wear or by a change in the patient's condition is covered when ordered by a physician. General provisions relating to the repair and replacement of durable medical equipment in §110.2 for the repair and replacement of prosthetic devices are applicable. (See the Medicare Benefit Policy Manual, Chapter 16, "General Exclusions from Coverage," §40.4, for payment for devices replaced under a warranty.) Replacement of conventional eyeglasses or contact lenses furnished in accordance with §120.B.3 is not covered.

Necessary supplies, adjustments, repairs, and replacements are covered even when the device had been in use before the user enrolled in Part B of the program, so long as the device continues to be medically required.

Pub. 100-2, Chapter 15, Section 130

Leg, Arm, Back, and Neck Braces, Trusses, and Artificial Legs, Arms, and Eyes

B3-2133, A3-3110.5, HO-228.5, AB-01-06 dated 1/18/01

These appliances are covered under Part B when furnished incident to physicians' services or on a physician's order. A brace includes rigid and semi-rigid devices which are used for the purpose of supporting a weak or deformed body member or restricting or eliminating motion in a diseased or injured part of the body. Elastic stockings, garter belts, and similar devices do not come within the scope of the definition of a brace. Back braces include, but are not limited to, special corsets, e.g., sacroiliac, sacrolumbar, dorsolumbar corsets, and belts. A terminal device (e.g., hand or hook) is covered under this provision whether an artificial limb is required by the patient. Stump stockings and harnesses (including replacements) are also covered when these appliances are essential to the effective use of the artificial limb.

Adjustments to an artificial limb or other appliance required by wear or by a change in the patient's condition are covered when ordered by a physician.

Adjustments, repairs and replacements are covered even when the item had been in use before the user enrolled in Part B of the program so long as the device continues to be medically required.

Pub. 100-2, Chapter 15, Section 140

Therapeutic Shoes for Individuals with Diabetes

B3-2134

Coverage of therapeutic shoes (depth or custom-molded) along with inserts for individuals with diabetes is available as of May 1, 1993. These diabetic shoes are covered if the requirements as specified in this section concerning certification and prescription are fulfilled. In addition, this benefit provides for a pair of diabetic shoes even if only one foot suffers from diabetic foot disease. Each shoe is equally equipped so that the affected limb, as well as the remaining limb, is protected. Claims for therapeutic shoes for diabetics are processed by the Durable Medical Equipment Regional Carriers (DMERCs).

Therapeutic shoes for diabetics are not DME and are not considered DME nor orthotics, but a separate category of coverage under Medicare Part B. (See §1861(s)(12) and §1833(o) of the Act.)

A. Definitions

The following items may be covered under the diabetic shoe benefit:

1. Custom-Molded Shoes

Custom-molded shoes are shoes that:

• Are constructed over a positive model of the patient's foot;

• Are made from leather or other suitable material of equal quality;

• Have removable inserts that can be altered or replaced as the patient's condition warrants; and

• Have some form of shoe closure.

2. Depth Shoes

Depth shoes are shoes that:

• Have a full length, heel-to-toe filler that, when removed, provides a minimum of 3/16 inch of additional depth used to accommodate custom-molded or customized inserts;

• Are made from leather or other suitable material of equal quality;

• Have some form of shoe closure; and

• Are available in full and half sizes with a minimum of three widths so that the sole is graded to the size and width of the upper portions of the shoes according to the American standard last sizing schedule or its equivalent. (The American standard last sizing schedule is the numerical shoe sizing system used for shoes sold in the United States.)

3. Inserts

Inserts are total contact, multiple density, removable inlays that are directly molded to the patient's foot or a model of the patient's foot and that are made of a suitable material with regard to the patient's condition.

B. Coverage

1. Limitations

For each individual, coverage of the footwear and inserts is limited to one of the following within one calendar year:

• No more than one pair of custom-molded shoes (including inserts provided with such shoes) and two additional pairs of inserts; or

• No more than one pair of depth shoes and three pairs of inserts (not including the noncustomized removable inserts provided with such shoes).

2. Coverage of Diabetic Shoes and Brace

Orthopedic shoes, as stated in the Medicare Claims Processing Manual, Chapter 20, "Durable Medical Equipment, Surgical Dressings and Casts, Orthotics and Artificial Limbs, and Prosthetic

Devices," generally are not covered. This exclusion does not apply to orthopedic shoes that are an integral part of a leg brace. In situations in which an individual qualifies for both diabetic shoes and a leg brace, these items are covered separately. Thus, the diabetic shoes may be covered if the requirements for this section are met, while the brace may be covered if the requirements of §130 are met.

3. Substitution of Modifications for Inserts

An individual may substitute modification(s) of custom-molded or depth shoes instead of obtaining a pair(s) of inserts in any combination. Payment for the modification(s) may not exceed the limit set for the inserts for which the individual is entitled. The following is a list of the most common shoe modifications available, but it is not meant as an exhaustive list of the modifications available for diabetic shoes:

• Rigid Rocker Bottoms - These are exterior elevations with apex positions for 51 percent to 75 percent distance measured from the back end of the heel. The apex is a narrowed or pointed end of an anatomical structure. The apex

must be positioned behind the metatarsal heads and tapered off sharply to the front tip of the sole. Apex height helps to eliminate pressure at the metatarsal heads. Rigidity is ensured by the steel in the shoe. The heel of the shoe tapers off in the back in order to cause the heel to strike in the middle of the heel;

• Roller Bottoms (Sole or Bar) - These are the same as rocker bottoms, but the heel is tapered from the apex to the front tip of the sole;

• Metatarsal Bars - An exterior bar is placed behind the metatarsal heads in order to remove pressure from the metatarsal heads. The bars are of various shapes, heights, and construction depending on the exact purpose;

• Wedges (Posting) - Wedges are either of hind foot, fore foot, or both and may be in the middle or to the side. The function is to shift or transfer weight bearing upon standing or during ambulation to the opposite side for added support, stabilization, equalized weight distribution, or balance; and

• Offset Heels - This is a heel flanged at its base either in the middle, to the side, or a combination, that is then extended upward to the shoe in order to stabilize extreme positions of the hind foot.

Other modifications to diabetic shoes include, but are not limited to flared heels, Velcro closures, and inserts for missing toes.

4. Separate Inserts

Inserts may be covered and dispensed independently of diabetic shoes if the supplier of the shoes verifies in writing that the patient has appropriate footwear into which the insert can be placed. This footwear must meet the definitions found above for depth shoes and custom-molded shoes.

C. Certification

The need for diabetic shoes must be certified by a physician who is a doctor of medicine or a doctor of osteopathy and who is responsible for diagnosing and treating the patient's diabetic systemic condition through a comprehensive plan of care. This managing physician must:

• Document in the patient's medical record that the patient has diabetes;

• Certify that the patient is being treated under a comprehensive plan of care for diabetes, and that the patient needs diabetic shoes; and

• Document in the patient's record that the patient has one or more of the following conditions:

o Peripheral neuropathy with evidence of callus formation;

o History of pre-ulcerative calluses;

o History of previous ulceration;

o Foot deformity;

o Previous amputation of the foot or part of the foot; or

o Poor circulation.

D. Prescription

Following certification by the physician managing the patient's systemic diabetic condition, a podiatrist or other qualified physician who is knowledgeable in the fitting of diabetic shoes and inserts may prescribe the particular type of footwear necessary.

E. Furnishing Footwear

The footwear must be fitted and furnished by a podiatrist or other qualified individual such as a pedorthist, an orthotist, or a prosthetist. The certifying physician may not furnish the diabetic shoes unless the certifying physician is the only qualified individual in the area. It is left to the discretion of each carrier to determine the meaning of "in the area."

Pub. 100-2, Chapter 15, Section 150

Dental Services

B3-2136

As indicated under the general exclusions from coverage, items and services in connection with the care, treatment, filling, removal, or replacement of teeth or structures directly supporting the teeth are not covered. "Structures directly supporting the teeth" means the periodontium, which includes the gingivae, dentogingival junction, periodontal membrane, cementum of the teeth, and alveolar process.

In addition to the following, see Pub 100-01, the Medicare General Information, Eligibility, and Entitlement Manual, Chapter 5, Definitions and Pub 3, the Medicare National Coverage Determinations Manual for specific services which may be covered when furnished by a dentist. If an otherwise noncovered procedure or service is performed by a dentist as incident to and as an integral part of a covered procedure or service performed by the dentist, the total service performed by the dentist on such an occasion is covered.

EXAMPLE 1:

The reconstruction of a ridge performed primarily to prepare the mouth for dentures is a noncovered procedure. However, when the reconstruction of a ridge is performed as a result of and at the same time as the surgical removal of a tumor (for other than dental purposes), the totality of surgical procedures is a covered service.

EXAMPLE 2:

Medicare makes payment for the wiring of teeth when this is done in connection with the reduction of a jaw fracture.

The extraction of teeth to prepare the jaw for radiation treatment of neoplastic disease is also covered. This is an exception to the requirement that to be covered, a noncovered procedure or service performed by a dentist must be an incident to and an integral part of a covered procedure or service performed by the dentist. Ordinarily, the dentist extracts the patient's teeth, but another physician, e.g., a radiologist, administers the radiation treatments.

When an excluded service is the primary procedure involved, it is not covered, regardless of its complexity or difficulty. For example, the extraction of an impacted tooth is not covered. Similarly, an alveoplasty (the surgical improvement of the shape and condition of the alveolar process) and a frenectomy are excluded from coverage when either of these procedures is performed in connection with an excluded service, e.g., the preparation of the mouth for dentures. In a like manner, the removal of a torus palatinus (a bony protuberance of the hard palate) may be a covered service. However, with rare exception, this surgery is performed in connection with an excluded service, i.e., the preparation of the mouth for dentures. Under such circumstances, Medicare does not pay for this procedure.

Dental splints used to treat a dental condition are excluded from coverage under 1862(a)(12) of the Act. On the other hand, if the treatment is determined to be a covered medical condition (i.e., dislocated upper/lower jaw joints), then the splint can be covered.

Whether such services as the administration of anesthesia, diagnostic x-rays, and other related procedures are covered depends upon whether the primary procedure being performed by the dentist is itself covered. Thus, an x-ray taken in connection with the reduction of a fracture of the jaw or facial bone is covered. However, a single x-ray or x-ray survey taken in connection with the care or treatment of teeth or the periodontium is not covered.

Medicare makes payment for a covered dental procedure no matter where the service is performed. The hospitalization or nonhospitalization of a patient has no direct bearing on the coverage or exclusion of a given dental procedure.

Payment may also be made for services and supplies furnished incident to covered dental services. For example, the services of a dental technician or nurse who is under the direct supervision of the dentist or physician are covered if the services are included in the dentist's or physician's bill.

Pub. 100-2, Chapter 15, Section 230

Language Pathology

Pub. 100-2, Chapter 15, Section 280.1

Glaucoma Screening

A. Conditions of Coverage

The regulations implementing the Benefits Improvements and Protection Act of 2000, §102, provide for annual coverage for glaucoma screening for beneficiaries in the following high risk categories:

- Individuals with diabetes mellitus;

- Individuals with a family history of glaucoma; or

- African Americans age 50 and over.

In addition, beginning with dates of service on or after January 1, 2006, 42 CFR 410.23(a)(2), revised, the definition of an eligible beneficiary in a high-risk category is expanded to include:

- Hispanic-Americans age 65 and over.

Medicare will pay for glaucoma screening examinations where they are furnished by or under the direct supervision in the office setting of an ophthalmologist or optometrist, who is legally authorized to perform the services under State law.

Screening for glaucoma is defined to include:

- A dilated eye examination with an intraocular pressure measurement; and

- A direct ophthalmoscopy examination, or a slit-lamp biomicroscopic examination.

Payment may be made for a glaucoma screening examination that is performed on an eligible beneficiary after at least 11 months have passed following the month in which the last covered glaucoma screening examination was performed.

The following HCPCS codes apply for glaucoma screening:

G0117 - Glaucoma screening for high-risk patients furnished by an optometrist or ophthalmologist; and

G0118 - Glaucoma screening for high-risk patients furnished under the direct supervision of an optometrist or ophthalmologist.

The type of service for the above G codes is: TOS Q.

For providers who bill intermediaries, applicable types of bill for screening glaucoma services are 13X, 22X, 23X, 71X, 73X, 75X, and 85X. The following revenue codes should be reported when billing for screening glaucoma services:

- Comprehensive outpatient rehabilitation facilities (CORFs), critical access hospitals (CAHs), skilled nursing facilities (SNFs), independent and provider-based RHCs and free standing and provider-based FQHCs bill for this service under revenue code 770. CAHs electing the optional method of payment for outpatient services report this service under revenue codes 96X, 97X, or 98X.

- Hospital outpatient departments bill for this service under any valid/appropriate revenue code. They are not required to report revenue code 770.

B. Calculating the Frequency

Once a beneficiary has received a covered glaucoma screening procedure, the beneficiary may receive another procedure after 11 full months have passed. To determine the 11-month period, start the count beginning with the month after the month in which the previous covered screening procedure was performed.

C. Diagnosis Coding Requirements

Providers bill glaucoma screening using screening ("V") code V80.1 (Special Screening for Neurological, Eye, and Ear Diseases, Glaucoma). Claims submitted without a screening diagnosis code may be returned to the provider as unprocessable.

D. Payment Methodology

1. Carriers

Contractors pay for glaucoma screening based on the Medicare physician fee schedule. Deductible and coinsurance apply. Claims from physicians or other providers where assignment was not taken are subject to the Medicare limiting charge (refer to the Medicare Claims Processing Manual, Chapter 12,

"Physician/Non-physician Practitioners," for more information about the Medicare limiting charge).

2. Intermediaries

Payment is made for the facility expense as follows:

- Independent and provider-based RHC/free standing and provider-based FQHC - payment is made under the all inclusive rate for the screening glaucoma service based on the visit furnished to the RHC/FQHC patient;

- CAH - payment is made on a reasonable cost basis unless the CAH has elected the optional method of payment for outpatient services in which case, procedures outlined in the Medicare Claims Processing Manual, Chapter 3, §30.1.1, should be followed;

- CORF - payment is made under the Medicare physician fee schedule;

- Hospital outpatient department - payment is made under outpatient prospective payment system (OPPS);

- Hospital inpatient Part B - payment is made under OPPS;

- SNF outpatient - payment is made under the Medicare physician fee schedule (MPFS); and

- SNF inpatient Part B - payment is made under MPFS.

Deductible and coinsurance apply.

E. Special Billing Instructions for RHCs and FQHCs

Screening glaucoma services are considered RHC/FQHC services. RHCs and FQHCs bill the contractor under bill type 71X or 73X along with revenue code 770 and HCPCS codes G0117 or G0118 and RHC/FQHC revenue code 520 or 521 to report the related visit. Reporting of revenue code 770 and HCPCS codes G0117 and G0118 in addition to revenue code 520 or 521 is required for this service in order for CWF to perform frequency editing.

Payment should not be made for a screening glaucoma service unless the claim also contains a visit code for the service. Therefore, the contractor installs an edit in its system to assure payment is not made for revenue code 770 unless the claim also contains a visit revenue code (520 or 521).

Pub. 100-2, Chapter 15, Section 290

Foot Care

A3-3158, B3-2323, HO-260.9, B3-4120.1

A. Treatment of Subluxation of Foot

Subluxations of the foot are defined as partial dislocations or displacements of joint surfaces, tendons ligaments, or muscles of the foot. Surgical or nonsurgical treatments undertaken for the sole purpose of correcting a subluxated structure in the foot as an isolated entity are not covered.

However, medical or surgical treatment of subluxation of the ankle joint (talo-crural joint) is covered. In addition, reasonable and necessary medical or surgical services, diagnosis, or treatment for medical conditions that have resulted from or are associated with partial displacement of structures is covered. For example, if a patient has osteoarthritis that has resulted in a partial displacement of joints in the foot, and the primary treatment is for the osteoarthritis, coverage is provided.

B. Exclusions from Coverage

The following foot care services are generally excluded from coverage under both Part A and Part B. (See §290.F and §290.G for instructions on applying foot care exclusions.)

1. Treatment of Flat Foot

The term "flat foot" is defined as a condition in which one or more arches of the foot have flattened out. Services or devices directed toward the care or correction of such conditions, including the prescription of supportive devices, are not covered.

2. Routine Foot Care

Except as provided above, routine foot care is excluded from coverage. Services that normally are considered routine and not covered by Medicare include the following:

• The cutting or removal of corns and calluses;

• The trimming, cutting, clipping, or debriding of nails; and

• Other hygienic and preventive maintenance care, such as cleaning and soaking the feet, the use of skin creams to maintain skin tone of either ambulatory or bedfast patients, and any other service performed in the absence of localized illness, injury, or symptoms involving the foot.

3. Supportive Devices for Feet

Orthopedic shoes and other supportive devices for the feet generally are not covered. However, this exclusion does not apply to such a shoe if it is an integral part of a leg brace, and its expense is included as part of the cost of the brace. Also, this exclusion does not apply to therapeutic shoes furnished to diabetics.

C. Exceptions to Routine Foot Care Exclusion

1. Necessary and Integral Part of Otherwise Covered Services

In certain circumstances, services ordinarily considered to be routine may be covered if they are performed as a necessary and integral part of otherwise covered services, such as diagnosis and treatment of ulcers, wounds, or infections.

2. Treatment of Warts on Foot

The treatment of warts (including plantar warts) on the foot is covered to the same extent as services provided for the treatment of warts located elsewhere on the body.

3. Presence of Systemic Condition

The presence of a systemic condition such as metabolic, neurologic, or peripheral vascular disease may require scrupulous foot care by a professional that in the absence of such condition(s) would be considered routine (and, therefore, excluded from coverage). Accordingly, foot care that would otherwise be considered routine may be covered when systemic condition(s) result in severe circulatory embarrassment or areas of diminished sensation in the individual's legs or feet. (See subsection A.)

In these instances, certain foot care procedures that otherwise are considered routine (e.g., cutting or removing corns and calluses, or trimming, cutting, clipping, or debriding nails) may pose a hazard when performed by a nonprofessional person on patients with such systemic conditions. (See §290.G for procedural instructions.)

4. Mycotic Nails

In the absence of a systemic condition, treatment of mycotic nails may be covered.

The treatment of mycotic nails for an ambulatory patient is covered only when the physician attending the patient's mycotic condition documents that (1) there is clinical evidence of mycosis of the toenail, and (2) the patient has marked limitation of ambulation, pain, or secondary infection resulting from the thickening and dystrophy of the infected toenail plate.

The treatment of mycotic nails for a nonambulatory patient is covered only when the physician attending the patient's mycotic condition documents that (1) there is clinical evidence of mycosis of the toenail, and (2) the patient suffers from pain or secondary infection resulting from the thickening and dystrophy of the infected toenail plate.

For the purpose of these requirements, documentation means any written information that is required by the carrier in order for services to be covered. Thus, the information submitted with claims must be substantiated by information found in the patient's medical record. Any information, including that contained in a form letter, used for documentation purposes is subject to carrier verification in order to ensure that the information adequately justifies coverage of the treatment of mycotic nails.

D. Systemic Conditions That Might Justify Coverage

Although not intended as a comprehensive list, the following metabolic, neurologic, and peripheral vascular diseases (with synonyms in parentheses) most commonly represent the underlying conditions that might justify coverage for routine foot care.

Diabetes mellitus *

Arteriosclerosis obliterans (A.S.O., arteriosclerosis of the extremities, occlusive peripheral arteriosclerosis)

Buerger's disease (thromboangiitis obliterans)

Chronic thrombophlebitis *

Peripheral neuropathies involving the feet -

Associated with malnutrition and vitamin deficiency *

• Malnutrition (general, pellagra)

• Alcoholism

• Malabsorption (celiac disease, tropical sprue)

• Pernicious anemia

Associated with carcinoma *

Associated with diabetes mellitus *

Associated with drugs and toxins *

Associated with multiple sclerosis *

Associated with uremia (chronic renal disease) *

Associated with traumatic injury

Associated with leprosy or neurosyphilis

Associated with hereditary disorders

• Hereditary sensory radicular neuropathy

• Angiokeratoma corporis diffusum (Fabry's)

• Amyloid neuropathy

When the patient's condition is one of those designated by an asterisk (*), routine procedures are covered only if the patient is under the active care of a doctor of medicine or osteopathy who documents the condition.

E. Supportive Devices for Feet

Orthopedic shoes and other supportive devices for the feet generally are not covered. However, this exclusion does not apply to such a shoe if it is an integral part of a leg brace, and its expense is included as part of the cost of the brace. Also, this exclusion does not apply to therapeutic shoes furnished to diabetics.

F. Presumption of Coverage

In evaluating whether the routine services can be reimbursed, a presumption of coverage may be made where the evidence available discloses certain physical and/or clinical

findings consistent with the diagnosis and indicative of severe peripheral involvement. For purposes of applying this presumption the following findings are pertinent:

Class A Findings

Nontraumatic amputation of foot or integral skeletal portion thereof.

Class B Findings

Absent posterior tibial pulse;

Advanced trophic changes as: hair growth (decrease or absence) nail changes (thickening) pigmentary changes (discoloration) skin texture (thin, shiny) skin color (rubor or redness) (Three required); and

Absent dorsalis pedis pulse.

Class C Findings

Claudication;

Temperature changes (e.g., cold feet);

Edema;

Paresthesias (abnormal spontaneous sensations in the feet); and

Burning.

The presumption of coverage may be applied when the physician rendering the routine foot care has identified:

1. A Class A finding;

2. Two of the Class B findings; or

3. One Class B and two Class C findings.

Cases evidencing findings falling short of these alternatives may involve podiatric treatment that may constitute covered care and should be reviewed by the intermediary's medical staff and developed as necessary.

For purposes of applying the coverage presumption where the routine services have been rendered by a podiatrist, the contractor may deem the active care requirement met if the claim or other evidence available discloses that the patient has seen an M.D. or D.O. for treatment and/or evaluation of the complicating disease process during the 6-month period prior to the rendition of the routine-type services. The intermediary may also accept the podiatrist's statement that the diagnosing and treating M.D. or D.O. also concurs with the podiatrist's findings as to the severity of the peripheral involvement indicated.

Services ordinarily considered routine might also be covered if they are performed as a necessary and integral part of otherwise covered services, such as diagnosis and treatment of diabetic ulcers, wounds, and infections.

G. Application of Foot Care Exclusions to Physician's Services

The exclusion of foot care is determined by the nature of the service. Thus, payment for an excluded service should be denied whether performed by a podiatrist, osteopath, or a doctor of medicine, and without regard to the difficulty or complexity of the procedure.

When an itemized bill shows both covered services and noncovered services not integrally related to the covered service, the portion of charges attributable to the noncovered services should be denied. (For example, if an itemized bill shows surgery for an ingrown toenail and also removal of calluses not necessary for the performance of toe surgery, any additional charge attributable to removal of the calluses should be denied.)

In reviewing claims involving foot care, the carrier should be alert to the following exceptional situations:

1. Payment may be made for incidental noncovered services performed as a necessary and integral part of, and secondary to, a covered procedure. For example, if trimming of toenails is required for application of a cast to a fractured foot, the carrier need not allocate and deny a portion of the charge for the trimming of the nails. However, a separately itemized charge for such excluded service should be disallowed. When the primary procedure is covered the administration of anesthesia necessary for the performance of such procedure is also covered.

2. Payment may be made for initial diagnostic services performed in connection with a specific symptom or complaint if it seems likely that its treatment would be covered even though the resulting diagnosis may be one requiring only noncovered care.

The name of the M.D. or D.O. who diagnosed the complicating condition must be submitted with the claim. In those cases, where active care is required, the approximate date the beneficiary was last seen by such physician must also be indicated.

NOTE: Section 939 of P.L. 96-499 removed "warts" from the routine foot care exclusion effective July 1, 1981.

Relatively few claims for routine-type care are anticipated considering the severity of conditions contemplated as the basis for this exception. Claims for this type of foot care should not be paid in the absence of convincing evidence that nonprofessional performance of the service would have been hazardous for the beneficiary because of an underlying systemic disease. The mere statement of a diagnosis such as those mentioned in §D above does not of itself indicate the severity of the condition. Where development is indicated to verify diagnosis and/or severity the carrier should follow existing claims processing practices which may include review of carrier's history and medical consultation as well as physician contacts.

The rules in §290.F concerning presumption of coverage also apply.

Codes and policies for routine foot care and supportive devices for the feet are not exclusively for the use of podiatrists. These codes must be used to report foot care services regardless of the specialty of the physician who furnishes the services. Carriers must instruct physicians to use the most appropriate code available when billing for routine foot care.

Pub. 100-2, Chapter 16, Section 10

General Exclusions From Coverage
A3-3150, HO-260, HHA-232, B3-2300

No payment can be made under either the hospital insurance or supplementary medical insurance program for certain items and services, when the following conditions exist:

- Not reasonable and necessary (§20);
- No legal obligation to pay for or provide (§40);
- Paid for by a governmental entity (§50);
- Not provided within United States (§60);
- Resulting from war (§70);
- Personal comfort (§80);
- Routine services and appliances (§90);
- Custodial care (§110);
- Cosmetic surgery (§120);
- Charges by immediate relatives or members of household (§130);
- Dental services (§140);
- Paid or expected to be paid under workers' compensation (§150);
- Nonphysician services provided to a hospital inpatient that were not provided directly or arranged for by the hospital (§170);
- Services Related to and Required as a Result of Services Which are not Covered Under Medicare (§180);
- Excluded foot care services and supportive devices for feet (§30); or
- Excluded investigational devices (See Chapter 14, §30).

Pub. 100-2, Chapter 16, Section 20

Services Not Reasonable and Necessary
A3-3151, HO-260.1, B3-2303, AB-00-52 - 6/00

Items and services which are not reasonable and necessary for the diagnosis or treatment of illness or injury or to improve the functioning of a malformed body member are not covered, e.g., payment cannot be made for the rental of a special hospital bed to be used by the patient in their home unless it was a reasonable and necessary part of the patient's treatment. See also §80.

A health care item or service for the purpose of causing, or assisting to cause, the death of any individual (assisted suicide) is not covered. This prohibition does not apply to the provision of an item or service for the purpose of alleviating pain or discomfort, even if such use may increase the risk of death, so long as the item or service is not furnished for the specific purpose of causing death.

Pub. 100-2, Chapter 16, Section 90

Routine Services and Appliances
A3-3157, HO-260.7, B3-2320, R-1797A3 - 5/00

Routine physical checkups; eyeglasses, contact lenses, and eye examinations for the purpose of prescribing, fitting, or changing eyeglasses; eye refractions by whatever practitioner and for whatever purpose performed; hearing aids and examinations for hearing aids; and immunizations are not covered.

The routine physical checkup exclusion applies to (a) examinations performed without relationship to treatment or diagnosis for a specific illness, symptom, complaint, or injury; and (b) examinations required by third parties such as insurance companies, business establishments, or Government agencies.

If the claim is for a diagnostic test or examination performed solely for the purpose of establishing a claim under title IV of Public Law 91-173, "Black Lung Benefits," the service is not covered under Medicare and the claimant should be advised to contact their Social Security office regarding the filing of a claim for reimbursement under the "Black Lung" program.

The exclusions apply to eyeglasses or contact lenses, and eye examinations for the purpose of prescribing, fitting, or changing eyeglasses or contact lenses for refractive errors. The exclusions do not apply to physicians' services (and services incident to a physicians' service) performed in conjunction with an eye disease, as for example, glaucoma or cataracts, or to post-surgical prosthetic lenses which are customarily used during convalescence from eye surgery in which the lens of the eye was removed, or to permanent prosthetic lenses required by an individual lacking the organic lens of the eye, whether by surgical removal or congenital disease. Such prosthetic lens is a replacement for an internal body organ - the lens of the eye. (See the Medicare Benefit Policy Manual, Chapter 15, "Covered Medical and Other Health Services," §120).

Expenses for all refractive procedures, whether performed by an ophthalmologist (or any other physician) or an optometrist and without regard to the reason for performance of the refraction, are excluded from coverage.

A. Immunizations

Vaccinations or inoculations are excluded as immunizations unless they are either

- Directly related to the treatment of an injury or direct exposure to a disease or condition, such as antirabies treatment, tetanus antitoxin or booster vaccine, botulin antitoxin, antivenin sera, or immune globulin.(In the absence of injury or direct exposure, preventive immunization (vaccination or inoculation) against such diseases as smallpox, polio, diphtheria, etc., is not covered.); or

- Specifically covered by statute, as described in the Medicare Benefit Policy Manual, Chapter 15, "Covered Medical and Other Health Services," §50.

B. Antigens

Prior to the Omnibus Reconciliation Act of 1980, a physician who prepared an antigen for a patient could not be reimbursed for that service unless the physician also administered the antigen to the patient. Effective January 1, 1981, payment may be made for a reasonable supply of antigens that have been prepared for a particular patient even though they have not been administered to the patient by the same physician who prepared them if:

- The antigens are prepared by a physician who is a doctor of medicine or osteopathy, and

- The physician who prepared the antigens has examined the patient and has determined a plan of treatment and a dosage regimen.

A reasonable supply of antigens is considered to be not more than a 12-week supply of antigens that has been prepared for a particular patient at any one time. The purpose of the reasonable supply limitation is to assure that the antigens retain their potency and effectiveness over the period in which they are to be administered to the patient. (See the Medicare Benefit Policy Manual, Chapter 15, "Covered Medical and Other Health Services," §50.4.4.2)

Pub. 100-2, Chapter 16, Section 140

Dental Services Exclusion
A3-3162, HO-260.13, B3-2336

Items and services in connection with the care, treatment, filling, removal, or replacement of teeth, or structures directly supporting the teeth are not covered. Structures directly supporting the teeth mean the periodontium, which includes the gingivae, dentogingival junction, periodontal membrane, cementum, and alveolar process. However, payment may be made for certain other services of a dentist. (See the Medicare Benefit Policy Manual, Chapter 15, "Covered Medical and Other Health Services," §150.)

The hospitalization or nonhospitalization of a patient has no direct bearing on the coverage or exclusion of a given dental procedure. When an excluded service is the primary procedure involved, it is not covered regardless of its complexity or difficulty. For example, the extraction of an impacted tooth is not covered. Similarly, an alveoplasty (the surgical improvement of the shape and condition of the alveolar process) and a frenectomy are excluded from coverage when either of these procedures is performed in connection with an excluded service, i.e., the preparation of the mouth for dentures. In like manner, the removal of the torus palatinus (a bony protuberance of the hard palate) could be a covered service. However, with rare exception, this surgery is performed in connection with an excluded service, i.e., the preparation of the mouth for dentures. Under such circumstances, reimbursement is not made for this purpose.

The extraction of teeth to prepare the jaw for radiation treatments of neoplastic disease is also covered. This is an exception to the requirement that to be covered, a noncovered procedure or service performed by a dentist must be an incident to and an integral part of a covered procedure or service performed by the dentist. Ordinarily, the dentist extracts the patient's teeth, but another physician, e.g., a radiologist, administers the radiation treatments.

Whether such services as the administration of anesthesia, diagnostic x-rays, and other related procedures are covered depends upon whether the primary procedure being performed by the dentist is covered. Thus, an x-ray taken in connection with the reduction of a fracture of the jaw or facial bone is covered. However, a single x-ray or xray survey taken in connection with the care or treatment of teeth or the periodontium is not covered.

See also the Medicare Benefit Policy Manual, Chapter 1, "Inpatient Hospital Services," §70, and Chapter 15, "Covered Medical and Other Health Services," §150 for additional information on dental services.

Pub. 100-3, Section 20.8

Cardiac Pacemakers

Cardiac pacemakers are covered as prosthetic devices under the Medicare program, subject to the following conditions and limitations. While cardiac pacemakers have been covered under

Medicare for many years, there were no specific guidelines for their use other than the general Medicare requirement that covered services be reasonable and necessary for the treatment of the condition. Services rendered for cardiac pacing on or after the effective dates of this instruction are subject to these guidelines, which are based on certain assumptions regarding the clinical goals of cardiac pacing. While some uses of pacemakers are relatively certain or unambiguous, many other uses require considerable expertise and judgment.

Consequently, the medical necessity for permanent cardiac pacing must be viewed in the context of overall patient management. The appropriateness of such pacing may be conditional on other diagnostic or therapeutic modalities having been undertaken. Although significant complications and adverse side effects of pacemaker use are relatively rare, they cannot be ignored when considering the use of pacemakers for dubious medical conditions, or marginal clinical benefit.

These guidelines represent current concepts regarding medical circumstances in which permanent cardiac pacing may be appropriate or necessary. As with other areas of medicine, advances in knowledge and techniques in cardiology are expected. Consequently, judgments about the medical necessity and acceptability of new uses for cardiac pacing in new classes of patients may change as more more conclusive evidence becomes available. This instruction applies only to permanent cardiac pacemakers, and does not address the use of temporary, non-implanted pacemakers.

The two groups of conditions outlined below deal with the necessity for cardiac pacing for patients in general. These are intended as guidelines in assessing the medical necessity for pacing therapies, taking into account the particular circumstances in each case. However, as a general rule, the two groups of current medical concepts may be viewed as representing:

Group I: Single-Chamber Cardiac Pacemakers - a) conditions under which single chamber pacemaker claims may be considered covered without further claims development; and b) conditions under which single-chamber pacemaker claims would be denied unless further claims development shows that they fall into the covered category, or special medical circumstances exist of the sufficiency to convince the contractor that the claim should be paid.

Group II: Dual-Chamber Cardiac Pacemakers - a) conditions under which dual-chamber pacemaker claims may be considered covered without further claims development, and b) conditions under which dual-chamber pacemaker claims would be denied unless further claims development shows that they fall into the covered categories for single- and dual-chamber pacemakers, or special medical circumstances exist sufficient to convince the contractor that the claim should be paid.

CMS opened the NCD on Cardiac Pacemakers to afford the public an opportunity to comment on the proposal to revise the language contained in the instruction. The revisions transfer the focus of the NCD from the actual pacemaker implantation procedure itself to the reasonable and necessary medical indications that justify cardiac pacing. This is consistent with our findings that pacemaker implantation is no longer considered routinely harmful or an experimental procedure.

Group I: Single-Chamber Cardiac Pacemakers (Effective March 16, 1983)

A. Nationally Covered Indications

Conditions under which cardiac pacing is generally considered acceptable or necessary, provided that the conditions are chronic or recurrent and not due to transient causes such as acute myocardial infarction, drug toxicity, or electrolyte imbalance. (In cases where there is a rhythm disturbance, if the rhythm disturbance is chronic or recurrent, a single episode of a symptom such as syncope or seizure is adequate to establish medical necessity.)

1. Acquired complete (also referred to as third-degree) AV heart block.

2. Congenital complete heart block with severe bradycardia (in relation to age), or significant physiological deficits or significant symptoms due to the bradycardia.

3. Second-degree AV heart block of Type II (i.e., no progressive prolongation of P-R interval prior to each blocked beat. P-R interval indicates the time taken for an impulse to travel from the atria to the ventricles on an electrocardiogram).

4. Second-degree AV heart block of Type I (i.e., progressive prolongation of P-R interval prior to each blocked beat) with significant symptoms due to hemodynamic instability associated with the heart block.

5. Sinus bradycardia associated with major symptoms (e.g., syncope, seizures, congestive heart failure; or substantial sinus bradycardia (heart rate less than 50) associated with dizziness or confusion. The correlation between symptoms and bradycardia must be documented, or the symptoms must be clearly attributable to the bradycardia rather than to some other cause.

6. In selected and few patients, sinus bradycardia of lesser severity (heart rate 50-59) with dizziness or confusion. The correlation between symptoms and bradycardia must be documented, or the symptoms must be clearly attributable to the bradycardia rather than to some other cause.

7. Sinus bradycardia is the consequence of long-term necessary drug treatment for which there is no acceptable alternative when accompanied by significant symptoms (e.g., syncope, seizures, congestive heart failure, dizziness or confusion). The correlation between symptoms and bradycardia must be documented, or the symptoms must be clearly attributable to the bradycardia rather than to some other cause.

8. Sinus node dysfunction with or without tachyarrhythmias or AV conduction block (i.e., the bradycardia-tachycardia syndrome, sino-atrial block, sinus arrest) when accompanied by significant symptoms (e.g., syncope, seizures, congestive heart failure, dizziness or confusion).

9. Sinus node dysfunction with or without symptoms when there are potentially life-threatening ventricular arrhythmias or tachycardia secondary to the bradycardia (e.g., numerous premature ventricular contractions, couplets, runs of premature ventricular contractions, or ventricular tachycardia).

10. Bradycardia associated with supraventricular tachycardia (e.g., atrial fibrillation, atrial flutter, or paroxysmal atrial tachycardia) with high-degree AV block which is unresponsive to appropriate pharmacological management and when the bradycardia is associated with significant symptoms (e.g., syncope, seizures, congestive heart failure, dizziness or confusion).

11. The occasional patient with hypersensitive carotid sinus syndrome with syncope due to bradycardia and unresponsive to prophylactic medical measures.

12. Bifascicular or trifascicular block accompanied by syncope which is attributed to transient complete heart block after other plausible causes of syncope have been reasonably excluded.

13. Prophylactic pacemaker use following recovery from acute myocardial infarction during which there was temporary complete (third-degree) and/or Mobitz Type II second-degree AV block in association with bundle branch block.

14. In patients with recurrent and refractory ventricular tachycardia, "overdrive pacing" (pacing above the basal rate) to prevent ventricular tachycardia.

(Effective May 9, 1985)

15. Second-degree AV heart block of Type I with the QRS complexes prolonged.

B. Nationally Noncovered Indications

Conditions which, although used by some physicians as a basis for permanent cardiac pacing, are considered unsupported by adequate evidence of benefit and therefore should not generally be considered appropriate uses for single-chamber pacemakers in the absence of the above indications. Contractors should review claims for pacemakers with these indications to determine the need for further claims development prior to denying the claim, since additional claims development may be required. The object of such further development is to establish whether the particular claim actually meets the conditions in a) above. In claims where this is not the case or where such an event appears unlikely, the contractor may deny the claim.

1. Syncope of undetermined cause.

2. Sinus bradycardia without significant symptoms.

3. Sino-atrial block or sinus arrest without significant symptoms.

4. Prolonged P-R intervals with atrial fibrillation (without third-degree AV block) or with other causes of transient ventricular pause.

5. Bradycardia during sleep.

6. Right bundle branch block with left axis deviation (and other forms of fascicular or bundle branch block) without syncope or other symptoms of intermittent AV block).

7. Asymptomatic second-degree AV block of Type I unless the QRS complexes are prolonged or electrophysiological studies have demonstrated that the block is at or beyond the level of the His bundle (a component of the electrical conduction system of the heart).

Effective October 1, 2001

8. Asymptomatic bradycardia in post-mycardial infarction patients about to initiate long-term beta-blocker drug therapy.

Group II: Dual-Chamber Cardiac Pacemakers - (Effective May 9, 1985)

A. Nationally Covered Indications

Conditions under dual-chamber cardiac pacing are considered acceptable or necessary in the general medical community unless conditions 1 and 2 under Group II. B., are present:

1. Patients in who single-chamber (ventricular pacing) at the time of pacemaker insertion elicits a definite drop in blood pressure, retrograde conduction, or discomfort.

2. Patients in whom the pacemaker syndrome (atrial ventricular asynchrony), with significant symptoms, has already been experienced with a pacemaker that is being replaced.

3. Patients in whom even a relatively small increase in cardiac efficiency will importantly improve the quality of life, e.g., patients with congestive heart failure despite adequate other medical measures.

4. Patients in whom the pacemaker syndrome can be anticipated, e.g., in young and active people, etc.

Dual-chamber pacemakers may also be covered for the conditions, as listed in Group I. A., if the medical necessity is sufficiently justified through adequate claims development. Expert physicians differ in their judgments about what constitutes appropriate criteria for dual-chamber pacemaker use. The judgment that such a pacemaker is warranted in the patient meeting accepted criteria must be based upon the individual needs and characteristics of that patient, weighing the magnitude and likelihood of anticipated benefits against the magnitude and likelihood of disadvantages to the patient.

B. Nationally Noncovered Indications

Whenever the following conditions (which represent overriding contraindications) are present, dual-chamber pacemakers are not covered:

1. Ineffective atrial contractions (e.g., chronic atrial fibrillation or flutter, or giant left atrium.

2. Frequent or persistent supraventricular tachycardias, except where the pacemaker is specifically for the control of the tachycardia.

3. A clinical condition in which pacing takes place only intermittently and briefly, and which is not associated with a reasonable likelihood that pacing needs will become prolonged, e.g., the occasional patient with hypersensitive carotid sinus syndrome with syncope due to bradycardia and unresponsive to prophylactic medical measures.

4. Prophylactic pacemaker use following recovery from acute myocardial infarction during which there was temporary complete (third-degree) and/or Type II second-degree AV block in association with bundle branch block.

C. Other

All other indications for dual-chamber cardiac pacing for which CMS has not specifically indicated coverage remain nationally noncovered, ecept for Category B IDE clinical trails, or as routine costs of dual-chamber cardiac pacing associated with clinical trials, in accordance with section 310.1 of the NCD Manual.

(This NCD last reviewed June 2004.)

Pub. 100-3, Section 20.8.1

Cardiac Pacemaker Evaluation Services

Medicare covers a variety of services for the post-implant follow-up and evaluation of implanted cardiac pacemakers. The following guidelines are designed to assist contractors in identifying and processing claims for such services.

NOTE: These new guidelines are limited to lithium battery-powered pacemakers, because mercury-zinc battery-powered pacemakers are no longer being manufactured and virtually all have been replaced by lithium units. Contractors still receiving claims for monitoring such units should continue to apply the guidelines published in 1980 to those units until they are replaced.

One fact of which contractors should be aware is that many dual-chamber units may be programmed to pace only the ventricles; this may be done either at the time the pacemaker is implanted or at some time afterward. In such cases, a dual-chamber unit, when programmed or reprogrammed for ventricular pacing, should be treated as a single-chamber pacemaker in applying screening guidelines.

The decision as to how often any patient's pacemaker should be monitored is the responsibility of the patient's physician who is best able to take into account the condition and circumstances of the individual patient. These may vary over time, requiring modifications of the frequency with which the patient should be monitored. In cases where monitoring is done by some entity other than the patient's physician, such as a commercial monitoring service or hospital outpatient department, the physician's prescription for monitoring is required and should be periodically renewed (at least annually) to assure that the frequency of monitoring is proper for the patient. When a patient is monitored both during clinica visits and transtelephonically, the contractor should be sure to include frequency data on both ypes of monitoring in evaluating the reasonableness of the frequency of monitoring services received by the patient.

Since there are over 200 pacemaker models in service at any given point, and a variety of patient conditions that give rise to the need for pacemakers, the question of the appropriate frequency of monitorings is a complex one. Nevertheless, it is possible to develop guidelines within which the vast majority of pacemaker monitorings will fall and contractors should do this, using their own data and experience, as well as the frequency guidelines which follow, in order to limit extensive claims development to those cases requiring special attention.

Pub. 100-3, Section 20.8.2

Self-Contained Pacemaker Monitors

Self-contained pacemaker monitors are accepted devices for monitoring cardiac pacemakers. Accordingly, program payment may be made for the rental or purchase of either of the following pacemaker monitors when it is prescribed by a physician for a patient with a cardiac pacemaker:

A. Digital Electronic Pacemaker Monitor.--This device provides the patient with an instantaneous digital readout of his pacemaker pulse rate. Use of this device does not involve professional services until there has been a change of five pulses (or more) per minute above or below the initial rate of the pacemaker; when such change occurs, the patient contacts his physician.

B. Audible/Visible Signal Pacemaker Monitor.--This device produces an audible and visible signal which indicates the pacemaker rate. Use of this device does not involve professional services until a change occurs in these signals; at such time, the patient contacts his physician.

NOTE: The design of the self-contained pacemaker monitor makes it possible for the patient to monitor his pacemaker periodically and minimizes the need for regular visits to the outpatient department of the provider.Therefore, documentation of the medical necessity for pacemaker evaluation in the outpatient department of the provider should be obtained where such evaluation is employed in addition to the self-contained pacemaker monitor used by the patient in his home.

Pub. 100-3, Section 20.9

Artificial Hearts and Related Devices

A. Covered Indications

1. Post-cardiotomy (effective for services performed on or after October 18, 1993)

Post-cardiotomy is the period following open-heart surgery. VADs used for support of blood circulation post-cardiotomy are covered only if they have received approval from the Food and Drug Administration (FDA) for that purpose, and the VADs are used according to the FDA-approved labeling instructions.

2. Bridge-to-Transplant (effective for services performed on or after January 22, 1996)

VADs used for bridge-to-transplant are covered only if they have received approval from the FDA for that purpose, and the VADs are used according to the FDA-approved labeling instructions. All of the following criteria must be fulfilled in order for Medicare coverage to be provided for a VAD used as a bridge-to-transplant:

a. The patient is approved and listed as a candidate for heart transplantation by a Medicare-approved heart transplant center; and,

b. The implanting site, if different than the Medicare-approved transplant center, must receive written permission from the Medicare-approved heart transplant center under which the patient is listed prior to implantation of the VAD.

The Medicare-approved heart transplant center should make every reasonable effort to transplant patients on such devices as soon as medically reasonable. Ideally, the Medicare-approved heart transplant centers should determine patient-specific timetables for transplantation, and should not maintain such patients on VADs if suitable hearts become available.

3. Destination Therapy (effective for services performed on or after October 1, 2003)

Destination therapy is for patients that require permanent mechanical cardiac support. VADs used for destination therapy are covered only if they have received approval from the FDA for that purpose, and the device is used according to the FDA-approved labeling instructions. VADs are covered for patients who have chronic end-stage heart failure (New York Heart Association Class IV end-stage left ventricular failure for at least 90 days with a life expectancy of less than 2 years), are not candidates for heart transplantation, and meet all of the following conditions:

a. The patient's Class IV heart failure symptoms have failed to respond to optimal medical management, including dietary salt restriction, diuretics, digitalis, beta-blockers, and ACE inhibitors (if tolerated) for at least 60 of the last 90 days;

b. The patient has a left ventricular ejection fraction (LVEF) < 25%,

c. The patient has demonstrated functional limitation with a peak oxygen consumption of < 12 ml/kg/min; or the patient has a continued need for intravenous inotropic therapy owing to symptomatic hypotension, decreasing renal function, or worsening pulmonary congestion; and

d. The patient has the appropriate body size > to support the VAD implantation.

In addition, the Centers for Medicare & Medicaid Services (CMS) has determined that VAD implantation as destination therapy is reasonable and necessary only when the procedure is performed in a Medicare-approved heart transplant facility that, between January 1, 2001, and September 30, 2003, implanted at least 15 VADs as a bridge-to-transplant or as destination therapy. These devices must have been approved by the FDA for destination therapy or as a bridge-to-transplant, or have been implanted as part of an FDA investigational device exemption (IDE) trial for one of these two indications. VADs implanted for other investigational indications or for support of blood circulation post-cardiotomy do not satisfy the volume requirement for this purpose. Since the relationship between volume and outcomes has not been well-established for VAD use, facilities that have minimal deficiencies in meeting this standard may apply and include a request for an exception based upon additional factors. Some of the factors CMS will consider are geographic location of the center, number of destination procedures performed, and patient outcomes from VAD procedures completed.

Also, this facility must be an active, continuous member of a national, audited registry that requires submission of health data on all VAD destination therapy patients from the date of implantation throughout the remainder of their lives. This registry must have the ability to accommodate data related to any device approved by the FDA for destination therapy regardless of manufacturer. The registry must also provide such routine reports as may be specified by CMS, and must have standards for data quality and timeliness of data submissions such that hospitals failing to meet them will be removed from membership. CMS believes that the registry sponsored by the International Society for Heart and Lung Transplantation is an example of a registry that meets these characteristics.

Hospitals also must have in place staff and procedures that ensure that prospective VAD recipients receive all information necessary to assist them in giving appropriate informed consent for the procedure so that they and their families are fully aware of the aftercare requirements and potential limitations, as well as benefits, following VAD implantation.

CMS plans to develop accreditation standards for facilities that implant VADs and, when implemented, VAD implantation will be considered reasonable and necessary only at accredited facilities.

A list of facilities eligible for Medicare reimbursement for VADs as destination therapy will be maintained on our website and available at www.cms.hhs.gov/coverage/lvadfacility.asp. In order to be placed on this list, facilities must submit a letter to the Director, Coverage and Analysis Group, 7500 Security Blvd, Mailstop C1-09-06, Baltimore, MD 21244. This letter must be received by CMS within 90 days of the issue date on this transmittal. The letter must include the following information:

Facility's name and complete address

Facility's Medicare provider number

List of all implantations between Jan. 1, 2001, and Sept. 30, 2003, with the following information:

Date of implantation

Indication for implantation (only destination and bridge-to-transplant can be reported; post-cardiotomy VAD implants are not to be included)

Device name and manufacturer, and

Date of device removal and reason (e.g., transplantation, recovery, device malfunction), or date and cause of patient's death

Point-of-contact for questions with telephone number

Registry to which patient information will be submitted; and

Signature of a senior facility administrative official.

Facilities not meeting the minimal standards and requesting exception should, in addition to supplying the information above, include the factors that they deem critical in requesting the exception to the standards.

CMS will review the information contained in the above letters. When the review is complete, all necessary information is received, and criteria are met, CMS will include the name of the newly Medicare-approved facility on the CMS web site. No reimbursement for destination therapy will be made for implantations performed before the date the facility is added to the CMS web site. Each newly approved facility will also receive a formal letter from CMS stating the official approval date it was added to the list.

B. Noncovered Indications (effective for services performed on or after May 19, 1986)

1.Artificial Heart

Since there is no authoritative evidence substantiating the safety and effectiveness of a VAD used as a replacement for the human heart, Medicare does not cover this device when used as an artificial heart.

2. All other indications for the use of VADs not otherwise listed remain noncovered, except in the context of Category B IDE clinical trials (42 CFR 405) or as a routine cost in clinical trials defined under section 310.1 of the NCD manual (old CIM 30-1).

(This NCD last reviewed October 2003.)

Pub. 100-3, Section 20.15

Electrocardiographic Services

B.Nationally Covered IndicationsThe following indications are covered nationally unless otherwise indicated:

a.Computer analysis of EKGs when furnished in a setting and under the circumstances required for coverage of other EKG services.

b.EKG services rendered by an independent diagnostic testing facility (IDTF), including physician review and interpretation. Separate physician services are not covered unless he/she is the patient's attending or consulting physician.

c.Emergency EKGs (i.e., when the patient is or may be experiencing a lifethreatening event) performed as a laboratory or diagnostic service by a portable x-ray supplier only when a physician is in attendance at the time the service is performed or immediately thereafter.

d.Home EKG services with documentation of medical necessity.

e.Trans-telephonic EKG transmissions (effective March 1, 1980) as a diagnostic service for the indications described below, when performed with equipment meeting the standards described below, subject to the limitations and conditions specified below. Coverage is further limited to the amounts payable with respect to the physician's service in interpreting the results of such transmissions, including charges for rental of the equipment. The device used by the beneficiary is part of a total diagnostic system and is not considered DME separately. Covered uses are to:

a.Detect, characterize, and document symptomatic transient arrhythmias;

b.Initiate, revise, or discontinue arrhythmic drug therapy; or,

c.Carry out early post-hospital monitoring of patients discharged after myocardial infarction (MI); (only if 24-hour coverage is provided, see C.5. below). Certain uses other than those specified above may be covered if, in the judgment of the local contractor, such use is medically necessary.Additionally, the transmitting devices must meet at least the following criteria:

a.They must be capable of transmitting EKG Leads, I, II, or III; and,

b.The tracing must be sufficiently comparable to a conventional EKG.24-hour attended coverage used as early post-hospital monitoring of patients discharged after MI is only covered if provision is made for such 24-hour attended coverage in the manner described below:24-hour attended coverage means there must be, at a monitoring site or central data center, an EKG technician or other non-physician, receiving calls and/or EKG data; tape recording devices do not meet this requirement. Further, such technicians should have immediate, 24-hour access to a physician to review transmitted data and make clinical decisions regarding the patient. The technician should also be instructed as to when and how to contact available facilities to assist the patient in case of emergencies.

C.Nationally Non-covered Indications. The following indications are non-covered nationally unless otherwise specified below:

a.The time-sampling mode of operation of ambulatory EKG cardiac event monitoring/recording.

b.Separate physician services other than those rendered by an IDTF unless rendered by the patient's attending or consulting physician.

c.Home EKG services without documentation of medical necessity.

d.Emergency EKG services by a portable x-ray supplier without a physician in attendance at the time of service or immediately thereafter.

e.24-hour attended coverage used as early post-hospital monitoring of patients discharged after MI unless provision is made for such 24-hour attended coverage in the manner described in section B.5. above.

f.Any marketed Food and Drug Administration (FDA)-approved ambulatory cardiac monitoring device or service that cannot be categorized according to the framework below.

D.OtherAmbulatory cardiac monitoring performed with a marketed, FDA-approved device, is eligible for coverage if it can be categorized according to the framework below. Unless there is a specific NCD for that device or service, determination as to whether a device or service that fits into the framework is reasonable and necessary is according to local contractor discretion.

Electrocardiographic Services Framework

Patient/Event-ActivatedIntermittent Recorders

Non-ActivatedContinuous Recorders/__

Pre-symptom memory loopo Insertableo Non-insertable

Post-symptom (no memory loop)

Dynamic Electrocardiography(e.g., Holter TM Monitor)<___

AttendedNon-attended

Non-attended

Non-attended

(This NCD last reviewed December 2004.)

Pub. 100-3, Section 20.19

Ambulatory Blood Pressure Monitoring

ABPM must be performed for at least 24 hours to meet coverage criteria.

ABPM is only covered for those patients with suspected white coat hypertension. Suspected white coat hypertension is defined as

1) office blood pressure >140/90 mm Hg on at least three separate clinic/office visits with two separate measurements made at each visit;

2) at least two documented blood pressure measurements taken outside the office which are <140/90 mm Hg; and

3) no evidence of end-organ damage.

The information obtained by ABPM is necessary in order to determine the appropriate management of the patient. ABPM is not covered for any other uses. In the rare circumstance that ABPM needs to be performed more than once in a patient, the qualifying criteria described above must be met for each subsequent ABPM test.

For those patients that undergo ABPM and have an ambulatory blood pressure of <135/85 with no evidence of end-organ damage, it is likely that their cardiovascular risk is similar to that of normotensives. They should be followed over time. Patients for which ABPM demonstrates a blood pressure of >135/85 may be at increased cardiovascular risk, and a physician may wish to consider antihypertensive therapy.

Pub. 100-3, Section 20.20

External Counterpulsation (ECP) for Severe Angina

Indications and Limitations of Coverage B. Nationally Covered Indications Effective for services performed on or after July 1, 1999, coverage is provided for the use of ECP for patients who have been diagnosed with disabling angina (Class III or Class IV, Canadian Cardiovascular Society Classification or equivalent classification) who, in the opinion of a cardiologist or cardiothoracic surgeon, are not readily amenable to surgical intervention, such as PTCA or cardiac bypass, because: Their condition is inoperable, or at high risk of operative complications or post-operative failure; Their coronary anatomy is not readily amenable to such procedures; or They have co-morbid states which create excessive risk. A full course of therapy usually consists of 35 one-hour treatments, which may be offered once or twice daily, usually 5 days per week. The patient is placed on a treatment table where their lower trunk and lower extremities are wrapped in a series of three compressive air cuffs which inflate and deflate in synchronization with the patient's cardiac cycle. During diastole the three sets of air cuffs are inflated sequentially (distal to proximal) compressing the vascular beds within the muscles of the calves, lower thighs and upper thighs. This action results in an increase in diastolic pressure, generation of retrograde arterial blood flow and an increase in venous return. The cuffs are deflated simultaneously just prior to systole, which produces a rapid drop in vascular impedance, a decrease in ventricular workload and an increase in cardiac output. The augmented diastolic pressure and retrograde aortic flow appear to improve myocardial perfusion, while systolic unloading appears to reduce cardiac workload and oxygen requirements. The increased venous return coupled with enhanced systolic flow appears to increase cardiac output. As a result of this treatment, most patients experience increased time until onset of ischemia, increased exercise tolerance, and a reduction in the number and severity of anginal episodes. Evidence was presented that this effect lasted well beyond the immediate post-treatment phase, with patients symptom-free for several months to two years. This procedure must be done under direct supervision of a physician. C. Nationally Non-Covered Indications All other cardiac conditions not otherwise specified as nationally covered for the use of ECP remain nationally non-covered. (This NCD last reviewed March 2006.) Transmittal Number 50 Transmittal Link http://www.cms.hhs.gov/transmittals/downloads/R50NCD.pdf Revision History 04/1999 - Revised existing noncoverage policy to limited coverage for use in patients with stable angina pectoris and designated CPT code for billing. Effective date 07/01/1999. (TN 111) 07/1999 - Changed CPT code. Effective date 07/01/1999. (TN 118) 02/2000 - Changed acronym from EECP to ECP, removed requirement limiting coverage to specific ECP systems, and changed CPT code. Effective and implementation dates 04/01/2000. (TN 122) (CR 1087) 10/2001 - Amended to indicate that policy only pertains to ECP devices intended for treatment of cardiac conditions. Effective and implementation dates 11/15/2001. (TN 146) (CR 1884) 03/2006 - Current coverage remains in effect. Effective Date: 03/20/2006 Implementation Date: 04/03/2006. (TN 50) (CR 4350)

Pub. 100-3, Section 20.21

Chelation Therapy for Treatment of Atherosclerosis

The application of chelation therapy using ethylenediamine-tetra-acetic acid (EDTA) for the treatment and prevention of atherosclerosis is controversial. There is no widely accepted rationale to explain the beneficial effects attributed to this therapy. Its safety is questioned and its clinical effectiveness has never been established by well designed, controlled clinical trials. It is not widely accepted and practiced by American physicians. EDTA chelation therapy for atherosclerosis is considered experimental. For these reasons, EDTA chelation therapy for the treatment or prevention of atherosclerosis is not covered.

Some practitioners refer to this therapy as chemoendarterectomy and may also show a diagnosis other than atherosclerosis, such as arteriosclerosis or calcinosis. Claims employing such variant terms should also be denied under this section.

Pub. 100-3, Section 20.22

Ethylenediamine-Tetra-Acetic (EDTA) Chelation Therapy for Treatment of Atherosclerosis

The use of EDTA as a chelating agent to treat atherosclerosis, arteriosclerosis, calcinosis, or similar generalized condition not listed by the FDA as an approved use is not covered. Any such use of EDTA is considered experimental.

APPENDIX 4 — PUB 100 REFERENCES

Pub. 100-3, Section 20.23

Fabric Wrapping of Abdominal Aneurysms

Fabric wrapping of abdominal aneurysms is not a covered Medicare procedure. This is a treatment for abdominal aneurysms which involves wrapping aneurysms with cellophane or fascia lata. This procedure has not been shown to prevent eventual rupture. In extremely rare instances, external wall reinforcement may be indicated when the current accepted treatment (excision of the aneurysm and reconstruction with synthetic materials) is not a viable alternative, but external wall reinforcement is not fabric wrapping. Accordingly, fabric wrapping of abdominal aneurysms is not considered reasonable and necessary within the meaning of §1862(a)(1) of the Act.

Pub. 100-3, Section 20.24

Displacement Cardiography

A.-Cardiokymography

Cardiokymography is covered for services rendered on or after October 12, 1998.

Cardiokymography is a covered service only when it is used as an adjunct to electrocardiographic stress testing in evaluating coronary artery disease and only when the following clinical indications are present:

For male patients, atypical angina pectoris or nonischemic chest pain; or:

For female patients, angina, either typical or atypical. :

B. Photokymography-NOT COVERED

Photokymography remains excluded from coverage

Pub. 100-3, Section 20.29

Hyperbaric Oxygen Therapy

A. Covered Conditions

Program reimbursement for HBO therapy will be limited to that which is administered in a chamber (including the one man unit) and is limited to the following conditions:

1. Acute carbon monoxide intoxication,
2. Decompression illness,
3. Gas embolism,
4. Gas gangrene,
5. Acute traumatic peripheral ischemia. HBO therapy is a valuable adjunctive treatment to be used in combination with accepted standard therapeutic measures when loss of function, limb, or life is threatened.
6. Crush injuries and suturing of severed limbs. As in the previous conditions, HBO therapy would be an adjunctive treatment when loss of function, limb, or life is threatened.
7. Progressive necrotizing infections (necrotizing fasciitis),
8. Acute peripheral arterial insufficiency,
9. Preparation and preservation of compromised skin grafts (not for primary management of wounds),
10. Chronic refractory osteomyelitis, unresponsive to conventional medical and surgical management,
11. Osteoradionecrosis as an adjunct to conventional treatment,
12. Soft tissue radionecrosis as an adjunct to conventional treatment,
13. Cyanide poisoning,
14. Actinomycosis, only as an adjunct to conventional therapy when the disease process is refractory to antibiotics and surgical treatment,
15. Diabetic wounds of the lower extremities in patients who meet the following three criteria:

a. Patient has type I or type II diabetes and has a lower extremity wound that is due to diabetes;

b. Patient has a wound classified as Wagner grade III or higher; and

c. Patient has failed an adequate course of standard wound therapy.

The use of HBO therapy is covered as adjunctive therapy only after there are no measurable signs of healing for at least 30 -days of treatment with standard wound therapy and must be used in addition to standard wound care. Standard wound care in patients with diabetic wounds includes: assessment of a patient's vascular status and correction of any vascular problems in the affected limb if possible, optimization of nutritional status, optimization of glucose control, debridement by any means to remove devitalized tissue, maintenance of a clean, moist bed of granulation tissue with appropriate moist dressings, appropriate off-loading, and necessary treatment to resolve any infection that might be present. Failure to respond to standard wound care occurs when there are no measurable signs of healing for at least 30 consecutive days. Wounds must be evaluated at least every 30 days during administration of HBO therapy. Continued treatment with HBO therapy is not covered if measurable signs of healing have not been demonstrated within any 30-day period of treatment.

B. Noncovered Conditions

All other indications not specified under §270.4(A) are not covered under the Medicare program. No program payment may be made for any conditions other than those listed in §270.4(A).

No program payment may be made for HBO in the treatment of the following conditions:

1. Cutaneous, decubitus, and stasis ulcers.
2. Chronic peripheral vascular insufficiency.
3. Anaerobic septicemia and infection other than clostridial.
4. Skin burns (thermal).
5. Senility.
6. Myocardial infarction.
7. Cardiogenic shock.
8. Sickle cell anemia.
9. Acute thermal and chemical pulmonary damage, i.e., smoke inhalation with pulmonary insufficiency.
10. Acute or chronic cerebral vascular insufficiency.
11. Hepatic necrosis.
12. Aerobic septicemia.
13. Nonvascular causes of chronic brain syndrome (Pick's disease, Alzheimer's disease, Korsakoff's disease).
14. Tetanus.
15. Systemic aerobic infection.
16. Organ transplantation.
17. Organ storage.
18. Pulmonary emphysema.
19. Exceptional blood loss anemia.
20. Multiple Sclerosis.
21. Arthritic Diseases.
22. Acute cerebral edema.

C. Topical Application of Oxygen

This method of administering oxygen does not meet the definition of HBO therapy as stated above. Also, its clinical efficacy has not been established. Therefore, no Medicare reimbursement may be made for the topical application of oxygen.

Pub. 100-3, Section 30.1

Biofeedback Therapy

Biofeedback therapy is covered under Medicare only when it is reasonable and necessary for the individual patient for muscle re-education of specific muscle groups or for treating pathological muscle abnormalities of spasticity, incapacitating muscle spasm, or weakness, and more conventional treatments (heat, cold, massage, exercise, support) have not been successful. This therapy is not covered for treatment of ordinary muscle tension states or for psychosomatic conditions. (See the Medicare Benefit Policy Manual, Chapter 15, for general coverage requirements about physical therapy requirements.)

Pub. 100-3, Section 30.1.1

Biofeedback Therapy for the Treatment of Urinary Incontinence

This policy applies to biofeedback therapy rendered by a practitioner in an office or other facility setting.

Biofeedback is covered for the treatment of stress and/or urge incontinence in cognitively intact patients who have failed a documented trial of pelvic muscle exercise (PME)training. Biofeedback is not a treatment, per se, but a tool to help patients learn how to perform PME. Biofeedback-assisted PME incorporates the use of an electronic or mechanical device to relay visual and/or auditory evidence of pelvic floor muscle tone, in order to improve awareness of pelvic floor musculature and to assist patients in the performance of PME.

A failed trial of PME training is defined as no clinically significant improvement in urinary incontinence after completing 4 weeks of an ordered plan of pelvic muscle exercises to increase periurethral muscle strength.

Contractors may decide whether or not to cover biofeedback as an initial treatment modality.

Home use of biofeedback therapy is not covered.

Pub. 100-3, Section 30.7

Laetrile and Related Substances

The FDA has determined that neither Laetrile nor any other drug called by the various terms mentioned above, nor any other product which might be characterized as a "nitriloside" is generally recognized (by experts qualified by scientific training and experience to evaluate the safety and effectiveness of drugs) to be safe and effective for any therapeutic use. Therefore, use of this drug cannot be considered to be reasonable and necessary within the meaning of §1862(a)(1) of the Act and program payment may not be made for its use or any services furnished in connection with its administration.

A hospital stay only for the purpose of having laetrile (or any other drug called by the terms mentioned above) administered is not covered. Also, program payment may not be made for laetrile (or other drug noted above) when it is used during the course of an otherwise covered hospital stay, since the FDA has found such drugs to not be safe and effective for any therapeutic purpose.

Pub. 100-3, Section 30.8

Cellular Therapy

Accordingly, cellular therapy is not considered reasonable and necessary within the meaning of section 1862(a)(1) of the law.

Pub. 100-3, Section 40.2

Home Blood Glucose Monitors

Indications and Limitations of Coverage

Blood glucose monitors are meter devices that read color changes produced on specially treated reagent strips by glucose concentrations in the patient's blood. The patient, using a disposable sterile lancet, draws a drop of blood, places it on a reagent strip and, following instructions which may vary with the device used, inserts it into the device to obtain a reading. Lancets, reagent strips, and other supplies necessary for the proper functioning of the device are also covered for patients for whom the device is indicated. Home blood glucose monitors enable certain patients to better control their blood glucose levels by frequently checking and appropriately contacting their attending physician for advice and treatment. Studies indicate that the patient's ability to carefully follow proper procedures is critical to obtaining satisfactory results with these devices. In addition, the cost of the devices, with their supplies, limits economical use to patients who must make frequent checks of their blood glucose levels. Accordingly, coverage of home blood glucose monitors is limited to patients meeting the following conditions:

1. The patient has been diagnosed as having diabetes; The patient's physician states that the patient is capable of being trained to use the particular device prescribed in an appropriate manner. In some cases, the patient may not be able to perform this function, but a responsible individual can be trained to use the equipment and monitor the patient to assure that the intended effect is achieved. This is permissible if the record is properly documented by the patient's physician; and

2. The device is designed for home rather than clinical use.

3. There is also a blood glucose monitoring system designed especially for use by those with visual impairments. The monitors used in such systems are identical in terms of reliability and sensitivity to the standard blood glucose monitors described above. They differ by having such features as voice synthesizers, automatic timers, and specially designed arrangements of supplies and materials to enable the visually impaired to use the equipment without assistance. These special blood glucose monitoring systems are covered under Medicare if the following conditions are met:

The patient and device meet the three conditions listed above for coverage of standard home blood glucose monitors; and

The patient's physician certifies that he or she has a visual impairment severe enough to require use of this special monitoring system.

The additional features and equipment of these special systems justify a higher reimbursement amount than allowed for standard blood glucose monitors. Separately identify claims for such devices and establish a separate reimbursement amount for them.

Transmittal Number 48 Transmittal Link http://www.cms.hhs.gov/transmittals/downloads/R48NCD.pdf Revision History 07/1988 - Changed coverage criteria from insulin-dependent diabetic to insulin treated, and provided that if patient unable to be trained to properly use device, coverage may still be granted if attending physician indicates that a responsible family member can be trained to use device and monitor patient. Effective date 07/15/1988. (TN 27) 04/1995 - Eliminated requirement that patient must be subject to poor diabetic control, and revised policy to allow any responsible individual, not just family member, to be trained to use device and monitor patient. Effective date 04/27/1995. (TN 75) 11/2002 - Implemented NCD under §1862(a)(1)(A) and §1861(n) of the Act. Effective and implementation dates NA. (TN 163) (CR 2445) 03/2006 - Technical Corrections to the NCD Manual. Effective and Implementation dates 06/19/2006. (TN 48) (CR 4278) National Coverage Analyses (NCAs) This NCD has been or is currently being reviewed under the National Coverage Determination process. The following are existing associations with NCAs, from the National Coverage Analyses database. Original consideration for Home Blood Glucose Monitors (CAG-00161N) Other Versions Home Blood Glucose Monitors - Version 1, Effective between 04/27/1995 - 06/19/2006

Pub. 100-3, Section 40.5

Treatment of Obesity

B. Nationally Covered Indications

Certain designated surgical services for the treatment of obesity are covered for Medicare beneficiaries who have a BMI >35, have at least one co-morbidity related to obesity and have been previously unsuccessful with the medical treatment of obesity. See §100.1.

C. Nationally Noncovered Indications

1. Treatments for obesity alone remain non-covered.

2. Supplemented fasting is not covered under the Medicare program as a general treatment for obesity (see section D. below for discretionary local coverage).

D. Other

Where weight loss is necessary before surgery in order to ameliorate the complications posed by obesity when it coexists with pathological conditions such as cardiac and respiratory diseases, diabetes, or hypertension (and other more conservative techniques to achieve this end are not regarded as appropriate), supplemented fasting with adequate monitoring of the patient is eligible for coverage on a case-by-case basis or pursuant to a local coverage determination. The risks associated with the achievement of rapid weight loss must be carefully balanced against the risk posed by the condition requiring surgical treatment.

(This NCD last reviewed February 2006.)

Pub. 100-3, Section 50.1

Speech Generating Devices

Effective January 1, 2001, augmentative and alternative communication devices or communicators, which are hereafter referred to as "speech generating devices" are now considered to fall within the DME benefit category established by §1861(n) of the Social Security Act. They may be covered if the contractor's medical staff determines that the patient suffers from a severe speech impairment and that the medical condition warrants the use of a device based on the following definitions.

Pub. 100-3, Section 50.2

Electronic Speech Aids

Electronic speech aids are covered under Part B as prosthetic devices when the patient has had a laryngectomy or his larynx is permanently inoperative.

Pub. 100-3, Section 50.3

Cochlear Implantation

B. Nationally Covered Indications

1.Effective for services performed on or after April 4, 2005, cochlear implantation may be covered for treatment of bilateral pre- or post-linguistic, sensorineural, moderate-to-profound hearing loss in individuals who demonstrate limited benefit from amplification. Limited benefit from amplification is defined by test scores of less than or equal to 40% correct in the best-aided listening condition on tape-recorded tests of open-set sentence cognition. Medicare coverage is provided only for those patients who meet all of the following selection guidelines.

Diagnosis of bilateral moderate-to-profound sensorineural hearing impairment with limited benefit from appropriate hearing (or vibrotactile) aids; :

Cognitive ability to use auditory clues and a willingness to undergo an extended program of rehabilitation; :

Freedom from middle ear infection, an accessible cochlear lumen that is structurally suited to implantation, and freedom from lesions in the auditory nerve and acoustic areas of the central nervous system; :

No contraindications to surgery; and :

The device must be used in accordance with Food and Drug Administration (FDA)-approved labeling. :

2.Effective for services performed on or after April 4, 2005, cochlear implantation may be covered for individuals meeting the selection guidelines above and with hearing test scores of greater than 40% and less than or equal to 60% only when the provider is participating in, and patients are enrolled in, either an FDA-approved category B investigational device exemption clinical trial as defined at 42 CFR 405.201, a trial under the Centers for Medicare & Medicaid (CMS) Clinical Trial Policy as defined at section 310.1 of the National Coverage Determinations Manual, or a prospective, controlled comparative trial approved by CMS as consistent with the evidentiary requirements for National Coverage Analyses and meeting specific quality standards.

C. Nationally Noncovered Indications

Medicare beneficiaries not meeting all of the coverage criteria for cochlear implantation listed are deemed not eligible for Medicare coverage under section 1862(a)(1)(A) of the Social Security Act.

D. Other

All other indications for cochlear implantation not otherwise indicated as nationally covered or non-covered above remain at local contractor discretion.

(This NCD last reviewed May 2005.)

Pub. 100-3, Section 50.4

Tracheostomy Speaking Valve

A trachea tube has been determined to satisfy the definition of a prosthetic device, and the tracheostomy speaking valve is an add on to the trachea tube which may be considered a medically necessary accessory that enhances the function of the tube. In other words, it makes the system a better prosthesis. As such, a tracheostomy speaking valve is covered as an element of the trachea tube which makes the tube more effective.

Pub. 100-3, Section 70.2.1

Services Provided for the Diagnosis and Treatment of Diabetic Sensory Neuropathy with Loss of Protective Sensation (AKA Diabetic Peripheral Neuropathy)

Diabetic sensory neuropathy with LOPS is a localized illness of the feet and falls within the regulation's exception to the general exclusionary rule [see 42 CFR §411.15(l)(1)(i)]. Foot exams for people with diabetic sensory neuropathy with LOPS are reasonable and necessary to allow for early intervention in serious complications that typically afflict diabetics with the disease.

Effective for services furnished on or after July 1, 2002, Medicare covers, as a physician service, an evaluation (examination and treatment) of the feet no more often than every six months for individuals with a documented diagnosis of diabetic sensory neuropathy and LOPS, as long as the beneficiary has not seen a foot care specialist for some other reason in the interim. LOPS shall be diagnosed through sensory testing with the 5.07 monofilament using established guidelines, such as those developed by the National Institute of Diabetes and Digestive and Kidney Diseases guidelines. Five sites should be tested on the plantar surface of each foot, according to the National Institute of Diabetes and Digestive and Kidney Diseases guidelines. The areas must be tested randomly since the loss of protective sensation may be patchy in distribution, and the patient may get clues if the test is done rhythmically. Heavily callused areas should be avoided. As suggested by the American Podiatric Medicine Association, an absence of sensation at two or more sites out of 5 tested on either foot when tested with the 5.07 Semmes-Weinstein monofilament must be present and documented to diagnose peripheral neuropathy with loss of protective sensation.

A.The examination includes:

1) a patient history, and

2) a physical examination that must consist of at least the following elements:

a.visual inspection of forefoot and hindfoot (including toe web spaces);

b.evaluation of protective sensation;

c.evaluation of foot structure and biomechanics;

d.evaluation of vascular status and skin integrity;

e.evaluation of the need for special footwear; and

3) patient education.

B.Treatment includes, but is not limited to:

1) local care of superficial wounds;

2) debridement of corns and calluses; and

3) trimming and debridement of nails.

The diagnosis of diabetic sensory neuropathy with LOPS should be established and documented prior to coverage of foot care. Other causes of peripheral neuropathy should be considered and investigated by the primary care physician prior to initiating or referring for foot care for persons with LOPS.

Pub. 100-3, Section 80.1

Hydrophilic Contact Lens For Corneal Bandage

Payment may be made under §1861(s)(2) of the Act for a hydrophilic contact les approved by the Food and Drug Administration (FDA) and used as a supply incident to a pphysician's service. Payment for the lens is included in the payment for the physician's service to which the lens is incident. Contractors are authorized to accept an FDA letter of approval or other FDA published material as evidence of FDA approval. (See §80.4 of the NCD Manual for coverage of a hydrophilic contact lens as prosthetic device.)

Pub. 100-3, Section 80.2

Ocular Photodynamic Therapy

B - Covered Indications

Effective April 1, 2004, OPT with verteporfin continues to be approved for a diagnosis of neovascular AMD with predominantly classic subfoveal CNV lesions (where the area of classic CNV occupies ≥50% of the area of the entire lesion) at the initial visit as determined by a fluorescein angiogram. (CNV lesions are comprised of classic and/or occult components.) Subsequent follow-up visits require a fluorescein angiogram prior to treatment. There are no requirements regarding visual acuity, lesion size, and number of re-treatments when treating predominantly classic lesions.

In addition, after thorough review and reconsideration of the August 20, 2002, noncoverage policy, CMS determines that the evidence is adequate to conclude that OPT with verteporfin is reasonable and necessary for treating:

1.Subfoveal occult with no classic CNV associated with AMD; and,

2.Subfoveal minimally classic CNV (where the area of classic CNV occupies <50% of the area of the entire lesion) associated with AMD.

The above 2 indications are considered reasonable and necessary only when:

1.The lesions are small (4 disk areas or less in size) at the time of initial treatment or within the 3 months prior to initial treatment; and,

2.The lesions have shown evidence of progression within the 3 months prior to initial treatment. Evidence of progression must be documented by deterioration of visual acuity (at least 5 letters on a standard eye examination chart), lesion growth (an increase in at least 1 disk area), or the appearance of blood associated with the lesion.

C - Noncovered Indications

Other uses of OPT with verteporfin to treat AMD not already addressed by CMS will continue to be noncovered. These include, but are not limited to, the following AMD indications:

Juxtafoveal or extrafoveal CNV lesions (lesions outside the fovea), :

Inability to obtain a fluorescein angiogram, :

Atrophic or "dry" AMD. :

D - Other

OPT with verteporfin for other ocular indications, such as pathologic myopia or presumed ocular histoplasmosis syndrome, continue to be eligible for local coverage determinations through individual contractor discretion.

Pub. 100-3, Section 80.3

Verteporfin

B - Covered Indications

Effective April 1, 2004, OPT with verteporfin is covered for patients with a diagnosis of neovascular age-related macular degeneration (AMD) with:

Predominately classic subfoveal choroidal neovascularization (CNV) lesions (where the area of classic CNV occupies ≥ 50% of the area of the entire lesion) at the initial visit as determined by a fluorescein angiogram. (CNV lesions are comprised of classic and/or occult components.) Subsequent follow-up visits require a fluorescein angiogram prior to treatment. There are no requirements regarding visual acuity, lesion size, and number of retreatments when treating predominantly classic lesions. :

Subfoveal occult with no classic associated with AMD. :

Subfoveal minimally classic CNV CNV (where the area of classic CNV occupies <50% of the area of the entire lesion) associated with AMD. :

The above 2 indications are considered reasonable and necessary only when:

1.The lesions are small (4 disk areas or less in size) at the time of initial treatment or within the 3 months prior to initial treatment; and,

2.The lesions have shown evidence of progression within the 3 months prior to initial treatment. Evidence of progression must be documented by deterioration of visual acuity (at least 5 letters on a standard eye examination chart), lesion growth (an increase in at least 1 disk area), or the appearance of blood associated with the lesion.

C - Noncovered Indications

Other uses of OPT with verteporfin to treat AMD not already addressed by CMS will continue to be noncovered. These include, but are not limited to, the following AMD indications: juxtafoveal or extrafoveal CNV lesions (lesions outside the fovea), inability to obtain a fluorescein angiogram, or atrophic or "dry" AMD.

D - Other

OPT with verteporfin for other ocular indications, such as pathologic myopia or presumed ocular histoplasmosis syndrome, continue to be eligible for local coverage determinations through individual contractor discretion.

Pub. 100-3, Section 80.4

Hydrophilic Contact Lenses

Hydrophilic contact lenses are eyeglasses within the meaning of the exclusion in §1862(a)(7) of the Act and are not covered when used in the treatment of nondiseased eyes with spherical ametrophia, refractive astigmatism, and/or corneal astigmatism. Payment may be made under the prosthetic device benefit, however, for hydrophilic contact lenses when prescribed for an aphakic patient.

Contractors are authorized to accept an FDA letter of approval or other FDA published material as evidence of FDA approval. (See §80.1 of the NCD Manual for coverage of a hydrophilic lens as a corneal bandage.)

Pub. 100-3, Section 80.5

Scleral Shell

A scleral shell fits over the entire exposed surface of the eye as opposed to a corneal contact lens which covers only the central non-white area encompassing the pupil and iris. Where an eye has been rendered sightless and shrunken by inflammatory disease, a scleral shell may, among other things, obviate the need for surgical enucleation and prosthetic implant and act to support the surrounding orbital tissue.

In such a case, the device serves essentially as an artificial eye. In this situation, payment may be made for a scleral shell under §1861(s)(8) of the Act.

Scleral shells are occasionally used in combination with artificial tears in the treatment of "dry eye" of diverse etiology. Tears ordinarily dry at a rapid rate, and are continually replaced by the lacrimal gland. When the lacrimal gland fails, the half-life of artificial tears may be greatly prolonged by the use of the scleral contact lens as a protective barrier against the drying action of the atmosphere. Thus, the difficult and sometimes hazardous process of frequent installation of artificial tears may be avoided. The lens acts in this instance to substitute, in part, for the functioning of the diseased lacrimal gland and would be covered as a prosthetic device in the rare case when it is used in the treatment of "dry eye."

Pub. 100-3, Section 100.6

Gastric Freezing

Since the procedure is now considered obsolete, it is not covered.

Pub. 100-3, Section 110.2

Certain Drugs Distributed by the National Cancer Institute

A physician is eligible to receive Group C drugs from the Divison of Cancer Treatment only if the following requirements are met:

A physician must be registered with the NCI as an investigator by having completed an FD-Form 1573; :

A written request for the drug, indicating the disease to be treated, must be submitted to the NCI; :

The use of the drug must be limited to indications outlined in the NCI's guidelines; and :

All adverse reactions must be reported to the Investigational Drug Branch of the Division of Cancer Treatment. :

In view of these NCI controls on distribution and use of Group C drugs, intermediaries may assume, in the absence of evidence to the contrary, that a Group C drug and the related hospital stay are covered if all other applicable coverage requirements are satisfied.

If there is reason to question coverage in a particular case, the matter should be resolved with the assistance of the Quality improvemetn organization (QIO), or if there is none, the assistance of your medical consultants.

Information regarding those drugs which are classified as Group C drugs may be obtained from:

Office of the Chief, Investigational Drug BranchDivision of Cancer Treatment, CTEP, Landow BuildingRoom 4C09, National Cancer InstituteBethesda, Maryland 20205

Appendix 4 — Pub 100 References

Pub. 100-3, Section 110.3

Anti-Inhibitor Coagulant Complex (AICC)

Anti-inhibitor coagulant complex, AICC, is a drug used to treat hemophilia in patients with factor VIII inhibitor antibodies. AICC has been shown to be safe and effective and has Medicare coverage when furnished to patients with hemophilia A and inhibitor antibodies to factor VIII who have major bleeding episodes and who fail to respond to other, less expensive therapies.

Pub. 100-3, Section 110.13

Cytotoxic Food Tests

Prior to August 5, 1985, Medicare covered cytotoxic food tests as an adjunct to in vivo clinical allergy tests in complex food allergy problems. Effective August 5, l985, cytotoxic leukocyte tests for food allergies are excluded from Medicare coverage because available evidence does not show that these tests are safe and effective. This exclusion was published as a CMS Ruling in the "Federal Register" on July 5, 1985.

Pub. 100-3, Section 130.5

Treatment of Alcoholism and Drug Abuse in a Freestanding Clinic

Coverage is available for alcoholism or drug abuse treatment services (such as drug therapy, psychotherapy, and patient education) that are provided incident to a physician's professional service in a freestanding clinic to patients who, for example, have been discharged from an inpatient hospital stay for the treatment of alcoholism or drug abuse or to individuals who are not in the acute stages of alcoholism or drug abuse but require treatment. The coverage available for these services is subject to the same rules generally applicable to the coverage of clinic services. Of course, the services also must be reasonable and necessary for the diagnosis or treatment of the individual's alcoholism or drug abuse. The Part B psychiatric limitation would apply to alcoholism or drug abuse treatment services furnished by physicians to individuals who are not hospital inpatients.

Pub. 100-3, Section 130.6

Treatment of Drug Abuse (Chemical Dependency)

Accordingly, when it is medically necessary for a patient to receive detoxification and/or rehabilitation for drug substance abuse as a hospital inpatient, coverage for care in that setting is available. Coverage is also available for treatment services that are provided in the outpatient department of a hospital to patients who, for example, have been discharged from an inpatient stay for the treatment of drug substance abuse or who require treatment but do not require the availability and intensity of services found only in the inpatient hospital setting. The coverage available for these services is subject to the same rules generally applicable to the coverage of outpatient hospital services. The services must also be reasonable and necessary for treatment of the individual's condition. Decisions regarding reasonableness and necessity of treatment, the need for an inpatient hospital level of care, and length of treatment should be made by intermediaries based on accepted medical practice with the advice of their medical consultant. (In hospitals under QIO review, QIO determinations of medical necessity of services and appropriateness of the level of care at which services are provided are binding on the title XVIII fiscal intermediaries for purposes of adjudicating claims for payment.)

Pub. 100-3, Section 140.2

Breast Reconstruction Following Mastectomy

Reconstruction of the affected and the contralateral unaffected breast following a medically necessary mastectomy is considered a relatively safe and effective noncosmetic procedure. Accordingly, program payment may be made for breast reconstruction surgery following removal of a breast for any medical reason.

Program payment may not be made for breast reconstruction for cosmetic reasons. (Cosmetic surgery is excluded from coverage under §l862(a)(l0) of the Social Security Act.)

Pub. 100-3, Section 150.2

Osteogenic Stimulators

Electrical Osteogenic Stimulators

B. Nationally Covered Indications

1. Noninvasive Stimulator.

The noninvasive stimulator device is covered only for the following indications:

Nonunion of long bone fractures; :

Failed fusion, where a minimum of nine months has elapsed since the last surgery; :

Congenital pseudarthroses; and :

Effective July 1, 1996, as an adjunct to spinal fusion surgery for patients at high risk of pseudarthrosis due to previously failsed spinal fusion at the same site or for those undergoing multiple level fusion. A multiple level fusion involves 3 or more vertebrae (e.g., L3-L5, L4-S1, etc).

Effective September 15, 1980, nonunion of long bone fractures is considered to exist only after 6 or more months have elapsed without healing of the fracture. :

Effective April 1, 2000, nonunion of long bone fractures is considered to exist only when serial radiographs have confirmed that fracture healing has ceased for 3 or more months prior to starting treatment with the electrical osteogenic stimulator. Serial radiographs must include a minimum of 2 sets of radiographs, each including multiple views of the fracture site, separated by a minimum of 90 days.:

2. Invasive (Implantable) Stimulator.

The invasive stimulator device is covered only for the following indications:

Nonunion of long bone fractures :

Effective July 1, 1996, as an adjunct to spinal fusion surgery for patients at high risk of pseudarthrosis due to previously failed spinal fusion at the same site or for those undergoing multiple level fusion. A multiple level fusion involves 3 or more vertebrae (e.g., L3-5, L4-S1, etc.)

Effective September 15, 1980, nonunion of long bone fractures is considered to exist only after 6 or more months have elapsed without healing of the fracture. :

Effective April 1, 2000, non union of long bone fractures is considered to exist only when serial radiographs have confirmed that fracture healing has ceased for 3 or more months prior to starting treatment with the electrical osteogenic stimulator. Serial radiographs must include a minimum of 2 sets of radiographs, each including multiple views of the fracture site, separated by a minimum of 90 days. :

Effective for services performed on or after January 1, 2001, ultrasonic osteogenic stimulators are covered as medically reasonable and necessary for the treatment of non-union fractures. In demonstrating nonunion of fractures, we would expect:

A minimum of two sets of radiographs obtained prior to starting treatment with the osteogenic stimulator, separated by a minimum of 90 days. Each radiograph must include multiple views of the fracture site accompanied with a written interpretation by a physician stating that there has been no clinically significant evidence of fracture healing between the two sets of radiographs. :

Indications that the patient failed at least one surgical intervention for the treatment of the fracture. :

Effective April 27, 2005, upon the recommendation of the ultrasound stimulation for nonunion fracture healing, CMS determins that the evidence is adequate to condlude that noninvasive ultrasound stimulation for the treatment of nonunion bone fractures prior to surfical intervention is reasonable and necessary. In demonstrating non-union fracturs, CMS expects::

A minimum of 2 sets of radiographs, obtained prior to starting treating with the osteogenic stimulator, separated by a minimum of 90 days. Each radiograph set must include multiple views of the fracture site accompanied with a written interpretation by a physician stating that there has been no clinically significant evidence of fracture healing between the 2 sets of radiographs.:

C. Nationally Non-Covered Indications

Nonunion fractures of the skull, vertebrae and those that are tumor-related are excluded from coverage.

Ultrasonic osteogenic stimulators may not be used concurrently with other non-invasive osteogenic devices.

Ultrasonic osteogenic stimulators for fresh fracturs and delayed unions remain non-covered.

(This NCD last reviewed June 2005)

Pub. 100-3, Section 150.3

Bone (Mineral) Density Studies

The Following Bone (Mineral) Density Studies Are Covered Under Medicare:

A. Single Photon Absorptiometry

A non-invasive radiological technique that measures absorption of a monochromatic photon beam by bone material. The device is placed directly on the patient, uses a low dose of radionuclide, and measures the mass absorption efficiency of the energy used. It provides a quantitative measurement of the bone mineral of cortical and trabecular bone, and is used in assessing an individual's treatment response at appropriate intervals.

Single photon absorptiometry is covered under Medicare when used in assessing changes in bone density of patients with osteodystrophy or osteoporosis when performed on the same individual at intervals of 6 to 12 months.

B. Bone Biopsy

A physiologic test which is a surgical, invasive procedure. A small sample of bone (usually from the ilium) is removed, generally by a biopsy needle. The biopsy sample is then examined histologically, and provides a qualitative measurement of the bone mineral of trabecular bone. This procedure is used in ascertaining a differential diagnosis of bone disorders and is used primarily to differentiate osteomalacia from osteoporosis.

Bone biopsy is covered under Medicare when used for the qualitative evaluation of bone no more than four times per patient, unless there is special justification given. When used more than four times on a patient, bone biopsy leaves a defect in the pelvis and may produce some patient discomfort.

C. Photodensitometry(radiographic absorptiometry)

A noninvasive radiological procedure that attempts to assess bone mass by measuring the optical density of extremity radiographs with a photodensitometer, usually with a reference to a standard density wedge placed on the film at the time of exposure. This procedure provides a quantitative measurement of the bone mineral of bone, and is used for monitoring gross bone change.

The Following Bone (Mineral) Density Study Is Not Covered Under Medicare:

D. Dual Photon Absorptiometry

A noninvasive radiological technique that measures absorption of a dichromatic beam by bone material. This procedure is not covered under Medicare because it is still considered to be in the investigational stage.

Pub. 100-3, Section 150.6

Vitamin B12 Injections to Strengthen Tendons, Ligaments, etc., of the Foot

Vitamin B12 injections to strengthen tendons, ligaments, etc., of the foot are not covered under Medicare because (1) there is no evidence that vitamin B12 injections are effective for the purpose of strengthening weakened tendons and ligaments, and (2) this is nonsurgical treatment under the subluxation exclusion. Accordingly, vitamin B12 injections are not considered reasonable and necessary within the meaning of §1862(a)(1) of the Act.

Pub. 100-3, Section 150.7

Prolotherapy, Joint Sclerotherapy, and Ligamentous Injections with Sclerosing Agents

The medical effectiveness of the above therapies has not been verified by scientifically controlled studies. Accordingly, reimbursement for these modalities should be denied on the ground that they are not reasonable and necessary as required by §1862(a)(1) of the Act.

Pub. 100-3, Section 160.2

Treatment of Motor Function Disorders with Electric Nerve Stimulation

Where electric nerve stimulation is employed to treat motor function disorders, no reimbursement may be made for the stimulator or for the services related to its implantation since this treatment cannot be considered reasonable and necessary.

Note: For Medicare coverage of deep brain stimulation for essential tremor and Parkinson's disease, see §160.24 of the NCD Manual.

Pub. 100-3, Section 160.6

Carotid Sinus Nerve Stimulator

Implantation of the carotid sinus nerve stimulator is indicated for relief of angina pectoris in carefully selected patients who are refractory to medical therapy and who after undergoing coronary angiography study either are poor candidates for or refuse to have coronary bypass surgery. In such cases, Medicare reimbursement may be made for this device and for the related services required for its implantation.

However, the use of the carotid sinus nerve stimulator in the treatment of paroxysmal supraventricular tachycardia is considered investigational and is not in common use by the medical community. The device and related services in such cases cannot be considered as reasonable and necessary for the treatment of an illness or injury or to improve the functioning of a malformed body member as required by §1862(a)(1) of the Act.

Pub. 100-3, Section 160.7

Electrical Nerve Stimulators

Two general classifications of electrical nerve stimulators are employed to treat chronic intractable pain: peripheral nerve stimulators and central nervous system stimulators.

A-Implanted Peripheral Nerve Stimulators

Payment may be made under the prosthetic device benefit for implanted peripheral nerve stimulators. Use of this stimulator involves implantation of electrodes around a selected peripheral nerve. The stimulating electrode is connected by an insulated lead to a receiver unit which is implanted under the skin at a depth not greater than 1/2 inch. Stimulation is induced by a generator connected to an antenna unit which is attached to the skin surface over the receiver unit. Implantation of electrodes requires surgery and usually necessitates an operating room.

NOTE: Peripheral nerve stimulators may also be employed to assess a patient's suitability for continued treatment with an electric nerve stimulator. As explained in §160.7.1, such use of the stimulator is covered as part of the total diagnostic service furnished to the beneficiary rather than as a prosthesis.

B-Central Nervous System Stimulators (Dorsal Column and Depth Brain Stimulators).The implantation of central nervous system stimulators may be covered as therapies for the relief of chronic intractable pain, subject to the following conditions:

1-Types of Implantations

There are two types of implantations covered by this instruction:

Dorsal Column (Spinal Cord) Neurostimulation.--The surgical implantation of neurostimulator electrodes within the dura mater (endodural) or the percutaneous insertion of electrodes in the epidural space is covered. :

Depth Brain Neurostimulation.--The stereotactic implantation of electrodes in the deep brain (e.g., thalamus and periaqueductal gray matter) is covered. :

2-Conditions for Coverage

No payment may be made for the implantation of dorsal column or depth brain stimulators or services and supplies related to such implantation, unless all of the conditions listed below have been met:

The implantation of the stimulator is used only as a late resort (if not a last resort) for patients with chronic intractable pain; :

With respect to item a, other treatment modalities (pharmacological, surgical, physical, or psychological therapies) have been tried and did not prove satisfactory, or are judged to be unsuitable or contraindicated for the given patient; :

Patients have undergone careful screening, evaluation and diagnosis by a multidisciplinary team prior to implantation. (Such screening must include psychological, as well as physical evaluation); :

All the facilities, equipment, and professional and support personnel required for the proper diagnosis, treatment training, and followup of the patient (including that required to satisfy item c) must be available; and :

Demonstration of pain relief with a temporarily implanted electrode precedes permanent implantation. :

Contractors may find it helpful to work with QIOs to obtain the information needed to apply these conditions to claims.

Pub. 100-3, Section 160.7.1

Assessing Patient's Suitability for Electrical Nerve Stimulation Therapy

Indications and Limitations of Coverage

CIM 35-46

Electrical nerve stimulation is an accepted modality for assessing a patient's suitability for ongoing treatment with a transcutaneous or an implanted nerve stimulator.

Accordingly, program payment may be made for the following techniques when used to determine the potential therapeutic usefulness of an electrical nerve stimulator:

A. Transcutaneous Electrical Nerve Stimulation(TENS)

This technique involves attachment of a transcutaneous nerve stimulator to the surface of the skin over the peripheral nerve to be stimulated. It is used by the patient on a trial basis and its effectiveness in modulating pain is monitored by the physician, or physical therapist. Generally, the physician or physical therapist is able to determine whether the patient is likely to derive a significant therapeutic benefit from continuous use of a transcutaneous stimulator within a trial period of 1 month; in a few cases this determination may take longer to make. Document the medical necessity for such services which are furnished beyond the first month. (See §160.13 for an explanation of coverage of medically necessary supplies for the effective use of TENS.)

If TENS significantly alleviates pain, it may be considered as primary treatment; if it produces no relief or greater discomfort than the original pain electrical nerve stimulation therapy is ruled out. However, where TENS produces incomplete relief, further evaluation with percutaneous electrical nerve stimulation may be considered to determine whether an implanted peripheral nerve stimulator would provide significant relief from pain.

Usually, the physician or physical therapist providing the services will furnish the equipment necessary for assessment. Where the physician or physical therapist advises the patient to rent the TENS from a supplier during the trial period rather than supplying it himself/herself, program payment may be made for rental of the TENS as well as for the services of the physician or physical therapist who is evaluating its use. However, the combined program payment which is made for the physician's or physical therapist's services and the rental of the stimulator from a supplier should not exceed the amount which would be payable for the total service, including the stimulator, furnished by the physician or physical therapist alone.

B. Percutaneous Electrical Nerve Stimulation (PENS)

This diagnostic procedure which involves stimulation of peripheral nerves by a needle electrode inserted through the skin is performed only in a physician's office, clinic, or hospital outpatient department. Therefore, it is covered only when performed by a physician or incident to physician's service. If pain is effectively controlled by percutaneous stimulation, implantation of electrodes is warranted.

As in the case of TENS (described in subsection A), generally the physician should be able to determine whether the patient is likely to derive a significant therapeutic benefit from continuing use of an implanted nerve stimulator within a trial period of 1 month. In a few cases, this determination may take longer to make. The medical necessity for such diagnostic services which are furnished beyond the first month must be documented.

NOTE: Electrical nerve stimulators do not prevent pain but only alleviate pain as it occurs. A patient can be taught how to employ the stimulator, and once this is done, can use it safely and effectively without direct physician supervision. Consequently, it is inappropriate for a patient to visit his/her physician, physical therapist, or an outpatient clinic on a continuing basis for treatment of pain with electrical nerve stimulation. Once it is determined that electrical nerve stimulation should be continued as therapy and the patient has been trained to use the stimulator, it is expected that a stimulator will be implanted or the patient will employ the TENS on a continual basis in his/her home. Electrical nerve stimulation treatments furnished by a physician in his/her office, by a physical therapist or outpatient clinic are excluded from coverage by §1862(a)(1) of the Act. (See §160.7 for an explanation of coverage of the therapeutic use of implanted peripheral nerve stimulators under the prosthetic devices benefit. See §280.13 for an explanation of coverage of the therapeutic use of TENS under the durable medical equipment benefit.)

Pub. 100-3, Section 160.12

Neuromuscular Electrical Stimulaton (NMES)

Indications and Limitations of Coverage

Treatment of Muscle Atrophy

Coverage of NMES to treat muscle atrophy is limited to the treatment of disuse atrophy where nerve supply to the muscle is intact, including brain, spinal cord and peripheral nerves, and other non-neurological reasons for disuse atrophy. Some examples would be casting or splinting of a limb, contracture due to scarring of soft tissue as in burn lesions, and hip replacement surgery (until orthotic training begins). (See §160.13 of the NCD Manual for an explanation of coverage of medically necessary supplies for the effective use of NMES.)

Use for Walking in Patients with Spinal Cord Injury (SCI)

The type of NMES that is use to enhance the ability to walk of SCI patients is commonly referred to as functional electrical stimulation (FES). These devices are surface units that use electrical impulses to activate paralyzed or weak muscles in precise sequence. Coverage for the use of NMES/FES is limited to SCI patients for walking, who have completed a training program which consists of at least 32 physical therapy sessions with the device over a period of three months. The trial period of physical therapy will enable the physician treating the patient for his or her spinal cord injury to properly evaluate the person's ability to use these devices frequently and for the long term. Physical therapy necessary to perform this training must be directly performed by the physical therapist as part of a one-on-one training program.

The goal of physical therapy must be to train SCI patients on the use of NMES/FES devices to achieve walking, not to reverse or retard muscle atrophy.

Coverage for NMES/FES for walking will be covered in SCI patients with all of the following characteristics:

1.Persons with intact lower motor unite (L1 and below) (both muscle and peripheral nerve);

2.Persons with muscle and joint stability for weight bearing at upper and lower extremities that can demonstrate balance and control to maintain an upright support posture independently;

3.Persons that demonstrate brisk muscle contraction to NMES and have sensory perception electrical stimulation sufficient for muscle contraction;

4.Persons that possess high motivation, commitment and cognitive ability to use such devices for walking;

5.Persons that can transfer independently and can demonstrate independent standing tolerance for at least 3 minutes;

6.Persons that can demonstrate hand and finger function to manipulate controls;

7.Persons with at least 6-month post recovery spinal cord injury and restorative surgery;

8.Persons with hip and knee degenerative disease and no history of long bone fracture secondary to osteoporosis; and

9.Persons who have demonstrated a willingness to use the device long-term.

NMES/FES for walking will not be covered in SCI patient with any of the following:

1.Persons with cardiac pacemakers;

2.Severe scoliosis or severe osteoporosis;

3.Skin disease or cancer at area of stimulation;

4.Irreversible contracture; or

5.Autonomic dysflexia.

The only settings where therapists with the sufficient skills to provide these services are employed, are inpatient hospitals; outpatient hospitals; comprehensive outpatient rehabilitation facilities; and outpatient rehabilitation facilities. The physical therapy necessary to perform this training must be part of a one-on-one training program.

Additional therapy after the purchase of the DME would be limited by our general policies in converge of skilled physical therapy.

Pub. 100-3, Section 160.13

Supplies Used in the Delivery of Transcutaneous Electrical Nerve Stimulation (TENS) and Neuromuscular Electrical Stimulation (NMES)

A form-fitting conductive garment (and medically necessary related supplies) may be covered under the program only when:

1. It has received permission or approval for marketing by the Food and Drug Administration;

2. It has been prescribed by a physician for use in delivering covered TENS or NMES treatment; and

3. One of the medical indications outlined below is met:

The patient cannot manage without the conductive garment because there is such a large area or so many sites to be stimulated and the stimulation would have to be delivered so frequently that it is not feasible to use conventional electrodes, adhesive tapes and lead wires;:

The patient cannot manage without the conductive garment for the treatment of chronic intractable pain because the areas or sites to be stimulated are inaccessible with the use of conventional electrodes, adhesive tapes and lead wires;:

The patient has a documented medical condition such as skin problems that preclude the application of conventional electrodes, adhesive tapes and lead wires;:

The patient requires electrical stimulation beneath a cast either to treat disuse atrophy, where the nerve supply to the muscle is intact, or to treat chronic intractable pain; or:

The patient has a medical need for rehabilitation strengthening (pursuant to a written plan of rehabilitation) following an injury where the nerve supply to the muscle is intact.:

A conductive garment is not covered for use with a TENS device during the trial period specified in §35-46 unless:

4. The patient has a documented skin problem prior to the start of the trial period; and

5. The carrier's medical consultants are satisfied that use of such an item is medically necessary for the patient.

Pub. 100-3, Section 160.23

Sensory Nerve Conduction Threshold Test (sNCT)

B.Nationally Covered Indications

Not applicable.

C. Nationally Noncovered Indications

All uses of sNCT to diagnose sensory neuropathies or radiculopathies are noncovered.

(This NCD last reviewed June 2004.)

Pub. 100-3, Section 180.2

Enteral and Parenteral Nutritional Therapy

Coverage of nutritional therapy as a Part B benefit is provided under the prosthetic device benefit provision which requires that the patient must have a permanently inoperative internal body organ or function thereof. Therefore, enteral and parenteral nutritional therapy are not covered under Part B in situations involving temporary impairments. Coverage of such therapy, however,

does not require a medical judgment that the impairment giving rise to the therapy will persist throughout the patient's remaining years. If the medical record, including the judgment of the attending physician, indicates that the impairment will be of long and indefinite duration, the test of permanence is considered met.

If the coverage requirements for enteral or parenteral nutritional therapy are met under the prosthetic device benefit provision, related supplies, equipment and nutrients are also covered under the conditions in the following paragraphs and the Medicare Benefit Policy Manual, Chapter 15, "Covered Medical and Other Health Services," §120.

Parenteral Nutrition Therapy

Daily parenteral nutrition is considered reasonable and necessary for a patient with severe pathology of the alimentary tract which does not allow absorption of sufficient nutrients to maintain weight and strength commensurate with the patient's general condition.

Since the alimentary tract of such a patient does not function adequately, an indwelling catheter is placed percutaneously in the subclavian vein and then advanced into the superior vena cava where intravenous infusion of nutrients is given for part of the day. The catheter is then plugged by the patient until the next infusion. Following a period of hospitalization which is required to initiate parenteral nutrition and to train the patient in catheter care, solution preparation, and infusion technique, the parenteral nutrition can be provided safely and effectively in the patient's home by nonprofessional persons who have undergone special training. However, such persons cannot be paid for their services, nor is payment available for any services furnished by nonphysician professionals except as services furnished incident to a physician's service.

For parenteral nutrition therapy to be covered under Part B, the claim must contain a physician's written order or prescription and sufficient medical documentation to permit an independent conclusion that the requirements of the prosthetic device benefit are met and that parenteral nutrition therapy is medically necessary. An example of a condition that typically qualifies for coverage is a massive small bowel resection resulting in severe nutritional deficiency in spite of adequate oral intake. However, coverage of parenteral nutrition therapy for this and any other condition must be approved on an individual, case-by-case basis initially and at periodic intervals of no more than three months by the carrier's medical consultant or specially trained staff, relying on such medical and other documentation as the carrier may require. If the claim involves an infusion pump, sufficient evidence must be provided to support a determination of medical necessity for the pump. Program payment for the pump is based on the reasonable charge for the simplest model that meets the medical needs of the patient as established by medical documentation.

Nutrient solutions for parenteral therapy are routinely covered. However, Medicare pays for no more than one month's supply of nutrients at any one time. Payment for the nutrients is based on the reasonable charge for the solution components unless the medical record, including a signed statement from the attending physician, establishes that the beneficiary, due to his/her physical or mental state, is unable to safely or effectively mix the solution and there is no family member or other person who can do so. Payment will be on the basis of the reasonable charge for more expensive premixed solutions only under the latter circumstances.

Enteral Nutrition Therapy

Enteral nutrition is considered reasonable and necessary for a patient with a functioning gastrointestinal tract who, due to pathology to, or nonfunction of, the structures that normally permit food to reach the digestive tract, cannot maintain weight and strength commensurate with his or her general condition. Enteral therapy may be given by nasogastric, jejunostomy, or gastrostomy tubes and can be provided safely and effectively in the home by nonprofessional persons who have undergone special training. However, such persons cannot be paid for their services, nor is payment available for any services furnished by nonphysician professionals except as services furnished incident to a physician's service.

Typical examples of conditions that qualify for coverage are head and neck cancer with reconstructive surgery and central nervous system disease leading to interference with the neuromuscular mechanisms of ingestion of such severity that the beneficiary cannot be maintained with oral feeding. However, claims for Part B coverage of enteral nutrition therapy for these and any other conditions must be approved on an individual, case-by-case basis. Each claim must contain a physician's written order or prescription and sufficient medical documentation (e.g., hospital records, clinical findings from the attending physician) to permit an independent conclusion that the patient's condition meets the requirements of the prosthetic device benefit and that enteral nutrition therapy is medically necessary. Allowed claims are to be reviewed at periodic intervals of no more than 3 months by the contractor's medical consultant or specially trained staff, and additional medical documentation considered necessary is to be obtained as part of this review.

Medicare pays for no more than one month's supply of enteral nutrients at any one time.

If the claim involves a pump, it must be supported by sufficient medical documentation to establish that the pump is medically necessary, i.e., gravity feeding is not satisfactory due to aspiration, diarrhea, dumping syndrome. Program payment for the pump is based on the reasonable charge for the simplest model that meets the medical needs of the patient as established by medical documentation.

Nutritional Supplementation

Some patients require supplementation of their daily protein and caloric intake. Nutritional supplements are often given as a medicine between meals to boost protein-caloric intake or the mainstay of a daily nutritional plan. Nutritional supplementation is not covered under Medicare Part B.

Pub. 100-3, Section 190.2

Diagnostic Pap Smears

A diagnostic pap smear and related medically necessary services are covered under Medicare Part B when ordered by a physician under one of the following conditions:

Previous cancer of the cervix, uterus, or vagina that has been or is presently being treated; :

Previous abnormal pap smear; :

Any abnormal findings of the vagina, cervix, uterus, ovaries, or adnexa; :

Any significant complaint by the patient referable to the female reproductive system; or :

Any signs or symptoms that might in the physician's judgment reasonably be related to a gynecologic disorder. :

Screening Pap Smears and Pelvic Examinations for Early Detection of Cervical or Vaginal Cancer. (See section 210.2.)

Pub. 100-3, Section 190.6

Hair Analysis

Indications and Limitations of Coverage

Hair analysis to detect mineral traces as an aid in diagnosing human disease is not a covered service under Medicare.

The correlation of hair analysis to the chemical state of the whole body is not possible at this time, and therefore this diagnostic procedure cannot be considered to be reasonable and necessary under §1862(a)(1) of the Act.

Pub. 100-3, Section 210.1

Prostate Cancer Screening Tests

Indications and Limitations of Coverage

CIM 50-55

Covered

A. General

Section 4103 of the Balanced Budget Act of 1997 provides for coverage of certain prostate cancer screening tests subject to certain coverage, frequency, and payment limitations. Medicare will cover prostate cancer screening tests/procedures for the early detection of prostate cancer. Coverage of prostate cancer screening tests includes the following procedures furnished to an individual for the early detection of prostate cancer:

Screening digital rectal examination; and :

Screening prostate specific antigen blood test :

B. Screening Digital Rectal Examinations

Screening digital rectal examinations are covered at a frequency of once every 12 months for men who have attained age 50 (at least 11 months have passed following the month in which the last Medicare-covered screening digital rectal examination was performed). Screening digital rectal examination means a clinical examination of an individual's prostate for nodules or other abnormalities of the prostate. This screening must be performed by a doctor of medicine or osteopathy (as defined in §1861(r)(1) of the Act), or by a physician assistant, nurse practitioner, clinical nurse specialist, or certified nurse midwife (as defined in §1861(aa) and §1861(gg) of the Act) who is authorized under State law to perform the examination, fully knowledgeable about the beneficiary's medical condition, and would be responsible for using the results of any examination performed in the overall management of the beneficiary's specific medical problem.

C. Screening Prostate Specific Antigen Tests

Screening prostate specific antigen tests are covered at a frequency of once every 12 months for men who have attained age 50 (at least 11 months have passed following the month in which the last Medicare-covered screening prostate specific antigen test was performed). Screening prostate specific antigen tests (PSA) means a test to detect the marker for adenocarcinoma of prostate. PSA is a reliable immunocytochemical marker for primary and metastatic adenocarcinoma of prostate. This screening must be ordered by the beneficiary's physician or by the beneficiary's physician assistant, nurse practitioner, clinical nurse specialist, or certified nurse midwife (the term "attending physician" is defined in §1861(r)(1) of the Act to mean a doctor of medicine or osteopathy and the terms "physician assistant, nurse practitioner, clinical nurse specialist, or certified nurse midwife" are defined in §1861(aa) and §1861(gg) of the Act) who is fully knowledgeable about the beneficiary's medical condition, and who would be responsible for using the results of any examination (test) performed in the overall management of the beneficiary's specific medical problem.

Pub. 100-3, Section 220.6

PET Scans

The following indications may be covered for PET under certain circumstances. Details of Medicare PET coverage are discussed later in this section. Unless otherwise indicated, the clinical conditions below are covered when PET utilizes FDG as a tracer.

NOTE: This manual section 220.6 lists all Medicare-covered uses of PET scans. Except as set forth below in cancer indications listed as "Coverage with Evidence Development", a particular use of PET scans is not covered unless this manual specifically provides that such use is covered. Although this section 220.6 lists some non-covered uses of PET scans, it does not constitute an exhaustive list of all non-covered uses.

Clinical Condition	Effective Date	Coverage
Solitary Pulmonary Nodules (SPNs)	January 1, 1998	Characterization
Lung Cancer (Non Small Cell)	January 1, 1998	Initial staging
Lung Cancer (Non Small Cell)	July 1, 2001	Diagnosis, staging, restaging
Esophageal Cancer	July 1, 2001	Diagnosis, staging, restaging

Clinical Condition	Effective Date	Coverage
Colorectal Cancer	July 1, 1999	Determining location of tumors if rising CEA level suggests recurrence
Colorectal Cancer	July 1, 2001	Diagnosis, staging, restaging
Lymphoma	July 1, 1999	Staging and restaging only when used as alternative to Gallium scan
Lymphoma	July 1, 2001	Diagnosis, staging and restaging
Melanoma	July 1, 1999	Evaluating recurrence prior to surgery as alternative to Gallium scan
Melanoma	July 1, 2001	Diagnosis, staging, restaging; Non-covered for evaluating regional node
Breast Cancer	October 1, 2002	As an adjunct to standard imaging modalities for staging patients with distant metastasis or restaging patients with loco-regional recurrence or metastasis; as an adjunct to standard imaging modalities for monitoring tumor response to treatment for women with locally advanced and metastatic breast cancer when a change in therapy is anticipated
Head and Neck Cancers (excluding CNS and thyroid)	July 1, 2001	Diagnosis, staging, restaging
Thyroid Cancer	October 1, 2003	Restaging of recurrent or residual thyroid cancers of follicular cell origin previously treated by thyroidectomy and radioiodine ablation and have a serum thyroglobulin >10ng/ml and negative I-131 whole body scan performed
Myocardial Viability	July 1, 2001 to September 30, 2002	Only following inconclusive SPECT
Myocardial Viability	October 1, 2002	Primary or initial diagnosis, or following an inconclusive SPECT prior to revascularization. SPECT may not be used following an inconclusive PET scan
Refractory Seizures	July 1, 2001	Pre-surgical evaluation only
Perfusion of the heart using Rubidium 82* tracer	March 14, 1995	Noninvasive imaging of the perfusion of the heart
Perfusion of the heart using ammonia N-13* tracer	October 1, 2003	Noninvasive imaging of the perfusion of the heart

*Not FDG-PET.

EFFECTIVE JANUARY 28, 2005: This manual section lists Medicare-covered uses of PET scans effective for services performed on or after January 28, 2005. Except as set forth below in cancer indications listed as "coverage with evidence development", a particular use of PET scans is not covered unless this manual specifically provides that such use is covered. Although this section 220.6 lists some non-covered uses of PET scans, it does not constitute an exhaustive list of all non-covered uses.

For cancer indications listed as "coverage with evidence development" CMS determines that the evidence is sufficient to conclude that an FDG PET scan is reasonable and necessary only when the provider is participating in, and patients are enrolled in, one of the following types of prospective clinical studies that is designed to collect additional information at the time of the scan to assist in patient management:

A clinical trial of FDG PET that meets the requirements of Food and Drug Administration (FDA) category B investigational device exemption (42 CFR 405.201); :

An FDG PET clinical study that is designed to collect additional information at the time of the scan to assist in patient management. Qualifying clinical studies must ensure that specific hypotheses are addressed; appropriate data elements are collected; hospitals and providers are qualified to provide the PET scan and interpret the results; participating hospitals and providers accurately report data on all enrolled patients not included in other qualifying trials through adequate auditing mechanisms; and, all patient confidentiality, privacy, and other Federal laws must be followed. :

Effective January 28, 2005: For PET services identified as "Coverage with Evidence Development. Medicare shall notify providers and beneficiaries where these services can be accessed, as they become available, via the following:

Federal Register Notice :

CMS coverage Web site at: www.cms.gov/coverage:

Indication	Covered 1	NationallyNon-covered 2	Coverage with Evidence Development 3
Brain			X
Breast-Diagnosis-Initial staging of axillary nodes-Staging of distant metastasis-Restaging, monitoring *	XX	XX	
Cervical-Staging as adjunct to conventional imaging-Other staging-Diagnosis, restaging, monitoring *	X		XX
Colorectal-Diagnosis, staging, restaging-Monitoring *	X		X
Esophagus-Diagnosis, staging, restaging-Monitoring *	X		X
Head and Neck (non-CNS/thyroid)-Diagnosis, staging, restaging-Monitoring *	X		X
Lymphoma-Diagnosis, staging, restaging-Monitoring *	X		X
Melanoma-Diagnosis, staging, restaging-Monitoring *	X		X
Non-Small Cell Lung-Diagnosis, staging, restaging-Monitoring *	X		X
Ovarian			X
Pancreatic			X
Small Cell Lung			X
Soft Tissue Sarcoma			X
Solitary Pulmonary Nodule (characterization)	X		
Thyroid-Staging of follicular cell tumors-Restaging of medullary cell tumors-Diagnosis, other staging & restaging-Monitoring *	X		XXX
Testicular			X
All other cancers not listed herein (all indications)			X

1 Covered nationally based on evidence of benefit. Refer to National Coverage Determination Manual Section 220.6 in its entirety for specific coverage language and limitations for each indication.

2 Non-covered nationally based on evidence of harm or no benefit.

3 Covered only in specific settings discussed above if certain patient safeguards are provided. Otherwise, non-covered nationally based on lack of evidence sufficient to establish either benefit or harm or no prior decision addressing this cancer. Medicare shall notify providers and beneficiaries where these services can be accessed, as they become available, via the following:

Federal Register Notice :

CMS coverage Web site at: www.cms.gov/coverage :

* Monitoring = monitoring response to treatment when a change in therapy is anticipated.

II. General Conditions of Coverage for FDG PET

Allowable FDG PET Systems

A. Definitions: For purposes of this section:

"Any FDA-approved" means all systems approved or cleared for marketing by the Food and Drug Administration (FDA) to image radionuclides in the body. :

"FDA-approved" means that the system indicated has been approved or cleared for marketing by the FDA to image radionuclides in the body. :

"Certain coincidence systems" refers to the systems that have all the following features:

Crystal at least 5/8-inch thick; :

Techniques to minimize or correct for scatter and/or randoms; and :

Digital detectors and iterative reconstruction. :Scans performed with gamma camera PET systems with crystals thinner than 5/8" will not be covered by Medicare. In addition, scans performed with systems with crystals greater than or equal to 5/8" in thickness, but that do not meet the other listed design characteristics are not covered by Medicare. :

B. Allowable PET systems by covered clinical indication:

Allowable Type of FDG PET System

Covered Clinical Condition	Prior toJuly 1, 2001	July 1, 2001 through December 31, 2001	On or afterJanuary 1, 2002
Characterization of single pulmonary nodules	Effective 1/1/1998, any FDA-approved	Any FDA-approved	FDA-approved: Full/Partial ring, certain coincidence systems
Initial staging of lung cancer (non small cell)	Effective 1/1/1998, any FDA-approved	Any FDA-approved	FDA-approved: Full/Partial ring, certain coincidence systems
Determining location of colorectal tumors if rising CEA level suggests recurrence	Effective 7/1/1999, any FDA-approved	Any FDA-approved	FDA approved: Full/Partial ring, certain coincidence systems
Staging or restaging of lymphoma only when used as alternative to gallium scan	Effective 7/1/1999, any FDA-approved	Any FDA-approved	FDA-approved: Full/Partial ring, certain coincidence systems
Evaluating recurrence of melanoma prior to surgery as alternative to gallium scan	Effective 7/1/1999, any FDA-approved.	Any FDA-approved	FDA-approved: Full/Partial ring, certain coincidence systems
Diagnosis, staging, restaging of colorectal cancer	Not covered by Medicare	Full ring	FDA-approved: Full/Partial ring
Diagnosis, staging, restaging of esophageal cancer	Not covered by Medicare	Full ring	FDA-approved: Full/Partial ring
Diagnosis, staging, restaging of head and neck cancers (excluding CNS and thyroid)	Not covered by Medicare	Full ring	FDA-approved: Full/Partial ring
Diagnosis, staging, restaging of lung cancer (non small cell)	Not covered by Medicare	Full ring	FDA-approved: Full/Partial ring
Diagnosis, staging, restaging of lymphoma	Not covered by Medicare	Full ring	FDA-approved: Full/Partial ring
Diagnosis, staging, restaging of melanoma (non-covered for evaluating regional nodes)	Not covered by Medicare	Full ring	FDA-approved: Full/Partial ring

Allowable Type of FDG PET System

Determination of myocardial viability only following inconclusive SPECT	Not covered by Medicare	Full ring	FDA-approved: Full/Partial ring
Pre-surgical evaluation of refractory seizures	Not covered by Medicare	Full ring	FDA-approved: Full ring
Breast Cancer	Not covered	Not covered	Effective October 1, 2002, Full/Partial ring
Thyroid Cancer	Not covered	Not covered	Effective October 1, 2003, Full/Partial ring
Myocardial Viability Primary or initial diagnosis prior to revascularization	Not covered	Not covered	Effective October 1, 2002, Full/Partial ring
All other oncology indications not previously specified	Not covered	Not covered	Effective January 28, 2005, Full/Partial ring

C. Regardless of any other terms or conditions, all uses of FDG PET scans, in order to be covered by the Medicare program, must meet the following general conditions prior to June 30, 2001:

Submission of claims for payment must include any information Medicare requires to ensure the PET scans performed were: (a) medically necessary, (b) did not unnecessarily duplicate other covered diagnostic tests, and (c) did not involve investigational drugs or procedures using investigational drugs, as determined by the FDA. :

The PET scan entity submitting claims for payment must keep such patient records as Medicare requires on file for each patient for whom a PET scan claim is made. :

Regardless of any other terms or conditions, all uses of FDG PET scans, in order to be covered by the Medicare program, must meet the following general conditions as of July 1, 2001:

The provider of the PET scan should maintain on file the doctor's referral and documentation that the procedure involved only FDA-approved drugs and devices, as is normal business practice. :

The ordering physician is responsible for documenting the medical necessity of the study and ensuring that it meets the conditions specified in the instructions. The physician should have documentation in the beneficiary's medical record to support the referral to the PET scan provider. :

III. Covered Indications for PET Scans and Limitations/Requirements for Usage

For all uses of PET relating to malignancies the following conditions apply:

A. Diagnosis: PET is covered only in clinical situations in which: (1) the PET results may assist in avoiding an invasive diagnostic procedure, or in which (2) the PET results may assist in determining the optimal anatomical location to perform an invasive diagnostic procedure. In general, for most solid tumors, a tissue diagnosis is made prior to the performance of PET scanning. PET scans following a tissue diagnosis are generally performed for staging rather than diagnosis.

PET is not covered as a screening test (i.e., testing patients without specific signs and symptoms of disease).

B. Staging: PET is covered for staging in clinical situations in which: (1)(a) the stage of the cancer remains in doubt after completion of a standard diagnostic workup, including conventional imaging (computed tomography (CT), magnetic resonance imaging (MRI), or ultrasound), or (1)(b) it could potentially replace one or more conventional imaging studies when it is expected that conventional study information is insufficient for the clinical management of the patient, and 2) clinical management of the patient would differ depending on the stage of the cancer identified.

C. Restaging: PET is covered for restaging: (1) after completion of treatment for the purpose of detecting residual disease, (2) for detecting suspected recurrence or metastasis, (3) to determine the extent of a known recurrence, or (4) if it could potentially replace one or more conventional imaging studies when it is expected that conventional study information is insufficient for the clinical management of the patient. Restaging applies to testing after a course of treatment is completed, and is covered subject to the conditions above.

D. Monitoring: This refers to use of PET to monitor tumor response to treatment during the planned course of therapy (i.e., when a change in therapy is anticipated).

NOTE: In the absence of national frequency limitations, contractors, should, if necessary, develop frequency requirements on any or all of the indications covered on and after July 1, 2001.

(This NCD last reviewed December 2004.)

Pub. 100-3, Section 230.1

Treatment of Kidney Stones

In addition to the traditional surgical/endoscopic techniques for the treatment of kidney stones, the following lithotripsy techniques are also covered for services rendered on or after March 15, 1985.

A.Extracorporeal Shock Wave Lithotripsy.--Extracorporeal Shock Wave Lithotripsy (ESWL) is a non-invasive method of treating kidney stones using a device called a lithotriptor. The lithotriptor uses shock waves generated outside of the body to break up upper urinary tract stones. It focuses the shock waves specifically on stones under X-ray visualization, pulverizing them by

repeated shocks. ESWL is covered under Medicare for use in the treatment of upper urinary tract kidney stones.

B.Percutaneous Lithotripsy.--Percutaneous lithotripsy (or nephrolithotomy) is an invasive method of treating kidney stones by using ultrasound, electrohydraulic or mechanical lithotripsy. A probe is inserted through an incision in the skin directly over the kidney and applied to the stone. A form of lithotripsy is then used to fragment the stone. Mechanical or electrohydraulic lithotripsy may be used as an alternative or adjunct to ultrasonic lithotripsy. Percutaneous lithotripsy of kidney stones by ultrasound or by the related techniques of electrohydraulic or mechanical lithotripsy is covered under Medicare.

The following is covered for services rendered on or after January 16, 1988.

C.Transurethral Ureteroscopic Lithotripsy.--Transurethral ureteroscopic lithotripsy is a method of fragmenting and removing ureteral and renal stones through a cystoscope. The cystoscope is inserted through the urethra into the bladder. Catheters are passed through the scope into the opening where the ureters enter the bladder. Instruments passed through this opening into the ureters are used to manipulate and ultimately disintegrate stones, using either mechanical crushing, transcystoscopic electrohydraulic shock waves, ultrasound or laser. Transurethral ureteroscopic lithotripsy for the treatment of urinary tract stones of the kidney or ureter is covered under Medicare.

Pub. 100-3, Section 230.5

Gravlee Jet Washer

The use of this device is indicated where the patient exhibits clinical symptoms or signs suggestive of endometrial disease, such as irregular or heavy vaginal bleeding.

Program payment cannot be made for the washer or the related diagnostic services when furnished in connection with the examination of an asymptomatic patient. Payment for routine physical checkups is precluded under the statute. (See§1862(a)(7) of the Act.)

Pub. 100-3, Section 230.6

Vabra Aspirator

Program payment cannot be made for the aspirator or the related diagnostic services when furnished in connection with the examination of an asymptomatic patient. Payment for routine physical checkups is precluded under the statute (§1862(a)(7) of the Act).

Pub. 100-3, Section 230.7

Water Purification and Softening Systems Used in Conjunction with Home Dialysis

A - Water Purification Systems

Water used for home dialysis should be chemically free of heavy trace metals and/or organic contaminants which could be hazardous to the patient. It should also be as free of bacteria as possible but need not be biologically sterile. Since the characteristics of natural water supplies in most areas of the country are such that some type of water purification system is needed, such a system used in conjunction with a home dialysis (either peritoneal or hemodialysis) unit is covered under Medicare.

There are two types of water purification systems which will satisfy these requirements:

Deionization - The removal of organic substances, mineral salts of magnesium and calcium (causing hardness), compounds of fluoride and chloride from tap water using the process of filtration and ion exchange; or :

Reverse Osmosis - The process used to remove impurities from tap water utilizing pressure to force water through a porous membrane. :

Use of both a deionization unit and reverse osmosis unit in series, theoretically to provide the advantages of both systems, has been determined medically unnecessary since either system can provide water which is both chemically and bacteriologically pure enough for acceptable use in home dialysis. In addition, spare deionization tanks are not covered since they are essentially a precautionary supply rather than a current requirement for treatment of the patient.

Activated carbon filters used as a component of water purification systems to remove unsafe concentrations of chlorine and chloramines are covered when prescribed by a physician.

B - Water Softening System

Except as indicated below, a water softening system used in conjunction with home dialysis is excluded from coverage under Medicare as not being reasonable and necessary within the meaning of §1862(a)(1) of the Act. Such a system, in conjunction with a home dialysis unit, does not adequately remove the hazardous heavy metal contaminants (such as arsenic) which may be present in trace amounts.

A water softening system may be covered when used to pretreat water to be purified by a reverse osmosis (RO) unit for home dialysis where:

The manufacturer of the RO unit has set standards for the quality of water entering the RO (e.g., the water to be purified by the RO must be of a certain quality if the unit is to perform as intended); :

The patient's water is demonstrated to be of a lesser quality than required; and :

The softener is used only to soften water entering the RO unit, and thus, used only for dialysis. (The softener need not actually be built into the RO unit, but must be an integral part of the dialysis system.) :

C - Developing Need When a Water Softening System is Replaced with a Water Purification Unit in an Existing Home Dialysis System

The medical necessity of water purification units must be carefully developed when they replace water softening systems in existing home dialysis systems. A purification system may be ordered under these circumstances for a number of reasons. For example, changes in the medical community's opinions regarding the quality of water necessary for safe dialysis may lead the

Appendix 4 — Pub 100 References

physician to decide the quality of water previously used should be improved, or the water quality itself may have deteriorated. Patients may have dialyzed using only an existing water softener previous to Medicare ESRD coverage because of inability to pay for a purification system. On the other hand, in some cases, the installation of a purification system is not medically necessary. Thus, when such a case comes to your attention, ask the physician to furnish the reason for the changes. Supporting documentation, such as the supplier's recommendations or water analysis, may be required. All such cases should be reviewed by your medical consultants.

Pub. 100-3, Section 230.8

Non-Implantable Pelvic Floor Electrical Stimulator

Pelvic floor electrical stimulation with a non-implantable stimulator is covered for the treatment of stress and/or urge urinary incontinence in cognitively intact patients who have failed a documented trial of pelvic muscle exercise (PME) training.

A failed trial of PME training is defined as no clinically significant improvement in urinary continence after completing 4 weeks of an ordered plan of pelvic muscle exercises designed to increase periurethral muscle strength.

Pub. 100-3, Section 230.10

Incontinence Control Devices

A.Mechanical/Hydraulic Incontinence Control Devices.--Mechanical/hydraulic incontinence control devices are accepted as safe and effective in the management of urinary incontinence in patients with permanent anatomic and neurologic dysfunctions of the bladder. This class of devices achieves control of urination by compression of the urethra. The materials used and the success rate may vary somewhat from device to device. Such a device is covered when its use is reasonable and necessary for the individual patient.

B.Collagen Implant.--A collagen implant, which is injected into the submucosal tissues of the urethra and/or the bladder neck and into tissues adjacent to the urethra, is a prosthetic device used in the treatment of stress urinary incontinence resulting from intrinsic sphincter deficiency (ISD). ISD is a cause of stress urinary incontinence in which the urethral sphincter is unable to contract and generate sufficient resistance in the bladder, especially during stress maneuvers.

Prior to collagen implant therapy, a skin test for collagen sensitivity must be administered and evaluated over a 4 week period.

In male patients, the evaluation must include a complete history and physical examination and a simple cystometrogram to determine that the bladder fills and stores properly. The patient then is asked to stand upright with a full bladder and to cough or otherwise exert abdominal pressure on his bladder. If the patient leaks, the diagnosis of ISD is established.

In female patients, the evaluation must include a complete history and physical examination (including a pelvic exam) and a simple cystometrogram to rule out abnormalities of bladder compliance and abnormalities of urethral support. Following that determination, an abdominal leak point pressure (ALLP) test is performed. Leak point pressure, stated in cm H2O, is defined as the intra-abdominal pressure at which leakage occurs from the bladder (around a catheter) when the bladder has been filled with a minimum of 150 cc fluid. If the patient has an ALLP of less than 100 cm H2O, the diagnosis of ISD is established.

To use a collagen implant, physicians must have urology training in the use of a cystoscope and must complete a collagen implant training program.

Coverage of a collagen implant, and the procedure to inject it, is limited to the following types of patients with stress urinary incontinence due to ISD:

Male or female patients with congenital sphincter weakness secondary to conditions such as myelomeningocele or epispadias; :

Male or female patients with acquired sphincter weakness secondary to spinal cord lesions; :

Male patients following trauma, including prostatectomy and/or radiation; and :

Female patients without urethral hypermobility and with abdominal leak point pressures of 100 cm H2O or less. :

Patients whose incontinence does not improve with 5 injection procedures (5 separate treatment sessions) are considered treatment failures, and no further treatment of urinary incontinence by collagen implant is covered. Patients who have a reoccurrence of incontinence following successful treatment with collagen implants in the past (e.g., 6-12 months previously) may benefit from additional treatment sessions. Coverage of additional sessions may be allowed but must be supported by medical justification.

C.Non-Implantable Pelvic Floor Electrical Stimulator.--(See §60-24.)

Pub. 100-3, Section 230.12

Dimethyl Sulfoxide (DMSO)

The Food and Drug Administration has determined that the only purpose for which DMSO is safe and effective for humans is in the treatment of the bladder condition, interstitial cystitis. Therefore, the use of DMSO for all other indications is not considered to be reasonable and necessary. Payment may be made for its use only when reasonable and necessary for a patient in the treatment of interstitial cystitis.

Pub. 100-3, Section 230.16

Bladder Stimulators (Pacemakers)

The use of spinal cord electrical stimulators, rectal electrical stimulators, and bladder wall stimulators is not considered reasonable and necessary. Therefore, no program payment may be made for these devices or for their implantation.

Pub. 100-3, Section 230.17

Urinary Drainage Bags

Urinary collection and retention system are covered as prosthetic devices that replace bladder function in the case of permanent urinary incontinence. There is insufficient evidence to support the medical necessity of a single use system bag rather than the multi-use bag. Therefore, a single use drainage system is subject to the same coverage parameters as the multi-use drainage bags.

Pub. 100-3, Section 240.2

Home Use of Oxygen

A - General

Medicare coverage of home oxygen and oxygen equipment under the durable medical equipment (DME) benefit (see §1861(s)(6) of the Act) is considered reasonable and necessary only for patients with significant hypoxemia who meet the medical documentation, laboratory evidence, and health conditions specified in subsections B, C, and D. This section also includes special coverage criteria for portable oxygen systems. Finally, a statement on the absence of coverage of the professional services of a respiratory therapist under the DME benefit is included in subsection F.

B - Medical Documentation

Initial claims for oxygen services must include a completed span Form CMS-484 (Certificate of Medical Necessity: Oxygen)to establish whether coverage criteria are met and to ensure that the oxygen services provided are consistent with the physician's prescription or other medical documentation. The treating physician's prescription or other medical documentation must indicate that other forms of treatment (e.g., medical and physical therapy directed at secretions, bronchospasm and infection) have been tried, have not been sufficiently successful, and oxygen therapy is still required. While there is no substitute for oxygen therapy, each patient must receive optimum therapy before long-term home oxygen therapy is ordered. Use Form CMS-484 for recertifications. (See the Medicare Program Integrity Manual, Chapter 5, for completion of Form CMS-484.)

The medical and prescription information in section B of Form CMS-484 can be completed only by the treating physician, the physician's employee, or another clinician (e.g., nurse, respiratory therapist, etc.) as long as that person is not the DME supplier. Although hospital discharge coordinators and medical social workers may assist in arranging for physician-prescribed home oxygen, they do not have the authority to prescribe the services. Suppliers may not enter this information. While this section may be completed by nonphysician clinician or a physician employee, it must be reviewed and the form CMS-484 signed by the attending physician.

A physician's certification of medical necessity for oxygen equipment must include the results of specific testing before coverage can be determined.

Claims for oxygen must also be supported by medical documentation in the patient's record. Separate documentation is used with electronic billing. (See Medicare Carriers Manual, Part 3, §4105.5.) This documentation may be in the form of a prescription written by the patient's attending physician who has recently examined the patient (normally within a month of the start of therapy) and must specify:

A diagnosis of the disease requiring home use of oxygen; :

The oxygen flow rate; and :

An estimate of the frequency, duration of use (e.g., 2 liters per minute, 10 minutes per hour, 12 hours per day), and duration of need (e.g., 6 months or lifetime). :

NOTE: A prescription for "Oxygen PRN" or "Oxygen as needed" does not meet this last requirement. Neither provides any basis for determining if the amount of oxygen is reasonable and necessary for the patient.

A member of the carrier's medical staff should review all claims with oxygen flow rates of more than 4 liters per minute before payment can be made.

The attending physician specifies the type of oxygen delivery system to be used (i.e., gas, liquid, or concentrator) by signing the completed form CMS-484. In addition the supplier or physician may use the space in section C for written confirmation of additional details of the physician's order. The additional order information contained in section C may include the means of oxygen delivery (mask, nasal, cannula, etc.), the specifics of varying flow rates, and/or the noncontinuous use of oxygen as appropriate. The physician confirms this order information with their signature in section D.

New medical documentation written by the patient's attending physician must be submitted to the carrier in support of revised oxygen requirements when there has been a change in the patient's condition and need for oxygen therapy.

Carriers are required to conduct periodic, continuing medical necessity reviews on patients whose conditions warrant these reviews and on patients with indefinite or extended periods of necessity as described in the Medicare Program Integrity Manual, Chapter 5, "Items and Services Having Special DMERC Review Considerations." When indicated, carriers may also request documentation of the results of a repeat arterial blood gas or oximetry study.

NOTE: Section 4152 of OBRA 1990 requires earlier recertification and retesting of oxygen patients who begin coverage with an arterial blood gas result at or above a partial pressure of 55 or an arterial oxygen saturation percentage at or above 89. (See the Medicare Claims Processing Manual, Chapter 20, "Durable Medical Equipment, Prosthetics and Orthotics, and Supplies (DMEPOS)," §100.2.3 for certification and retesting schedules.)

C - Laboratory Evidence

Initial claims for oxygen therapy must also include the results of a blood gas study that has been ordered and evaluated by the attending physician. This is usually in the form of a measurement of the partial pressure of oxygen (PO 2) in arterial blood. (See Medicare Carriers Manual, Part 3, §2070.1 for instructions on clinical laboratory tests.) A measurement of arterial oxygen saturation obtained by ear or pulse oximetry, however, is also acceptable when ordered and evaluated by the attending physician and performed under his or her supervision or when performed by a qualified provider or supplier of laboratory services. When the arterial blood gas and the oximetry studies are both used to document the need for home oxygen therapy and the results are conflicting, the arterial blood gas study is the preferred source of documenting medical need. A DME supplier is not considered a qualified provider or supplier of laboratory services for purposes of these guidelines. This prohibition does not extend to the results of blood gas test conducted by a hospital certified to do such tests. The conditions under which the laboratory tests are performed must be specified in writing and submitted with the initial claim, i.e., at rest, during exercise, or during sleep.

The preferred sources of laboratory evidence are existing physician and/or hospital records that reflect the patient's medical condition. Since it is expected that virtually all patients who qualify for home oxygen coverage for the first time under these guidelines have recently been discharged from a hospital where they submitted to arterial blood gas tests, the carrier needs to request that such test results be submitted in support of their initial claims for home oxygen. If more than one arterial blood gas test is performed during the patient's hospital stay, the test result obtained closest to, but no earlier than 2 days prior to the hospital discharge date is required as evidence of the need for home oxygen therapy.

For those patients whose initial oxygen prescription did not originate during a hospital stay, blood gas studies should be done while the patient is in the chronic stable state, i.e., not during a period of an acute illness or an exacerbation of their underlying disease.

Carriers may accept a attending physician's statement of recent hospital test results for a particular patient, when appropriate, in lieu of copies of actual hospital records.

A repeat arterial blood gas study is appropriate when evidence indicates that an oxygen recipient has undergone a major change in their condition relevant to home use of oxygen. If the carrier has reason to believe that there has been a major change in the patient's physical condition, it may ask for documentation of the results of another blood gas or oximetry study.

D   Health Conditions

Coverage is available for patients with significant hypoxemia in the chronic stable state if:

1.The attending physician has determined that the patient has a health condition outlined in subsection D.1,

2.The patient meets the blood gas evidence requirements specified in subsection D.3, and

3.The patient has appropriately tried other alternative treatment measures without complete success. (See subsection B.)

1 - Conditions for Which Oxygen Therapy May Be Covered

A severe lung disease, such as chronic obstructive pulmonary disease, diffuse interstitial lung disease, whether of known or unknown etiology; cystic fibrosis bronchiectasis; widespread pulmonary neoplasm; or :

Hypoxia-related symptoms or findings that might be expected to improve with oxygen therapy. Examples of these symptoms and findings are pulmonary hypertension, recurring congestive heart failure due to chronic cor pulmonale, erythrocytosis, impairment of the cognitive process, nocturnal restlessness, and morning headache. :

2 - Conditions for Which Oxygen Therapy Is Not Covered

Angina pectoris in the absence of hypoxemia. This condition is generally not the result of a low oxygen level in the blood, and there are other preferred treatments; :

Breathlessness without cor pulmonale or evidence of hypoxemia. Although intermittent oxygen use is sometimes prescribed to relieve this condition, it is potentially harmful and psychologically addicting; :

Severe peripheral vascular disease resulting in clinically evident desaturation in one or more extremities. There is no evidence that increased PO 2 improves the oxygenation of tissues with impaired circulation; or :

Terminal illnesses that do not affect the lungs. :

3 - Covered Blood Gas Values

If the patient has a condition specified in subsection D.1, the carrier must review the medical documentation and laboratory evidence that has been submitted for a particular patient (see subsections B and C) and determine if coverage is available under one of the three group categories outlined below.

a.Group I - Except as modified in subsection d, coverage is provided for patients with significant hypoxemia evidenced by any of the following:

An arterial PO 2 at or below 55 mm Hg, or an arterial oxygen saturation at or below 88 percent, taken at rest, breathing room air. :

An arterial PO 2 at or below 55 mm Hg, or an arterial oxygen saturation at or below 88 percent, taken during sleep for a patient who demonstrates an arterial PO 2 at or above 56 mm Hg, or an arterial oxygen saturation at or above 89 percent, while awake; or a greater than normal fall in oxygen level during sleep (a decrease in arterial PO 2 more than 10 mm Hg, or decrease in arterial oxygen saturation more than 5 percent) associated with symptoms or signs reasonably attributable to hypoxemia (e.g., impairment of cognitive processes and nocturnal restlessness or insomnia). In either of these cases, coverage is provided only for use of oxygen during sleep, and then only one type of unit will be covered. Portable oxygen, therefore, would not be covered in this situation. :

An arterial PO 2 at or below 55 mm Hg or an arterial oxygen saturation at or below 88 percent, taken during exercise for a patient who demonstrates an arterial PO 2 at or above 56 mm Hg, or an arterial oxygen saturation at or above 89 percent, during the day while at rest. In this case, supplemental oxygen is provided for during exercise if there is evidence the use of oxygen improves the hypoxemia that was demonstrated during exercise when the patient was breathing room air. :

b.Group II - Except as modified in subsection d, coverage is available for patients whose arterial PO 2 is 56-59 mm Hg or whose arterial blood oxygen saturation is 89 percent, if there is evidence of:

Dependent edema suggesting congestive heart failure; :

Pulmonary hypertension or cor pulmonale, determined by measurement of pulmonary artery pressure, gated blood pool scan, echocardiogram, or "P" pulmonale on EKG (P wave greater than 3 mm in standard leads II, III, or AVFL; or

Erythrocythemia with a hematocrit greater than 56 percent. :

c.Group III - Except as modified in subsection d, carriers must apply a rebuttable presumption that a home program of oxygen use is not medically necessary for patients with arterial PO 2 levels at or above 60 mm Hg, or arterial blood oxygen saturation at or above 90 percent. In order for claims in this category to be reimbursed, the carrier's reviewing physician needs to review any documentation submitted in rebuttal of this presumption and grant specific approval of the claims. CMS expects few claims to be approved for coverage in this category.

d.Variable Factors That May Affect Blood Gas Values - In reviewing the arterial PO 2 levels and the arterial oxygen saturation percentages specified in subsections D.3.a, b and c, the carrier's medical staff must take into account variations in oxygen measurements that may result from such factors as the patient's age, the altitude level, or the patient's decreased oxygen carrying capacity.

E - Portable Oxygen Systems

A patient meeting the requirements specified below may qualify for coverage of a portable oxygen system either (1) by itself or (2) to use in addition to a stationary oxygen system. A portable oxygen system is covered for a particular patient if:

The claim meets the requirements specified in subsections A-D, as appropriate; and :

The medical documentation indicates that the patient is mobile in the home and would benefit from the use of a portable oxygen system in the home. Portable oxygen systems are not covered for patients who qualify for oxygen solely based on blood gas studies obtained during sleep. :

F - Respiratory Therapists

Respiratory therapists' services are not covered under the provisions for coverage of oxygen services under the Part B durable medical equipment benefit as outlined above. This benefit provides for coveravge of home use of oxygen and oxygen equipment, but does not include a professional component in the delivery of such services.

Pub. 100-3, Section 240.4

Continuous Positive Airway Pressure (CPAP)

B. Nationally Covered Indications

The use of CPAP is covered under Medicare when used in adult patients with moderate or severe OSA for whom surgery is a likely alternative to CPAP. The use of CPAP devices must be ordered and prescribed by the licensed treating physician to be used in adult patients with moderate to severe OSA if either of the following criterion using the Apnea-Hypopnea Index (AHI) are met:

AHI greater than or equal to 15 events per hour, or:

AHI greater than or equal to 5 and less than or equal to 14 events per hour with documented symptoms of excessive daytime sleepiness, impaired cognition, mood disorders or insomnia, or documented hypertension, ischemic heart disease, or history of stroke.:

The AHI is equal to the average number of episodes of apnea and hypopnea per hour and must be based on a minimum of 2 hours of sleep recorded by polysomnography using actual recorded hours of sleep (i.e., the AHI may not be extrapolated or projected).

Apnea is defined as cessation of airflow for least 10 seconds. Hypopnea is defined as an abnormal respiratory event lasting at least 10 seconds with at least 30 percent reduction in thoracoabdominal movement or aiflow as compared to baseline, and with at least a 4 percent oxygen desaturation.

The polysomnography must be performed in a facility - based sleep study laboratory, and not in the home or in a mobile facility.

Initial claims must be supported by medical documentation (separate documentation where electronic billing is used), such as prescription written by the patient's attending physician that specifies:

A diagnosis of moderate or severe obstructive sleep apnea, and:

Surgery is a likely alternative.:

The claim must also certify that the documentation supporting a diagnosis of OSA (described above) is available.

C. Nationally Non-covered Indications

Effective April 4, 2005, the Centers for Medicare & Medicaid Services determined that upon reconsideration of the current policy, there is not sufficient evidence to conclude that unattended portable multi-channel sleep study testing is reasonable and necessary in the diagnosis of OSA for CPAP therapy, and these tests will remain noncovered for this purpose.

D. Other

N/A

(This NCD last reviewed April 2005)

Pub. 100-3, Section 240.5

Intrapulmonary Percussive Ventilator (IPV)

Studies do not demonstrate any advantage of IPV over that achieved with good pulmonary care in the hospital environment and there are no studies in the home setting. There are no data to support the effectiveness of the device. Therefore, IPV in the home setting is not covered.

Pub. 100-3, Section 260.3

Pancreas Transplants

B. National Covered Indications

CMS determines that whole organ pancreas transplantation will be nationally covered by Medicare only when performed siumltaneous with or after a kidney transplant. If the pancreas transplant occurs after the kidney transplant, immunosuppressive therapy will begin with the date of discharge from the inpatient stay for the pancrease transplant.

C. Nationally Noncovered Indications

CMS determines that the following procedures are not considered reasonable and necessary within the meaning of section 1862(a)(1)(A) of the Social Security Act:

1. Pancreas transplantation for diabetic patients who have not experienced end stage renal failure secondary to diabetes.

2. Transplantation of partial pancreatic tissue or islet cells (except in the context of a clinical trial (see section 260.3.1 of the NCD Manual)).

D. Other

Not applicable

(This NCD last reviewed July 2004.)

Pub. 100-3, Section 260.6

Dental Examination Prior to Kidney Transplantation

Despite the "dental services exclusion" in §1862(a)(12) of the Act (see the Medicare Benefit Policy Manual,Chapter 16, "General Exclusions from Coverage" §140), an oral or dental examination performed on an inpatient basis as part of a comprehensive workup prior to renal transplant surgery is a covered service. This is because the purpose of the examination is not for the care of the teeth or structures directly supporting the teeth. Rather, the examination is for the identification, prior to a complex surgical procedure, of existing medical problems where the increased possibility of infection would not only reduce the chances for successful surgery but would also expose the patient to additional risks in undergoing such surgery.

Such a dental or oral examination would be covered under Part A of the program if performed by a dentist on the hospital's staff, or under Part B if performed by a physician. (When performing a dental or oral examination, a dentist is not recognized as a physician under §1861(r) of the law.)(See the Mediacre Geneal Information, Eligibility and Entitlement Manual, Chapter 15, "Covered Medical and Other Health Services," §150)

Pub. 100-3, Section 260.7

Lymphocyte Immune Globulin, Anti-Thymocyte Globulin (Equine)

The FDA has approved one lymphocyte immune globulin preparation for marketing, lymphocyte immune globulin, anti-thymocyte globulin (equine). This drug is indicated for the management of allograft rejection episodes in renal transplantation. It is covered under Medicare when used for this purpose. Other forms of lymphocyte globulin preparation which the FDA approves for this indication in the future may be covered under Medicare.

Pub. 100-3, Section 270.1

Electrical Stimulation (ES) and Electromagnetic Therapy for the Treatment of Wounds

A. Nationally Covered Indications

The use of ES and electromagnetic therapy for the treatment of wounds are considered adjunctive therapies, and will only be covered for chronic Stage III or Stage IV pressure ulcers, arterial ulcers, diabetic ulcers, and venous stasis ulcers. Chronic ulcers are defined as ulcers that have not healed within 30 days of occurrence. ES or electromagnetic therapy will be covered only after appropriate standard wound care has been tried for at least 30 days and there are no measurable signs of improved healing. This 30-day period may begin while the wound is acute.

Standard wound care includes: optimization of nutritional status, debridement by any means to remove devitalized tissue, maintenance of a clean, moist bed of granulation tissue with appropriate moist dressings, and necessary treatment to resolve any infection that may be present. Standard wound care based on the specific type of wound includes: frequent repositioning of a patient with pressure ulcers (usually every 2 hours), offloading of pressure and good glucose control for diabetic ulcers, establishment of adequate circulation for arterial ulcers, and the use of a compression system for patients with venous ulcers.

Measurable signs of improved healing include: a decrease in wound size (either surface area or volume), decrease in amount of exudates, and decrease in amount of necrotic tissue. ES or electromagnetic therapy must be discontinued when the wound demonstrates 100% epitheliliazed wound bed.

ES and electromagnetic therapy services can only be covered when performed by a physician, physical therapist, or incident to a physician service. Evaluation of the wound is an integral part of wound therapy. When a physician, physical therapist, or a clinician incident to a physician, performs ES or electromagnetic therapy, the practitioner must evaluate the wound and contact the treating physician if the wound worsens. If ES or electromagnetic therapy is being used, wounds must be evaluated at least monthly by the treating physician.

B. Nationally Noncovered Indications

1. ES and electromagnetic therapy will not be covered as an initial treatment modality.

2. Continued treatment with ES or electromagnetic therapy is not covered if measurable signs of healing have not been demonstrated within any 30-day period of treatment.

3. Unsupervised use of ES or electromagnetic therapy for wound therapy will not be covered, as this use has not been found to be medically reasonable and necessary.

C. Other

All other uses of ES and electromagnetic therapy not otherwise specified for the treatment of wounds remain at local contractor discretion.

(This NCD last reviewed March 2004.)

Pub. 100-3, Section 270.2

Noncontact Normothermic Wound Therapy (NNWT)

There is insufficient scientific or clinical evidence to consider this device as reasonable and necessary for the treatment of wounds within the meaning of §1862(a)(1)(A) of the Social Security Act and will not be covered by Medicare.

Pub. 100-3, Section 280.1

Durable Medical Equipment Reference List

Durable Medical Equipment Reference List

Air Cleaners	Deny--environmental control equipment; not primarily medical in nature (§1861(n) of the Act).
Air Conditioners	Deny--environmental control equipment; not primarily medical in nature (§1861 (n) of the Act).
Air-Fluidized Bed s	(See Air-Fluidized Beds, §280.8 of the NCD Manual.)
Alternating Pressure Pads, Mattresses and Lambs Wool Pads	Covered if patient has, or is highly susceptible to, decubitus ulcers and the patient's physician specifies that he/she has specified that he will be supervising the course of treatment.
Audible/Visible Signal/Pacemaker Monitors	(See Self-Contained Pacemaker Monitors.)
Augmentative Communication Devices	(See Speech Generating Devices, §50.1 of the NCD Manual.)
Bathtub Lifts	Deny--convenience item; not primarily medical in nature (§1861(n) of the Act).
Bathtub Seats	Deny--comfort or convenience item; hygienic equipment; not primarily medical in nature (§1861(n) of the Act).
Bead Beds	(See §280.8 of the NCD Manual.)
Bed Baths (home type)	Deny--hygienic equipment; not primarily medical in nature (§1861(n) of the Act).
Bed Lifter s (bed elevators)	Deny--not primarily medical in nature (§1861(n) of the Act).
Bedboards	Deny--not primarily medical in nature (§1861(n) of the Act).
Bed Pans (autoclavable hospital type)	Covered if patient is bed confined.
Bed Side Rails	(See Hospital Beds, §280.7 of the NCD Manual.)
Beds-Lounge s (power or manual)	Deny--not a hospital bed; comfort or convenience item; not primarily medical in nature (§1861(n) of the Act).
Beds--Oscillating	Deny--institutional equipment; inappropriate for home use.
Bidet Toilet Seats	(See Toilet Seats.)
Blood Glucose Analyzers -- Reflectance Colorimeter	Deny--unsuitable for home use (see §40.2 of the NCD Manual).
Blood Glucose Monitors	Covered if patient meets certain conditions (see §40.2 of the NCD Manual).
Braille Teaching Texts	Deny--educational equipment; not primarily medical in nature (§1861(n) of the Act).
Canes	Covered if patient meets Mobility Assistive Equipment clinical criteria (see §280.3 of the NCD Manual).
Carafes	Deny--convenience item; not primarily medical in nature (§1861(n) of the Act).
Catheters	Deny--nonreusable disposable supply (§1861(n) of the Act). (See The Medicare Claims Processing Manual, Chapter 20, DMEPOS).
Commodes	Covered if patient is confined to bed or room.NOTE: The term "room confined" means that the patient's condition is such that leaving the room is medically contraindicated. The accessibility of bathroom facilities generally would not be a factor in this determination. However, confinement of a patient to a home in a case where there are no toilet facilities in the home may be equated to room confinement. Moreover, payment may also be made if a patient's medical condition confines him to a floor of the home and there is no bathroom located on that floor.

Communicators (See §50.1 of the NCD Manual, "Speech Generating Devices.")	
Continuous Passive Motion Devices	Continuous passive motion devices are devices Covered for patients who have received a total knee replacement. To qualify for coverage, use of the device must commence within 2 days following surgery. In addition, coverage is limited to that portion of the 3-week period following surgery during which the device is used in the patient's home. There is insufficient evidence to justify coverage of these devices for longer periods of time or for other applications.
Continuous Positive Airway Pressure (CPAP) Devices	(See §240.4 of the NCD Manual.)
Crutches	Covered if patient meets Mobility Assistive Equipment clinical criteria (see section 280.3 of the NCD Manual).
Cushion Lift Power Seats	(See Seat Lifts.)
Dehumidifiers (room or central heating system type)	Deny--environmental control equipment; not primarily medical in nature (§1861(n) of the Act).
Diathermy Machines (standard pulses wave types)	Deny--inappropriate for home use (see §150.5 of the NCD Manual).
Digital Electronic Pacemaker Monitors	(See Self-Contained Pacemaker Monitor s .)
Disposable Sheets and Bags	Deny--nonreusable disposable supplies (§1861(n) of the Act).
Elastic Stockings	Deny--nonreusable supply; not rental-type items (§1861(n) of the Act). (See §270.5 of the NCD Manual.)
Electric Air Cleaners	Deny--(See Air Cleaners.) (§1861(n) of the Act).
Electric Hospital Beds	(See Hospital Beds §280.7 of the NCD Manual.)
Electrical Stimulation for Wounds	Deny--inappropriate for home use. (See §270.1 of the NCD Manual.)
Electrostatic Machines	Deny--(See Air Cleaners and Air Conditioners.) (§1861(n) of the Act).
Elevators	Deny--convenience item; not primarily medical in nature (§1861(n) of the Act).
Emesis Basins	Deny--convenience item; not primarily medical in nature (§1861(n) of the Act).
Esophageal Dilators	Deny--physician instrument; inappropriate for patient use.
Exercise Equipment	Deny--not primarily medical in nature (§1861(n) of the Act).
Fabric Supports	Deny--nonreusable supplies; not rental-type items (§1861(n) of the Act).
Face Masks (oxygen)	Covered if oxygen is covered. (See §240.2 of the NCD Manual.)
Face Masks (surgical)	Deny--nonreusable disposable items (§1861(n) of the Act).
Flowmeters	(See Medical Oxygen Regulators.) (See §240.2 of the NCD Manual.)
Fluidic Breathing Assisters	(See Intermittent Positive Pressure Breathing Machines.)
Fomentation Devices	(See Heating Pads.)
Gel Flotation Pads and Mattresses	(See Alternating Pressure Pads and Mattresses.)
Grab Bars	Deny--self-help device; not primarily medical in nature (§1861(n) of the Act).
Heat and Massage Foam Cushion Pads	Deny--notprimarily medical in nature; personal comfort item (§§1861(n) and 1862(a)(6) of the Act).
Heating and Cooling Plants	Deny--environmental control equipment not primarily medical in nature (§1861(n) of the Act).
Heating Pads	Covered if the contractor's medical staff determines patient's medical condition is one for which the application of heat in the form of a heating pad is therapeutically effective.

Heat Lamps	Covered if the contractor's medical staff determines patient's medical condition is one for which the application of heat in the form of a heat lamp is therapeutically effective.
Hospital Beds	(See §280.7 of the NCD Manual.)
Hot Packs	(See Heating Pads.)
Humidifiers (oxygen)	(See Oxygen Humidifiers.)
Humidifiers (room or central heating system types)	Deny--environmental control equipment; not medical in nature (§1861(n) of the Act).
Hydraulic Lift s	(See Patient Lifts.)
Incontinent Pads	Deny--nonreusable supply; hygienic item (§1861(n) of the Act).
Infusion Pumps	For external and implantable pumps, see §40.2 of the NCD Manual. If the pump is used with an enteral or parenteral nutritional therapy system. (See §180.2 of the NCD Manual for special coverage rules.)
Injectors (hypodermic jet	Deny--not covered self-administered drug supply;pressure powered devices (§1861(s)(2)(A) of the Act) for injection of insulin.
Intermittent Positive Pressure Breathing Machines	Covered if patient's ability to breathe is severely impaired.
Iron Lungs	(See Ventilators.)
Irrigating Kit s	Deny--nonreusable supply; hygienic equipment (§1861(n) of the Act).
Lambs Wool Pads	(See Alternating Pressure Pads, Mattresses, and Lamb s Wool Pads.)
Leotards	Deny--(See Pressure Leotards.) (§1861(n) of the Act).
Lymphedema Pumps	Covered--(See Pneumatic Compression Devices, §280.6 of the NCD Manual.)
Massage Devices	Deny--personal comfort items; not primarily medical in nature (§§1861(n) and 1862(a)(6) of the Act).
Mattresses	Covered only where hospital bed is medically necessary. (Separate Charge for replacement mattress should not be allowed where hospital bed with mattress is rented.) (See §280.7 of the NCD Manual.)
Medical Oxygen Regulators	Covered if patient's ability to breathe is severely impaired. (See §240.2 of the NCD Manual.)
Mobile Geriatric Chairs	Covered if patient meets Mobility Assistive Equipment clinical criteria (see §280.3 of the NCD Manual).
Motorized Wheelchairs	Covered if patient meets Mobility Assistive Equipment clinical criteria (see §280.3 of the NCD manual).
Muscle Stimulators	Covered for certain conditions. (See §250.4 of the NCD Manual.)
Nebulizers	Covered if patient's ability to breathe is severely impaired.
Oscillating Beds	Deny--institutional equipment - inappropriate for home use.
Overbed Tables	Deny--convenience item; not primarily medical in nature (§1861(n) of the Act).
Oxygen	Covered if the oxygen has been prescribed for use in connection with medically necessary DME . (See §240.2 of the NCD Manual.)
Oxygen Humidifiers	Covered if the oxygen has been prescribed for use in connection with medically necessary DME for purposes of moisturizing oxygen. (See §240.2 of the NCD Manual.)
Oxygen Regulators (Medical)	(See Medical Oxygen Regulators.)
Oxygen Tents	(See §240.2 of the NCD Manual.)
Paraffin Bath Units (Portable)	(See Portable Paraffin Bath Units.)
Paraffin Bath Units (Standard)	Deny--institutional equipment; inappropriate for home use.
Parallel Bars	Deny--support exercise equipment; primarily for institutional use; in the home setting other devices (e.g., walkers) satisfy the patient's need.

Appendix 4 — Pub 100 References

Patient Lifts	Covered if contractor's medical staff determines patient's condition is such that periodic movement is necessary to effect improvement or to arrest or retard deterioration in his condition.
Percussors	Covered for mobilizing respiratory tract secretions in patients with chronic obstructive lung disease, chronic bronchitis, or emphysema, when patient or operator of powered percussor receives appropriate training by a physician or therapist, and no one competent to administer manual therapy is available.
Portable Oxygen Systems	1. Regulated Covered (adjustable Covered under conditions specified in a flow rate). Refer all claims to medical staff for this determination.2. Preset Deny (flow rate Deny emergency, first-aid, or not adjustable) precautionary equipment; essentially not therapeutic in nature.
Portable Paraffin Bath Units	Covered when the patient has undergone a successful trial period of paraffin therapy ordered by a physician and the patient's condition is expected to be relieved by long term use of this modality.
Portable Room Heaters	Deny--environmental control equipment; not primarily medical in nature (§1861(n) of the Act).
Portable Whirlpool Pumps	Deny--not primarily medical in nature; personal comfort items (§§1861(n) and 1862(a)(6) of the Act).
Postural Drainage Boards	Covered if patient has a chronic pulmonary condition.
Preset Portable Oxygen Units	Deny--emergency, first-aid, or precautionary equipment; essentially not therapeutic in nature.
Pressure Leotards	Deny--non-reusable supply, not rental-type item (§1861(n) of the Act).
Pulse Tachometers	Deny--not reasonable or necessary for monitoring pulse of homebound patient with or without a cardiac pacemaker.
Quad-Canes	Covered if patient meets Mobility Assistive Equipment clinical criteria (see §280.3 of the NCD Manual).
Raised Toilet Seats	Deny--convenience item; hygienic equipment; not primarily medical in nature (§1861(n) of the Act).
Reflectance Colorimeters	(See Blood Glucose Analyzers.)
Respirators	(See Ventilators.)
Rolling Chairs	Covered if patient meets Mobility Assistive Equipment clinical criteria (see §280.3 of the NCD Manual). Coverage is limited to those roll-about chairs having casters of at least 5 inches in diameter and specifically designed to meet the needs of ill, injured, or otherwise impaired individuals. Coverage is denied for the wide range of chairs with smaller casters as are found in general use in homes, offices, and institutions for many purposes not related to the care/treatment of ill/injured persons. This type is not primarily medical in nature. (§1861(n) of the Act.)
Safety Rollers	Covered if patient meets Mobility Assistive Equipment clinical criteria (see §280.3 of the NCD Manual).
Sauna Baths	Deny--not primarily medical in nature; personal comfort items (§§1861(n) and 1862(a)(6) of the Act).
Seat Lifts	Covered under the conditions specified in §280.4 of the NCD Manual. Refer all to medical staff for this determination.
Self Contained Pacemaker Monitors	Covered when prescribed by a physician for a patient with a cardiac pacemaker. (See §§20.8.1 and 280.2 of the NCD Manual.)
Sitz Baths	Covered if the contractor's medical staff determines patient has an infection or injury of the perineal area and the item has been prescribed by the patient's physician as a part of his planned regimen of treatment in the patient's home.
Spare Tanks of Oxygen	Deny--convenience or precautionary supply.
Speech Teaching Machines	Deny--education equipment; not primarily medical in nature (§1861(n) of the Act).
Stairway Elevators	Deny--(See Elevators.) (§1861(n) of the Act).
Standing Tables	Deny--convenience item; not primarily medical in nature (§1861(n) of the Act).
Steam Packs	These packs are Covered under the same condition s as heating pad s . (See Heating Pads.)
Suction Machines	Covered if the contractor's medical staff determines that the machine specified in the claim is medically required and appropriate for home use without technical or professional supervision.
Support Hose	Deny (See Fabric Supports.) (§1861(n) of the Act).
Surgical Leggings	Deny--non-reusable supply; not rental-type item (§1861(n) of the Act).
Telephone Alert Systems	Deny--these are emergency communications systems and do not serve a diagnostic or therapeutic purpose
Toilet Seats	Deny--not medical equipment (§1861(n) of the Act).
Traction Equipment	Covered if patient has orthopedic impairment requiring traction equipment that prevents ambulation during the period of use (Consider covering devices usable during ambulation; e.g., cervical traction collar, under the brace provision).
Trapeze Bars	Covered if patient is bed confined and the patient needs a trapeze bar to sit up because of respiratory condition, to change body position for other medical reasons, or to get in and out of bed.
Treadmill Exercisers	Deny--exercise equipment; not primarily medical in nature (§1861(n) of the Act).
Ultraviolet Cabinets	Covered for selected patients with generalized intractable psoriasis. Using appropriate consultation, the contractor should determine whether medical and other factors justify treatment at home rather than at alternative sites, e.g., outpatient department of a hospital.
Urinals autoclavable	Covered if patient is bed confined hospital type.
Vaporizers	Covered if patient has a respiratory illness.
Ventilators	Covered for treatment of neuromuscular diseases, thoracic restrictive diseases, and chronic respiratory failure consequent to chronic obstructive pulmonary disease. Includes both positive and negative pressure types. (See §240.5 of the NCD Manual.)
Walkers	Covered if patient meets Mobility Assistive Equipment clinical criteria (see §280.3 of the NCD Manual).
Water and Pressure Pads and Mattresses	(See Alternating Pressure Pads, Mattresses and Lamb Wool Pads.)
Wheelchairs (manual)	Covered if patient meets Mobility Assistive Equipment clinical criteria (see §280.3 of the NCD Manual).
Wheelchairs (power operated)	Covered if patient meets Mobility Assistive Equipment clinical criteria (see §280.3 of the NCD Manual).
Wheelchairs (scooter/POV)	Covered if patient meets Mobility Assistive Equipment clinical criteria (see §280.3 of the NCD Manual).
Wheelchairs (specially-sized)	Covered if patient meets Mobility Assistive Equipment clinical criteria (see §280.3 of the NCD Manual).
Whirlpool Bath Equipment	Covered if patient is homebound and has a (standard)condition for which the whirlpool bath can be expected to provide substantial therapeutic benefit justifying its cost. Where patient is not homebound but has such a condition, payment is restricted to the cost of providing the services elsewhere; e.g., an outpatient department of a participating hospital, if that alternative is less costly. In all cases, refer claim to medical staff for a determination.
Whirlpool Pumps	Deny--(See Portable Whirlpool Pumps.) (§1861(n) of the Act).
White Canes	Deny--(See §280.2 of the NCD Manual.) (Not considered Mobility Assistive Equipment)

Pub. 100-3, Section 280.2

White Cane For Use By A Blind Person

A white cane for use by a blind person is more an identifying and self-help device rather than an item which makes a meaningful contribution in the treatment of an illness or injury.

Pub. 100-3, Section 280.3

Mobility Assistive Equipment

B. Nationally Covered Indications

Effective May 5, 2005, CMS finds that the evidence is adequate to determine that MAE is reasonable and necessary for beneficiaries who have a personal mobility deficit sufficient to impair their participation in mobility-related activities of daily living (MRADLs) such as toileting, feeding, dressing, grooming, and bathing in customary locations within the home. Determination of the presence of a mobility deficit will be made by an algorithmic process, Clinical Criteria for MAE Coverage, to provide the appropriate MAE to correct the mobility deficit.

Clinical Criteria for MAE Coverage

The beneficiary, the beneficiary's family or other caregiver, or a clinician, will usually initiate the discussion and consideration of MAE use. Sequential consideration of the questions below provides clinical guidance for the coverage of equipment of appropriate type and complexity to restore the beneficiary's ability to participate in MRADLs such as toileting, feeding, dressing, grooming, and bathing in customary locations in the home. These questions correspond to the numbered decision points on the accompanying flow chart. In individual cases where the beneficiary's condition clearly and unambiguously precludes the reasonable use of a device, it is not necessary to undertake a trial of that device for that beneficiary.

1.Does the beneficiary have a mobility limitation that significantly impairs his/her ability to participate in one or more MRADLs in the home? A mobility limitation is one that:

a.Prevents the beneficiary from accomplishing the MRADLs entirely, or,

b.Places the beneficiary at reasonably determined heightened risk of morbidity or mortality secondary to the attempts to participate in MRADLs, or,

c.Prevents the beneficiary from completing the MRADLs within a reasonable time frame.

2.Are there other conditions that limit the beneficiary's ability to participate in MRADLs at home?

a.Some examples are significant impairment of cognition or judgment and/or vision.

b.For these beneficiaries, the provision of MAE might not enable them to participate in MRADLs if the comorbidity prevents effective use of the wheelchair or reasonable completion of the tasks even with MAE.

3.If these other limitations exist, can they be ameliorated or compensated sufficiently such that the additional provision of MAE will be reasonably expected to significantly improve the beneficiary's ability to perform or obtain assistance to participate in MRADLs in the home?

a.A caregiver, for example a family member, may be compensatory, if consistently available in the beneficiary's home and willing and able to safely operate and transfer the beneficiary to and from the wheelchair and to transport the beneficiary using the wheelchair. The caregiver's need to use a wheelchair to assist the beneficiary in the MRADLs is to be considered in this determination.

b.If the amelioration or compensation requires the beneficiary's compliance with treatment, for example medications or therapy, substantive non-compliance, whether willing or involuntary, can be grounds for denial of MAE coverage if it results in the beneficiary continuing to have a significant limitation. It may be determined that partial compliance results in adequate amelioration or compensation for the appropriate use of MAE.

4.Does the beneficiary or caregiver demonstrate the capability and the willingness to consistently operate the MAE safely?

a.Safety considerations include personal risk to the beneficiary as well as risk to others. The determination of safety may need to occur several times during the process as the consideration focuses on a specific device.

b.A history of unsafe behavior in other venues may be considered.

5.Can the functional mobility deficit be sufficiently resolved by the prescription of a cane or walker?

a.The cane or walker should be appropriately fitted to the beneficiary for this evaluation.

b.Assess the beneficiary's ability to safely use a cane or walker.

6.Does the beneficiary's typical environment support the use of wheelchairs including scooters/power-operated vehicles (POVs)?

a.Determine whether the beneficiary's environment will support the use of these types of MAE.

b.Keep in mind such factors as physical layout, surfaces, and obstacles, which may render MAE unusable in the beneficiary's home.

7.Does the beneficiary have sufficient upper extremity function to propel a manual wheelchair in the home to participate in MRADLs during a typical day? The manual wheelchair should be optimally configured (seating options, wheelbase, device weight, and other appropriate accessories) for this determination.

a.Limitations of strength, endurance, range of motion, coordination, and absence or deformity in one or both upper extremities are relevant.

b.A beneficiary with sufficient upper extremity function may qualify for a manual wheelchair. The appropriate type of manual wheelchair, i.e. light weight, etc., should be determined based on the beneficiary's physical characteristics and anticipated intensity of use.

c.The beneficiary's home should provide adequate access, maneuvering space and surfaces for the operation of a manual wheelchair.

d.Assess the beneficiary's ability to safely use a manual wheelchair.NOTE: If the beneficiary is unable to self-propel a manual wheelchair, and if there is a caregiver who is available, willing, and able to provide assistance, a manual wheelchair may be appropriate.

8.Does the beneficiary have sufficient strength and postural stability to operate a POV/scooter?

a.A POV is a 3- or 4-wheeled device with tiller steering and limited seat modification capabilities. The beneficiary must be able to maintain stability and position for adequate operation.

b.The beneficiary's home should provide adequate access, maneuvering space and surfaces for the operation of a POV.

c.Assess the beneficiary's ability to safely use a POV/scooter.

9.Are the additional features provided by a power wheelchair needed to allow the beneficiary to participate in one or more MRADLs?

a.The pertinent features of a power wheelchair compared to a POV are typically control by a joystick or alternative input device, lower seat height for slide transfers, and the ability to accommodate a variety of seating needs.

b.The type of wheelchair and options provided should be appropriate for the degree of the beneficiary's functional impairments.

c.The beneficiary's home should provide adequate access, maneuvering space and surfaces for the operation of a power wheelchair.

d.Assess the beneficiary's ability to safely use a power wheelchair.NOTE: If the beneficiary is unable to use a power wheelchair, and if there is a caregiver who is available, willing, and able to provide assistance, a manual wheelchair is appropriate. A caregiver's inability to operate a manual wheelchair can be considered in covering a power wheelchair so that the caregiver can assist the beneficiary. Flow chart

C. Nationally Non-Covered Indications

Medicare beneficiaries not meeting the clinical criteria for prescribing MAE as outlined above, and as documented by the beneficiary's physician, would not be eligible for Medicare coverage of the MAE.

D. Other

All other durable medical equipment (DME) not meeting the definition of MAE as described in this instruction will continue to be covered, or noncovered, as is currently described in the NCD Manual, in Section 280, Medical and Surgical Supplies. Also, all other sections not altered here and the corresponding policies regarding MAEs which have not been discussed here remain unchanged.

(This NCD last reviewed May 2005).

Pub. 100-3, Section 280.4

Seat Lift

Reimbursement may be made for the rental or purchase of a medically necessary seat lift when prescribed by a physician for a patient with severe arthritis of the hip or knee and patients with muscular dystrophy or other neuromuscular diseases when it has been determined the patient can benefit therapeutically from use of the device. In establishing medical necessity for the seat lift, the evidence must show that the item is included in the physician's course of treatment, that it is likely to effect improvement, or arrest or retard deterioration in the patient's condition, and that the severity of the condition is such that the alternative would be chair or bed confinement.

Coverage of seat lifts is limited to those types which operate smoothly, can be controlled by the patient, and effectively assist a patient in standing up and sitting down without other assistance. Excluded from coverage is the type of lift which operates by a spring release mechanism with a sudden, catapult-like motion and jolts the patient from a seated to a standing position. Limit the payment for units which incorporate a recliner feature along with the seat lift to the amount payable for a seat lift without this feature.

Pub. 100-3, Section 280.5

Safety Roller

Indications and Limitations of Coverage

They may be appropriate, and therefore covered, for some patients who are obese, have severe neurological disorders, or restricted use of one hand, which makes it impossible to use a wheeled walker that does not have the sophisticated braking system found on safety rollers.

In order to assure that payment is not made for a safety roller when a less expensive standard wheeled walker would satisfy the patient's medical needs, carriers refer safety roller claims to their medical consultants. The medical consultant determines whether some or all of the features provided in a safety roller are necessary, and therefore covered and reimbursable. If it is determined that the patient could use a standard wheeled walker, the charge for the safety roller is reduced to the charge of a standard wheeled walker.

Some obese patients who could use a standard wheeled walker if their weight did not exceed the walker's strength and stability limits can have it reinforced and its wheel base expanded. Such modifications are routine mechanical adjustments and justify a moderate surcharge. In these cases the carrier reduces the charge for the safety roller to the charge for the standard wheeled walker plus the surcharge for modifications.

In the case of patients with medical documentation showing severe neurological disorders or restricted use of one hand which makes it impossible for them to use a wheeled walker that does not have a sophisticated braking system, a reasonable charge for the safety roller may be determined without relating it to the reasonable charge for a standard wheeled walker. (Such reasonable charge should be developed in accordance with the instructions in Medicare Claims Processing Manual, Chapter 23.)

Pub. 100-3, Section 280.6

Pneumatic Compression Devices

Pneumatic devices are covered for the treatment of lymphedema or for the treatment of chronic venous insufficiency with venous stasis ulcers.

Lymphedema

Lymphedema is the swelling of subcutaneous tissues due to the accumulation of excessive lymph fluid. The accumulation of lymph fluid results from impairment to the normal clearing function of the lymphatic system and/or from an excessive production of lymph. Lymphedema is divided into two broad classes according to etiology. Primary lymphedema is a relatively uncommon, chronic condition which may be due to such causes as Milroy's Disease or congenital anomalies. Secondary lymphedema, which is much more common, results from the destruction of or damage to formerly functioning lymphatic channels, such as surgical removal of lymph nodes or post radiation fibrosis, among other causes.

Pneumatic compression devices are covered in the home setting for the treatment of lymphedema if the patient has undergone a four-week trial of conservative therapy and the treating physician determines that there has been no significant improvement or if significant symptoms remain after the trial. The trial of conservative therapy must include use of an appropriate compression bandage system or compression garment, exercise, and elevation of the limb. The garment may be prefabricated or custom-fabricated but must provide adequate graduated compression.

Chronic Venous Insufficiency With Venous Stasis Ulcers

Chronic venous insufficiency (CVI) of the lower extremities is a condition caused by abnormalities of the venous wall and valves, leading to obstruction or reflux of blood flow in the veins. Signs of CVI include hyperpigmentation, stasis dermatitis, chronic edema, and venous ulcers.

Pneumatic compression devices are covered in the home setting for the treatment of CVI of the lower extremities only if the patient has one or more venous stasis ulcer(s) which have failed to heal after a 6 month trial of conservative therapy directed by the treating physician. The trial of conservative therapy must include a compression bandage system or compression garment, appropriate dressings for the wound, exercise, and elevation of the limb.

General Coverage Criteria

Pneumatic compression devices are covered only when prescribed by a physician and when they are used with appropriate physician oversight, i.e., physician evaluation of the patient's condition to determine medical necessity of the device, assuring suitable instruction in the operation of the machine, a treatment plan defining the pressure to be used and the frequency and duration of use, and ongoing monitoring of use and response to treatment.

The determination by the physician of the medical necessity of a pneumatic compression device must include (1) the patient's diagnosis and prognosis; (2) symptoms and objective findings, including measurements which establish the severity of the condition; (3) the reason the device is required, including the treatments which have been tried and failed; and (4) the clinical response to an initial treatment with the device. The clinical response includes the change in pre-treatment measurements, ability to tolerate the treatment session and parameters, and ability of the patient (or caregiver) to apply the device for continued use in the home.

The only time that a segmented, calibrated gradient pneumatic compression device (HCPCs code E0652) would be covered is when the individual has unique characteristics that prevent them from receiving satisfactory pneumatic compression treatment using a nonsegmented device in conjunction with a segmented appliance or a segmented compression device without manual control of pressure in each chamber.

Pub. 100-3, Section 280.7

Hospital Beds

A. General Requirements for Coverage of Hospital Beds.--A physician's prescription, and such additional documentation as the contractors' medical staffs may consider necessary, including medical records and physicians' reports, must establish the medical necessity for a hospital bed due to one of the following reasons:

The patient's condition requires positioning of the body; e.g., to alleviate pain, promote good body alignment, prevent contractures, avoid respiratory infections, in ways not feasible in an ordinary bed; or:

The patient's condition requires special attachments that cannot be fixed and used on an ordinary bed.:

B. Physician's Prescription.--The physician's prescription, which must accompany the initial claim, and supplementing documentation when required, must establish that a hospital bed is medically necessary. If the stated reason for the need for a hospital bed is the patient's condition requires positioning, the prescription or other documentation must describe the medical condition, e.g., cardiac disease, chronic obstructive pulmonary disease, quadriplegia or paraplegia, and also the severity and frequency of the symptoms of the condition, that necessitates a hospital bed for positioning.

If the stated reason for requiring a hospital bed is the patient's condition requires special attachments, the prescription must describe the patient's condition and specify the attachments that require a hospital bed.

C. Variable Height Feature.--In well documented cases, the contractors' medical staffs may determine that a variable height feature of a hospital bed, approved for coverage under subsection A above, is medically necessary and, therefore, covered, for one of the following conditions:

Severe arthritis and other injuries to lower extremities; e.g., fractured hip. The condition requires the variable height feature to assist the patient to ambulate by enabling the patient to place his or her feet on the floor while sitting on the edge of the bed;:

Severe cardiac conditions. For those cardiac patients who are able to leave bed, but who must avoid the strain of "jumping" up or down;:

Spinal cord injuries, including quadriplegic and paraplegic patients, multiple limb amputee and stroke patients. For those patients who are able to transfer from bed to a wheelchair, with or without help; or:

Other severely debilitating diseases and conditions, if the variable height feature is required to assist the patient to ambulate.:

D. Electric Powered Hospital Bed Adjustments.--Electric powered adjustments to lower and raise head and foot may be covered when the contractor's medical staff determines that the patient's condition requires frequent change in body position and/or there may be an immediate need for a change in body position (i.e., no delay can be tolerated) and the patient can operate the controls and cause the adjustments. Exceptions may be made to this last requirement in cases of spinal cord injury and brain damaged patients.

E. Side Rails.--If the patient's condition requires bed side rails, they can be covered when an integral part of, or an accessory to, a hospital bed.

Pub. 100-3, Section 280.8

Air-Fluidized Bed

Indications and Limitations of Coverage

Air fluidized beds are covered for services rendered on or after: July 30, 1990.

Medicare payment for home use of the air-fluidized bed for treatment of pressure sores can be made if such use is reasonable and necessary for the individual patient.

A decision that use of an air-fluidized bed is reasonable and necessary requires that:

The patient has a stage 3 (full thickness tissue loss) or stage 4 (deep tissue destruction) pressure sore; :

The patient is bedridden or chair bound as a result of severely limited mobility; :

In the absence of an air-fluidized bed, the patient would require institutionalization; :

The air-fluidized bed is ordered in writing by the patient's attending physician based upon a comprehensive assessment and evaluation of the patient after completion of a course of conservative treatment designed to optimize conditions that promote wound healing. This course of treatment must have been at least one month in duration without progression toward wound healing. This month of prerequisite conservative treatment may include some period in an institution as long as there is documentation available to verify that the necessary conservative treatment has been rendered. :

Use of wet-to-dry dressings for wound debridement, begun during the period of conservative treatment and which continue beyond 30 days, will not preclude coverage of air-fluidized bed. Should additional debridement again become necessary, while a patient is using an air-fluidized bed (after the first 30-day course of conservative treatment) that will not cause the air-fluidized bed to become non-covered. In all instances documentation verifying the continued need for the bed must be available.

A trained adult caregiver is available to assist the patient with activities of daily living, fluid balance, dry skin care, repositioning, recognition and management of altered mental status, dietary needs, prescribed treatments, and management and support of the air-fluidized bed system and its problems such as leakage; :

A physician directs the home treatment regimen, and reevaluates and recertifies the need for the air-fluidized bed on a monthly basis; and :

All other alternative equipment has been considered and ruled out. :

Conservative treatment must include:

Frequent repositioning of the patient with particular attention to relief of pressure over bony prominences (usually every 2 hours); :

Use of a specialized support surface (Group II) designed to reduce pressure and shear forces on healing ulcers and to prevent new ulcer formation; :

Necessary treatment to resolve any wound infection; :

Optimization of nutrition status to promote wound healing; :

Debridement by any means (including wet to dry dressings-which does not require an occulsive covering) to remove devitalized tissue from the wound bed;

Maintenance of a clean, moist bed of granulation tissue with appropriate moist dressings protected by an occlusive covering, while the wound heals. :

Home use of the air-fluidized bed is not covered under any of the following circumstances:

The patient has coexisting pulmonary disease (the lack of firm back support makes coughing ineffective and dry air inhalation thickens pulmonary secretions); :

The patient requires treatment with wet soaks or moist wound dressings that are not protected with an impervious covering such as plastic wrap or other occlusive material; an air-fluidized bed;

The caregiver is unwilling or unable to provide the type of care required by the patient on an air-fluidized bed; :

Structural support is inadequate to support the weight of the air-fluidized bed system (it generally weighs 1600 pounds or more); :

Electrical system is insufficient for the anticipated increase in energy consumption; or :

Other known contraindications exist. :

Coverage of an air-fluidized bed is limited to the equipment itself. Payment for this covered item may only be made if the written order from the attending physician is furnished to the supplier prior to the delivery of the equipment. Payment is not included for the caregiver or for architectural adjustments such as electrical or structural improvement.

Pub. 100-3, Section 280.9

Power-Operated Vehicles That May Be Used as Wheelchairs

Power-operated vehicles that may be appropriately used as wheelchairs are covered under the durable medical equipment provision.

These vehicles have been appropriately used in the home setting for vocational rehabilitation and to improve the ability of chronically disabled persons to cope with normal domestic, vocational and social activities. They may be covered if a wheelchair is medically necessary and the patient is unable to operate a wheelchair manually.

A specialist in physical medicine, orthopedic surgery, neurology, or rheumatology must provide an evaluation of the patient's medical and physical condition and a prescription for the vehicle to assure that the patient requires the vehicle and is capable of using it safely. When an intermediary determines that such a specialist is not reasonably accessible, e.g., more than 1 day's round trip from the beneficiary's home, or the patient's condition precludes such travel, a prescription from the beneficiary's physician is acceptable.

The intermediary's medical staff reviews all claims for a power-operated vehicle, including the specialists' or other physicians' prescriptions and evaluations of the patient's medical and physical conditions, to insure that all coverage requirements are met.

Pub. 100-3, Section 280.11

Corset Used as Hernia Support

A hernia support (whether in the form of a corset or truss) which meets the definition of a brace is covered under Part B under §1861(s)(9) of the Act.

Pub. 100-3, Section 280.12

Sykes Hernia Control

Based on professional advice, it has been determined that the sykes hernia control (a spring-type, U-shaped, strapless truss) is not functionally more beneficial than a conventional truss. Make program reimbursement for this device only when an ordinary truss would be covered. (Like all trusses, it is only of benefit when dealing with a reducible hernia). Thus, when a charge for this item is substantially in excess of that which would be reasonable for a conventional truss used for the same condition, base reimbursement on the reasonable charges for the conventional truss.

Pub. 100-3, Section 280.14

Infusion Pumps

B. Nationally Covered Indications

The following indications for treatment using infusion pumps are covered under Medicare:

1.External Infusion Pumps

a.Iron Poisoning (Effective for Services Performed On or After September 26, 1984)When used in the administration of deferoxamine for the treatment of acute iron poisoning and iron overload, only external infusion pumps are covered.

b.Thromboembolic Disease (Effective for Services Performed On or After September 26, 1984)When used in the administration of heparin for the treatment of thromboembolic disease and/or pulmonary embolism, only external infusion pumps used in an institutional setting are covered.

c.Chemotherapy for Liver Cancer (Effective for Services Performed On or After January 29, 1985)The external chemotherapy infusion pump is covered when used in the treatment of primary hepatocellular carcinoma or colorectal cancer where this disease is unresectable; OR, where the patient refuses surgical excision of the tumor.

d.Morphine for Intractable Cancer Pain (Effective for Services Performed On or After April 22, 1985)Morphine infusion via an external infusion pump is covered when used in the treatment of intractable pain caused by cancer (in either an inpatient or outpatient setting, including a hospice).

e.Continuous Subcutaneous Insulin Infusion (CSII) Pumps (Effective for Services Performed On or after December 17, 2004)Continuous subcutaneous insulin infusion (CSII) and related drugs/supplies are covered as medically reasonable and necessary in the home setting for the treatment of diabetic patients who: (1) either meet the updated fasting C-Peptide testing requirement, or, are beta cell autoantibody positive; and, (2) satisfy the remaining criteria for insulin pump therapy as described below. Patients must meet either Criterion A or B as follows:Criterion A: The patient has completed a comprehensive diabetes education program, and has been on a program of multiple daily injections of insulin (i.e., at least 3 injections per day), with frequent self-adjustments of insulin doses for at least 6 months prior to initiation of the insulin pump, and has documented frequency of glucose self-testing an average of at least 4 times per day during the 2 months prior to initiation of the insulin pump, and meets one or more of the following criteria while on the multiple daily injection regimen:

Glycosylated hemoglobin level (HbAlc) > 7.0 percent; :

History of recurring hypoglycemia; :

Wide fluctuations in blood glucose before mealtime; :

Dawn phenomenon with fasting blood sugars frequently exceeding 200 mg/dl; or, :

History of severe glycemic excursions. :Criterion B: The patient with diabetes has been on a pump prior to enrollment in Medicare and has documented frequency of glucose self-testing an average of at least 4 times per day during the month prior to Medicare enrollment.General CSII CriteriaIn addition to meeting Criterion A or B above, the following general requirements must be met:The patient with diabetes must be insulinopenic per the updated fasting C-peptide testing requirement, or, as an alternative, must be beta cell autoantibody positive.Updated fasting C-peptide testing requirement:

Insulinopenia is defined as a fasting C-peptide level that is less than or equal to 110% of the lower limit of normal of the laboratory's measurement method.:

For patients with renal insufficiency and creatinine clearance (actual or calculated from age, gender, weight, and serum creatinine) <50 ml/minute, insulinopenia is defined as a fasting C-peptide level that is less than or equal to 200% of the lower limit of normal of the laboratory's measurement method.:

Fasting C-peptide levels will only be considered valid with a concurrently obtained fasting glucose <225 mg/dL.:

Levels only need to be documented once in the medical records.:Continued coverage of the insulin pump would require that the patient be seen and evaluated by the treating physician at least every 3 months.The pump must be ordered by and follow-up care of the patient must be managed by a physician who manages multiple patients with CSII and who works closely with a team including nurses, diabetes educators, and dietitians who are knowledgeable in the use of CSII.Other Uses of CSIIThe CMS will continue to allow coverage of all other uses of CSII in accordance with the Category B investigational device exemption (IDE) clinical trials regulation

(42 CFR 405.201) or as a routine cost under the clinical trials policy (Medicare National Coverage Determinations (NCD) Manual 310.1).

f.Other UsesOther uses of external infusion pumps are covered if the contractor's medical staff verifies the appropriateness of the therapy and the prescribed pump for the individual patient.

NOTE: Payment may also be made for drugs necessary for the effective use of a covered external infusion pump as long as the drug being used with the pump is itself reasonable and necessary for the patient's treatment.

2.Implantable Infusion Pumps

a.Chemotherapy for Liver Cancer (Effective for Services Performed On or After September 26, 1984)

The implantable infusion pump is covered for intra-arterial infusion of 5-FUdR for the treatment of liver cancer for patients with primary hepatocellular carcinoma or Duke's Class D colorectal cancer, in whom the metastases are limited to the liver, and where: (1) the disease is unresectable, or (2) the patient refuses surgical excision of the tumor.

b.Anti-Spasmodic Drugs for Severe Spasticity

An implantable infusion pump is covered when used to administer anti-spasmodic drugs intrathecally (e.g., baclofen) to treat chronic intractable spasticity in patients who have proven unresponsive to less invasive medical therapy as determined by the following criteria:As indicated by at least a 6-week trial, the patient cannot be maintained on noninvasive methods of spasm control, such as oral anti-spasmodic drugs, either because these methods fail to control adequately the spasticity or produce intolerable side effects, and prior to pump implantation, the patient must have responded favorably to a trial intrathecal dose of the anti-spasmodic drug.

c.Opioid Drugs for Treatment of Chronic Intractable Pain

An implantable infusion pump is covered when used to administer opioid drugs (e.g., morphine) intrathecally or epidurally for treatment of severe chronic intractable pain of malignant or nonmalignant origin in patients who have a life expectancy of at least 3 months, and who have proven unresponsive to less invasive medical therapy as determined by the following criteria:The patient's history must indicate that he/she would not respond adequately to noninvasive methods of pain control, such as systemic opioids (including attempts to eliminate physical and behavioral abnormalities which may cause an exaggerated reaction to pain); and a preliminary trial of intraspinal opioid drug administration must be undertaken with a temporary intrathecal/epidural catheter to substantiate adequately acceptable pain relief and degree of side effects (including effects on the activities of daily living) and patient acceptance.

d.Coverage of Other Uses of Implanted Infusion Pumps

Determinations may be made on coverage of other uses of implanted infusion pumps if the contractor's medical staff verifies that:

The drug is reasonable and necessary for the treatment of the individual patient;

It is medically necessary that the drug be administered by an implanted infusion pump; and, :

The Food and Drug Administration (FDA)-approved labeling for the pump must specify that the drug being administered and the purpose for which it is administered is an indicated use for the pump. :

e.Implantation of Infusion Pump Is Contraindicated

The implantation of an infusion pump is contraindicated in the following patients:

With a known allergy or hypersensitivity to the drug being used (e.g., oral baclofen, morphine, etc.); :

Who have an infection; :

Whose body size is insufficient to support the weight and bulk of the device; and,

With other implanted programmable devices since crosstalk between devices may inadvertently change the prescription.

NOTE: Payment may also be made for drugs necessary for the effective use of an implantable infusion pump as long as the drug being used with the pump is itself reasonable and necessary for the patient's treatment.

C. Nationally Noncovered Indications

The following indications for treatment using infusion pumps are not covered under Medicare:

1.External Infusion Pumps

a.Vancomycin (Effective for Services Beginning On or After September 1, 1996)

Medicare coverage of vancomycin as a durable medical equipment infusion pump benefit is not covered. There is insufficient evidence to support the necessity of using an external infusion pump, instead of a disposable elastomeric pump or the gravity drip method, to administer vancomycin in a safe and appropriate manner.

2.Implantable Infusion Pump

a.Thromboembolic Disease (Effective for Services Performed On or After September 26, 1984)

According to the Public Health Service, there is insufficient published clinical data to support the safety and effectiveness of the heparin implantable pump. Therefore, the use of an implantable infusion pump for infusion of heparin in the treatment of recurrent thromboembolic disease is not covered.

b.Diabetes

An implanted infusion pump for the infusion of insulin to treat diabetes is not covered. The data does not demonstrate that the pump provides effective administration of insulin.

D. Other

Appendix 4 — Pub 100 References

Not applicable.

(This NCD last reviewed January 2005.)

Pub. 100-3, Section 300.1

Obsolete or Unreliable Diagnostic Tests

Indications and Limitations of Coverage

CIM 50-34

A. Diagnostic TestsDo not routinely pay for the following diagnostic tests because they are obsolete and have been replaced by more advanced procedures. The listed tests may be paid for only if the medical need for the procedure is satisfactorily justified by the physician who performs it. When the services are subject to the Quality Improvement Organization (QIO) Review, the QIO is responsible for determining that satisfactory medical justification exists. When the services are not subject to QIO review, the intermediary or carrier is responsible for determining that satisfactory medical justification exists. This includes:

Amylase, blood isoenzymes, electrophoretic,

Chromium, blood,

Guanase, blood,

Zinc sulphate turbidity, blood,

Skin test, cat scratch fever,

Skin test, lymphopathia venereum,

Circulation time, one test,

Cephalin flocculation,

Congo red, blood,

Hormones, adrenocorticotropin quantitative animal tests,

Hormones, adrenocorticotropin quantitative bioassay,

Thymol turbidity, blood,

Skin test, actinomycosis,

Skin test, brucellosis,

Skin test, psittacosis,

Skin test, trichinosis,

Calcium, feces, 24-hour quantitative,

Starch, feces, screening,

Chymotrypsin, duodenal contents,

Gastric analysis, pepsin,

Gastric analysis, tubeless,

Calcium saturation clotting time,

Capillary fragility test (Rumpel-Leede),

Colloidal gold,

Bendien's test for cancer and tuberculosis,

Bolen's test for cancer,

Rehfuss test for gastric acidity, and

Serum seromucoid assay for cancer and other diseases.

B. Cardiovascular Tests

Do not pay for the following phonocardiography and vectorcardiography diagnostic tests because they have been determined to be outmoded and of little clinical value. They include:

Phonocardiogram with or without ECG lead; with supervision during recording with interpretation and report (when equipment is supplied by the physician),

Phonocardiogram; tracing only, without interpretation and report (e.g., when equipment is supplied by the hospital, clinic),

Phonocardiogram; interpretation and report,

Phonocardiogram with ECG lead, with indirect carotid artery and/or jugular vein tracing, and/or apex cardiogram; with interpretation and report,

Phonocardiogram; without interpretation and report,

Phonocardiogram; interpretation and report only,

Intracardiac,

Vectorcardiogram (VCG), with or without ECG; with interpretation and report,

Vectorcardiogram; tracing only, without interpretation and report, and

Vectorcardiogram; interpretation and report only.

Transmittal Number48 Transmittal Linkhttp://www.cms.hhs.gov/transmittals/downloads/R48NCD.pdfRevision History04/01/1997 - Excluded coverage of 10 phonocardiography and vectorcardiography diagnostic tests. Effective 1/1/1997. (TN 96)03/2006 - Delete coding information. Effective/Implementation date: 06/19/2006. (TN 48) (CR4278)Other VersionsObsolete or Unreliable Diagnostic Tests - Version 1, Effective between 01/01/1997 - 06/19/2006-

Pub. 100-4, Chapter 1, Section 10.1.4.1

Physician and Ambulance Services Furnished in Connection With Covered Foreign Inpatient Hospital Services

Payment is made for necessary physician and ambulance services that meet the other coverage requirements of the Medicare program, and are furnished in connection with and during a period of covered foreign hospitalization.

A. Coverage of Physician and Ambulance Services Furnished Outside the U.S.

Where inpatient services in a foreign hospital are covered, payment may also be made for

• Physicians' services furnished to the beneficiary while he/she is an inpatient,

• Physicians' services furnished to the beneficiary outside the hospital on the day of his/her admission as an inpatient, provided the services were for the same condition for which the beneficiary was hospitalized (including the services of a Canadian ship's physician who furnishes emergency services in Canadian waters on the day the patient is admitted to a Canadian hospital for a covered emergency stay and,

• Ambulance services, where necessary, for the trip to the hospital in conjunction with the beneficiary's admission as an inpatient. Return trips from a foreign hospital are not covered.

In cases involving foreign ambulance services, the general requirements in Chapter 15 are also applicable, subject to the following special rules:

• If the foreign hospitalization was determined to be covered on the basis of emergency services, the medical necessity requirements outlined in Chapter 15 are considered met.

• The definition of "physician," for purposes of coverage of services furnished outside the U.S., is expanded to include a foreign practitioner, provided the practitioner is legally licensed to practice in the country in which the services are furnished.

• Only the enrollee can file for Part B benefits; the assignment method may not be used.

• Where the enrollee is deceased, the rules for settling Part B underpayments are applicable. Payment is made to the foreign physician or foreign ambulance company on an unpaid bill provided the physician or ambulance company accepts the payment as the full charge for the service, or payment an be made to a person who has agreed to assume legal liability to pay the physician or supplier. Where the bill is paid, payment may be made in accordance with Medicare regulations. The regular deductible and coinsurance requirements apply to physicians' and ambulance services furnished outside the U.S.

Pub. 100-4, Chapter 1, Section 30.3.5

Effect of Assignment Upon Purchase of Cataract Glasses From Participating Physician or Supplier on Claims Submitted to Carriers

B3-3045.4

A pair of cataract glasses is comprised of two distinct products: a professional product (the prescribed lenses) and a retail commercial product (the frames). The frames serve not only as a holder of lenses but also as an article of personal apparel. As such, they are usually selected on the basis of personal taste and style. Although Medicare will pay only for standard frames, most patients want deluxe frames. Participating physicians and suppliers cannot profitably furnish such deluxe frames unless they can make an extra (noncovered) charge for the frames even though they accept assignment.

Therefore, a participating physician or supplier (whether an ophthalmologist, optometrist, or optician) who accepts assignment on cataract glasses with deluxe frames may charge the Medicare patient the difference between his/her usual charge to private pay patients for glasses with standard frames and his/her usual charge to such patients for glasses with deluxe frames, in addition to the applicable deductible and coinsurance on glasses with standard frames, if all of the following requirements are met:

A. The participating physician or supplier has standard frames available, offers them for sale to the patient, and issues and ABN to the patient that explains the price and other differences between standard and deluxe frames. Refer to Chapter 30.

B. The participating physician or supplier obtains from the patient (or his/her representative) and keeps on file the following signed and dated statement:

_____

Name of Patient Medicare Claim Number

Having been informed that an extra charge is being made by the physician or supplier for deluxe frames, that this extra charge is not covered by Medicare, and that standard frames are available for purchase from the physician or supplier at no extra charge, I have chosen to purchase deluxe frames. _____ Signature Date

C. The participating physician or supplier itemizes on his/her claim his/her actual charge for the lenses, his/her actual charge for the standard frames, and his/her actual extra charge for the deluxe frames (charge differential).

Once the assigned claim for deluxe frames has been processed, the carrier will follow the ABN instructions as described in §60.

Pub. 100-4, Chapter 3, Section 10.4

Payment of Nonphysician Services for Inpatients

HO-407

All items and nonphysician services furnished to inpatients must be furnished directly by the hospital or billed through the hospital under arrangements. This provision applies to all hospitals, regardless of whether they are subject to PPS.

A. Other Medical Items, Supplies, and Services

The following medical items, supplies, and services furnished to inpatients are covered under Part A. Consequently, they are covered by the prospective payment rate or reimbursed as reasonable costs under Part A to hospitals excluded from PPS.

• Laboratory services (excluding anatomic pathology services and certain clinical pathology services);

• Pacemakers and other prosthetic devices including lenses, and artificial limbs, knees, and hips;

• Radiology services including computed tomography (CT) scans furnished to inpatients by a physician's office, other hospital, or radiology clinic;

• Total parenteral nutrition (TPN) services; and

• Transportation, including transportation by ambulance, to and from another hospital or freestanding facility to receive specialized diagnostic or therapeutic services not available at the facility where the patient is an inpatient.

The hospital must include the cost of these services in the appropriate ancillary service cost center, i.e., in the cost of the diagnostic or therapeutic service. It must not show them separately under revenue code 0540.

EXCEPTIONS:

• Pneumococcal Vaccine - is payable under Part B only and is billed by the hospital on the Form CMS-1450.

• Ambulance Service - For purposes of this section "hospital inpatient" means a beneficiary who has been formally admitted it does not include a beneficiary who is in the process of being transferred from one hospital to another. Where the patient is transferred from one hospital to another, and is admitted as an inpatient to the second, the ambulance service is payable under only Part B. If transportation is by a hospital owned and operated ambulance, the hospital bills separately on Form CMS-1450 as appropriate. Similarly, if the hospital arranges for the ambulance transportation with an ambulance operator, including paying the ambulance operator, it bills separately. However, if the hospital does not assume any financial responsibility, the billing is to the carrier by the ambulance operator or beneficiary, as appropriate, if an ambulance is used for the transportation of a hospital inpatient to another facility for diagnostic tests or special treatment the ambulance trip is considered part of the DRG, and not separately billable, if the resident hospital is under PPS.

• Part B Inpatient Services - Where Part A benefits are not payable, payment may be made to the hospital under Part B for certain medical and other health services. See Chapter 4 for a description of Part B inpatient services

• Anesthetist Services "Incident to" Physician Services - If a physician's practice was to employ anesthetists and to bill on a reasonable charge basis for these services and that practice was in effect as of the last day of the hospital's most recent 12-month cost reporting period ending before September 30, 1983, the physician may continue that practice through cost reporting periods beginning October 1, 1984. However, if the physician chooses to continue this practice, the hospital may not add costs of the anesthetist's service to its base period costs for purposes of its transition payment rates. If it is the existing or new practice of the physician to employ certified registered nurse anesthetists (CRNAs) and other qualified anesthetists and include charges for their services in the physician bills for anesthesiology services for the hospital's cost report periods beginning on or after October 1, 1984, and before October 1, 1987, the physician may continue to do so.

B. Exceptions/Waivers

These provisions were waived before cost reporting periods beginning on or after October 1, 1986, under certain circumstances. The basic criteria for waiver was that services furnished by outside suppliers are so extensive that a sudden change in billing practices would threaten the stability of patient care. Specific criteria for waiver and processing procedures are in §2804 of the Provider Reimbursement Manual (CMS Pub. 15-1).

Pub. 100-4, Chapter 3, Section 20.7.3

Payment for Blood Clotting Factor Administered to Hemophilia Inpatients

Section 6011 of Public Law (P.L.) 101-239 amended §1886(a)(4) of the Social Security Act (the Act) to provide that prospective payment system (PPS) hospitals receive an additional payment for the costs of administering blood clotting factor to Medicare hemophiliacs who are hospital inpatients. Section 6011(b) of P.L. 101.239 specified that the payment be based on a predetermined price per unit of clotting factor multiplied by the number of units provided. This add-on payment originally was effective for blood clotting factors furnished on or after June 19, 1990, and before December 19, 1991. Section 13505 of P. L. 103-66 amended §6011 (d) of P.L. 101-239 to extend the period covered by the add-on payment for blood clotting factors administered to Medicare inpatients with hemophilia through September 30, 1994. Section 4452 of P.L. 105-33 amended §6011(d) of P.L. 101-239 to reinstate the add-on payment for the costs of administering blood-clotting factor to Medicare beneficiaries who have hemophilia and who are hospital inpatients for discharges occurring on or after October 1, 1998.

Local carriers shall process non-institutional blood clotting factor claims.

The FIs shall process institutional blood clotting factor claims payable under either Part A or Part B.

A. Inpatient Bills

Under the Inpatient Prospective Payment System (PPS), hospitals receive a special add-on payment for the costs of furnishing blood clotting factors to Medicare beneficiaries with hemophilia, admitted as inpatients of PPS hospitals. The clotting factor add-on payment is calculated using the number of units (as defined in the HCPCS code long descriptor) billed by the provider under special instructions for units of service.

The PPS Pricer software does not calculate the payment amount. The Fiscal Intermediary Standard System (FISS) calculates the payment amount and subtracts the charges from those submitted to Pricer so that the clotting factor charges are not included in cost outlier computations.

Blood clotting factors not paid on a cost or PPS basis are priced as a drug/biological under the Medicare Part B Drug Pricing File effective for the specific date of service. As of January 1, 2005, the average sales price (ASP) plus 6 percent shall be used.

If a beneficiary is in a covered Part A stay in a PPS hospital, the clotting factors are paid in addition to the DRG/HIPPS payment (For FY 2004, this payment is based on 95 percent of average wholesale price.) For a SNF subject to SNF/PPS, the payment is bundled into the SNF/PPS rate.

For SNF inpatient Part A, there is no add-on payment for blood clotting factors.

The codes for blood-clotting factors are found on the Medicare Part B Drug Pricing File. This file is distributed on a quarterly basis.

For discharges occurring on or after October 1, 2000, and before December 31, 2005, report HCPCS Q0187 based on 1 billing unit per 1.2 mg. Effective January 1, 2006, HCPCS code J7189 replaces Q0187 and is defined as 1 billing unit per 1 microgram (mcg).

The examples below include the HCPCS code and indicate the dosage amount specified in the descriptor of that code. Facilities use the units field as a multiplier to arrive at the dosage amount.

EXAMPLE 1

HCPCS	Drug	Dosage
J7189	Factor VIIa	1 mcg

Actual dosage: 13,365 mcg

On the bill, the facility shows J7189 and 13,365 in the units field (13,365 mcg divided by 1 mcg = 13,365 units).

NOTE: The process for dealing with one international unit (IU) is the same as the process of dealing with one microgram.

EXAMPLE 2

HCPCS	Drug	Dosage
J9355	Trastuzumab	10 mg

Actual dosage: 140 mg

On the bill, the facility shows J9355 and 14 in the units field (140 mg divided by 10mg = 14 units).

When the dosage amount is greater than the amount indicated for the HCPCS code, the facility rounds up to determine units. When the dosage amount is less than the amount indicated for the HCPCS code, use 1 as the unit of measure.

EXAMPLE 3

HCPCS	Drug	Dosage
J3100	Tenecteplase	50 mg

Actual Dosage: 40 mg

The provider would bill for 1 unit, even though less than 1 full unit was furnished.

At times, the facility provides less than the amount provided in a single use vial and there is waste, i.e.; some drugs may be available only in packaged amounts that exceed the needs of an individual patient. Once the drug is reconstituted in the hospital's pharmacy, it may have a limited shelf life. Since an individual patient may receive less than the fully reconstituted amount, we encourage hospitals to schedule patients in such a way that the hospital can use the drug most efficiently. However, if the hospital must discard the remainder of a vial after administering part of it to a Medicare patient, the provider may bill for the amount of drug discarded plus the amount administered.

Example 1:

Drug X is available only in a 100-unit size. A hospital schedules three Medicare patients to receive drug X on the same day within the designated shelf life of the product. An appropriate hospital staff member administers 30 units to each patient. The remaining 10 units are billed to Medicare on the account of the last patient. Therefore, 30 units are billed on behalf of the first patient seen and 30 units are billed on behalf of the second patient seen. Forty units are billed on behalf of the last patient seen because the hospital had to discard 10 units at that point.

Example 2:

An appropriate hospital staff member must administer 30 units of drug X to a Medicare patient, and it is not practical to schedule another patient who requires the same drug. For example, the hospital has only one patient who requires drug X, or the hospital sees the patient for the first time and did not know the patient's condition. The hospital bills for 100 units on behalf of the patient, and Medicare pays for 100 units.

When the number of units of blood clotting factor administered to hemophiliac inpatients exceeds 99,999, the hospital reports the excess as a second line for revenue code 0636 and repeats the HCPCS code. One hundred thousand fifty (100,050) units are reported on one line as 99,999, and another line shows 1,051.

Revenue Code 0636 is used. It requires HCPCS. Some other inpatient drugs continue to be billed without HCPCS codes under pharmacy.

No changes in beneficiary notices are required. Coverage is applicable to hospital Part A claims only. Coverage is also applicable to inpatient Part B services in SNFs and all types of hospitals, including CAHs. Separate payment is not made to SNFs for beneficiaries in an inpatient Part A stay.

B. FI Action

The FI is responsible for the following:

• It accepts HCPCS codes for inpatient services;

• It edits to require HCPCS codes with Revenue Code 0636. Multiple iterations of the revenue code are possible with the same or different HCPCS codes. It does not edit units except to ensure a numeric value;

• It reduces charges forwarded to Pricer by the charges for hemophilia clotting factors in revenue code 0636. It retains the charges and revenue and HCPCS codes for CWF; and

• It modifies data entry screens to accept HCPCS codes for hospital (including CAH) swing bed, and SNF inpatient claims (bill types 11X, 12X, 18x, 21x and, 22x).

The September 1, 1993, IPPS final rule (58 FR 46304) states that payment will be made for the blood clotting factor only if an ICD-9-CM diagnosis code for hemophilia is included on the bill.

Since inpatient blood-clotting factors are covered only for beneficiaries with hemophilia, the FI must ensure that one of the following hemophilia diagnosis codes is listed on the bill before payment is made:

286.0	Congenital factor VIII disorder
286.1	Congenital factor IX disorder
286.2	Congenital factor IX disorder
286.3	Congenital deficiency of other clotting factor
286.4	von Willebrands' disease

Effective for discharges on or after August 1, 2001, payment may also be made if one of the following diagnosis codes is reported:

286.5	Hemorrhagic disorder due to circulating anticoagulants
286.7	Acquired coagulation factor deficiency

C. Part A Remittance Advice

1. X12.835 Ver. 003030M

For remittance reporting PIP and/or non-PIP payments, the Hemophilia Add on will be reported in a claims level 2-090-CAS segment (CAS is the element identifier) exhibiting an "OA" Group Code and adjustment reason code "97" (payment is included in the allowance for the basic service/procedure) followed by the associated dollar amount (POSITIVE) and units of service. For this version of the 835, "OA" group coded line level CAS segments are informational and are not included in the balancing routine. The Hemophilia Add On amount will always be included in the 2-010-CLP04 Claim Payment Amount.

For remittance reporting PIP payments, the Hemophilia Add On will also be reported in the provider level adjustment (element identifier PLB) segment with the provider level adjustment reason code "CA" (Manual claims adjustment) followed by the associated dollar amount (NEGATIVE).

NOTE: A data maintenance request will be submitted to ANSI ASC X12 for a new PLB adjustment reason code specifically for PIP payment Hemophilia Add On situations for future use. However, continue to use adjustment reason code "CA" until further notice.

The FIs enter MA103 (Hemophilia Add On) in an open MIA (element identifier) remark code data element. This will alert the provider that the reason code 97 and PLB code "CA" adjustments are related to the Hemophilia Add On.

2. X12.835 Ver. 003051

For remittances reporting PIP and/or non-PIP payments, Hemophilia Add On information will be reported in the claim level 2-062-AMT and 2-064-QTY segments. The 2-062-AMT01 element will carry a "ZK" (Federal Medicare claim MANDATE - Category 1) qualifier code followed by the total claim level Hemophilia Add On amount (POSITIVE). The 2-064QTY01 element will carry a "FL" (Units) qualifier code followed by the number of units approved for the Hemophilia Add On for the claim. The Hemophilia Add On amount will always be included in the 2-010-CLP04 Claim Payment Amount.

NOTE: A data maintenance request will be submitted to ANSI ASC X12 for a new AMT qualifier code specifically for the Hemophilia Add On for future use. However, continue to use adjustment reason code "ZK" until further notice.

For remittances reporting PIP payments, the Hemophilia Add On will be reported in the provider level adjustment PLB segment with the provider level adjustment reason "ZZ" followed by the associated dollar amount (NEGATIVE).

NOTE: A data maintenance request will be submitted to ANSI ASC X12 for a new PLB, adjustment reason code specifically for the Hemophilia Add On for future use. However, continue to use PLB adjustment reason code "ZZ" until further notice.

The FIs enter MA103 (Hemophilia Add On) in an open MIA remark code data element. This will alert the provider that the ZK, FL and ZZ entries are related to the Hemophilia Add On. (Effective with version 4010 of the 835, report ZK in lieu of FL in the QTY segment.)

3. Standard Hard Copy Remittance Advice

For paper remittances reporting non-PIP payments involving Hemophilia Add On, add a "Hemophilia Add On" category to the end of the "Pass Thru Amounts" listings in the "Summary"

section of the paper remittance. Enter the total of the Hemophilia Add On amounts due for the claims covered by this remittance next to the Hemophilia Add On heading.

The FIs add the Remark Code "MA103" (Hemophilia Add On) to the remittance advice under the REM column for those claims that qualify for Hemophilia Add On payments.

This will be the full extent of Hemophilia Add On reporting on paper remittance notices; providers wishing more detailed information must subscribe to the Medicare Part A specifications for the ANSI ASC X12N 835, where additional information is available.

See chapter 22, for detailed instructions and definitions.

Pub. 100-4, Chapter 3, Section 40.2.2

Charges to Beneficiaries for Part A Services

The hospital submits a bill even where the patient is responsible for a deductible which covers the entire amount of the charges for non-PPS hospitals, or in PPS hospitals, where the DRG payment amount will be less than the deductible.

A beneficiary's liability for payment is governed by the limitation on liability notification rules in Chapter 30 where the admission is found not to be reasonable and necessary and no payment will be made for the stay under limitation on liability. A hospital receiving payment for a covered hospital stay (or PPS hospital that includes at least one covered day, or one treated as covered under guarantee of payment or limitation on liability) may charge the beneficiary, or other person, for items and services furnished during the stay only as described in subsections A through H.

A - Deductible and Coinsurance

The hospital may charge the beneficiary or other person for applicable deductible and coinsurance amounts. The deductible is satisfied only by charges for covered services. The FI deducts the deductible and coinsurance first from the PPS payment. Where the deductible exceeds the PPS amount, the excess will be applied to a subsequent payment to the hospital. (See Chapter 3 of the Medicare General Information, Eligibility, and Entitlement Manual for specific policies.)

B - Blood Deductible

The Part A blood deductible provision applies and reporting of the number of pints is applicable to both PPS and non-PPS hospitals. (See Chapter 3 of the Medicare General Information, Eligibility, and Entitlement Manual for specific policies.)

C - Inpatient Care No Longer Required

The hospital may charge for services that are not reasonable and necessary or that constitute custodial care, furnished on or after the third day following the date of the written notification when the following requirements are met:

• The hospital (acting directly or through its URC) determined that the beneficiary no longer required inpatient hospital care. (For this purpose, a beneficiary is considered to require inpatient hospital care if the beneficiary needed a SNF level of care but an SNF-level bed was unavailable.) The hospital cannot issue a notice of noncoverage if a bed is not available. Medicare pays for days awaiting placement until a bed is available and it is documented in the medical record that SNF placement is actively being sought.

• The attending physician agreed with the hospital's determination in writing, i.e., by issuing a written discharge order. Or, if the physician disagreed with the hospital's determination, the hospital requested a review by the QIO and the QIO concurred with the hospitals' notice.

Prior to charging for the noncovered period, the hospital (acting directly or through the URC) notified the beneficiary (or person acting on the beneficiary's behalf) in writing that:

• In its opinion and with the concurrence of the attending physician (or of the QIO), the beneficiary no longer requires inpatient hospital care (See §§130 for coordination with a QIO); or

• Customary charges will be made for continued hospital care beginning with the third day following the date of the notice.

The beneficiary may request that the QIO make a formal determination on the validity of the hospital's finding if the beneficiary remains in the hospital after becoming liable for charges. If the beneficiary wants an immediate review by the QIO, the beneficiary must request it within 3 days of receiving the hospital's notice. Any patient during the course of a stay will receive the QIO decision within 2 workdays.

The determination of the QIO may be appealed if it is unfavorable to the beneficiary in any way and the QIO decision will be made within 30 days.

To the extent that a finding is made that the beneficiary required continued hospital care beyond the point indicated by the hospital, the charges for the continued care will be invalidated and any money paid by the beneficiary, or on the beneficiary's behalf, refunded.

The manner in which the hospital gives the notice to the beneficiary is in Chapter 30.

If a hospital furnishing covered inpatient hospital services is able to determine in advance that the beneficiary will not require inpatient hospital care as of a certain date, it may give the notice in advance of that date, but ordinarily no earlier than 3 days before that date. If a hospital determines, however, that a beneficiary needs (or by the third day thereafter, will need) only a SNF-level of care but a SNF bed is not or will not be available, it may notify the beneficiary (or the beneficiary's representative) that the beneficiary will be subject to charges beginning with the third day after the date of the notice that the SNF bed becomes available. This can be done as an advance beneficiary notice. The hospital needs to notify the beneficiary or representative the day the bed becomes available or has knowledge of the bed available.

The beneficiary has the same right to appeal the QIO's determination that the beneficiary no longer required inpatient hospital care as of a certain date as applies to QIO determinations regarding medical necessity. The hospital also has the right to appeal a QIO's determination that is unfavorable to the beneficiary.

When the hospital appeals in such cases the following entries are required on the bill:

• Occurrence code 3I (and date) to indicate the date the hospital notified the patient in accordance with the first bullet above;

• Occurrence span code 76 (and dates) to indicate the period of noncovered care for which it is charging the beneficiary;

• Occurrence span code 77 (and dates) to indicate the period of noncovered care for which the provider is liable, when it is aware of this prior to billing; and

• Value code 3I (and amount) to indicate the amount of charges it may bill the beneficiary for days for which inpatient care was no longer required. They are included as noncovered charges on the bill.

D - Change in the Beneficiary's Condition

If the beneficiary remains in the hospital after receiving notice as described in subsection C, and the hospital, the physician who concurred in the hospital's determination, or the QIO, subsequently determines that the beneficiary again requires inpatient hospital care, the hospital may not charge the beneficiary or other person for services furnished after the beneficiary again required inpatient hospital care until the conditions in subsection C. are again met. If a patient who needs only a SNF level of care remains in the hospital after the SNF bed becomes available, and the bed ceases to be available, the hospital may continue to charge the beneficiary. It need not provide the beneficiary with a subsequent notice when the patient chose not to be discharged to the SNF bed.

E - Admission Denied

If the entire hospital admission is determined to be not reasonable or necessary:

• If the beneficiary was notified in writing prior to, or upon admission, the hospital may charge for the entire period of hospitalization.

• If the beneficiary was notified in writing on the day following the admission or subsequently, the hospital may charge the beneficiary for the hospitalization beginning with the day following the day the written notice was given. In this circumstance, the provider is liable for the period between admission and the day after the beneficiary was notified.

The notice to the beneficiary must state:

• The basis of the determination that inpatient hospital care is not necessary or reasonable (e.g., coverage exclusions);

• That customary charges will be made for hospital care beginning with the day following the day on which the notice is given to either the beneficiary or to a representative on his behalf;

• The beneficiary may request that the QIO make a formal determination on the validity of the hospital's finding if the beneficiary remains in the hospital. If the beneficiary wishes immediate QIO review, it must be requested within 3 days of receiving the hospital's notice;

• The beneficiary may appeal the determination of the QIO if it is unfavorable to the beneficiary in any way. The hospital also has the right to appeal a QIO's decision; and

• If a finding is made that the beneficiary required the hospitalization, the charges for the hospital stay will be invalidated, and money paid by the beneficiary or on his behalf will be refunded.

In such cases the following entries are required on the bill:

• Occurrence code 3I (and date) to indicate the date the hospital notified the beneficiary.

• Occurrence span code 76 (and dates) to indicate the period of noncovered care for which the hospital is charging the beneficiary.

• Occurrence span code 77 (and dates) to indicate any period of noncovered care for which the provider is liable (e.g., the period between issuing the notice and the time it may charge the beneficiary) when the provider is aware of this prior to billing.

• Value code 3I (and amount) to indicate the amount of charges the hospital may bill the beneficiary for hospitalization that was not necessary or reasonable. They are included as noncovered charges on the bill.

F - Procedures, Studies and Courses of Treatment That Are Not Reasonable or Necessary

If diagnostic procedures, studies, therapeutic studies and courses of treatment are excluded from coverage as not reasonable and necessary (even though the beneficiary requires inpatient hospital care) the hospital may charge the beneficiary or other person for the services or care under the following circumstances:

• If the beneficiary was notified in writing prior to receipt of the care or services that the hospital may charge for the excluded care or services; and

• The notice to the beneficiary must state:

-The basis of the determination that inpatient hospital care is not necessary or reasonable (i.e., coverage exclusions);

-The determination is the hospital's opinion. (If the hospital obtained concurrence from the FI or the QIO this may be stated);

-Customary charges will be made if the beneficiary receives the services;

-The beneficiary may request the FI, or the QIO when medical necessity is involved, to make a formal determination on the validity of the hospital's finding if the beneficiary receives the items or services. If the beneficiary wants immediate QIO review, the beneficiary must request it within 3 days of receiving the hospital's notice;

-The FI's determination, or the QIO's where a medical necessity determination is involved, may be appealed by the beneficiary if unfavorable to the beneficiary in any way. The hospital also has the right to appeal the FI's or the QIO's decision; and

-The charges for the services will be invalidated and refunded if they are found to be covered.

The hospital may consult with the FI (on coverage exclusions) or the QIO (on medical necessity determinations) prior to issuing the notice to the beneficiary.

The following bill entries apply to these circumstances:

• Occurrence code 32 (and date) to indicate the date the hospital provided the notice to the beneficiary.

• Value code 3I (and amount) to indicate the amount of such charges to be billed to the beneficiary. They are included as noncovered charges on the bill.

G - Nonentitlement Days and Days after Benefits Exhausted

If a hospital stay exceeds the day outlier threshold, the hospital may charge for some, or all, of the days on which the patient is not entitled to Medicare Part A, or after the Part A benefits are exhausted (i.e., the hospital may charge its customary charges for services furnished on those days). It may charge the beneficiary for the lesser of:

• The number of days on which the patient was not entitled to benefits or after the benefits were exhausted; or

• The number of outlier days. (Day outliers were discontinued at the end of FY 1997.)

If the number of outlier days exceeds the number of days on which the patient was not entitled to benefits, or after benefits were exhausted, the hospital may charge for all days on which the patient was not entitled to benefits or after benefits were exhausted. If the number of days on which the beneficiary was not entitled to benefits, or after benefits were exhausted, exceeds the number of outlier days, the hospital determines the days for which it may charge by starting with the last day of the stay (i.e., the day before the day of discharge) and identifying and counting off in reverse order, days on which the patient was not entitled to benefits or after the benefits were exhausted, until the number of days counted off equals the number of outlier days. The days counted off are the days for which the hospital may charge.

H - Contractual Exclusions

In addition to receiving the basic prospective payment, the hospital may charge the beneficiary for any services that are excluded from coverage for reasons other than, or in addition to, absence of medical necessity, provision of custodial care, non-entitlement to Part A, or exhaustion of benefits. For example, it may charge for most cosmetic and dental surgery.

I - Private Room Care

Payment for medically necessary private room care is included in the prospective payment. Where the beneficiary requests private room accommodations, the hospital must inform the beneficiary of the additional charge. (See the Medicare Benefit Policy Manual, Chapter 1.) When the beneficiary accepts the liability, the hospital will supply the service, and bill the beneficiary directly. If the beneficiary believes the private room was medically necessary, the beneficiary has a right to a determination and may initiate a Part A appeal.

J - Deluxe Item or Service

Where a beneficiary requests a deluxe item or service, i.e., an item or service which is more expensive than is medically required for the beneficiary's condition, after the hospital informs the beneficiary of the additional charge, it may collect the additional charge. That charge is the difference between the customary charge for the item or service most commonly furnished by the hospital to private pay patients with the beneficiary's condition, and the charge for the more expensive item or service requested. If the beneficiary believes that the more expensive item or service was medically necessary, the beneficiary has a right to a determination and may initiate a Part A appeal.

K - Inpatient Acute Care Hospital Admission Followed By a Death or Discharge Prior To Room Assignment

A patient of an acute care hospital is considered an inpatient upon issuance of written doctor's orders to that effect. If a patient either dies or is discharged prior to being assigned and/or occupying a room, a hospital may enter an appropriate room and board charge on the claim. If a patient leaves of their own volition prior to being assigned and/or occupying a room, a hospital may enter an appropriate room and board charge on the claim as well as a patient status code 07 which indicates they left against medical advice. A hospital is not required to enter a room and board charge, but failure to do so may have a minimal impact on future DRG weight calculations.

Pub. 100-4, Chapter 3, Section 40.3

Outpatient Services Treated as Inpatient Services
A3-3610.3, HO-415.6, HO-400D, A-03-008, A-03-013, A-03-054

A Outpatient Services Followed by Admission Before Midnight of the Following Day (Effective For Services Furnished Before October 1, 1991)

When a beneficiary receives outpatient hospital services during the day immediately preceding the hospital admission, the outpatient hospital services are treated as inpatient services if the beneficiary has Part A coverage. Hospitals and FIs apply this provision only when the beneficiary is admitted to the hospital before midnight of the day following receipt of outpatient services. The day on which the patient is formally admitted as an inpatient is counted as the first inpatient day.

When this provision applies, services are included in the applicable PPS payment and not billed separately. When this provision applies to hospitals and units excluded from the hospital PPS, services are shown on the bill and included in the Part A payment. See Chapter 1 for FI requirements for detecting duplicate claims in such cases.

B Preadmission Diagnostic Services (Effective for Services Furnished On or After January 1, 1991)

Diagnostic services (including clinical diagnostic laboratory tests) provided to a beneficiary by the admitting hospital, or by an entity wholly owned or wholly operated by the admitting hospital (or by another entity under arrangements with the admitting hospital), within 3 days prior to and including the date of the beneficiary's admission are deemed to be inpatient services and included in the inpatient payment, unless there is no Part A coverage. For example, if a patient is admitted on a Wednesday, outpatient services provided by the hospital on Sunday, Monday, Tuesday, or Wednesday are included in the inpatient Part A payment.

This provision does not apply to ambulance services and maintenance renal dialysis services (see the Medicare Benefit Policy Manual, Chapters 10 and 11, respectively). Additionally, Part A services furnished by skilled nursing facilities, home health agencies, and hospices are excluded from the payment window provisions.

For services provided before October 31, 1994, this provision applies to both hospitals subject to the hospital inpatient prospective payment system (IPPS) as well as those hospitals and units excluded from IPPS.

For services provided on or after October 31, 1994, for hospitals and units excluded from IPPS, this provision applies only to services furnished within one day prior to and including the date of the beneficiary's admission. The hospitals and units that are excluded from IPPS are: psychiatric hospitals and units; inpatient rehabilitation facilities (IRF) and units; long-term care hospitals (LTCH); children's hospitals; and cancer hospitals.

Critical access hospitals (CAHs) are not subject to the 3-day (nor 1-day) DRG payment window.

An entity is considered to be "wholly owned or operated" by the hospital if the hospital is the sole owner or operator. A hospital need not exercise administrative control over a facility in order to operate it. A hospital is considered the sole operator of the facility if the hospital has exclusive responsibility for implementing facility policies (i.e., conducting or overseeing the facility's routine operations), regardless of whether it also has the authority to make the policies.

For this provision, diagnostic services are defined by the presence on the bill of the following revenue and/or HCPCS codes:

0254 - Drugs incident to other diagnostic services

0255 - Drugs incident to radiology

030X - Laboratory

031X - Laboratory pathological

032X - Radiology diagnostic

0341 - Nuclear medicine, diagnostic

035X - CT scan

0371 - Anesthesia incident to Radiology

0372 - Anesthesia incident to other diagnostic services

040X - Other imaging services

046X - Pulmonary function

0471 - Audiology diagnostic

048X - Cardiology, with HCPCS codes 93015, 93307, 93308, 93320, 93501, 93503, 93505, 93510, 93526, 93541, 93542, 93543, 93544 - 93552, 93561, or 93562

053X - Osteopathic services

061X - MRT

062X - Medical/surgical supplies, incident to radiology or other diagnostic services

073X - EKG/ECG

074X - EEG

092X - Other diagnostic services

The CWF rejects services furnished January 1, 1991, or later when outpatient bills for diagnostic services with through dates or last date of service (occurrence span code 72) fall on the day of admission or any of the 3 days immediately prior to admission to an IPPS or IPPS-excluded hospital. This reject applies to the bill in process, regardless of whether the outpatient or inpatient bill is processed first. Hospitals must analyze the two bills and report appropriate corrections. For services on or after October 31, 1994, for hospitals and units excluded from IPPS, CWF will reject outpatient diagnostic bills that occur on the day of or one day before admission. For IPPS hospitals, CWF will continue to reject outpatient diagnostic bills for services that occur on the day of or any of the 3 days prior to admission.

Hospitals in Maryland that are under the jurisdiction of the Health Services Cost Review Commission are subject to the 3-day payment window.

C Other Preadmission Services (Effective for Services Furnished On or After October 1, 1991)

Nondiagnostic outpatient services that are related to a patient's hospital admission and that are provided by the hospital, or by an entity wholly owned or wholly operated by the admitting hospital (or by another entity under arrangements with the admitting hospital), to the patient during the 3 days immediately preceding and including the date of the patient's admission are deemed to be inpatient services and are included in the inpatient payment. Effective March 13, 1998, we defined nondiagnostic preadmission services as being related to the admission only when

there is an exact match (for all digits) between the ICD-9-CM principal diagnosis code assigned for both the preadmission services and the inpatient stay. Thus, whenever Part A covers an

admission, the hospital may bill nondiagnostic preadmission services to Part B as outpatient services only if they are not related to the admission. The FI shall assume, in the absence of evidence to the contrary, that such bills are not admission related and, therefore, are not deemed to be inpatient (Part A) services. If there are both diagnostic and nondiagnostic preadmission services and the nondiagnostic services are unrelated to the admission, the hospital may separately bill the nondiagnostic preadmission services to Part B. This provision applies only when the patient has Part A coverage. This provision does not apply to ambulance services and maintenance renal dialysis. Additionally, Part A services furnished by skilled nursing facilities, home health agencies, and hospices are excluded from the payment window provisions.

For services provided before October 31, 1994, this provision applies to both hospitals subject to IPPS as well as those hospitals and units excluded from IPPS (see section B above).

For services provided on or after October 31, 1994, for hospitals and units excluded from IPPS, this provision applies only to services furnished within one day prior to and including the date of the beneficiary's admission.

Critical access hospitals (CAHs) are not subject to the 3-day (nor 1-day) DRG payment window.

Hospitals in Maryland that are under the jurisdiction of the Health Services Cost Review Commission are subject to the 3-day payment window.

Pub. 100-4, Chapter 4, Section 10.12

Through Payment Status Under the Hospital Outpatient Prospective Payment System

http://www.cms.hhs.gov/regulations/hopps/newcatapp11602final1.pdf

This describes in detail the process and information required for applications requesting additional categories for medical devices that may be eligible for transitional pass-through payment under the Medicare hospital outpatient prospective payment system (OPPS). This applies solely to requests for additional categories of medical devices.

The CMS makes information used in the rate setting process under the OPPS available to the public for analysis. Any information submitted, including commercial or financial data, is subject to disclosure for this purpose.

The CMS accepts category applications on an ongoing basis. However, CMS must receive applications sufficiently in advance of the calendar quarter in which a category would be established to allow time for analysis, decision-making, and computer programming. Therefore, the following schedule applies:

Complete Application Must Be Received by No Later Than...	For Consideration for Implementation Beginning...
December 3	March 1
March 1	July 1
June 1	October 1
September 3	January 1

A longer evaluation period may be required if an application is incomplete or if further information is required upon which to base a determination of eligibility.

An application is not considered complete until:

• All required information has been submitted; and

• All questions related to such information have been answered.

Applicants submitting amended requests to establish a new medical device category should attach a statement indicating that the amended application is intended to replace or to supplement a previous filing. The applicant should also submit a copy of the previous filing. We can act only on applications that fully address the criteria and requirements set forth in this announcement.

Device manufacturers, hospitals, or other interested parties may apply for a new device category for transitional pass-through payments. The law requires that:

• New categories be established in such a way that no medical device is described by more than one category; and

• The average cost of devices included in a new category be "not insignificant" relative to the payment amount for the procedure(s) or service(s) with which the device is associated. The definition of "not insignificant" cost is described below.

To be included in a category a device must meet all applicable criteria that were previously established for a device eligible for transitional pass-through payments. Those criteria are the following:

1. If required by the FDA, the device must have received FDA approval or clearance. (This requirement is met if a device has received an FDA investigational device exemption (IDE) and has been classified as a Category B device by the FDA in accordance with 405.203 through 405.207 and 405.211 through 405.215 of Title 42 of the Code of Federal Regulations or has received another appropriate FDA exemption.)

2. The device is determined to be reasonable and necessary for the diagnosis or treatment of an illness or injury or to improve the functioning of a malformed body part

(as required by §1862(a)(1)(A) of the Act.) Note that neither assignment of a HCPCS code nor approval of a device for transitional pass-through payment assures coverage of the specific item or service in a given case. To receive transitional pass-through payments, qualified devices must be considered reasonable and necessary; each use of a qualified device is subject to medical review for determination of whether its use was reasonable and necessary.

3. The device must:

a. Be an integral and subordinate part of the service furnished;

b. Be used for one patient only;

c. Come in contact with human tissue; and

d. Be surgically implanted or inserted whether or not the device remains with the patient when the patient is released from the hospital.

4. The device is not any of the following:

a. Equipment, an instrument, apparatus, implement, or item of this type for which depreciation and financing expenses are recovered as depreciable assets as defined in Chapter 1 of the Medicare Provider Reimbursement Manual (CMS Pub. 15-1);

b. A material or supply furnished incident to a service (for example, a suture, customized surgical kit, scalpel, or clip, other than radiological site marker); and

c. A material that may be used to replace human skin (for example, a biological or synthetic material).

Pub. 100-4, Chapter 4, Section 20.5

HCPCS/Revenue Code Chart

A-01-93, A-01-50, A-03-066

The following chart reflects HCPCS coding to be reported under OPPS by hospital outpatient departments. This chart is intended only as a guide to be used by hospitals to assist them in reporting services rendered. Hospitals that are currently utilizing different revenue/HCPCS reporting may continue to do so. They are not required to change the way they currently report their services to agree with this chart. Note that this chart does not represent all HCPCS coding subject to OPPS.

Revenue Code	HCPCS Code	Description
*	10040-69990	Surgical Procedure
*	92950-92961	Cardiovascular
*	96570, 96571	Photodynamic Therapy
*	99170, 99185, 99186	Other Services and Procedures
*	99291-99292	Critical Care
*	99440	Newborn Care
*	90782-90799	Therapeutic or Diagnostic Injections
*	D0150, D0240-D0274, D0277, D0460, D0472- D0999, D1510-D1550, D2970, D2999, D3460, D3999, D4260-D4264, D4270-D4273, D4355-D4381, D5911-D5912, D5983-D5985, D5987, D6920, D7110-D7260, D7291, D7940, D9630, D9930, D9940, D9950-D9952	Dental Services
*	92502-92596, 92599	Otorhinolaryngologic Services (ENT)
0278	E0749, E0782, E0783, E0785	Implanted Durable Medical Equipment
0278	E0751, E0753, L8600, L8603, L8610, L8612, L8613, L8614, L8630, L8641, L8642, L8658, L8670, L8699	Implanted Prosthetic Devices
0302	86485-86586	Immunology
0305	85060-85102, 86077-86079	Hematology
031X	80500-80502	Pathology - Lab
0310	88300-88365, 88399	Surgical Pathology
0311	88104-88125, 88160-88199	Cytopathology
032X	70010-76092, 76094-76999	Diagnostic Radiology
0333	77261-77799	Radiation Oncology
034X	78000-79999	Nuclear Medicine
037X	99141-99142	Anesthesia
045X	99281-99285, 99291	Emergency
046X	94010-94799	Pulmonary Function

Revenue Code	HCPCS Code	Description
0480	93600-93790, 93799, G0166	Intra Electrophysiological Procedures and Other Vascular Studies
0481	93501-93572	Cardiac Catheterization
0482	93015-93024	Stress Test
0483	93303-93350	Echocardiography
051X	92002-92499	Ophthalmological Services
051X	99201-99215, 99241-99245, 99271-99275	Clinic Visit
0510, 0517, 0519	95144-95149, 95165, 95170, 95180, 95199	Allergen Immunotherapy
0519	95805-95811	Sleep Testing
0530	98925-98929	Osteopathic Manipulative Procedures
0636	A4642, A9500, A9605	Radionucleides
0636	90476-90665, 90675-90749	Vaccines, Toxoids
0636	90296-90379, 90385, 90389-90396	Immune Globulins
073X	G0004-G0006, G0015	Event Recording ECG
0730	93005-93009, 93011-93013, 93040-93224, 93278	Electrocardiograms (ECGs)
0731	93225-93272	Holter Monitor
074X	95812-95827, 95950-95962	Electroencephalogram (EEG)
0771	G0008-G0010	Vaccine Administration
088X	90935-90999	Non-ESRD Dialysis
0900	90801, 90802, 90865,90899	Behavioral Health Treatment/Services
0901	90870, 90871	Psychiatry
0903	90910, 90911, 90812-90815, 90823, 90824, 90826-90829	Psychiatry
0909	90880	Psychiatry
0914	90804-90809, 90816-90819, 90821, 90822, 90845, 90862	Psychiatry
0915	90853, 90857	Psychiatry
0916	90846,90847, 90849	Psychiatry
0917	90901-90911	Biofeedback
0918	96100-96117	Central Nervous System Assessments/Tests
092X	95829-95857, 95900-95937, 95970-95999	Miscellaneous Neurological Procedures
0920, 0929	93875-93990	Non Invasive Vascular Diagnosis Studies
0922	95858-95875	Electromyography (EMG)
0924	95004-95078	Allergy Test
0940	96900-96999	Special Dermatological Procedures
0940	98940-98942	Chiropractic Manipulative Treatment
0940	99195	Other Services and Procedures
0943	93797-93798	Cardiac Rehabilitation

*Revenue codes have not been identified for these procedures, as they can be performed in a number of revenue centers within a hospital, such as emergency room (0450), operating room (0360), or clinic (0510). Hospitals are to report these HCPCS codes under the revenue center where they were performed.

NOTE: The listing of HCPCS codes contained in the above chart does not assure coverage on the specific service. Current coverage criteria apply. FIs are not to install additional edits for matching of revenue codes and HCPCS codes.

20.5.1 - Appropriate Revenue Codes to Report Medical Devices That Have Been Granted Pass-Through Status

A-03-035

The FIs shall instruct their hospitals to use an appropriate HCPCS code and one of the following revenue codes:

0272, 0275, 0276, 0278, 0279, 0280, 0289 or 0624 to bill implantable devices that have been granted pass-through status under the OPPS. Devices eligible for pass-through payment, as designated by payment status indicator "H," should not be reported utilizing any other revenue code series or subcategories.

The FIs shall instruct their hospitals to report implantable orthotic and prosthetic devices and implantable durable medical equipment (DME) under another revenue code such as 0278- other implants. Hospitals are not to use revenue codes 0274 or 0290 to report implantable orthotic and prosthetic devices or implantable DME. Similar requirements apply to reporting revenue codes for non-pass-through devices.

Pub. 100-4, Chapter 4, Section 61.1

Requirement that Hospitals Report Device Codes on Claims on Which They Report Specified Procedures

Effective January 1, 2005, hospitals paid under the OPPS (bill types 12X and 13X) that report procedure codes that require the use of devices must also report the applicable HCPCS codes and charges for all devices that are used to perform the procedures where such codes exist. This is necessary so that the OPPS payment for these procedures will be correct in future years in which the claims are used to create the APC payment amounts. Current HCPCS codes for devices are found at http://www.cms.hhs.gov/medicare/HCPCS.

Pub. 100-4, Chapter 4, Section 61.2

Edits for Claims on Which Specified Procedures are to be Reported With Device Codes

The OCE will return to the provider any claim that reports a HCPCS code for a procedure listed in the table of device edits that does not also report at least one device HCPCS code required for that procedure as listed on the CMS Web site at http://www.cms.hhs.gov/providers/hopps/. The table shows the effective date for each edit. If the claim is returned to the provider for failure to pass the edits, the hospital will need to modify the claim by either correcting the procedure code or ensuring that one of the required device codes is on the claim before resubmission. While all devices that have device HCPCS codes, and that were used in a given procedure should be reported on the

claim, where more than one device code is listed for a given procedure code, only one of the possible device codes is required to be on the claim for payment to be made, unless otherwise specified.

Device edits do not apply to the specified procedure code if the provider reports one of the following modifiers with the procedure code:

52 - Reduced Services;

73 -- Discontinued outpatient procedure prior to anesthesia administration; and

74 -- Discontinued outpatient procedure after anesthesia administration.

Where a procedure that normally requires a device is interrupted, either before or after the administration of anesthesia if anesthesia is required or at any point if anesthesia is not required, and the device is not used, hospitals should report modifier 52, 73 or 74 as applicable. The device edits are not applied in these cases.

Pub. 100-4, Chapter 4, Section 160

Coding for Clinic and Emergency Visits

A-01-93

The OPPS hospitals previously reported CPT code 99201 to indicate a visit of any type. Under OPPS, 31 codes are used to indicate visits, with payment differentials for more or less intense services.

Hospitals code the site of the visit and the level of intensity, using the following codes:

92002, 92004, 92012, 92014, 99201, 99202, 99203, 99204, 99205, 99211, 99212, 99213, 99214, 99215, 99241, 99242, 99243, 99244, 99245, 99271, 99272, 99273, 99274, 99275, 99281, 99282, 99283, 99284, 99285, 99291, and G0175.

Because CPT is more descriptive of practitioner than of facility services, hospitals must use CPT guidelines when applicable, or crosswalk hospital coding structures to CPT. For example, a hospital that has eight levels of emergency and trauma care, depending on nursing ratios, should crosswalk those eight levels to the CPT codes for emergency care.

Pub. 100-4, Chapter 4, Section 190

Implanted DME, Prosthetic Devices and Diagnostic Devices

Implanted DME, implanted prosthetic devices, and implanted diagnostic devices are paid under OPPS and therefore are no longer payable under the DME Orthotic/Prosthetic fee schedules. The following are the appropriate HCPCS codes for payment under OPPS:

- Implanted DME: E0749, E0782, E0783, E0785

- Implanted Prosthetic Devices: E0751, E0753, L8600, L8603, L8610, L8612, L8613, L8614, L8630, L8641, L8642, L8658, L8670, L8699

- Implanted Diagnostic Device: C1361

Effective with claims with dates of service on or after August 1, 2000, hospitals under OPPS do not bill the local carrier for these services.

Pub. 100-4, Chapter 4, Section 220.3

Billing for Linear Accelerator (Gantry or Image Directed) SR Planning and Delivery

Effective for services furnished on or after April 1, 2002, hospitals must bill for gantry or image directed linear accelerator SR using G0242 for planning. Hospitals must bill G0173 for delivery if the delivery occurs in one session, and G0251 for delivery per session (not to exceed five sessions) if delivery occurs during multiple sessions.

G0173   Linear accelerator based stereotactic radiosurgery, delivery including collimator changes and custom plugging, complete course of treatment in one session, all lesions.

G0251   Linear accelerator based stereotactic radiosurgery, delivery including collimator changes and custom plugging, fractionated treatment, all lesions, per session, maximum 5 sessions per course of treatment.

NOTE: Although Code G0251 is effective on April 1, 2002, the Outpatient Code Editor or the OPPS Pricer will not recognize the code until July 1, 2002. Therefore, FIs instruct hospitals to either hold all bills that contain this code and submit the bills after July 1, 2002, or submit bills but omit this code and submit an adjustment bill reflecting this service after July 1, 2002.

Pub. 100-4, Chapter 4, Section 230.1

Coding and Payment for Drugs and Biologicals

This section provides hospitals with coding instructions and payment information for drugs paid under OPPS.

Pub. 100-4, Chapter 4, Section 230.2.1

Administration of Drugs Via Implantable or Portable Pumps

Table 2: CY 2006 OPPS Drug Administration Codes for Implantable or Portable Pumps

2005 CPT	Final CY 2006 OPPS	2005 CPT	2005 Descrip	Code	Descrip
SI	APC	n/a	n/a	C8957	Intravenous infusion for therapy/diagnosis; initiation of prolonged infusion (more than 8 hours), requiring use of portable or implantable pump
S	0120	96414	Chemotherapy administration, intravenous; infusion technique, initiation of prolonged infusion (more than 8 hours), requiring the use of a portable or implantable pump	96416	Chemotherapy administration, intravenous infusion technique; initiation of prolonged chemotherapy infusion (more than 8 hours), requiring use of portable or implantable pump
S	0117	96425	Chemotherapy administration, infusion technique, initiation of prolonged infusion (more than 8 hours), requiring the use of a portable or implantable pump)	96425	Chemotherapy administration, intra-arterial; infusion technique, initiation of prolonged infusion (more than 8 hours), requiring the use of a portable or implantable pump
S	0117	96520	Refilling and maintenance of portable pump	96521	Refilling and maintenance of portable pump

2005 CPT	Final CY 2006 OPPS	2005 CPT	2005 Descrip	Code	Descrip
T	0125	SI	APC	96530	Refilling and maintenance of implantable pump or reservoir for drug delivery, systemic (e.g. Intravenous, intra-arterial)
96522	Refilling and maintenance of implantable pump or reservoir for drug delivery, systemic (e.g., intravenous, intra-arterial)	T	0125	n/a	n/a
96523	Irrigation of implanted venous access device for drug delivery systems	N	-		

Hospitals are to report HCPCS code C8957 and CPT codes 96416 and 96425 to indicate the initiation of a prolonged infusion that requires the use of an implantable or portable pump. CPT codes 96521, 92522, and 96523 should be used by hospitals to indicate refilling and maintenance of drug delivery systems or irrigation of implanted venous access devices for such systems, and may be reported for the servicing of devices used for therapeutic drugs other than chemotherapy.

Pub. 100-4, Chapter 4, Section 230.2.3

Chemotherapy Drug Administration

A. Administration of Non-Chemotherapy Drugs by Intravenous Infusion

Table 5: CY 2006 OPPS Non-Chemotherapy Drug Administration -Intravenous Infusion Technique

2005 CPT	Final CY 2006 OPPS	2005 CPT	2005 Descrip	Code	Descrip
SI	APC	90780	Intravenous infusion for therapy/diagnosis, administered by physician or under direct supervision of physician; up to one hour	C8950	Intravenous infusion for therapy/diagnosis; up to 1 hour
S	0120	90781	Intravenous infusion for therapy/diagnosis, administered by physician or under direct supervision of physician; each additional hour, up to eight (8) hours (List separately in addition to code for primary procedure)	C8951	Intravenous infusion for therapy/diagnosis; each additional hour (List separately in addition to C8950)

2005 CPT	Final CY 2006 OPPS	2005 CPT	2005 Descrip	Code	Descrip
N	-	n/a	n/a	C8957	Intravenous infusion for therapy/diagnosis; initiation of prolonged infusion (more than 8 hours), requiring use of portable or implantable pump
S	0120				

Hospitals are to report HCPCS code C8950 to indicate an infusion of drugs other than anti-neoplastic drugs furnished on or after January 1, 2006 (except as noted at 230.2.2(A) above). HCPCS code C8951 should be used to report all additional infusion hours, with no limit on the number of hours billed per line. Medically necessary separate therapeutic or diagnostic hydration services should be reported with C8950 and C8951, as these are considered intravenous infusions for therapy/diagnosis.

HCPCS codes C8950 and C8951 should not be reported when the infusion is a necessary and integral part of a separately payable OPPS procedure.

When more than one nonchemotherapy drug is infused, hospitals are to code HCPCS codes C8950 and C8951 (if necessary) to report the total duration of an infusion, regardless of the number of substances or drugs infused. Hospitals are reminded to bill separately for each drug infused, in addition to the drug administration services.

The OCE pays one APC for each encounter reported by HCPCS code C8950, and only pays one APC for C8950 per day (unless Modifier 59 is used). Payment for additional hours of infusion reported by HCPCS code C8951 is packaged into the payment for the initial infusion. While no separate payment will be made for units of HCPCS code C8951, hospitals are instructed to report all codes that appropriately describe the services provided and the corresponding charges so that CMS may capture specific historical hospital cost data for future payment rate setting activities.

OCE logic assumes that all services for non-chemotherapy infusions billed on the same date of service were provided during the same encounter. Where a beneficiary makes two separate visits to the hospital for non-chemotherapy infusions in the same day, hospitals are to report modifier 59 for non-chemotherapy infusion codes during the second encounter that were also furnished in the first encounter. The OCE identifies modifier 59 and pays up to a maximum number of units per day, as listed in Table 1.

EXAMPLE 1

A beneficiary receives infused drugs that are not anti-neoplastic drugs (including hydrating solutions) for 2 hours. The hospital reports one unit of HCPCS code C8950 and one unit of HCPCS code C8951. The OCE will pay one unit of APC 0120. Payment for the unit of HCPCS code C8951 is packaged into the payment for one unit of APC 0120. (NOTE: See §230.1 for drug billing instructions.)

EXAMPLE 2

A beneficiary receives infused drugs that are not anti-neoplastic drugs (including hydrating solutions) for 12 hours. The hospital reports one unit of HCPCS code C8950 and eleven units of HCPCS code C8951. The OCE will pay one unit of APC 0120. Payment for the 11 units of HCPCS code C8951 is packaged into the payment for one unit of APC 0120. (NOTE: See §230.1 for drug billing instructions.)

EXAMPLE 3

A beneficiary experiences multiple attempts to initiate an intravenous infusion before a successful infusion is started 20 minutes after the first attempt. Once started, the infusion lasts one hour. The hospital reports one unit of HCPCS code C8950 to identify the 1 hour of infusion time. The 20 minutes spent prior to the infusion attempting to establish an IV line are not separately billable in the OPPS. The OCE pays one unit of APC 0120. (NOTE: See §230.1 for drug billing instructions.)

B. Administration of Non-Chemotherapy Drugs by a Route Other Than Intravenous Infusion

Table 6: CY 2006 OPPS Non-Chemotherapy Drug Administration -Route Other Than Intravenous Infusion

2005 CPT	Final CY 2006 OPPS	2005 CPT	2005 Descrip	Code	Descrip
SI	APC	90784	Therapeutic, prophylactic or diagnostic injection (specify material injected); intravenous	C8952	Therapeutic, prophylactic or diagnostic injection; intravenous push

2005 CPT	Final CY 2006 OPPS	2005 CPT	2005 Descrip	Code	Descrip
X	0359	90782	Therapeutic, prophylactic or diagnostic injection (specify material injected); subcutaneous or intramuscular	90772	Therapeutic, prophylactic or diagnostic injection (specify substance or drug); subcutaneous or intramuscular
X	0353	90783	Therapeutic, prophylactic or diagnostic injection (specify material injected); intra-arterial	90773	Therapeutic, prophylactic or diagnostic injection (specify substance or drug); intra-arterial
X	0359	90779	Unlisted therapeutic, prophylactic or diagnostic intravenous or intra-arterial, injection or infusion	90779	Unlisted therapeutic, prophylactic or diagnostic intravenous or intra-arterial injection or infusion
X	0352				

Pub. 100-4, Chapter 4, Section 240

Inpatient Part B Hospital Services

Inpatient Part B services which are paid under OPPS include:

• Diagnostic x-ray tests, and other diagnostic tests (excluding clinical diagnostic laboratory tests);

• X-ray, radium, and radioactive isotope therapy, including materials and services of technicians;

• Surgical dressings applied during an encounter at the hospital and splints, casts, and other devices used for reduction of fractures and dislocations (splints and casts, etc., include dental splints);

• Implantable prosthetic devices;

• Hepatitis B vaccine and its administration, and certain preventive screening services (pelvic exams, screening sigmoidoscopies, screening colonoscopies, bone mass measurements, and prostate screening.)

• Bone Mass measurements;

• Prostate screening;

• Immunosuppressive drugs;

• Oral anti-cancer drugs;

• Oral drug prescribed for use as an acute anti-emetic used as part of an anti-cancer chemotherapeutic regimen; and

• Epoetin Alfa (EPO)

NOTE: Payment for some of these services is packaged into the payment rate of other separately payable services.

Inpatient Part B services paid under other payment methods include:

• Clinical diagnostic laboratory tests, prosthetic devices other than implantable ones and other than dental which replace all or part of an internal body organ (including contiguous tissue), or all or part of the function of a permanently inoperative or malfunctioning internal body organ, including replacement or repairs of such devices;

• Leg, arm, back and neck braces; trusses and artificial legs; arms and eyes including adjustments, repairs, and replacements required because of breakage, wear, loss, or a change in the patient's physical condition; take home surgical dressings;

outpatient physical therapy; outpatient occupational therapy; and outpatient speech pathology services;

• Ambulance services;

• Screening pap smears, screening colorectal tests, and screening mammography;

• Influenza virus vaccine and its administration, pneumococcal vaccine and its administration;

• Diabetes self-management;

• Hemophilia clotting factors for hemophilia patients competent to use these factors without supervision).

See Chapter 6 of the Medicare Benefit Policy Manual for a discussion of the circumstances under which the above services may be covered as Part B Inpatient services.

Pub. 100-4, Chapter 4, Section 290.4.1

Billing and Payment for All Hospital Observation Services Furnished On or After January 1, 2006

Beginning January 1, 2006, two new G-codes are to be used to report observation services and direct admission for observation care. The OPPS claims processing logic will determine the payment status of the observation and direct admission services, that is, whether they are packaged or separately payable. Thus, hospitals are able to provide consistent coding and billing under all circumstances in which they deliver observation care.

Beginning January 1, 2006, hospitals should not report CPT codes 99217-99220 or 99234-99236 for observation services. In addition, the following HCPCS codes are discontinued as of January 1, 2006: G0244 (Observation care by facility to patient), G0263 (Direct Admission with congestive heart failure, chest pain or asthma), and G0264 (Assessment other than congestive heart failure, chest pain, or asthma).

The three discontinued G-codes and the CPT codes that are no longer recognized are replaced by two new G-codes to be used by hospitals to report all observation services, whether separately payable or packaged, and direct admission for observation care, whether separately payable or packaged:

• G0378- Hospital observation services, per hour; and

• G0379- Direct admission of patient for hospital observation care.

The OPPS claims processing logic will determine whether observation services billed as units of G0378 are separately payable under APC 0339 (Observation) or whether payment for observation services will be packaged into the payment for other services provided by the hospital in the same encounter. Therefore, hospitals should bill HCPCS code G0378 when observation services are provided to any patient in "observation status," regardless of the patient's condition. The units of service should equal the number of hours the patient is in observation status.

Hospitals should report G0379 when observation services are the result of a direct admission to "observation status" without an associated emergency room visit, hospital outpatient clinic visit, or critical care service on the day of initiation of observation services. Hospitals should only report HCPCS code G0379 when a patient is admitted directly to observation care after being seen by a physician in the community (see §290.4.2 below)

Change Request 4047, issued on November 25, 2005, (Transmittal 763), explains that some non-repetitive OPPS services provided on the same day by a hospital may be billed on different claims, provided that all charges associated with each procedure or service being reported are billed on the same claim with the HCPCS code which describes that service. It is vitally important that all of the charges that pertain to a non-repetitive, separately paid procedure or service be reported on the same claim with that procedure or service. It should also be emphasized that this relaxation of same day billing requirements for some non-repetitive services does not apply to non-repetitive services provided on the same day as either direct admission to observation care or observation services because the OCE claim-by-claim logic cannot function properly unless all services related to the episode of observation care, including diagnostic tests, lab services, hospital clinic visits, emergency department visits, critical care services, and ``T'' status procedures, are reported on the same claim. Additional guidance can be found in the Change Request cited above.

Pub. 100-4, Chapter 12, Section 30.4

93799)

A. Echocardiography Contrast Agents

Effective October 1, 2000, physicians may separately bill for contrast agents used in echocardiography. Physicians should use HCPCS Code A9700 (Supply of Injectable Contrast Material for Use in Echocardiography, per study). The type of service code is 9. This code will be carrier-priced.

B. Electronic Analyses of Implantable Cardioverter-defibrillators and Pacemakers

The CPT codes 93731, 93734, 93741 and 93743 are used to report electronic analyses of single or dual chamber pacemakers and single or dual chamber implantable cardioverter-defibrillators. In the office, a physician uses a device called a programmer to obtain information about the status and performance of the device and to evaluate the patient's cardiac rhythm and response to the implanted device.

Advances in information technology now enable physicians to evaluate patients with implanted cardiac devices without requiring the patient to be present in the physician's office. Using a manufacturer's specific monitor/transmitter, a patient can send complete device data and specific cardiac data to a distant receiving station or secure Internet server. The electronic analysis of cardiac device data that is remotely obtained provides immediate and long-term data on the device and clinical data on the patient's cardiac functioning equivalent to that obtained during an in-office evaluation. Physicians should report the electronic analysis of an implanted cardiac device using remotely obtained data as described above with CPT code 93731, 93734, 93741 or 93743, depending on the type of cardiac device implanted in the patient.

Pub. 100-4, Chapter 12, Section 30.6.1.1

Initial Preventive Physical Examination (HCPCS Codes G0344, G0366, G0367 and G0368)

A. Definition

The initial preventive physical examination (IPPE), or "Welcome to Medicare Visit", is a preventive evaluation and management service (E/M) that includes: (1) review of the individual's medical and social history with attention to modifiable risk factors for disease detection, (2) review of the individual's potential (risk factors) for depression or other mood disorders, (3) review of the individual's functional ability and level of safety; (4) a physical examination to include measurement of the individual's height, weight, blood pressure, a visual acuity screen, and other factors as deemed appropriate by the examining physician or qualified nonphysician practitioner (NPP), (5) performance and interpretation of an electrocardiogram (EKG); (6) education, counseling, and referral, as deemed appropriate, based on the results of the review and evaluation services described in the previous 5 elements, and (7) education, counseling, and referral including a brief written plan (e.g., a checklist or alternative) provided to the individual for obtaining the appropriate screening and other preventive services, which are separately covered under Medicare Part B benefits. (For billing requirements, refer to Pub. 100-04, Chapter 18, Section 80.)

B. Who May Perform

The IPPE may be performed by a doctor of medicine or osteopathy as defined in section 1861 (r)(1) of the Social Security Act or by a qualified NPP (nurse practitioner, physician assistant and clinical nurse specialist). The carrier will pay the appropriate physician fee schedule amount based on the rendering UPIN/PIN.

C. Eligibility

Medicare will pay for one IPPE per beneficiary per lifetime. A beneficiary is eligible when he first enrolls in Medicare Part B on or after January 1, 2005, and receives the IPPE benefit within the first 6 months of the effective date of the initial Part B coverage period.

D. The EKG Component

If the physician or qualified NPP is not able to perform both the examination and the screening EKG, an arrangement may be made to ensure that another physician or entity performs the screening EKG and reports the EKG separately using the appropriate

HCPCS G code. The primary physician or qualified NPP shall document the results of the screening EKG into the beneficiary's medical record to complete and bill for the IPPE benefit. NOTE: Both components of the IPPE (the examination and the screening EKG) must be performed before the claims can be submitted by the physician, qualified NPP and/or entity.

E. Codes Used to Bill the IPPE

The physician or qualified NPP shall bill HCPCS code G0344 for the physical examination performed face-to-face and HCPCS code G0366 for performing a screening EKG that includes both the interpretation and report. If the primary physician or qualified NPP performs only the examination, he/she shall bill HCPCS code G0344 only. The physician or entity that performs the screening EKG that includes both the interpretation and report shall bill HCPCS code G0366. The physician or entity that performs the screening EKG tracing only (without interpretation and report) shall bill HCPCS code G0367. The physician or entity that performs the interpretation and report only (without the EKG tracing) shall bill HCPCS code G0368. Medicare will pay for a screening EKG only as part of the IPPE. NOTE: For an IPPE performed during the global period of surgery refer to section 30.6.6, chapter 12, Pub 100-04 for reporting instructions.

F. Documentation

The physician and qualified NPP shall use the appropriate screening tools typically used in routine physician practice. As for all E/M services, the 1995 and 1997 E/M documentation guidelines (http://www.cms.hhs.gov/medlearn/emdoc.asp) should be followed for recording the appropriate clinical information in the beneficiary's medical record. All referrals and a written medical plan must be included in this documentation.

G. Reporting A Medically Necessary E/M at Same IPPE Visit

When the physician or qualified NPP provide a medically necessary E/M service in addition to the IPPE, CPT codes 99201 - 99215 may be used depending on the clinical appropriateness of the circumstances. CPT Modifier -25 shall be appended to the medically necessary E/M service identifying this service as a separately identifiable service from the IPPE code G0344 reported. NOTE: Some of the components of a medically necessary E/M service (e.g., a portion of history or physical exam portion) may have been part of the IPPE and should not be included when determining the most appropriate level of E/M service to be billed for the medically necessary E/M service.

Pub. 100-4, Chapter 12, Section 70

Payment Conditions for Radiology Services
B3-15022

See chapter 13, for claims processing instructions for radiology.

Pub. 100-4, Chapter 12, Section 190

Medicare Payment for Telehealth Services
A3-3497, A3-3660.2, B3-4159, B3-15516

Pub. 100-4, Chapter 12, Section 210.1

Application of Limitation
B3-2472 - 2472.5

A. Status of Patient

The limitation is applicable to expenses incurred in connection with the treatment of an individual who is not an inpatient of a hospital. Thus, the limitation applies to mental health services furnished to a person in a physician's office, in the patient's home, in a skilled nursing facility, as an outpatient, and so forth. The term "hospital" in this context means an institution, which is primarily engaged in providing to inpatients, by or under the supervision of physician(s):

• Diagnostic and therapeutic services for medical diagnosis, treatment and care of injured, disabled, or sick persons;

• Rehabilitation services for injured, disabled, or sick persons; or

• Psychiatric services for the diagnosis and treatment of mentally ill patients.

B. Disorders Subject to Limitation

The term "mental, psychoneurotic, and personality disorders" is defined as the specific psychiatric conditions described in the American Psychiatric Association's (APA) "Diagnostic and Statistical Manual of Mental Disorders, Third Edition - Revised (DSM-III-R)."

When the treatment services rendered are both for a psychiatric condition as defined in the DSM-III-R and one or more nonpsychiatric conditions, separate the expenses for the psychiatric aspects of treatment from the expenses for the nonpsychiatric aspects of treatment. However, in any case in which the psychiatric treatment component is not readily distinguishable from the nonpsychiatric treatment component, all of the expenses are allocated to whichever component constitutes the primary diagnosis.

1. Diagnosis Clearly Meets Definition - If the primary diagnosis reported for a particular service is the same as or equivalent to a condition described in the APA's DSM-III-R, the expense for the service is subject to the limitation except as described in subsection D.

2. Diagnosis Does Not Clearly Meet Definition - When it is not clear whether the primary diagnosis reported meets the definition of mental, psychoneurotic, and personality disorders, it may be necessary to contact the practitioner to clarify the diagnosis. In deciding whether contact is necessary in a given case, give consideration to such factors as the type of services rendered, the diagnosis, and the individual's previous utilization history.

C. Services Subject to Limitation

Carriers apply the limitation to claims for professional services that represent mental health treatment furnished to individuals who are not hospital inpatients by physicians, clinical psychologists, clinical social workers, and other allied health professionals. Items and supplies furnished by physicians or other mental health practitioners in connection with treatment are also subject to the limitation. (The limitation also applies to CORF claims processed by intermediaries.)

Carriers apply the limitation only to treatment services. It does not apply to diagnostic services as described in subsection D. Testing services performed to evaluate a patient's progress during treatment are considered part of treatment and are subject to the limitation.

D. Services Not Subject to Limitation

1. Diagnosis of Alzheimer's Disease or Related Disorder - When the primary diagnosis reported for a particular service is Alzheimer's Disease (coded 331.0 in the "International Classification of Diseases, 9th Revision") or Alzheimer's or other disorders coded 290.XX in the APA's DSM-III-R, carriers look to the nature of the service that has been rendered in determining whether it is subject to the limitation. Typically, treatment provided to a patient with a diagnosis of Alzheimer's Disease or a related disorder represents medical management of the patient's condition (rather than psychiatric treatment) and is not subject to the limitation. However, when the primary treatment rendered to a patient with such a diagnosis is psychotherapy, it is subject to the limitation.

2. Brief Office Visits for Monitoring or Changing Drug Prescriptions - Brief office visits for the sole purpose of monitoring or changing drug prescriptions used in the treatment of mental, psychoneurotic and personality disorders are not subject to the limitation. These visits are reported using HCPCS code M0064 (brief office visit for the sole purpose of monitoring or changing drug prescriptions used in the treatment of mental, psychoneurotic, and personality disorders). Claims where the diagnosis reported is a mental, psychoneurotic, or personality disorder (other than a diagnosis specified in subsection A) are subject to the limitation except for the procedure identified by HCPCS code M0064.

3. Diagnostic Services - Carriers do not apply the limitation to tests and evaluations performed to establish or confirm the patient's diagnosis. Diagnostic services include psychiatric or psychological tests and interpretations, diagnostic consultations, and initial evaluations.

An initial visit to a practitioner for professional services often combines diagnostic evaluation and the start of therapy. Such a visit is neither solely diagnostic nor solely therapeutic. Therefore, carriers deem the initial visit to be diagnostic so that the limitation does not apply. Separating diagnostic and therapeutic components of a visit is not administratively feasible, unless the practitioner already has separately identified them on the bill. Determining the entire visit to be therapeutic is not justifiable since some diagnostic work must be done before even a tentative diagnosis can be made and certainly before therapy can be instituted. Moreover, the patient should not be disadvantaged because therapeutic as well as diagnostic services were provided in the initial visit. In the rare cases where a practitioner's diagnostic services take more than one visit, carriers do not apply the limitation to the additional visits. However, it is expected such cases are few. Therefore, when a practitioner bills for more than one visit for professional diagnostic services, carriers request documentation to justify the reason for more than one diagnostic visit.

4. Partial Hospitalization Services Not Directly Provided by Physician - The limitation does not apply to partial hospitalization services that are not directly provided by a physician. These services are billed by hospitals and community mental health centers (CMHCs) to intermediaries.

E. Computation of Limitation

Carriers determine the Medicare allowed payment amount for services subject to the limitation. They:

• Multiply this amount by 0.625;

• Subtract any unsatisfied deductible; and,

• Multiply the remainder by 0.8 to obtain the amount of Medicare payment.

The beneficiary is responsible for the difference between the amount paid by Medicare and the full allowed amount.

EXAMPLE A:

A beneficiary is referred to a Medicare participating psychiatrist who performs a diagnostic evaluation that costs $350. Those services are not subject to the limitation, and they satisfy the deductible. The psychiatrist then conducts 10 weekly therapy sessions for which he/she charges $125 each. The Medicare allowed amount is $90 each, for a total of $900.

Apply the limitation by multiplying 0.625 times $900, which equals $562.50.

Apply regular 20 percent coinsurance by multiplying 0.8 times $562.50, which equals $450 (the amount of Medicare payment).

The beneficiary is responsible for $450 (the difference between Medicare payment and the allowed amount).

EXAMPLE B:

A beneficiary was an inpatient of a psychiatric hospital and was discharged on January 1, 1992. During his/her inpatient stay he/she was diagnosed and therapy was begun under a treatment team that included a clinical psychologist. He/she received post-discharge therapy from the psychologist for 12 sessions, at which point the psychologist administered testing that showed the patient had recovered sufficiently to warrant termination of therapy. The allowed amount for the therapy sessions was $80 each, and the amount for the testing was $125, for a total of $1085. All services in 1992 were subject to the limitation, since the diagnosis had been completed in the hospital and the subsequent testing was a part of therapy.

Apply the limitation by multiplying 0.625 times $1085, which gives $678.13.

Since the deductible must be met for 1992, subtract $100 from $678.13, for a remainder of $578.13.

Determine Medicare payment by multiplying the remainder by 0.8, which equals $462.50.

The beneficiary is responsible for $622.50.

Pub. 100-4, Chapter 13, Section 20

Payment Conditions for Radiology Services
B3-15022

Pub. 100-4, Chapter 13, Section 40.1.2

HCPCS Coding Requirements
Providers must report HCPCS codes when submitting claims for MRA of the chest, abdomen, head, neck or peripheral vessels of lower extremities. The following HCPCS codes should be used to report these services:

MRA of head	70544, 70544-26, 70544-TC
MRA of head	70545, 70545-26, 70545-TC
MRA of head	70546, 70546-26, 70546-TC
MRA of neck	70547, 70547-26, 70547-TC
MRA of neck	70548, 70548-26, 70548-TC
MRA of neck	70549, 70549-26, 70549-TC
MRA of chest	71555, 71555-26, 71555-TC
MRA of pelvis	72198, 72198-26, 72198-TC
MRA of abdomen (dates of service on or after July 1, 2003) - see below.	74185, 74185-26, 74185-TC
MRA of peripheral vessels of lower extremities	73725, 73725-26, 73725-TC

Hospitals subject to OPPS should report the following C codes in place of the above HCPCS codes as follows:

- MRA of chest 71555: C8909 - C8911
- MRA of abdomen 74185: C8900 - C8902
- MRA of peripheral vessels of lower extremities 73725: C8912 - C8914

For claims with dates of service on or after July 1, 2003, coverage under this benefit has been expanded for the use of MRA for diagnosing pathology in the renal or aortoiliac arteries. The following HCPCS code should be used to report this expanded coverage of MRA:

- MRA, pelvis, with or without contrast material(s) 72198, 72198-26, 72198-TC

Hospitals subject to OPPS report the following C codes in place of HCPCS code 72198:

- MRA, pelvis, with or without contrast material(s) 72198: C8918 - C8920

Providers utilizing the UB-92 flat file, use record type 61, HCPCS code (Field No. 6) to report HCPCS/CPT code. Providers utilizing the hard copy UB-92, report the HCPCS/CPT code in FL 44 "HCPCS/Rates." Providers utilizing the Medicare A 837 Health Care Claim version 3051 implementations 3A.01 and 1A.C1, report the HCPCS/CPT in 2-395-SV202-02.

Pub. 100-4, Chapter 13, Section 60.3

PET Scan Qualifying Conditions and HCPCS Code Chart
Below is a summary of all covered PET scan conditions, with effective dates.

NOTE: The G codes below except those a # can be used to bill for PET Scan services through January 27, 2005. Effective for dates of service on or after January 28, 2005, providers must bill for PET Scan services using the appropriate CPT codes. See section 60.3.1. The G codes with a # can continue to be used for billing after January 28, 2005 and these remain non-covered by Medicare. (NOTE: PET Scanners must be FDA-approved.)

Conditions	Coverage Effective Date	****HCPCS/ CPT
*Myocardial perfusion imaging (following previous PET G0030-G0047) single study, rest or stress (exercise and/or pharmacologic)	3/14/95	G0030
*Myocardial perfusion imaging (following previous PET G0030-G0047) multiple studies, rest or stress (exercise and/or pharmacologic)	3/14/95	G0031
*Myocardial perfusion imaging (following rest SPECT, 78464); single study, rest or stress (exercise and/or pharmacologic)	3/14/95	G0032
*Myocardial perfusion imaging (following rest SPECT 78464); multiple studies, rest or stress (exercise and/or pharmacologic)	3/14/95	G0033
*Myocardial perfusion (following stress SPECT 78465); single study, rest or stress (exercise and/or pharmacologic)	3/14/95	G0034
*Myocardial Perfusion Imaging (following stress SPECT 78465); multiple studies, rest or stress (exercise and/or pharmacologic)	3/14/95	G0035
*Myocardial Perfusion Imaging (following coronary angiography 93510-93529); single study, rest or stress (exercise and/or pharmacologic)	3/14/95	G0036
*Myocardial Perfusion Imaging, (following coronary angiography), 93510-93529); multiple studies, rest or stress (exercise and/or pharmacologic)	3/14/95	G0037
*Myocardial Perfusion Imaging (following stress planar myocardial perfusion, 78460); single study, rest or stress (exercise and/or pharmacologic)	3/14/95	G0038
*Myocardial Perfusion Imaging (following stress planar myocardial perfusion, 78460); multiple studies, rest or stress (exercise and/or pharmacologic)	3/14/95	G0039
*Myocardial Perfusion Imaging (following stress echocardiogram 93350); single study, rest or stress (exercise and/or pharmacologic)	3/14/95	G0040
*Myocardial Perfusion Imaging (following stress echocardiogram, 93350); multiple studies, rest or stress (exercise and/or pharmacologic)	3/14/95	G0041
*Myocardial Perfusion Imaging (following stress nuclear ventriculogram 78481 or 78483); single study, rest or stress (exercise and/or pharmacologic)	3/14/95	G0042
*Myocardial Perfusion Imaging (following stress nuclear ventriculogram 78481 or 78483); multiple studies, rest or stress (exercise and/or pharmacologic)	3/14/95	G0043
*Myocardial Perfusion Imaging (following stress ECG, 93000); single study, rest or stress (exercise and/or pharmacologic)	3/14/95	G0044
*Myocardial perfusion (following stress ECG, 93000), multiple studies; rest or stress (exercise and/or pharmacologic)	3/14/95	G0045
*Myocardial perfusion (following stress ECG, 93015), single study; rest or stress (exercise and/or pharmacologic)	3/14/95	G0046
*Myocardial perfusion (following stress ECG, 93015); multiple studies, rest or stress (exercise and/or pharmacologic)	3/14/95	G0047
PET imaging regional or whole body; single pulmonary nodule	1/1/98	G0125
Lung cancer, non-small cell (PET imaging whole body) Diagnosis, Initial Staging, Restaging	7/1/01	G0210, G0211, G0212
Colorectal cancer (PET imaging whole body) Diagnosis, Initial Staging, Restaging	7/1/01	G0213, G0214, G0215

Conditions	Coverage Effective Date	****HCPCS/ CPT
Melanoma (PET imaging whole body) Diagnosis, Initial Staging, Restaging	7/1/01	G0216, G0217, G0218
Melanoma for non-covered indications	7/1/01	#G0219
Lymphoma (PET imaging whole body) Diagnosis, Initial Staging, Restaging	7/1/01	G0220, G0221, G0222
Head and neck cancer; excluding thyroid and CNS cancers (PET imaging whole body or regional) Diagnosis, Initial Staging, Restaging	7/1/01	G0223, G0224, G0225
Esophageal cancer (PET imaging whole body) Diagnosis, Initial Staging, Restaging	7/1/01	G0226, G0227, G0228
Metabolic brain imaging for pre-surgical evaluation of refractory seizures	7/1/01	G0229
Metabolic assessment for myocardial viability following inconclusive SPECT study	7/1/01	G0230
Recurrence of colorectal or colorectal metastatic cancer (PET whole body, gamma cameras only)	1/1/02	G0231
Staging and characterization of lymphoma (PET whole body, gamma cameras only)	1/1/02	G0232
Recurrence of melanoma or melanoma metastatic cancer (PET whole body, gamma cameras only)	1/1/02	G0233
Regional or whole body, for solitary pulmonary nodule following CT, or for initial staging of non-small cell lung cancer (gamma cameras only)	1/1/02	G0234
Non-Covered Service PET imaging, any site not otherwise specified	1/28/05	#G0235
Non-Covered Service Initial diagnosis of breast cancer and/or surgical planning for breast cancer (e.g., initial staging of axillary lymph nodes), not covered (full- and partial-ring PET scanners only)	10/1/02	#G0252
Breast cancer, staging/restaging of local regional recurrence or distant metastases, i.e., staging/restaging after or prior to course of treatment (full- and partial-ring PET scanners only)	10/1/02	G0253
Breast cancer, evaluation of responses to treatment, performed during course of treatment (full- and partial-ring PET scanners only)	10/1/02	G0254
Myocardial imaging, positron emission tomography (PET), metabolic evaluation)	10/1/02	78459
Restaging or previously treated thyroid cancer of follicular cell origin following negative I-131 whole body scan (full- and partial-ring PET scanner only)	10/1/03	G0296
Tracer Rubidium**82 (Supply of Radiopharmaceutical Diagnostic Imaging Agent) (This is only billed through Outpatient Perspective Payment System, OPPS.) (Carriers must use HCPCS Code A4641).	10/1/03	Q3000
Supply of Radiopharmaceutical Diagnostic Imaging Agent, Ammonia N-13	01/1/04	A9526
PET imaging, brain imaging for the differential diagnosis of Alzheimer's disease with aberrant features vs. fronto-temporal dementia	09/15/04	Appropriate CPT Code from section 60.3.1
PET Cervical Cancer Staging as adjunct to conventional imaging, other staging, diagnosis, restaging, monitoring	1/28/05	Appropriate CPT Code from section 60.3.1

*NOTE: Carriers must report A4641 for the tracer Rubidium 82 when used with PET scan codes G0030 through G0047 for services performed on or before January 27, 2005

**NOTE: Not FDG PET

***NOTE: For dates of service October 1, 2003, through December 31, 2003, use temporary code Q4078 for billing this radiopharmaceutical.

Pub. 100-4, Chapter 13, Section 60.3.1

Appropriate CPT Codes Effective for PET Scans for Services Performed on or After January 28, 2005

NOTE: All PET scan services require the use of a radiopharmaceutical diagnostic imaging agent (tracer). The applicable tracer code should be billed when billing for a PET scan service. See section 60.3.2 below for applicable tracer codes.

CPT Code	Description
78459	Myocardial imaging, positron emission tomography (PET), metabolic evaluation
78491	Myocardial imaging, positron emission tomography (PET), perfusion, single study at rest or stress
78492	Myocardial imaging, positron emission tomography (PET), perfusion, multiple studies at rest and/or stress
78608	Brain imaging, positron emission tomography (PET); metabolic evaluation
78609	Brain imaging, positron emission tomography (PET); perfusion evaluation
78811	Tumor imaging, positron emission tomography (PET); limited area (e.g., chest, head/neck)
78812	Tumor imaging, positron emission tomography (PET); skull base to mid thigh
78813	Tumor imaging, positron emission tomography (PET); whole body
78814	Tumor imaging, positron emission tomography (PET) with concurrently acquired computed tomography (CT) for attenuation correction and anatomical localization; limited area (e.g., chest, head/neck)
78815	Tumor imaging, positron emission tomography (PET) with concurrently acquired computed tomography (CT) for attenuation correction and anatomical localization; skull base to mid thigh
78816	Tumor imaging, positron emission tomography (PET) with concurrently acquired computed tomography (CT) for attenuation correction and anatomical localization; whole body

Pub. 100-4, Chapter 13, Section 60.3.2

Tracer Codes Required for PET Scans

Tracer codes applicable to CPT 78491 and 78492:

Institutional providers billing the fiscal intermediary

HCPCS	Description
*A9555	Supply of Radiopharmaceutical Diagnostic Imaging Agent, Rubidium RB-82, Diagnostic, Per study dose, Up To 60 Millicuries
* Q3000 (Deleted effective 12/31/05)	Supply of Radiopharmaceutical Diagnostic Imaging Agent, Rubidium RB-82
A9526	Supply of Radiopharmaceutical Diagnostic Imaging Agent, Ammonia N-13

NOTE: For claims with dates of service prior to 1/01/06, providers report Q3000 for supply of radiopharmaceutical diagnostic imaging agent, Rubidium RB-82. For claims with dates of service 1/01/06 and later, providers report A9555 for radiopharmaceutical diagnostic imaging agent, Rubidium RB-82 in place of Q3000.

Physicians / practitioners billing the carrier:

HCPCS	Description
A4641	Supply of Radiopharmaceutical Diagnostic Imaging Agent, Not Otherwise Classified
A9526	Supply of Radiopharmaceutical Diagnostic Imaging Agent, Ammonia N-13
A9555	Supply of Radiopharmaceutical Diagnostic Imaging Agent, Rubidium RB-82, Diagnostic, Per study dose, Up To 60 Millicuries

Tracer codes applicable to CPT 78459, 78608, 78609, 78811-78816:

Institutional providers billing the fiscal intermediary:

HCPCS	Description
* A9552 (OPPS Only)	Supply of Radiopharmaceutical Diagnostic Imaging Agent, Fluorodeoxyglucose F18, FDG, Diagnostic, Per study dose, Up to 45 Millicuries

HCPCS	Description
* C1775 (Deleted effective 12/31/05)	Supply of Radiopharmaceutical Diagnostic Imaging Agent, Fluorodeoxyglucose F18
A4641	Supply of Radiopharmaceutical Diagnostic Imaging Agent, Not Otherwise Classified

* NOTE: For claims with dates of service prior to 1/01/06, OPPS hospitals report C1775 and other providers report A4641 for supply of radiopharmaceutical diagnostic imaging agent, Fluorodeoxyglucose F1. For claims with dates of service 1/01/06 and later, providers report A9552 for radiopharmaceutical diagnostic imaging agent, Fluorodeoxyglucose F18 in place of C1775 and A4641.

Physicians / practitioners billing the carrier:

HCPCS	Description
A4641	Supply of Radiopharmaceutical Diagnostic Imaging Agent, Not Otherwise Classified
A9552	Supply of Radiopharmaceutical Diagnostic Imaging Agent, Fluorodeoxyglucose F18, FDG, Diagnostic, Per study dose, Up to 45 Millicuries

Pub. 100-4, Chapter 13, Section 60.14

Covered Indications

For services performed on or after January 28, 2005, contractors shall accept claims with the following HCPCS code for non-covered PET indications:

- G0235: PET imaging, any site not otherwise specified

Short Descriptor: PET not otherwise specified

Type of Service: 4

NOTE: This code is for a non-covered service.

Pub. 100-4, Chapter 13, Section 90

Ray Suppliers

B3-2070.4, B3-15022.G, B3-4131, B3-4831

Services furnished by portable x-ray suppliers may have as many as four components. Carriers must follow the following rules.

Pub. 100-4, Chapter 13, Section 90.3

R0076)

This component represents the transportation of the equipment to the patient. Establish local RVUs for the transportation R codes based on carrier knowledge of the nature of the service furnished. Carriers shall allow only a single transportation payment for each trip the portable x-ray supplier makes to a particular location. When more than one Medicare patient is x-rayed at the same location, e.g., a nursing home, prorate the single fee schedule transportation payment among all patients receiving the services. For example, if two patients at the same location receive x-rays, make one-half of the transportation payment for each.

R0075 must be billed in conjunction with the CPT radiology codes (7000 series) and only when the x-ray equipment used was actually transported to the location where the x-ray was taken. R0075 would not apply to the x-ray equipment stored in the location where the x-ray was done (e.g., a nursing home) for use as needed.

Below are the definitions for each modifier that must be reported with R0075. Only one of these five modifiers shall be reported with R0075. NOTE: If only one patient is served, R0070 should be reported with no modifier since the descriptor for this code reflects only one patient seen.

UN - Two patients served

UP - Three patients served

UQ - Four patients served

UR - Five Patients served

US - Six or more patients served

Payment for the above modifiers must be consistent with the definition of the modifiers. Therefore, for R0075 reported with modifiers, -UN, -UP, -UQ, and -UR, the total payment for the service shall be divided by 2, 3, 4, and 5 respectively. For modifier -US, the total payment for the service shall be divided by 6 regardless of the number of patients served. For example, if 8 patients were served, R0075 would be reported with modifier -US and the total payment for this service would be divided by 6.

The units field for R0075 shall always be reported as "1" except in extremely unusual cases. The number in the units field should be completed in accordance with the provisions of 100-04, chapter 23, section 10.2 item 24 G which defines the units field as the number of times the patient has received the itemized service during the dates listed in the from/to field. The units field must never be used to report the number of patients served during a single trip. Specifically, the units field must reflect the number of services that the specific beneficiary received, not the number of services received by other beneficiaries.

As a carrier priced service, carriers must initially determine a payment rate for portable x-ray transportation services that is associated with the cost of providing the service. In order to determine an appropriate cost, the carrier should, at a minimum, cost out the vehicle, vehicle

modifications, gasoline and the staff time involved in only the transportation for a portable x-ray service. A review of the pricing of this service should be done every five years.

Direct costs related to the vehicle carrying the x-ray machine are fully allocable to determining the payment rate. This includes the cost of the vehicle using a recognized depreciation method, the salary and fringe benefits associated with the staff who drive the vehicle, the communication equipment used between the vehicle and the home office, the salary and fringe benefits of the staff who determine the vehicles route (this could be proportional of office staff), repairs and maintenance of the vehicle(s), insurance for the vehicle(s), operating expenses for the vehicles and any other reasonable costs associated with this service as determined by the carrier. The carrier will have discretion for allocating indirect costs (those costs that cannot be directly attributed to portable x-ray transportation) between the transportation service and the technical component of the x-ray tests.

Suppliers may send carriers unsolicited cost information. The carrier may use this cost data as a comparison to its carrier priced determination. The data supplied should reflect a year's worth (either calendar or corporate fiscal) of information. Each provider who submits such data is to be informed that the data is subject to verification and will be used to supplement other information that is used to determine Medicare's payment rate.

Carriers are required to update the rate on an annual basis using independently determined measures of the cost of providing the service. A number of readily available measures (e.g., ambulance inflation factor, the Medicare economic index) that are used by the Medicare program to adjust payment rates for other types of services may be appropriate to use to update the rate for years that the carrier does not recalibrate the payment. Each carrier has the flexibility to identify the index it will use to update the rate. In addition, the carrier can consider locally identified factors that are measured independently of CMS as an adjunct to the annual adjustment.

NOTE: No transportation charge is payable unless the portable x-ray equipment used was actually transported to the location where the x-ray was taken. For example, carriers do not allow a transportation charge when the x-ray equipment is stored in a nursing home for use as needed. However, a set-up payment (see §90.4, below) is payable in such situations. Further, for services furnished on or after January 1, 1997, carriers may not make separate payment under HCPCS code R0076 for the transportation of EKG equipment by portable x-ray suppliers or any other entity.

Pub. 100-4, Chapter 13, Section 90.4

Up Component (HCPCS Code Q0092)

Carriers must pay a set-up component for each radiologic procedure (other than retakes of the same procedure) during both single patient and multiple patient trips under Level II HCPCS code Q0092. Carriers do not make the set-up payment for EKG services furnished by the portable x-ray supplier.

Pub. 100-4, Chapter 13, Section 140

Bone Mass Measurements

SNF-533.5 B3-4181, A3-3631.n

Sections 1861(s)(15) and (rr)(1) of the Act (as added by §4106 of the Balanced Budget Act (BBA) of 1997) standardize Medicare coverage of medically necessary bone mass measurements by providing for uniform coverage under Medicare Part B. This coverage is effective for claims with dates of service furnished on or after July 1, 1998.

Pub. 100-4, Chapter 16, Section 10

Background

B3-2070, B3-2070.1, B3-4110.3, B3-5114

Diagnostic X-ray, laboratory, and other diagnostic tests, including materials and the services of technicians, are covered under the Medicare program. Some clinical laboratory procedures or tests require Food and Drug Administration (FDA) approval before coverage is provided.

A diagnostic laboratory test is considered a laboratory service for billing purposes, regardless of whether it is performed in:

• A physician's office, by an independent laboratory;

• By a hospital laboratory for its outpatients or nonpatients;

• In a rural health clinic; or

• In an HMO or Health Care Prepayment Plan (HCPP) for a patient who is not a member.

When a hospital laboratory performs laboratory tests for nonhospital patients, the laboratory is functioning as an independent laboratory, and still bills the fiscal intermediary (FI). Also, when physicians and laboratories perform the same test, whether manually or with automated equipment, the services are deemed similar.

Laboratory services furnished by an independent laboratory are covered under SMI if the laboratory is an approved Independent Clinical Laboratory. However, as is the case of all diagnostic services, in order to be covered these services must be related to a patient's illness or injury (or symptom or complaint) and ordered by a physician. A small number of laboratory tests can be covered as a preventive screening service.

See the Medicare Benefit Policy Manual, Chapter 15, for detailed coverage requirements.

See the Medicare Program Integrity Manual, Chapter 10, for laboratory/supplier enrollment guidelines.

See the Medicare State Operations Manual for laboratory/supplier certification requirements.

Pub. 100-4, Chapter 16, Section 10.1

Definitions

B3-2070.1, B3-2070.1.B, RHC-406.4

"Independent Laboratory" - An independent laboratory is one that is independent both of an attending or consulting physician's office and of a hospital that meets at least the requirements to qualify as an emergency hospital as defined in §1861(e) of the Social Security Act (the Act). (See the Medicare Benefits Policy Manual, Chapter 15, for detailed discussion.)

"Physician Office Laboratory" - A physician office laboratory is a laboratory maintained by a physician or group of physicians for performing diagnostic tests in connection with the physician practice.

"Clinical Laboratory" - See the Medicare Benefits Policy Manual, Chapter 15.

"Qualified Hospital Laboratory" - A qualified hospital laboratory is one that provides some clinical laboratory tests 24 hours a day, 7 days a week, to serve a hospital's emergency room that is also available to provide services 24 hours a day, 7 days a week. For the qualified hospital laboratory to meet this requirement, the hospital must have physicians physically present or available within 30 minutes through a medical staff call roster to handle emergencies 24 hours a day, 7 days a week; and hospital laboratory technologists must be on duty or on call at all times to provide testing for the emergency room.

"Hospital Outpatient" - See the Medicare Benefit Policy Manual, Chapter 2.

"Referring laboratory" - A Medicare-approved laboratory that receives a specimen to be tested and that refers the specimen to another laboratory for performance of the laboratory test.

"Reference laboratory" - A Medicare-enrolled laboratory that receives a specimen from another, referring laboratory for testing and that actually performs the test.

"Billing laboratory" - The laboratory that submits a bill or claim to Medicare.

"Service" - A clinical diagnostic laboratory test. Service and test are synonymous.

"Test" - A clinical diagnostic laboratory service. Service and test are synonymous.

"CLIA" - The Clinical Laboratory Improvement Act and CMS implementing regulations and processes.

"Certification" - A laboratory that has met the standards specified in the CLIA.

"Draw Station' - A place where a specimen is collected but no Medicare-covered clinical laboratory testing is performed on the drawn specimen.

"Medicare-approved laboratory - A laboratory that meets all of the enrollment standards as a Medicare provider including the certification by a CLIA certifying authority.

Pub. 100-4, Chapter 16, Section 60

Specimen Collection Fee and Travel Allowance
B3-5114.1

Pub. 100-4, Chapter 16, Section 110.4

Carrier Contacts With Independent Clinical Laboratories
B3-2070.1.F

An important role of the carrier is as a communicant of necessary information to independent clinical laboratories. Failure to inform independent laboratories of Medicare regulations and claims processing procedures may have an adverse effect on prosecution of laboratories suspected of fraudulent activities with respect to tests performed by, or billed on behalf of, independent laboratories. United States Attorneys often must prosecute under a handicap or may refuse to prosecute cases where there is no evidence that a laboratory has been specifically informed of Medicare regulations and claims processing procedures.

To assure that laboratories are aware of Medicare regulations and carrier's policy, notification must be sent to independent laboratories when any changes are made in coverage policy or claims processing procedures. Additionally, to completely document efforts to fully inform independent laboratories of Medicare policy and the laboratory's responsibilities, previously issued newsletters should be periodically re-issued to remind laboratories of existing requirements.

Some items which should be discussed are the requirements to have the same charges for Medicare and private patients, to document fully the medical necessity for collection of specimens from a skilled nursing facility or a beneficiary's home, and, in cases when a laboratory service is referred from one independent laboratory to another independent laboratory, to identify the laboratory actually performing the test.

Additionally, when carrier professional relations representatives make personal contacts with particular laboratories, they should prepare and retain reports of contact indicating dates, persons present, and issues discussed.

Pub. 100-4, Chapter 17, Section 80.1.1

HCPCS Service Coding for Oral Cancer Drugs
The following codes may be used for drugs other than Prodrugs, when covered:

Generic/Chemical Name	How Supplied	HCPCS
Busulfan	2 mg/ORAL	J8510
Capecitabine	150mg/ORAL	J8520
Capecitabine	500mg/ORAL	J8521
Methotrexate	2.5 mg/ORAL	J8610
Cyclophosphamide *	25 mg/ORAL	J8530

Generic/Chemical Name	How Supplied	HCPCS
Cyclophosphamide *	(Treat 50 mg. as 2 units) 50 mg/ORAL	J8530
Etoposide	50 mg/ORAL	J8560
Melphalan	2 mg/ORAL	J8600
Prescription Drug chemotherapeutic NOC	ORAL	J8999

Each tablet or capsule is equal to one unit, except for 50 mg./ORAL of cyclophosphamide (J8530), which is shown as 2 units. The 25m and 50 mg share the same code.

NOTE: HIPAA requires that drug claims submitted to DMERCs be identified by NDC.

Pub. 100-4, Chapter 17, Section 80.1.2

HCPCS and NDC Reporting for Prodrugs
FI claims

For oral anti-cancer Prodrugs HCPCS code J8999 is reported with revenue code 0636.

DMERC claims

The supplier reports the NDC code on the claim. The DMERC converts the NDC code to a "WW" HCPCS code for CWF. As new "WW" codes are established for oral anti-cancer drugs they will be communicated in a Recurring Update Notification.

Pub. 100-4, Chapter 17, Section 80.2

Emetic Drugs Used as Full Replacement for Intravenous Anti-Emetic Drugs as Part of a Cancer Chemotherapeutic Regimen
See the Medicare Benefits Policy Manual, Chapter 15, for detailed coverage requirements.

Effective for dates of service on or after January 1, 1998, FIs and carriers pay for oral anti-emetic drugs when used as full therapeutic replacement for intravenous dosage forms as part of a cancer chemotherapeutic regimen when the drug(s) is administered or prescribed by a physician for use immediately before, at, or within 48 hours after the time of administration of the chemotherapeutic agent.

The allowable period of covered therapy includes day one, the date of service of the chemotherapy drug (beginning of the time of treatment), plus a period not to exceed two additional calendar days, or a maximum period up to 48 hours. Some drugs are limited to 24 hours; some to 48 hours. The hour limit is included in the narrative description of the HCPCS code.

The oral anti-emetic drug(s) should be prescribed only on a per chemotherapy treatment basis. For example, only enough of the oral anti-emetic(s) for one 24- or 48-hour dosage regimen (depending upon the drug) should be prescribed/supplied for each incidence of chemotherapy treatment. These drugs may be supplied by the physician in the office, by an inpatient or outpatient provider (e.g., hospital, CAH, SNF), or through a supplier (e.g., a pharmacy).

The physician must indicate on the prescription that the beneficiary is receiving the oral anti-emetic drug(s) as full therapeutic replacement for an intravenous anti-emetic drug as part of a cancer chemotherapeutic regimen. Where the drug is provided by a facility, the beneficiary's medical record maintained by the facility must be documented to reflect that the beneficiary is receiving the oral anti-emetic drug(s) as full therapeutic replacement for an intravenous anti-emetic drug as part of a cancer chemotherapeutic regimen.

Payment for these drugs is made under Part B. Beginning 1/1/05, the payment allowance limit for these Part B drugs (the term "drugs" includes biologicals) will be based on the Average Sales Price (ASP) plus 6%. Payment allowances for drugs will be based on the lower of the submitted charge or the ASP file price. These drugs continue to be priced based on the date of service. The drug payment allowance limit pricing file will be distributed to contractors by CMS. CMS will update and provide this file quarterly. Carriers/DMERCs/SADMERCs shall develop payment allowance limits for covered drugs when CMS does not supply the payment allowance limit on the ASP drug pricing file.

The HCPCS codes shown in section 80.2.1 are used.

The CWF edits claims with these codes to assure that the beneficiary is receiving the oral anti-emetic(s) as part of a cancer chemotherapeutic regimen by requiring a diagnosis of cancer.

Most drugs furnished as an outpatient hospital service are packaged under OPPS. However, chemotherapeutic agents and the supportive and adjunctive drugs used with them are paid separately.

Effective for dates of service on or after April 4, 2005, coverage for the use of the oral anti-emetic 3-drug combination of aprepitant (Emend(tm)), a 5-HT3 antagonist, and dexamethasone is considered reasonable and necessary for only those patients who are receiving one or more of the following anti-cancer chemotherapeutic agents:

- Carmustine
- Cisplatin
- Cyclophosphamide
- Dacarbazine
- Mechlorethamine
- Streptozocin

Appendix 4 — Pub 100 References

- Doxorubicin
- Epirubicin
- Lomustine

Pub. 100-4, Chapter 17, Section 80.2.1

Emetic Drugs

The physician/supplier bills for these drugs on Form CMS-1500 or its electronic equivalent. The facility bills for these drugs on Form CMS-1450 or its electronic equivalent. The following HCPCS codes are assigned:

J8501 APREPITANT, 5mg, Oral (Code is Effective 1/1/05 but coverage is effective 4/4/05, Note: Aprepitant is only covered in combination with a 5-HT3 antagonist, and dexamethasone for beneficiaries who have received one or more of the specified anti-cancer chemotherapeutic agents.

Q0163 DIPHENHYDRAMINE HYDROCHLORIDE 50mg, oral, FDA-approved prescription anti-emetic, for use as a complete therapeutic substitute for an IV anti-emetic at time of chemotherapy treatment not to exceed a 48-hour dosage regimen.

Q0164 PROCHLORPERAZINE MALEATE 5mg, oral, FDA-approved prescription anti-emetic, for use as a complete therapeutic substitute for an IV anti-emetic at the time of chemotherapy treatment, not to exceed a 48-hour dosage regimen.

Q0165 PROCHLORPERAZINE MALEATE 10mg, oral, FDA-approved prescription anti-emetic, for use as a complete therapeutic substitute for an IV anti-emetic at the time of chemotherapy treatment, not to exceed a 48-hour dosage regimen.

Q0166 GRANISETRON HYDROCHLORIDE 1mg, oral, FDA-approved prescription anti-emetic, for use as a complete therapeutic substitute for an IV anti-emetic at the time of chemotherapy treatment, not to exceed a 24-hour dosage regimen.

Q0167 DRONABINOL 2.5mg, oral, FDA-approved prescription anti-emetic, for use as a complete therapeutic substitute for an IV anti-emetic at the time of chemotherapy treatment, not to exceed a 48-hour dosage regimen.

Q0168 DRONABINOL 5mg, oral, FDA-approved prescription anti-emetic, for use as a complete therapeutic substitute for an IV anti-emetic at the time of chemotherapy treatment, not to exceed a 48-hour dosage regimen.

Q0169 PROMETHAZINE HYDROCHLORIDE 12.5mg, oral, FDA-approved prescription anti-emetic, for use as a complete therapeutic substitute for an IV anti-emetic at the time of chemotherapy treatment, not to exceed a 48-hour dosage regimen.

Q0170 PROMETHAZINE HYDROCHLORIDE 25mg, oral, FDA-approved prescription anti-emetic, for use as a complete therapeutic substitute for an IV anti-emetic at the time of chemotherapy treatment, not to exceed a 48-hour dosage regimen.

Q0171 CHLORPROMAZINE HYDROCHLORIDE 10mg, oral, FDA-approved prescription anti-emetic, for use as a complete therapeutic substitute for an IV anti-emetic at the time of chemotherapy treatment, not to exceed a 48-hour dosage regimen.

Q0172 CHLORPROMAZINE HYDROCHLORIDE 25mg, oral, FDA-approved prescription anti-emetic, for use as a complete therapeutic substitute for an IV anti-emetic at the time of chemotherapy treatment, not to exceed a 48-hour dosage regimen.

Q0173 TRIMETHOBENZAMIDE HYDROCHLORIDE 250mg, oral, FDA-approved prescription anti-emetic, for use as a complete therapeutic substitute for an IV anti-emetic at the time of chemotherapy treatment, not to exceed a 48-hour dosage regimen.

Q0174 THIETHYLPERAZINE MALEATE 10mg, oral, FDA-approved prescription anti-emetic, for use as a complete therapeutic substitute for an IV anti-emetic at the time of chemotherapy treatment, not to exceed a 48-hour dosage regimen.

Q0175 PERPHENAZINE 4mg, oral, FDA-approved prescription anti-emetic, for use as a complete therapeutic substitute for an IV anti-emetic at the time of chemotherapy treatment, not to exceed a 48-hour dosage regimen.

Q0176 PERPHENAZINE 8mg, oral, FDA-approved prescription anti-emetic, for use as a complete therapeutic substitute for an IV anti-emetic at the time of chemotherapy treatment, not to exceed a 48-hours dosage regimen.

Q0177 HYDROXYZINE PAMOATE 25mg, oral, FDA-approved prescription anti-emetic, for use as a complete therapeutic substitute for an IV anti-emetic at the time of chemotherapy treatment, not to exceed a 48-hour dosage regimen.

Q0178 HYDROXYZINE PAMOATE 50mg, oral, FDA-approved prescription anti-emetic, for use as a complete therapeutic substitute for an IV anti-emetic at the time of chemotherapy treatment, not to exceed a 48-hour dosage regimen.

Q0179 ONDANSETRON HYDROCHLORIDE 8mg, oral, FDA-approved prescription anti-emetic, for use as a complete therapeutic substitute for an IV anti-emetic at the time of chemotherapy treatment, not to exceed a 48-hour dosage regimen.

Q0180 DOLASETRON MESYLATE 100mg, oral, FDA-approved prescription anti-emetic, for use as a complete therapeutic substitute for an IV anti-emetic at the time of chemotherapy treatment, not to exceed a 24-hour dosage regimen.

Q0181 UNSPECIFIED ORAL DOSAGE FORM, FDA-approved prescription anti-emetic, for use as a complete therapeutic substitute for an IV anti-emetic at the time of chemotherapy treatment, not to exceed a 48-hour dosage regimen.

NOTE: The 24-hour maximum drug supply limitation on dispensing, for HCPCS Codes Q0166 and Q0180, has been established to bring the Medicare benefit as it applies to these two therapeutic entities in conformity with the "Indications and Usage" section of currently FDA-approved product labeling for each affected drug product.

Pub. 100-4, Chapter 17, Section 80.2.4

Billing and Payment Instructions for FIs

Claims for the initial dose of the oral anti-emetic drug aprepitant must be billed to the FI on the ASC 837I or on hard copy Form CMS-1450 (UB-92) with the appropriate cancer diagnosis and HCPCS code or CPT code. The following payment methodologies apply when furnished to hospital and SNF outpatients:

- Based on APC for hospitals subject to OPPS;
- Under current payment methodologies for hospitals not subject to OPPS; or
- On a reasonable cost basis for SNFs.

Institutional providers bill for aprepitant under Revenue Code 0636 (Drugs requiring detailed coding).

Medicare contractors shall pay claims submitted for services provided by a CAH as follows: Method I technical services are paid at 101% of reasonable cost; Method II technical services are paid at 101% of reasonable cost, and, Professional services are paid at 115% of the Medicare Physician Fee Schedule Data Base.

NOTE: Inpatient claims submitted for oral anti-emetic drugs are processed under the current payment methodologies.

Pub. 100-4, Chapter 17, Section 80.3

Billing for Immunosuppressive Drugs

B3-4471, A3-3660.8, PM AB-01-10

Beginning January 1, 1987, Medicare pays for FDA approved immunosuppressive drugs and for drugs used in immunosuppressive therapy. (See the Medicare Benefit Policy Manual, Chapter 15 for detailed coverage requirements.) Generally, contractors pay for self-administered immunosuppressive drugs that are specifically labeled and approved for marketing as such by the FDA, or identified in FDA-approved labeling for use in conjunction with immunosuppressive drug therapy. This benefit is subject to the Part B deductible and coinsurance provision.

Contractors are expected to keep informed of FDA additions to the list of the immunosuppressive drugs and notify providers. Prescriptions for immunosuppressive drugs generally should be nonrefillable and limited to a 30-day supply. The 30-day guideline is necessary because dosage frequently diminishes over a period of time, and further, it is not uncommon for the physician to change the prescription from one drug to another. Also, these drugs are expensive and the coinsurance liability on unused drugs could be a financial burden to the beneficiary. Unless there are special circumstances, contractors will not consider a supply of drugs in excess of 30 days to be reasonable and necessary and should deny payment accordingly.

Entities that normally bill the carrier bill the DMERC. Entities that normally bill the FI continue to bill the FI, except for hospitals subject to OPPS, which must bill the DMERC.

Prior to December 21, 2000 coverage was limited to immunosuppressive drugs received within 36 months of a transplant. ESRD beneficiaries continue to be limited to 36 months of coverage after a Medicare covered kidney transplant. For all other beneficiaries, BBA '97 increased the length of time a beneficiary could receive immunosuppressives by a sliding method. So for the period 8/97 thru 12/00 a longer period of time MAY apply for a transplant. Effective with immunosuppressive drugs furnished on or after December 21, 2000, there is no time limit, but an organ transplant must have occurred for which immunosuppressive therapy is appropriate. That is, the time limit for immunosuppressive drugs was eliminated for transplant beneficiaries that will continue Medicare coverage after 36 months based on disability or age. The date of transplant is reported to the FI with occurrence code 36.

CWF will edit claim records to determine if a history of a transplant is on record. If not an error will be returned. See Chapter 27 for edit codes and resolution.

Pub. 100-4, Chapter 17, Section 80.3.1

Requirements for Billing FI for Immunosuppressive Drugs

Hospitals not subject to OPPS bill on a Form CMS-1450 with bill type 12x (hospital inpatient Part B) or 13x (hospital outpatient) as appropriate. For claims with dates of service prior to April 1, 2000, providers report the following entries:

- Occurrence code 36 and date in FL 32-35;
- Revenue code 0250 in FL 42; and
- Narrative description in FL 43.

For claims with dates of service on or after April 1. 2000, hospitals report

- Occurrence code 36 and date in FL 32-35;
- Revenue code 0636 in FL 42;
- HCPCS code of the immunosuppressive drug in FL 44; and
- Number of units in FL 46 (the number of units billed must accurately reflect the definition of one unit of service in each code narrative. E.g.: If fifty 10-mg. Prednisone tablets are dispensed, the hospital bills J7506, 100 units (1 unit of J7506 = 5 mg.).

The hospital completes the remaining items in accordance with regular billing instructions.

Pub. 100-4, Chapter 17, Section 80.4

Billing for Hemophilia Clotting Factors

Blood clotting factors not paid on a cost or prospective payment system basis are priced as a drug/biological under the drug pricing fee schedule effective for the specific date of service. As of January 1, 2005, the average sales price (ASP) plus 6 percent shall be used.

If a beneficiary is in a covered part A stay in a PPS hospital, the clotting factors are paid in addition to the DRG/HIPPS payment (For FY 2005, this payment is based on 95 percent of AWP). For a SNF subject to SNF/PPS, the payment is bundled into the SNF/PPS rate.

For hospitals subject to OPPS, the clotting factors, when paid under Part B, are paid the APC. For SNFs the clotting factors, when paid under Part B, are paid based on cost.

Local carriers shall process non-institutional blood clotting factor claims.

The FIs shall process institutional blood clotting factor claims (Part A and Part B institutional).

Pub. 100-4, Chapter 18, Section 60.1

Payment

Payment (carrier and FI) is under the MPFS except as follows:

Fecal occult blood tests (82270*(G0107*and G0328) are paid under the clinical diagnostic lab fee schedule except reasonable cost is paid to CAHs when submitted on TOB 85X. See section A below for payment to Maryland waiver on TOB 13X. Payment from all hospitals for non-patient laboratory specimens on TOB 14X will be based on the clinical diagnostic fee schedule, including CAHs and Maryland waiver hospitals.

Flexible sigmoidoscopy (code G0104) is paid under OPPS for hospital outpatient departments and on a reasonable cost basis for CAHs; or current payment methodologies for hospitals not subject to OPPS.

Colonoscopy (G0105) and barium enemas (G0106 and G0120) are paid under OPPS for hospital outpatient departments and on a reasonable costs basis for CAHs or current payment methodologies for hospitals not subject to OPPS. Also colonoscopies may be done in an Ambulatory Surgical Center (ASC) and when done in an ASC the ASC rate applies. The ASC rate is the same for diagnostic and screening colonoscopies.

The following screening codes must be paid at rates consistent with the diagnostic codes indicated.

A. Special Payment Instructions for TOB 13X Maryland Waiver Hospitals

For hospitals in Maryland under the jurisdiction of the Health Services Cost Review Commission, screening colorectal services HCPCS codes G0104, G0105, G0106, 82270*(G0107*) G0120, G0121 and G0328 are paid according to the terms of the waiver, that is 94% of submitted charges minus any unmet existing deductible, co-insurance and non-covered charges. Maryland Hospitals bill TOB 13X for outpatient colorectal cancer screenings.

B. Special Payment Instructions for Non-Patient Laboratory Specimen (TOB 14X) for all hospitals

Payment for colorectal cancer screenings (82270*(G0107*) and G0328) to a hospital for a non-patient laboratory specimen (TOB 14X), is the lesser of the actual charge, the fee schedule amount, or the National Limitation Amount (NLA), (including CAHs and Maryland Waiver hospitals). Part B deductible and coinsurance do not apply.

NOTE: For claims with dates of service prior to January 1, 2007, physicians, suppliers, and providers report HCPCS code G0107. Effective January 1, 2007, code G0107 is discontinued and replaced with CPT code 82270.

Pub. 100-4, Chapter 18, Section 60.2

HCPCS Codes, Frequency Requirements, and Age Requirements (If Applicable)

B3-4180.2, A3-3660.17.A, AB-03-114

Effective for services furnished on or after January 1, 1998, the following codes are used for colorectal cancer screening services:

82270*(G0107*) - Colorectal cancer screening; fecal-occult blood tests, 1-3 simultaneous determinations;

G0104 - Colorectal cancer screening; flexible sigmoidoscopy;

G0105 - Colorectal cancer screening; colonoscopy on individual at high risk;

G0106 - Colorectal cancer screening; barium enema; as an alternative to G0104, screening sigmoidoscopy;

G0120 - Colorectal cancer screening; barium enema; as an alternative to G0105, screening colonoscopy.

Effective for services furnished on or after July 1, 2001 the following codes are used for colorectal cancer screening services:

G0121 - Colorectal cancer screening; colonoscopy on individual not meeting criteria for high risk. Note that the description for this code has been revised to remove the term "noncovered."

G0122 - Colorectal cancer screening; barium enema (noncovered).

Effective for services furnished on or after January 1, 2004, the following code is used for colorectal cancer screening services as an alternative to 82270*(G0107*):

G0328 - Colorectal cancer screening; immunoassay, fecal-occult blood test, 1-3 simultaneous determinations

NOTE: For claims with dates of service prior to January 1, 2007, physicians, suppliers, and providers report HCPCS code G0107. Effective January 1, 2007, code G0107 is discontinued and replaced with CPT code 82270.

G0104 - Colorectal Cancer Screening; Flexible Sigmoidoscopy

Screening flexible sigmoidoscopies (code G0104) may be paid for beneficiaries who have attained age 50, when performed by a doctor of medicine or osteopathy at the frequencies noted below.

For claims with dates of service on or after January 1, 2002, contractors pay for screening flexible sigmoidoscopies (code G0104) for beneficiaries who have attained age 50 when these services were performed by a doctor of medicine or osteopathy, or by a physician assistant, nurse practitioner, or clinical nurse specialist (as defined in §1861(aa)(5) of the Act and in the Code of Federal Regulations at 42 CFR 410.74, 410.75, and 410.76) at the frequencies noted above. For claims with dates of service prior to January 1, 2002, contractors pay for these services under the conditions noted only when a doctor of medicine or osteopathy performs them.

For services furnished from January 1, 1998, through June 30, 2001, inclusive:

Once every 48 months (i.e., at least 47 months have passed following the month in which the last covered screening flexible sigmoidoscopy was done).

For services furnished on or after July 1, 2001:

Once every 48 months as calculated above unless the beneficiary does not meet the criteria for high risk of developing colorectal cancer (refer to §60.3 of this chapter) and he/she has had a screening colonoscopy (code G0121) within the preceding 10 years. If such a beneficiary has had a screening colonoscopy within the preceding 10 years, then he or she can have covered a screening flexible sigmoidoscopy only after at least 119 months have passed following the month that he/she received the screening colonoscopy (code G0121).

NOTE: If during the course of a screening flexible sigmoidoscopy a lesion or growth is detected which results in a biopsy or removal of the growth; the appropriate diagnostic procedure classified as a flexible sigmoidoscopy with biopsy or removal should be billed and paid rather than code G0104.

G0105 - Colorectal Cancer Screening, Colonoscopy on Individual at High Risk

Ref: AB-03-114

Screening colonoscopies (code G0105) may be paid when performed by a doctor of medicine or osteopathy at a frequency of once every 24 months for beneficiaries at high risk for developing colorectal cancer (i.e., at least 23 months have passed following the month in which the last covered G0105 screening colonoscopy was performed). Refer to §60.3 of this chapter for the criteria to use in determining whether or not an individual is at high risk for developing colorectal cancer.

NOTE: If during the course of the screening colonoscopy, a lesion or growth is detected which results in a biopsy or removal of the growth, the appropriate diagnostic procedure classified as a colonoscopy with biopsy or removal should be billed and paid rather than code G0105.

A. Colonoscopy Cannot be Completed Because of Extenuating Circumstances

1. FIs

When a covered colonoscopy is attempted but cannot be completed because of extenuating circumstances, Medicare will pay for the interrupted colonoscopy as long as the coverage conditions are met for the incomplete procedure. However, the frequency standards associated with screening colonoscopies will not be applied by CWF. When a covered colonoscopy is next attempted and completed, Medicare will pay for that colonoscopy according to its payment methodology for this procedure as long as coverage conditions are met, and the frequency standards will be applied by CWF. This policy is applied to both screening and diagnostic colonoscopies. When submitting a facility claim for the interrupted colonoscopy, providers are to suffix the colonoscopy HCPCS codes with a modifier of " – 73" or "– 74" as appropriate to indicate that the procedure was interrupted. Payment for covered incomplete screening colonoscopies shall be consistent with payment methodologies currently in place for complete screening colonoscopies, including those contained in 42 CFR 419.44(b). In situations where a critical access hospital (CAH) has elected payment Method II for CAH patients, payment shall be consistent with payment methodologies currently in place as outlined in Chapter 3. As such, instruct CAHs that elect Method II payment to use modifier " – 53" to identify an incomplete screening colonoscopy (physician professional service(s) billed in revenue code 096X, 097X, and/or 098X). Such CAHs will also bill the technical or facility component of the interrupted colonoscopy in revenue code 075X (or other appropriate revenue code) using the "-73" or "-74" modifier as appropriate.

Note that Medicare would expect the provider to maintain adequate information in the patient's medical record in case it is needed by the contractor to document the incomplete procedure.

2. Carriers

When a covered colonoscopy is attempted but cannot be completed because of extenuating circumstances (see Chapter 12), Medicare will pay for the interrupted colonoscopy at a rate consistent with that of a flexible sigmoidoscopy as long as coverage conditions are met for the incomplete procedure. When a covered colonoscopy is next attempted and completed, Medicare will pay for that colonoscopy according to its payment methodology for this procedure as long as coverage conditions are met. This policy is applied to both screening and diagnostic colonoscopies. When submitting a claim for the interrupted colonoscopy, professional providers are to suffix the colonoscopy code with a modifier of " – 53" to indicate that the procedure was interrupted. When submitting a claim for the facility fee associated with this procedure, Ambulatory Surgical Centers (ASCs) are to suffix the colonoscopy code with " – 73" or " – 74" as appropriate. Payment for covered screening colonoscopies, including that for the associated ASC facility fee when applicable, shall be consistent with payment for diagnostic colonoscopies, whether the procedure is complete or incomplete.

Note that Medicare would expect the provider to maintain adequate information in the patient's medical record in case it is needed by the contractor to document the incomplete procedure.

G0106 - Colorectal Cancer Screening; Barium Enema; as an Alternative to G0104, Screening Sigmoidoscopy

Screening barium enema examinations may be paid as an alternative to a screening sigmoidoscopy (code G0104). The same frequency parameters for screening sigmoidoscopies (see those codes above) apply.

Appendix 4 — Pub 100 References

In the case of an individual aged 50 or over, payment may be made for a screening barium enema examination (code G0106) performed after at least 47 months have passed following the month in which the last screening barium enema or screening flexible sigmoidoscopy was performed. For example, the beneficiary received a screening barium enema examination as an alternative to a screening flexible sigmoidoscopy in January 1999. Start counts beginning February 1999. The beneficiary is eligible for another screening barium enema in January 2003.

The screening barium enema must be ordered in writing after a determination that the test is the appropriate screening test. Generally, it is expected that this will be a screening double contrast enema unless the individual is unable to withstand such an exam. This means that in the case of a particular individual, the attending physician must determine that the estimated screening potential for the barium enema is equal to or greater than the screening potential that has been estimated for a screening flexible sigmoidoscopy for the same individual. The screening single contrast barium enema also requires a written order from the beneficiary's attending physician in the same manner as described above for the screening double contrast barium enema examination.

82270*(G0107*) - Colorectal Cancer Screening; Fecal-Occult Blood Test, 1-3 Simultaneous Determinations

Effective for services furnished on or after January 1, 1998, screening FOBT 82270*(G0107*) may be paid for beneficiaries who have attained age 50, and at a frequency of once every 12 months (i.e., at least 11 months have passed following the month in which the last covered screening FOBT was performed). This screening FOBT means a guaiac-based test for peroxidase activity, in which the beneficiary completes it by taking samples from two different sites of three consecutive stools. This screening requires a written order from the beneficiary's attending physician. (The term "attending physician" is defined to mean a doctor of medicine or osteopathy (as defined in §1861(r)(1) of the Act) who is fully knowledgeable about the beneficiary's medical condition, and who would be responsible for using the results of any examination performed in the overall management of the beneficiary's specific medical problem.)

Effective for services furnished on or after January 1, 2004, payment may be made for a immunoassay-based FOBT (G0328, described below) as an alternative to the guaiac-based FOBT, 82270*(G0107*).

Medicare will pay for only one covered FOBT per year, either82270*(G0107*)or G0328, but not both. *NOTE: For claims with dates of service prior to January 1, 2007, physicians, suppliers, and providers report HCPCS code G0107. Effective January 1, 2007, code G0107 is discontinued and replaced with CPT code 82270.

G0328 - Colorectal Cancer Screening; Immunoassay, Fecal-Occult Blood Test, 1-3 Simultaneous Determinations

Effective for services furnished on or after January 1, 2004, screening FOBT, (code G0328) may be paid as an alternative to 82270*(G0107*) for beneficiaries who have attained age 50. Medicare will pay for a covered FOBT (either82270*(G0107*) or G0328, but not both) at a frequency of once every 12 months (i.e., at least 11 months have passed following the month in which the last covered screening FOBT was performed). Screening FOBT, immunoassay, includes the use of a spatula to collect the appropriate number of samples or the use of a special brush for the collection of samples, as determined by the individual manufacturer's instructions. This screening requires a written order from the beneficiary's attending physician. (The term "attending physician" is defined to mean a doctor of medicine or osteopathy (as defined in §1861(r)(1) of the Act) who is fully knowledgeable about the beneficiary's medical condition, and who would be responsible for using the results of any examination performed in the overall management of the beneficiary's specific medical problem.)

G0120 - Colorectal Cancer Screening; Barium Enema; as an Alternative to or G0105, Screening Colonoscopy

Screening barium enema examinations may be paid as an alternative to a screening colonoscopy (code G0105) examination. The same frequency parameters for screening colonoscopies (see those codes above) apply.

In the case of an individual who is at high risk for colorectal cancer, payment may be made for a screening barium enema examination (code G0120) performed after at least 23 months have passed following the month in which the last screening barium enema or the last screening colonoscopy was performed. For example, a beneficiary at high risk for developing colorectal cancer received a screening barium enema examination (code G0120) as an alternative to a screening colonoscopy (code G0105) in January 2000. Start counts beginning February 2000. The beneficiary is eligible for another screening barium enema examination (code G0120) in January 2002.

The screening barium enema must be ordered in writing after a determination that the test is the appropriate screening test. Generally, it is expected that this will be a screening double contrast enema unless the individual is unable to withstand such an exam. This means that in the case of a particular individual, the attending physician must determine that the estimated screening potential for the barium enema is equal to or greater than the screening potential that has been estimated for a screening colonoscopy, for the same individual. The screening single contrast barium enema also requires a written order from the beneficiary's attending physician in the same manner as described above for the screening double contrast barium enema examination.

G0121 - Colorectal Screening; Colonoscopy on Individual Not Meeting Criteria for High Risk - Applicable On and After July 1, 2001

Effective for services furnished on or after July 1, 2001, screening colonoscopies (code G0121) performed on individuals not meeting the criteria for being at high risk for developing colorectal cancer (refer to §60.2 of this chapter) may be paid under the following conditions:

At a frequency of once every 10 years (i.e., at least 119 months have passed following the month in which the last covered G0121 screening colonoscopy was performed.)

If the individual would otherwise qualify to have covered a G0121 screening colonoscopy based on the above but has had a covered screening flexible sigmoidoscopy (code G0104), then he or she may have covered a G0121 screening colonoscopy only after at least 47 months have passed following the month in which the last covered G0104 flexible sigmoidoscopy was performed.

NOTE: If during the course of the screening colonoscopy, a lesion or growth is detected which results in a biopsy or removal of the growth, the appropriate diagnostic procedure classified as a colonoscopy with biopsy or removal should be billed and paid rather than code G0121.

G0122 - Colorectal Cancer Screening; Barium Enema

The code is not covered by Medicare.

Pub. 100-4, Chapter 18, Section 60.2.1

Common Working Files (CWF) Edits
Effective for dates of service January 1, 1998, and later, CWF will edit all colorectal screening claims for age and frequency standards. The CWF will also edit FI claims for valid procedure codes (G0104, G0105, G0106, 82270*(G0107*), G0120, G0121, G0122, and G0328) and for valid bill types. The CWF currently edits for valid HCPCS codes for carriers. (See §60.6 of this chapter for bill types.)

NOTE: For claims with dates of service prior to January 1, 2007, physicians, suppliers, and providers report HCPCS code G0107. Effective January 1, 2007, code G0107 is discontinued and replaced with CPT code 82270.

Pub. 100-4, Chapter 18, Section 60.6

Billing Requirements for Claims Submitted to FIs
Follow the general bill review instructions in Chapter 25. Hospitals use the ANSI X12N 837I to bill the FI or on the hardcopy Form CMS-1450. Hospitals bill revenue codes and HCPCS codes as follows:

82270***

(G0107)***

G0328

The appropriate revenue code when reporting any other surgical procedure.

14X is only applicable for non-patient laboratory specimens

For claims with dates of service prior to January 1, 2007, physicians, suppliers, and providers report HCPCS code G0107. Effective January 1, 2007, code G0107, is discontinued and replaced with CPT code 82270.

CAHs that elect Method II bill revenue code 096X, 097X, and/or 098X for professional services and 075X (or other appropriate revenue code) for the technical or facility component.

A - Special Billing Instructions for Hospital Inpatients

When these tests/procedures are provided to inpatients of a hospital, they are covered under this benefit. However, the provider bills on bill type 13X using the discharge date of the hospital stay to avoid editing in the Common Working File (CWF) as a result of the hospital bundling rules.

Pub. 100-4, Chapter 20, Section 20

Calculation and Update of Payment Rates
B3-5017, PM B-01-54, 2002 PEN Fee Schedule

Section1834 of the Act requires the use of fee schedules under Medicare Part B for reimbursement of durable medical equipment (DME) and for prosthetic and orthotic devices, beginning January 1 1989. Payment is limited to the lower of the actual charge for the equipment or the fee established.

Beginning with fee schedule year 1991, CMS calculates the updates for the fee schedules and national limitation amounts and provides the contractors with the revised payment amounts. The CMS calculates most fee schedule amounts and provides them to the carriers, DMERCs, FIs and RHHIs. However, for some services CMS asks carriers to calculate local fee amounts and to provide them to CMS to include in calculation of national amounts. These vary from update to update, and CMS issues special related instructions to carriers when appropriate.

Parenteral and enteral nutrition services paid on and after January 1, 2002 are paid on a fee schedule. This fee schedule also is furnished by CMS. Prior to 2002, payment amounts for PEN were determined under reasonable charge rules, including the application of the lowest charge level (LCL) restrictions.

The CMS furnishes fee schedule updates (DMEPOS, PEN, etc.) at least 30 days prior to the scheduled implementation. FIs use the fee schedules to pay for covered items, within their claims processing jurisdictions, supplied by hospitals, home health agencies, and other providers. FIs consult with DMERCs and where appropriate with carriers on filling gaps in fee schedules.

The CMS furnishes the fee amounts annually, or as updated if special updates should occur during the year, to carriers and FIs, including DMERCs and RHHIs, and to other interested parties (including the Statistical Analysis DMERC (SADMERC), Railroad Retirement Board (RRB), Indian Health Service, and United Mine Workers).

Pub. 100-4, Chapter 20, Section 20.4

Contents of Fee Schedule File
PM A-02-090

The fee schedule file provided by CMS contains HCPCS codes and related prices subject to the DMEPOS fee schedules, including application of any update factors and any changes to the national limited payment amounts. The file does not contain fees for drugs that are necessary for the effective use of DME. It also does not include fees for items for which fee schedule amounts are not established. See Chapter 23 for a description of pricing for these. The CMS releases via program issuance, the gap-filled amounts and the annual update factors for the various DMEPOS payment classes:

- IN = Inexpensive/routinely purchased...DME;
- FS = Frequency Service...DME;
- CR = Capped Rental... DME;
- OX = Oxygen and Oxygen Equipment... OXY;
- OS = Ostomy, Tracheostomy and Urologicals...P/O;
- S/D = Surgical Dressings...S/D;
- P/O = Prosthetics and Orthotics...P/O;
- SU = Supplies...DME; and
- TE = TENS...DME,

The RHHIs need to retrieve data from all of the above categories. Regular FIs need to retrieve data only from categories P/O, S/D and SU. FIs need to retrieve the SU category in order to be able to price supplies on Part B SNF claims.

Pub. 100-4, Chapter 20, Section 40.1

General
B3-5102.2.G, B3-5102.3

Contractors pay for maintenance and servicing of purchased equipment in the following classes:

- inexpensive or frequently purchased,
- customized items, other prosthetic and orthotic devices, and
- capped rental items purchased in accordance with §30.5.2 or §30.5.3.

They do not pay for maintenance and servicing of purchased items that require frequent and substantial servicing, or oxygen equipment. (Maintenance and servicing may be paid for purchased items in these two classes if they were purchased prior to June 1, 1989). Reasonable and necessary charges include only those made for parts and labor that are not otherwise covered under a manufacturer's or supplier's warranty. Contractors pay on a lump-sum, as needed basis based on their individual consideration for each item. Payment may not be made for maintenance and servicing of rented equipment other than maintenance and servicing for PEN pumps (under the conditions of §40.3) or the maintenance and servicing fee established for capped rental items in §40.2.

Servicing of equipment that a beneficiary is purchasing or already owns is covered when necessary to make the equipment serviceable. The service charge may include the use of "loaner" equipment where this is required. If the expense for servicing exceeds the estimated expense of purchasing or renting another item of equipment for the remaining period of medical need, no payment can be made for the amount of the excess. Contractors investigate and deny cases suggesting malicious damage, culpable neglect or wrongful disposition of equipment as discussed in BPM Chapter 15 where they determine that it is unreasonable to make program payment under the circumstances. Such cases are referred to the program integrity specialist in the RO.

Pub. 100-4, Chapter 20, Section 100

General Documentation Requirements
B3-4107.1, B3-4107.8, HHA-463, Medicare Handbook for New Suppliers: Getting Started, B-02-31

Benefit policies are set forth in the Medicare Benefit Policy Manual, Chapter 15, §§110-130.

Program integrity policies for DMEPOS are set forth in the Medicare Program Integrity Manual, Chapter 5.

See Chapter 21 for applicable MSN messages.

See Chapter 22 for Remittance Advice coding.

Pub. 100-4, Chapter 20, Section 100.2

Certificates of Medical Necessity (CMN)
B3-3312

For certain items or services billed to the DME Regional Carrier (DMERC), the supplier must receive a signed Certificate of Medical Necessity (CMN) from the treating physician. CMNs are not required for the same items when billed by HHAs to RHHIs. Instead, the items must be included in the physician's signed orders on the home health plan of care. See the Medicare Program Integrity Manual, Chapter 6.

The FI will inform other providers (see §01 for definition pf provider) of documentation requirements.

Contractors may ask for supporting documentation beyond a CMN.

Refer to the local DMERC Web site described in §10 for downloadable copies of CMN forms.

See the Medicare Program Integrity Manual, Chapter 5, for specific Medicare policies and instructions on the following topics:

- Requirements for supplier retention of original CMNs
- CMN formats, paper and electronic
- List of currently approved CMNs and items requiring CMNs
- Supplier requirements for submitting CMNs
- Requirements for CMNs to also serve as a physician's order
- Civil monetary penalties for violation of CMN requirements
- Supplier requirements for completing portions of CMNs

- Physician requirements for completing portions of CMNs

Pub. 100-4, Chapter 20, Section 100.2.2

Evidence of Medical Necessity for Parenteral and Enteral Nutrition (PEN) Therapy
B3-3324, B3-4450

The PEN coverage is determined by information provided by the treating physician and the PEN supplier. A completed certification of medical necessity (CMN) must accompany and support initial claims for PEN to establish whether coverage criteria are met and to ensure that the PEN therapy provided is consistent with the attending or ordering physician's prescription. Contractors ensure that the CMN contains pertinent information from the treating physician. Uniform specific medical data facilitate the review and promote consistency in coverage determinations and timelier claims processing.

The medical and prescription information on a PEN CMN can be most appropriately completed by the treating physician or from information in the patient's records by an employee of the physician for the physician's review and signature. Although PEN suppliers sometimes may assist in providing the PEN services, they cannot complete the CMN since they do not have the same access to patient information needed to properly enter medical or prescription information. Contractors use appropriate professional relations issuances, training sessions, and meetings to ensure that all persons and PEN suppliers are aware of this limitation of their role.

When properly completed, the PEN CMN includes the elements of a prescription as well as other data needed to determine whether Medicare coverage is possible. This practice will facilitate prompt delivery of PEN services and timely submittal of the related claim.

Pub. 100-4, Chapter 20, Section 130.2

Billing for Inexpensive or Other Routinely Purchased DME
A3-3629, B3-4107.8

This is equipment with a purchase price not exceeding $150, or equipment that the Secretary determines is acquired by purchase at least 75 percent of the time, or equipment that is an accessory used in conjunction with a nebulizer, aspirator, or ventilators that are either continuous airway pressure devices or intermittent assist devices with continuous airway pressure devices. Suppliers and providers other than HHAs bill the DMERC or, in the case of implanted DME only, the local carrier. HHAs bill the RHHI.

Effective for items and services furnished after January 1, 1991, Medicare DME does not include seat lift chairs. Only the seat lift mechanism is defined under Medicare as DME. Therefore, seat lift coverage is limited to the seat lift mechanism. If a seat lift chair is provided to a beneficiary, contractors pay only for the lift mechanism portion of the chair. Some lift mechanisms are equipped with a seat that is considered an integral part of the lift mechanism. Contractors do not pay for chairs (HCPCS code E0620) furnished on or after January 1, 1991. The appropriate HCPCS codes for seat lift mechanisms are E0627, E0628, and E0629.

For TENS, suppliers and providers other than HHAs bill the DMERC. HHAs bill the RHHI using revenue code 0291 for the 2-month rental period (see §30.1.2), billing each month as a separate line item and revenue code 0292 for the actual purchase along with the appropriate HCPCS code.

Pub. 100-4, Chapter 20, Section 130.3

Billing for Items Requiring Frequent and Substantial Servicing
A3-3629, B3-4107.8

These are items such as intermittent positive pressure breathing (IPPB) machines and ventilators, excluding ventilators that are either continuous airway pressure devices or intermittent assist devices with continuous airway pressure devices.

Suppliers and providers other than HHAs bill the DMERC. HHAs bill the RHHI.

Pub. 100-4, Chapter 20, Section 130.4

Billing for Certain Customized Items
A3-3629, B3-4107.8

Due to their unique nature (custom fabrication, etc.), certain customized DME cannot be grouped together for profiling purposes. Claims for customized items that do not have specific HCPCS codes are coded as E1399 (miscellaneous DME). This includes circumstances where an item that has a HCPCS code is modified to the extent that neither the original terminology nor the terminology of another HCPCS code accurately describes the modified item.

Suppliers and providers other than HHAs bill the DMERC or local carrier. HHAs bill their RHHI, using revenue code 0292 along with the HCPCS.

Pub. 100-4, Chapter 20, Section 130.5

Billing for Capped Rental Items (Other Items of DME)
A3-3629, B3-4107.8

These are DME items, other than oxygen and oxygen equipment, not covered by the above categories. Suppliers and providers other than HHAs bill the DMERC. HHAs bill the RHHIs.

Pub. 100-4, Chapter 20, Section 160.1

Billing for Total Parenteral Nutrition and Enteral Nutrition Furnished to Part B Inpatients
A3-3660.6, SNF-544, SNF-559, SNF-260.4, SNF-261, HHA-403, HO-438, HO-229

Inpatient Part A hospital or SNF care includes total parenteral nutrition (TPN) systems and enteral nutrition (EN).

For inpatients for whom Part A benefits are not payable (e.g., benefits are exhausted or the beneficiary is entitled to Part B only), total parenteral nutrition (TPN) systems and enteral nutrition (EN) delivery systems are covered by Medicare as prosthetic devices when the coverage criteria are met. When these criteria are met, the medical equipment and medical supplies (together with nutrients) being used comprise covered prosthetic devices for coverage purposes rather than durable medical equipment. However, reimbursement rules relating to DME continue to apply to such items.

When a facility supplies TPN or EN systems that meet the criteria for coverage as a prosthetic device to an inpatient whose care is not covered under Part A, the facility must bill one of the DMERCs. Additionally, HHAs, SNFs, and hospitals that provide PEN supplies, equipment and nutrients as a prosthetic device under Part B must use the CMS-1500 or the related NSF or ANSI ASC X12N 837 format to bill the appropriate DMERC. The DMERC is determined according to the residence of the beneficiary. Refer to §10 for jurisdiction descriptions.

FIs return claims containing PEN charges for Part B services where the bill type is 12x, 13x, 22x, 23x, 32x, 33x, or 34x with instructions to the provider to bill the DMERC.

Pub. 100-4, Chapter 20, Section 170

Billing for Splints and Casts

AB-01-60, AB-01-126

The cost of supplies used in creating casts are not included in the payment amounts for the CPT codes for fracture management and for casts and splints. Thus, for settings in which CPT codes are used to pay for services that include the provision of a cast or splint, supplies maybe billed with separate CPCS codes. The work and practice expenses involved with the creation of the cast or splint are included in the payment for the code for that service.

For claims with dates of service on or after July 1, 2001, jurisdiction for processing claims for splints transferred from the DMERCs to the local carriers. The local carriers have jurisdiction for processing claims for splints and casts, which includes codes for splints that may have previously been billed to the DMERCs.

Jurisdiction for slings is jointly maintained by the local carriers (for physician claims) and the DMERCs (for supplier claims). Notwithstanding the above where the beneficiary receives the service from any of the following providers claims jurisdiction is with the FI. An exception to this is hospital outpatient services and hospital inpatient Part B services, which are included in the OPPS payment and are billed on the Form CMS-1450 to the FI.

Other providers and suppliers that normally bill the FI for services bill the carrier for splints and casts.

Pub. 100-4, Chapter 32, Section 11.1

Electrical Stimulation

A. Coding Applicable to Carriers & Fiscal Intermediaries (FIs)

Effective April 1, 2003, a National Coverage Decision was made to allow for Medicare coverage of Electrical Stimulation for the treatment of certain types of wounds. The type of wounds covered are chronic Stage III or Stage IV pressure ulcers, arterial ulcers, diabetic ulcers and venous stasis ulcers. All other uses of electrical stimulation for the treatment of wounds are not covered by Medicare. Electrical stimulation will not be covered as an initial treatment modality.

The use of electrical stimulation will only be covered after appropriate standard wound care has been tried for at least 30 days and there are no measurable signs of healing. If electrical stimulation is being used, wounds must be evaluated periodically by the treating physician but no less than every 30 days by a physician. Continued treatment with electrical stimulation is not covered if measurable signs of healing have not been demonstrated within any 30-day period of treatment. Additionally, electrical stimulation must be discontinued when the wound demonstrates a 100% epithelialzed wound bed.

Coverage policy can be found in Pub. 100-03, Medicare National Coverage Determinations Manual, Chapter 1, Section 270.1 (http://www.cms.hhs.gov/manuals/103_cov_determ/ncd103index.asp)

The applicable Healthcare Common Procedure Coding System (HCPCS) code for Electrical Stimulation and the covered effective date is as follows:

HCPCS	Definition	Effective Date
G0281	Electrical Stimulation, (unattended), to one or more areas for chronic Stage III and Stage IV pressure ulcers, arterial ulcers, diabetic ulcers and venous stasis ulcers not demonstrating measurable signs of healing after 30 days of conventional care as part of a therapy plan of care.	04/01/2003

Medicare will not cover the device used for the electrical stimulation for the treatment of wounds. However, Medicare will cover the service. Unsupervised home use of electrical stimulation will not be covered.

B. FI Billing Instructions

The applicable types of bills acceptable when billing for electrical stimulation services are 12X, 13X, 22X, 23X, 71X, 73X, 74X, 75X, and 85X. Chapter 25 of this manual provides general billing instructions that must be followed for bills submitted to FIs. FIs pay for electrical stimulation services under the Medicare Physician Fee Schedule for a hospital, Comprehensive Outpatient Rehabilitation Facility (CORF), Outpatient Rehabilitation Facility (ORF), Outpatient Physical Therapy (OPT) and Skilled Nursing Facility (SNF).

Payment methodology for independent Rural Health Clinic (RHC), provider-based RHCs, free-standing Federally Qualified Health Center (FQHC) and provider based FQHCs is made under the all-inclusive rate for the visit furnished to the RHC/FQHC patient to obtain the therapy service. Only one payment will be made for the visit furnished to the RHC/FQHC patient to obtain the

therapy service. As of April 1, 2005, RHCs/FQHCs are no longer required to report HCPCS codes when billing for these therapy services.

Payment Methodology for a Critical Access Hospital (CAH) is on a reasonable cost basis unless the CAH has elected the Optional Method and then the FI pays115% of the MPFS amount for the professional component of the HCPCS code in addition to the technical component.

In addition, the following revenues code must be used in conjunction with the HCPCS code identified:

Revenue Code	Description
420	Physical Therapy
430	Occupational Therapy
520	Federal Qualified Health Center *
521	Rural Health Center *
977, 978	CriticalAccess Hospital-method II CAH professional services only

* NOTE: As of April 1, 2005, RHCs/FQHCs are no longer required to report HCPCS codes when billing for these therapy services.

C. Carrier Claims

Carriers pay for Electrical Stimulation services billed with HCPCS codes G0281 based on the MPFS. Claims for Electrical Stimulation services must be billed on Form CMS-1500 or the electronic equivalent following instructions in chapter 12 of this manual (http://www.cms.hhs.gov/manuals/104_claims/clm104c12.pdf).

D. Coinsurance and Deductible

The Medicare contractor shall apply coinsurance and deductible to payments for these therapy services except for services billed to the FI by FQHCs. For FQHCs, only co-insurance applies.

Pub. 100-4, Chapter 32, Section 11.2

Electromagnetic Therapy

A. HCPCS Coding Applicable to Carriers & Fiscal Intermediaries (FIs)

Effective July 1, 2004, a National Coverage Decision was made to allow for Medicare coverage of electromagnetic therapy for the treatment of certain types of wounds. The type of wounds covered are chronic Stage III or Stage IV pressure ulcers, arterial ulcers, diabetic ulcers and venous stasis ulcers. All other uses of electromagnetic therapy for the treatment of wounds are not covered by Medicare. Electromagnetic therapy will not be covered as an initial treatment modality.

The use of electromagnetic therapy will only be covered after appropriate standard wound care has been tried for at least 30 days and there are no measurable signs of healing. If electromagnetic therapy is being used, wounds must be evaluated periodically by the treating physician but no less than every 30 days by a physician. Continued treatment with electromagnetic therapy is not covered if measurable signs of healing have not been demonstrated within any 30-day period of treatment. Additionally, electromagnetic therapy must be discontinued when the wound demonstrates a 100% epithelialzed wound bed.

Coverage policy can be found in Pub. 100-03, Medicare National Coverage Determinations Manual, Chapter 1, Section 270.1. (www.cms.hhs.gov/manuals/103_cov_determ/ncd103index.asp)

The applicable Healthcare Common Procedure Coding System (HCPCS) code for Electrical Stimulation and the covered effective date is as follows:

HCPCS	Definition	Effective Date
G0329	ElectromagneticTherapy, to one or more areas for chronic Stage III and Stage IV pressure ulcers, arterial ulcers, diabetic ulcers and venous stasis ulcers not demonstrating measurable signs of healing after 30 days of conventional care as part of a therapy plan of care.	07/01/2004

Medicare will not cover the device used for the electromagnetic therapy for the treatment of wounds. However, Medicare will cover the service. Unsupervised home use of electromagnetic therapy will not be covered.

B. FI Billing Instructions

The applicable types of bills acceptable when billing for electromagnetic therapy services are 12X, 13X, 22X, 23X, 71X, 73X, 74X, 75X, and 85X. Chapter 25 of this manual provides general billing instructions that must be followed for bills submitted to FIs. FIs pay for electromagnetic therapy services under the Medicare Physician Fee Schedule for a hospital, CORF, ORF, and SNF.

Payment methodology for independent (RHC), provider-based RHCs, free-standing FQHC and provider based FQHCs is made under the all-inclusive rate for the visit furnished to the RHC/FQHC patient to obtain the therapy service. Only one payment will be made for the visit furnished to the RHC/FQHC patient to obtain the therapy service. As of April 1, 2005, RHCs/FQHCs are no longer required to report HCPCS codes when billing for the therapy service.

Payment Methodology for a CAH is payment on a reasonable cost basis unless the CAH has elected the Optional Method and then the FI pays pay 115% of the MPFS amount for the professional component of the HCPCS code in addition to the technical component.

In addition, the following revenues code must be used in conjunction with the HCPCS code identified:

Revenue Code	Description
420	Physical Therapy
430	Occupational Therapy
520	Federal Qualified Health Center *
521	Rural Health Center *
977, 978	CriticalAccess Hospital-method II CAH professional services only

* NOTE: As of April 1, 2005, RHCs/FQHCs are no longer required to report HCPCS codes when billing for the therapy service.

C. Carrier Claims

Carriers pay for Electromagnetic Therapy services billed with HCPCS codes G0329 based on the MPFS. Claims for electromagnetic therapy services must be billed on Form CMS-1500 or the electronic equivalent following instructions in chapter 12 of this manual (www.cms.hhs.gov/manuals/104_claims/clm104index.asp).

Payment information for HCPCS code G0329 will be added to the July 2004 update of the Medicare Physician Fee Schedule Database (MPFSD).

D. Coinsurance and Deductible

The Medicare contractor shall apply coinsurance and deductible to payments for electromagnetic therapy services except for services billed to the FI by FQHCs. For FQHCs only co-insurance applies.

Pub. 100-4, Chapter 32, Section 12

Use Cessation Counseling Services

Background: Effective for services furnished on or after March 22, 2005, a National Coverage Determination (NCD) provides for coverage of smoking and tobacco-use cessation counseling services. Conditions of Medicare Part A and Medicare Part B coverage for smoking and tobacco-use cessation counseling services are located in the Medicare National Coverage Determinations Manual, Publication 100-3, section 210.4.

Pub. 100-4, Chapter 32, Section 30.1

Billing Requirements for HBO Therapy for the Treatment of Diabetic Wounds of the Lower Extremities

Hyperbaric Oxygen Therapy is a modality in which the entire body is exposed to oxygen under increased atmospheric pressure. Effective April 1, 2003, a National Coverage Decision expanded the use of HBO therapy to include coverage for the treatment of diabetic wounds of the lower extremities. For specific coverage criteria for HBO Therapy, refer to the National Coverage Determinations Manual, chapter 1, section 20.29.

NOTE: Topical application of oxygen does not meet the definition of HBO therapy as stated above. Also, its clinical efficacy has not been established. Therefore, no Medicare reimbursement may be made for the topical application of oxygen.

I. Billing Requirements for Intermediaries

Claims for HBO therapy should be submitted on Form CMS-1450 or its electronic equivalent.

a. Applicable Bill Types

The applicable hospital bill types are 11X, 13X and 85X.

b. Procedural Coding

• 99183 - Physician attendance and supervision of hyperbaric oxygen therapy, per session.

• C1300 - Hyperbaric oxygen under pressure, full body chamber, per 30-minute interval.

The HCPCS codes are shown in FL 44 of the Form CMS-1450 or the electronic equivalent.

NOTE: Code C1300 is not available for use other than in a hospital outpatient department. In skilled nursing facilities (SNFs), HBO therapy is part of the SNF PPS payment for beneficiaries in covered Part A stays.

For hospital inpatients and critical access hospitals (CAHs) not electing Method I, HBO therapy is reported under revenue code 940 without any HCPCS code. For inpatient services, show ICD-9-CM procedure code 93.59 in FL 80 and 81.

For CAHs electing Method I, HBO therapy is reported under revenue code 940 along with HCPCS code 99183.

c. Payment Requirements for Intermediaries

Payment is as follows:

Intermediary payment is allowed for HBO therapy for diabetic wounds of the lower extremities when performed as a physician service in a hospital outpatient setting and for inpatients. Payment is allowed for claims with valid diagnostic ICD-9 codes as shown above with dates of service on or after April 1, 2003. Those claims with invalid codes should be denied as not medically necessary.

For hospitals, payment will be based upon the Ambulatory Payment Classification (APC) or the inpatient Diagnosis Related Group (DRG). Deductible and coinsurance apply.

Payment to Critical Access Hospitals (electing Method I) is made under cost reimbursement. For Critical Access Hospitals electing Method II, the technical component is paid under cost reimbursement and the professional component is paid under the Physician Fee Schedule.

II. Carrier Billing Requirements

Claims for this service should be submitted on Form CMS-1500 or its electronic equivalent.

The following HCPCS code applies:

• 99183 - Physician attendance and supervision of hyperbaric oxygen therapy, per session.

a. Payment Requirements for Carriers

Payment and pricing information will occur through updates to the Medicare Physician Fee Schedule Database (MPFSDB). Pay for this service on the basis of the MPFSDB. Deductible and coinsurance apply. Claims from physicians or other practitioners where assignment was not taken, are subject to the Medicare limiting charge.

III. Medicare Summary Notices (MSNs)

Use the following MSN Messages where appropriate:

In situations where the claim is being denied on the basis that the condition does not meet our coverage requirements, use one of the following MSN Messages:

"Medicare does not pay for this item or service for this condition." (MSN Message 16.48)

The Spanish version of the MSN message should read:

"Medicare no paga por este articulo o servicio para esta afeccion."

In situations where, based on the above utilization policy, medical review of the claim results in a determination that the service is not medically necessary, use the following MSN message:

"The information provided does not support the need for this service or item." (MSN Message 15.4)

The Spanish version of the MSN message should read:

"La informacion proporcionada no confirma la necesidad para este servicio o articulo."

IV. Remittance Advice Notices

Use appropriate existing remittance advice and reason codes at the line level to express the specific reason if you deny payment for HBO therapy for the treatment of diabetic wounds of lower extremities.

Pub. 100-4, Chapter 32, Section 50

Deep Brain Stimulation for Essential Tremor and Parkinson's Disease

Deep brain stimulation (DBS) refers to high-frequency electrical stimulation of anatomic regions deep within the brain utilizing neurosurgically implanted electrodes. These DBS electrodes are stereotactically placed within targeted nuclei on one (unilateral) or both (bilateral) sides of the brain. There are currently three targets for DBS -- the thalamic ventralis intermedius nucleus (VIM), subthalamic nucleus (STN) and globus pallidus interna (GPi).

Essential tremor (ET) is a progressive, disabling tremor most often affecting the hands. ET may also affect the head, voice and legs. The precise pathogenesis of ET is unknown. While it may start at any age, ET usually peaks within the second and sixth decades. Beta-adrenergic blockers and anticonvulsant medications are usually the first line treatments for reducing the severity of tremor. Many patients, however, do not adequately respond or cannot tolerate these medications. In these medically refractory ET patients, thalamic VIM DBS may be helpful for symptomatic relief of tremor.

Parkinson's disease (PD) is an age-related progressive neurodegenerative disorder involving the loss of dopaminergic cells in the substantia nigra of the midbrain. The disease is characterized by tremor, rigidity, bradykinesia and progressive postural instability. Dopaminergic medication is typically used as a first line treatment for reducing the primary symptoms of PD. However, after prolonged use, medication can become less effective and can produce significant adverse events such as dyskinesias and other motor function complications. For patients who become unresponsive to medical treatments and/or have intolerable side effects from medications, DBS for symptom relief may be considered.

Pub. 100-4, Chapter 32, Section 70

Billing Requirements for Islet Cell Transplantation for Beneficiaries in a National Institutes of Health (NIH) Clinical Trial

For services performed on or after October 1, 2004, Medicare will cover islet cell transplantation for patients with Type I diabetes who are participating in an NIH sponsored clinical trial. See Pub 100-04 (National Coverage Determinations Manual) section 260.3.1 for complete coverage policy.

The islet cell transplant may be done alone or in combination with a kidney transplant. Islet recipients will also need immunosuppressant therapy to prevent rejection of the transplanted islet cells. Routine follow-up care will be necessary for each trial patient. See Pub 100-04, section 310 for further guidance relative to routine care. All other uses for islet cell services will remain non-covered.

Pub. 100-4, Chapter 32, Section 100

Billing Requirements for Expanded Coverage of Cochlear Implantation

Effective for dates of services on and after April 4, 2005, the Centers for Medicare & Medicaid Services (CMS) has expanded the coverage for cochlear implantation to cover moderate-to-profound hearing loss in individuals with hearing test scores equal to or less than 40% correct in the best aided listening condition on tape-recorded tests of open-set sentence recognition and who demonstrate limited benefit from amplification. (See Publication 100-03, chapter 1, section 50.3, for specific coverage criteria).

In addition CMS is covering cochlear implantation for individuals with open-set sentence recognition test scores of greater than 40% to less than or equal to 60% correct but only when the provider is participating in, and patients are enrolled in, either:

• A Food and Drug Administration(FDA)-approved category B investigational device exemption (IDE) clinical trial; or

• A trial under the CMS clinical trial policy (see Pub. 100-03, section 310.1); or

A prospective, controlled comparative trial approved by CMS as consistent with the evidentiary requirements for national coverage analyses and meeting specific quality standards.

Pub. 100-8, Chapter 5, Section 5.1.1.2

Written Orders

Written orders are acceptable for all transactions involving DMEPOS. Written orders may take the form of a photocopy, facsimile image, electronically maintained, or original "pen-and-ink" document. (See Chapter 3, Section 3.4.1.1.B.)

All orders must clearly specify the start date of the order.

For items that are dispensed based on a verbal order, the supplier must obtain a written order that meets the requirements of this section.

If the written order is for supplies that will be provided on a periodic basis, the written order should include appropriate information on the quantity used, frequency of change, and duration of need. (For example, an order for surgical dressings might specify one 4 x 4 hydrocolloid dressing that is changed 1-2 times per week for 1 month or until the ulcer heals.)

The written order must be sufficiently detailed, including all options or additional features that will be separately billed or that will require an upgraded code. The description can be either a narrative description (e.g., lightweight wheelchair base) or a brand name/model number.

If the order is for a rented item or if the coverage criteria in a policy specify length of need, the order must include the length of need.

If the supply is a drug, the order must specify the name of the drug, concentration (if applicable), dosage, frequency of administration, and duration of infusion (if applicable).

Someone other than the physician may complete the detailed description of the item. However, the treating physician must review the detailed description and personally sign and date the order to indicate agreement.

If a supplier does not have a faxed, photocopied, electronic or pen & ink signed order in their records before they can submit a claim to Medicare (i.e., if there is no order or only a verbal order), the claim will be denied. If the item is one that requires a written order prior to delivery (see Section 5.1.1.2.1), the claim will be denied as not meeting the benefit category. If the claim is for an item for which an order is required by statute (e.g., therapeutic shoes for diabetics, oral anticancer drugs, oral antiemetic drugs which are a replacement for intravenous antiemetic drugs), the claim will be denied as not meeting the benefit category and is therefore not appealable by the supplier (see MCM Section 12000 for more information on appeals). For all other items, if the supplier does not have an order that has been both signed and dated by the treating physician before billing the Medicare program, the item will be denied as not reasonable and necessary

If an item requires a Certificate of Medical Necessity (CMN) and the supplier does not have a faxed, photocopied, electronic, or pen & ink signed CMN in their records before they submit a claim to Medicare, the claim will be denied. If the CMN is used to verify that statutory benefit requirements have been met, then the claim will be denied as not meeting the benefit category. If the CMN is used to verify that medical necessity criteria have been met, the claim will be denied as not reasonable and necessary.

Medical necessity information (e.g., an ICD-9-CM diagnosis code, narrative description of the patient's condition, abilities, limitations, etc.) is NOT in itself considered to be part of the order although it may be put on the same document as the order.

APPENDIX 5 — NEW, CHANGED, DELETED, AND REINSTATED HCPCS CODES FOR 2006

New Codes

A4461	A4463	A4559	A4600	A4601	A8000	A8001
A8002	A8003	A8004	A9279	A9527	A9568	C1821
C9232	C9233	C9234	C9235	C9350	C9351	C9727
D0145	D0273	D0360	D0362	D0363	D0486	D1206
D1555	D4230	D4231	D6012	D6091	D6092	D6093
D7292	D7293	D7294	D7951	D7998	D8693	D9120
D9612	E0676	E0936	E2373	E2374	E2375	E2376
E2377	E2381	E2382	E2383	E2384	E2385	E2386
E2387	E2388	E2389	E2390	E2391	E2392	E2393
E2394	E2395	E2396	G0380	G0381	G0382	G0383
G0384	G0389	G0390	G0392	G0393	G0394	G8191
G8192	G8193	G8194	G8195	G8196	G8197	G8198
G8199	G8200	G8201	G8202	G8203	G8204	G8205
G8206	G8207	G8208	G8209	G8210	G8211	G8212
G8213	G8214	G8215	G8216	G8217	G8218	G8219
G8220	G8221	G8222	G8223	G8224	G8225	G8226
G8227	G8228	G8229	G8230	G8231	G8232	G8234
G8235	G8236	G8237	G8238	G8239	G8240	G8241
G8242	G8243	G8245	G8246	G8247	G8248	G8249
G8250	G8251	G8252	G8253	G8254	G8255	G8256
G8257	G8258	G8259	G8260	G8261	G8262	G8263
G8264	G8265	G8266	G8267	G8268	G8269	G8270
G8271	G8272	G8273	G8274	G8275	G8276	G8277
G8278	G8279	G8280	G8281	G8282	G8283	G8284
G8285	G8286	G8287	G8288	G8289	G8290	G8291
G8292	G8293	G8294	G8295	G8296	G8297	G8298
G8299	G8300	G8301	G8302	G8303	G8304	G8305
G8306	G8307	G8308	G8309	G8310	G8311	G8312
G8313	G8314	G8315	G8316	G8317	G8318	G8319
G8320	G8321	G8322	G8323	G8324	G8325	G8326
G8327	G8328	G8329	G8330	G8331	G8332	G8333
G8334	G8335	G8336	G8337	G8338	G8339	G8340
G8341	G8342	G8343	G8344	G8345	G8346	G8347
G9131	G9132	G9133	G9134	G9135	G9136	G9137
G9138	G9139	H0049	H0050	J0129	J0348	J0364
J0594	J0894	J1324	J1458	J1562	J1740	J2170
J2248	J2315	J3243	J3473	J7187	J7311	J7319
J7345	J7346	J7607	J7609	J7610	J7615	J7634
J7645	J7647	J7650	J7657	J7660	J7667	J7670
J7685	J8650	J9261	K0733	K0734	K0735	K0736
K0737	K0738	K0800	K0801	K0802	K0806	K0807
K0808	K0812	K0813	K0814	K0815	K0816	K0820
K0821	K0822	K0823	K0824	K0825	K0826	K0827
K0828	K0829	K0830	K0831	K0835	K0836	K0837
K0838	K0839	K0840	K0841	K0842	K0843	K0848
K0849	K0850	K0851	K0852	K0853	K0854	K0855
K0856	K0857	K0858	K0859	K0860	K0861	K0862
K0863	K0864	K0868	K0869	K0870	K0871	K0877
K0878	K0879	K0880	K0884	K0885	K0886	K0890
K0891	K0898	K0899	L1001	L3806	L3808	L3915
L5993	L5994	L6611	L6624	L6639	L6703	L6704
L6706	L6707	L6708	L6709	L7007	L7008	L7009
L8690	L8691	L8695	Q4081	Q4082	Q5001	Q5002
Q5003	Q5004	Q5005	Q5006	Q5007	Q5008	Q5009
S0147	S0180	S0345	S0346	S0347	S2325	S2344
S3855	T4543					

Changed Codes

A4216	A4306	A4326	A4394	A4558	A5105	D0120
D0480	D2952	D2953	D6970	D6976	D7310	D7944
D7950	D9310	D9610	E0163	E0165	E0167	E0181
E0182	E0190	E0720	E0730	E0967	E2209	G0103
G8009	G8011	G8015	G8016	G8017	G8018	G8023
G8024	G8025	G8026	G8035	G8128	G8152	G8153
G8154	G9041	G9042	G9043	G9044	G9067	G9070
G9083	G9089	G9095	G9099	G9104	G9108	G9112
G9117	G9130	J7611	J7612	J7613	J7614	J7620
J7622	J7624	J7626	J7627	J7628	J7629	J7633
J7635	J7636	J7637	J7638	J7640	J7641	J7642
J7643	J7644	J7648	J7649	J7658	J7659	J7668
J7669	J7680	J7681	J7682	J7683	J7684	L0631
L5848	L5995	L6805	L6810	L6881	L6884	L7040
L7045	L8614	L8689	P9011	Q1003	Q4080	S0316
S1040	S2260	S2265	S2266	S2267	S5523	T5001

Deleted Codes

A0800	A4348	A4359	A4462	A4632	A9549	C1178
C2632	C8950	C8951	C8952	C8953	C8954	C8955
C9220	C9221	C9222	C9224	C9225	C9227	C9228
C9229	C9230	C9231	D1201	D1205	D6971	E0164
E0166	E0180	E0701	E0977	E0997	E0998	E0999
E2320	G0107	G0243	G9076	G9081	G9082	G9118
G9119	G9120	G9121	G9122	G9127	J2912	J7188
J7317	J7320	J7350	K0090	K0091	K0092	K0093
K0094	K0095	K0096	K0097	K0099	L0100	L0110
L3902	L3914	L6700	L6705	L6710	L6715	L6720
L6725	L6730	L6735	L6740	L6745	L6750	L6755
L6765	L6770	L6775	L6780	L6790	L6795	L6800
L6806	L6807	L6808	L6809	L6825	L6830	L6835
L6840	L6845	L6850	L6855	L6860	L6865	L6867
L6868	L6870	L6872	L6873	L6875	L6880	L7010
L7015	L7020	L7025	L7030	L7035	Q3019	Q3020
S0116	S0133	S0198	S2262	S2362	S2363	S3701
S4036	S8075	S8093	S8260	S9022		

Reinstated Codes

J1562	J1740	J2170	J7610	J7615	J7645	J7650
J7660	J7670	L8690				

APPENDIX 6 — PLACE OF SERVICE AND TYPE OF SERVICE

Place of Service Codes for Professional Claims

Database (last updated September 1, 2006)

Listed below are place of service codes and descriptions. These codes should be used on professional claims to specify the entity where service(s) were rendered. Check with individual payers (e.g., Medicare, Medicaid, other private insurance) for reimbursement policies regarding these codes. If you would like to comment on a code(s) or description(s), please send your request to posinfo@cms.hhs.gov.

Code	Name	Description
01	Pharmacy	A facility or location where drugs and other medically related items and services are sold, dispensed, or otherwise provided directly to patients.
02	Unassigned	N/A
03	School	A facility whose primary purpose is education.
04	Homeless Shelter	A facility or location whose primary purpose is to provide temporary housing to homeless individuals (e.g., emergency shelters, individual or family shelters).
05	Indian Health Service Free-standing Facility	A facility or location, owned and operated by the Indian Health Service, which provides diagnostic, therapeutic (surgical and non-surgical), and rehabilitation services to American Indians and Alaska Natives who do not require hospitalization.
06	Indian Health Service Provider-based Facility	A facility or location, owned and operated by the Indian Health Service, which provides diagnostic, therapeutic (surgical and non-surgical), and rehabilitation services rendered by, or under the supervision of, physicians to American Indians and Alaska Natives admitted as inpatients or outpatients.
07	Tribal 638 Free-standing Facility	A facility or location owned and operated by a federally recognized American Indian or Alaska Native tribe or tribal organization under a 638 agreement, which provides diagnostic, therapeutic (surgical and non-surgical), and rehabilitation services to tribal members who do not require hospitalization.
08	Tribal 638 Provider-based Facility	A facility or location owned and operated by a federally recognized American Indian or Alaska Native tribe or tribal organization under a 638 agreement, which provides diagnostic, therapeutic (surgical and non-surgical), and rehabilitation services to tribal members admitted as inpatients or outpatients.
09	Prison/Correctional Facility	A prison, jail, reformatory, work farm, detention center, or any other similar facility maintained by either Federal, State or local authorities for the purpose of confinement or rehabilitation of adult or juvenile criminal offenders. (effective July 1, 2006)
10	Unassigned	N/A
11	Office	Location, other than a hospital, skilled nursing facility (SNF), military treatment facility, community health center, State or local public health clinic, or intermediate care facility (ICF), where the health professional routinely provides health examinations, diagnosis, and treatment of illness or injury on an ambulatory basis.
12	Home	Location, other than a hospital or other facility, where the patient receives care in a private residence.
13	Assisted Living Facility	Congregate residential facility with self-contained living units providing assessment of each resident's needs and on-site support 24 hours a day, 7 days a week, with the capacity to deliver or arrange for services including some health care and other services.
14	Group Home	A residence, with shared living areas, where clients receive supervision and other services such as social and/or behavioral services, custodial service, and minimal services (e.g., medication administration).
15	Mobile Unit	A facility/unit that moves from place-to-place equipped to provide preventive, screening, diagnostic, and/or treatment services.
16-19	Unassigned	N/A
20	Urgent Care Facility	Location, distinct from a hospital emergency room, an office, or a clinic, whose purpose is to diagnose and treat illness or injury for unscheduled, ambulatory patients seeking immediate medical attention.
21	Inpatient Hospital	A facility, other than psychiatric, which primarily provides diagnostic, therapeutic (both surgical and nonsurgical), and rehabilitation services by, or under, the supervision of physicians to patients admitted for a variety of medical conditions.
22	Outpatient Hospital	A portion of a hospital which provides diagnostic, therapeutic (both surgical and nonsurgical), and rehabilitation services to sick or injured persons who do not require hospitalization or institutionalization.

23	Emergency Room - Hospital	A portion of a hospital where emergency diagnosis and treatment of illness or injury is provided.
24	Ambulatory Surgical Center	A freestanding facility, other than a physician's office, where surgical and diagnostic services are provided on an ambulatory basis.
25	Birthing Center	A facility, other than a hospital's maternity facilities or a physician's office, which provides a setting for labor, delivery, and immediate post-partum care as well as immediate care of new born infants.
26	Military Treatment Facility	A medical facility operated by one or more of the Uniformed Services. Military Treatment Facility (MTF) also refers to certain former U.S. Public Health Service (USPHS) facilities now designated as Uniformed Service Treatment Facilities (USTF).
27-30	Unassigned	N/A
31	Skilled Nursing Facility	A facility which primarily provides inpatient skilled nursing care and related services to patients who require medical, nursing, or rehabilitative services but does not provide the level of care or treatment available in a hospital.
32	Nursing Facility	A facility which primarily provides to residents skilled nursing care and related services for the rehabilitation of injured, disabled, or sick persons, or, on a regular basis, health-related care services above the level of custodial care to other than mentally retarded individuals.
33	Custodial Care Facility	A facility which provides room, board and other personal assistance services, generally on a long-term basis, and which does not include a medical component.
34	Hospice	A facility, other than a patient's home, in which palliative and supportive care for terminally ill patients and their families are provided.
35-40	Unassigned	N/A
41	Ambulance - Land	A land vehicle specifically designed, equipped and staffed for lifesaving and transporting the sick or injured.
42	Ambulance - Air or Water	An air or water vehicle specifically designed, equipped and staffed for lifesaving and transporting the sick or injured.
43-48	Unassigned	N/A
49	Independent Clinic	A location, not part of a hospital and not described by any other Place of Service code, that is organized and operated to provide preventive, diagnostic, therapeutic, rehabilitative, or palliative services to outpatients only.
50	Federally Qualified Health Center	A facility located in a medically underserved area that provides Medicare beneficiaries preventive primary medical care under the general direction of a physician.
51	Inpatient Psychiatric Facility	A facility that provides inpatient psychiatric services for the diagnosis and treatment of mental illness on a 24-hour basis, by or under the supervision of a physician.
52	Psychiatric Facility-Partial Hospitalization	A facility for the diagnosis and treatment of mental illness that provides a planned therapeutic program for patients who do not require full time hospitalization, but who need broader programs than are possible from outpatient visits to a hospital-based or hospital-affiliated facility.
53	Community Mental Health Center	A facility that provides the following services: outpatient services, including specialized outpatient services for children, the elderly, individuals who are chronically ill, and residents of the CMHC's mental health services area who have been discharged from inpatient treatment at a mental health facility; 24 hour a day emergency care services; day treatment, other partial hospitalization services, or psychosocial rehabilitation services; screening for patients being considered for admission to State mental health facilities to determine the appropriateness of such admission; and consultation and education services.
54	Intermediate Care Facility/Mentally Retarded	A facility which primarily provides health-related care and services above the level of custodial care to mentally retarded individuals but does not provide the level of care or treatment available in a hospital or SNF.
55	Residential Substance Abuse Treatment Facility	A facility which provides treatment for substance (alcohol and drug) abuse to live-in residents who do not require acute medical care. Services include individual and group therapy and counseling, family counseling, laboratory tests, drugs and supplies, psychological testing, and room and board.
56	Psychiatric Residential Treatment Center	A facility or distinct part of a facility for psychiatric care which provides a total 24-hour therapeutically planned and professionally staffed group living and learning environment.

Appendix 6 — Place of Service and Type of Service

57	Non-residential Substance Abuse Treatment Facility	A location which provides treatment for substance (alcohol and drug) abuse on an ambulatory basis. Services include individual and group therapy and counseling, family counseling, laboratory tests, drugs and supplies, and psychological testing.
58-59	Unassigned	N/A
60	Mass Immunization Center	A location where providers administer pneumococcal pneumonia and influenza virus vaccinations and submit these services as electronic media claims, paper claims, or using the roster billing method. This generally takes place in a mass immunization setting, such as, a public health center, pharmacy, or mall but may include a physician office setting.
61	Comprehensive Inpatient Rehabilitation Facility	A facility that provides comprehensive rehabilitation services under the supervision of a physician to inpatients with physical disabilities. Services include physical therapy, occupational therapy, speech pathology, social or psychological services, and orthotics and prosthetics services.
62	Comprehensive Outpatient Rehabilitation Facility	A facility that provides comprehensive rehabilitation services under the supervision of a physician to outpatients with physical disabilities. Services include physical therapy, occupational therapy, and speech pathology services.
63-64	Unassigned	N/A
65	End-Stage Renal Disease Treatment Facility	A facility other than a hospital, which provides dialysis treatment, maintenance, and/or training to patients or caregivers on an ambulatory or home-care basis.
66-70	Unassigned	N/A
71	Public Health Clinic	A facility maintained by either State or local health departments that provides ambulatory primary medical care under the general direction of a physician. (effective 10/1/03)
72	Rural Health Clinic	A certified facility which is located in a rural medically underserved area that provides ambulatory primary medical care under the general direction of a physician.
73-80	Unassigned	N/A
81	Independent Laboratory	A laboratory certified to perform diagnostic and/or clinical tests independent of an institution or a physician's office.
82-98	Unassigned	N/A
99	Other Place of Service	Other place of service not identified above.

Type of Service

Common Working File Type of Service (TOS) Indicators

For submitting a claim to the Common Working File (CWF), use the following table to assign the proper TOS. Some procedures may have more than one applicable TOS. CWF will reject alerts on codes with incorrect TOS designations. CWF is rejecting codes with incorrect TOS designations.

The only exceptions to this table are:

- Surgical services billed with the ASC facility service modifier SG must be reported as TOS F. The indicator F does not appear on the TOS table because its use is dependent upon the use of the SG modifier.

- Surgical services billed with an assistant-at-surgery modifier (80-82, AS,) must be reported with TOS 8. The 8 indicator does not appear on the TOS table because its use is dependent upon the use of the appropriate modifier. (See Medicare Claims Processing Manual, Chapter 12, "Physician/Practitioner Billing," for instructions on when assistant-at-surgery is allowable.)

- Psychiatric treatment services that are subject to the outpatient mental health treatment limitation should be reported with TOS T.

- TOS H appears in the list of descriptors. However, it does not appear in the table. In CWF, "H" is used only as an indicator for hospice. The carrier should not submit TOS H to CWF at this time.

- When these specific transfusion medicine codes appear on the claim (86880, 86885, 86886, 86900, 86903, 86904, 86905, and 86906 that also contains a blood product (P9010-P9022)), the transfusion medicine codes are paid under reasonable charge. When these services are to be paid under reasonable charge, use TOS 1. When paid under reasonable charge, tests are paid at 80 percent. Coinsurance and deductible also apply.

NOTE: For injection codes with more than one possible TOS designation, use the following guidelines when assigning the TOS:

When the choice is L or 1,

- Use TOS L when the drug is used related to ESRD; or
- Use TOS 1 when the drug is not related to ESRD and is administered in the office.

When the choice is G or 1:

- Use TOS G when the drug is an immunosuppressive drug; or
- Use TOS 1 when the drug is used for other than immunosuppression.

When the choice is P or 1,

- Use TOS P if the drug is administered through durable medical equipment (DME); or
- Use TOS 1 if the drug is administered in the office.

The place of service or diagnosis may be considered when determining the appropriate TOS. The descriptors for each of the TOS codes listed in the following table are:

0	Whole Blood
1	Medical Care
2	Surgery
3	Consultation
4	Diagnostic Radiology
5	Diagnostic Laboratory
6	Therapeutic Radiology
7	Anesthesia
8	Assistant at Surgery
9	Other Medical Items or Services
A	Used DME
B	High Risk Screening Mammography
C	Low Risk Screening Mammography
D	Ambulance
E	Enteral/Parenteral Nutrients/Supplies
F	Ambulatory Surgical Center (Facility Usage for Surgical Services)
G	Immunosuppressive Drugs
H	Hospice

J   Diabetic Shoes

K   Hearing Items and Services

L   ESRD Supplies

M   Monthly Capitation Payment for Dialysis

N   Kidney Donor

P   Lump Sum Purchase of DME, Prosthetics, Orthotics

Q   Vision Items or Services

R   Rental of DME

S   Surgical Dressings or Other Medical Supplies

T   Outpatient Mental Health Treatment Limitation

U   Occupational Therapy

V   Pneumococcal/Flu Vaccine

W   Physical Therapy

Berenson-Eggers Type of Service (BETOS) Codes

The BETOS coding system was developed primarily for analyzing the growth in Medicare expenditures. The coding system covers all HCPCS codes; assigns a HCPCS code to only one BETOS code; consists of readily understood clinical categories (as opposed to statistical or financial categories); consists of categories that permit objective assignment; is stable over time; and is relatively immune to minor changes in technology or practice patterns.

BETOS CODES AND DESCRIPTIONS:

1. Evaluation And Management

   1. M1A Office Visits—New
   2. M1B Office Visits—Established
   3. M2A Hospital Visit—Initial
   4. M2B Hospital Visit—Subsequent
   5. M2C Hospital Visit—Critical Care
   6. M3 Emergency Room Visit
   7. M4A Home Visit
   8. M4B Nursing Home Visit
   9. M5A Specialist—Pathology
   10. M5B Specialist—Psychiatry
   11. M5C Specialist—Ophthalmology
   12. M5D Specialist—Other
   13. M6 Consultations

2. Procedures

   1. P0 Anesthesia
   2. P1A Major Procedure—Breast
   3. P1B Major Procedure—Colectomy
   4. P1C Major Procedure—Cholecystectomy
   5. P1D Major Procedure—Turp
   6. P1E Major Procedure—Hysterectomy
   7. P1F Major Procedure—Explor/Decompr/Excisdisc
   8. P1G Major Procedure—Other
   9. P2A Major Procedure, Cardiovascular—CABG
   10. P2B Major Procedure, Cardiovascular—Aneurysm Repair
   11. P2C Major Procedure, Cardiovascular—Thromboendarterectomy
   12. P2D Major Procedure, Cardiovascular—Coronary Angioplasty (PTCA)
   13. P2E Major Procedure, Cardiovascular—Pacemaker Insertion
   14. P2F Major Procedure, Cardiovascular—Other
   15. P3Aa Major Procedure, Orthopedic—Hip Fracture Repair
   16. P3B Major Procedure, Orthopedic—Hip Replacement
   17. P3C Major Procedure, Orthopedic—Knee Replacement
   18. P3D Major Procedure, Orthopedic—Other
   19. P4A Eye Procedure—Corneal Transplant
   20. P4B Eye Procedure—Cataract Removal/Lens Insertion
   21. P4C Eye Procedure—Retinal Detachment
   22. P4D Eye Procedure—Treatment Of Retinal Lesions
   23. P4E Eye Procedure—Other
   24. P5A Ambulatory Procedures—Skin
   25. P5B Ambulatory Procedures—Musculoskeletal
   26. P5C Ambulatory Procedures—Inguinal Hernia Repair
   27. P5D Ambulatory Procedures—Lithotripsy
   28. P5E Ambulatory Procedures—Other
   29. P6A Minor Procedures—Skin
   30. P6B Minor Procedures—Musculoskeletal
   31. P6C Minor Procedures—Other (Medicare Fee Schedule)
   32. P6D Minor Procedures—Other (Non-Medicare Fee Schedule)
   33. P7A Oncology—Radiation Therapy
   34. P7B Oncology—Other
   35. P8A Endoscopy—Arthroscopy
   36. P8B Endoscopy—Upper Gastrointestinal
   37. P8C Endoscopy—Sigmoidoscopy
   38. P8D Endoscopy—Colonoscopy
   39. P8E Endoscopy—Cystoscopy
   40. P8F Endoscopy—Bronchoscopy
   41. P8G Endoscopy—Laparoscopic Cholecystectomy
   42. P8H Endoscopy—Laryngoscopy
   43. P8I Endoscopy—Other
   44. P9A Dialysis Services (Medicare Fee Schedule)
   45. P9B Dialysis Services (Non-Medicare Fee Schedule)

3. Imaging

   1. I1A Standard Imaging—Chest
   2. I1B Standard Imaging—Musculoskeletal
   3. I1C Standard Imaging—Breast
   4. I1D Standard Imaging—Contrast Gastrointestinal
   5. I1E Standard Imaging—Nuclear Medicine
   6. I1F Standard Imaging—Other
   7. I2A Advanced Imaging—CAT/CT/CTA; Brain/Head/Neck
   8. I2B Advanced Imaging—CAT/CT/CTA; Other
   9. I2C Advanced Imaging—MRI/MRA; Brain/Head/Neck
   10. I2D Advanced Imaging—MRI/MRA; Other
   11. I3A Echography—Eye

Appendix 6 — Place of Service and Type of Service

12. I3B Echography—Abdomen/Pelvis

13. I3C Echography—Heart

14. I3D Echography—Carotid Arteries

15. I3E Echography—Prostate, Transrectal

16. I3F Echography—Other

17. I4A Imaging/Procedure—Heart,Including Cardiac Catheterization

18. I4B Imaging/Procedure—Other

4. Tests

1. T1A Lab Tests—Routine Venipuncture (Non-Medicare Fee Schedule)

2. T1B Lab Tests—Automated General Profiles

3. T1C Lab Tests—Urinalysis

4. T1D Lab Tests—Blood Counts

5. T1E Lab Tests—Glucose

6. T1F Lab Tests—Bacterial Cultures

7. T1G Lab Tests—Other (Medicare Fee Schedule)

8. T1H Lab Tests—Other (Non-Medicare Fee Schedule)

9. T2A Other Tests—Electrocardiograms

10. T2B Other Tests—Cardiovascular Stress Tests

11. T2C Other Tests—Ekg Monitoring

12. T2D Other Tests—Other

5. Durable Medical Equipment

1. D1A Medical/Surgical Supplies

2. D1B Hospital Beds

3. D1C Oxygen And Supplies

4. D1D Wheelchairs

5. D1E Other DME

6. D1F Orthotic Devices

7. D1G Drugs Administered through DME

6. Other

1. O1A Ambulance

2. O1B Chiropractic

3. O1C Enteral And Parenteral

4. O1D Chemotherapy

5. O1E Other Drugs

6. O1F Vision, Hearing And Speech Services

7. O1G Influenza Immunization

7. Exceptions/Unclassified

1. Y1 Other—Medicare Fee Schedule

2. Y2 Other—Non-Medicare Fee Schedule

3. Z1 Local Codes

4. Z2 Undefined Codes

NOTES

NOTES

NOTES